OXFORD GEOGRAPHICAL AND ENVIRONMENTAL STUDIES

General Editors

Gordon Clark, Andrew Goudie, and Ceri Peach

War Epidemics

An Historical Geography of Infectious Diseases
in Military Conflict and Civil Strife, 1850–2000

M. R. Smallman-Raynor
and
A. D. Cliff

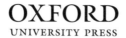

OXFORD

UNIVERSITY PRESS

Great Clarendon Street, Oxford OX2 6DP

Oxford University Press is a department of the University of Oxford.
It furthers the University's objective of excellence in research, scholarship,
and education by publishing worldwide in

Oxford New York

Auckland Bangkok Buenos Aires Cape Town Chennai
Dar es Salaam Delhi Hong Kong Istanbul Karachi Kolkata
Kuala Lumpur Madrid Melbourne Mexico City Mumbai Nairobi
São Paulo Shanghai Taipei Tokyo Toronto

Oxford is a registered trade mark of Oxford University Press
in the UK and in certain other countries

Published in the United States
by Oxford University Press Inc., New York

© M. R. Smallman-Raynor and A. D. Cliff 2004.

The moral rights of the authors have been asserted

Database right Oxford University Press (maker)

First published 2004

British Library Cataloguing in Publication Data

Data available

Library of Congress Cataloging in Publication Data

Data available

ISBN 0–19–823364–7

1 3 5 7 9 10 8 6 4 2

Typeset by SNP Best-set Typesetter Ltd., Hong Kong
Printed in Great Britain
on acid-free paper by
Biddles Ltd,
King's Lynn, Norfolk

For Peace

EDITORS' PREFACE

Geography and environmental studies are two closely related and burgeoning fields of academic enquiry. Both have grown rapidly over the past few decades. At once catholic in its approach and yet strongly committed to a comprehensive understanding of the world, geography has focused upon the interaction between global and local phenomena. Environmental studies, on the other hand, have shared with the discipline of geography an engagement with different disciplines, addressing wide-ranging and significant environmental issues in the scientific community and the policy community. From the analysis of climate change and physical environmental processes to the cultural dislocations of post-modernism across the landscape, these two fields of enquiry have been at the forefront of attempts to comprehend transformations taking place in the world, manifesting themselves at a variety of interrelated spatial scales.

The Oxford Geographical and Environmental Studies series aims to reflect this diversity and engagement. Our goal is to publish the best and original research in the two related fields and, in doing so, demonstrate the significance of geographical and environmental perspectives for understanding the contemporary world. As a consequence, our scope is deliberately international and ranges widely in terms of topics, approaches, and methodologies. Authors are welcome from all corners of the globe. We hope the series will assist in redefining the frontiers of knowledge and build bridges within the fields of geography and environmental studies. We hope also that it will cement links with issues and approaches that have originated outside the strict confines of these disciplines. In doing so, our publications contribute to the frontiers of research and knowledge while representing the fruits of particular and diverse scholarly traditions.

Gordon L. Clark
Andrew Goudie
Ceri Peach

PREFACE

The spectre of war and disease has loomed large throughout history. In looking forward to the end of the world, the Revelation of St John the Divine, the last book of the Bible, relates the story of the Four Horsemen of the Apocalypse. The 2000-year-old picture revealed by the opening of the seals is grim indeed, but the ideas encapsulated were old even when they were written. The first and second riders on their white and red horses represent wars of conquest and civil war. The third horseman with his black horse represents famine. The fourth horse, ridden by Death, is 'sickly pale'. Death has an additional right—to kill by pestilence: 'To him was given power over a quarter of the earth, with the right to kill by sword and by famine, by pestilence and wild beasts' (Rev. 6: 8).

And so, down the ages, it is accepted at least in the round that epidemics of infectious diseases arising as a consequence of war have caused more mortality than the weapons of the combatants. Thus, in his résumé of mortality in the armies of the American Civil War (1861–5), Friedrich Prinzing noted that typhoid fever spread as 'murderous epidemics', smallpox 'raged very extensively', measles and malaria were 'widespread', and dysentery was 'unusually prevalent'.[1] A decade earlier, in the Crimean War (1854–6), the French Army lost no less than 10 per cent of its maximum effective strength to epidemics of cholera, dysentery, and typhus fever whilst, during the American Revolutionary Wars (1808–26), malaria and yellow fever decimated the European forces.

Such epidemiological bombardments were not restricted to military personnel. So, during the South African (Great Boer) War (1899–1902) and the Philippine–American War (1899–1902), a plethora of infectious diseases—cholera, diphtheria, measles, malaria, mumps, typhoid fever, varicella, and whooping cough—spread rapidly through the civilian concentration 'camps' and 'zones'. Likewise, in the course of the Cuban Insurrection of 1895–8, simultaneous epidemics of smallpox and enteric fever contributed to a civilian death toll of upwards of 200,000.

There is a vast literature on war and disease, and it includes some great historical works: Joseph J. Woodward's *Outlines of the Chief Camp Diseases of the United States Armies* (1863); August Hirsch's *Handbook of Geographical and Historical Pathology* (1883); Friedrich Prinzing's *Epidemics Resulting from Wars* (1916); Hans Zinsser's *Rats, Lice and History* (1935); and Ralph H. Major's *War and Disease* (1940). It has been with some trepidation that we have approached this subject, especially since the detailed nature of the conjunc-

---

[1] Prinzing (1916: 177–80).

tions between war and disease has caused controversy among historians and demographers alike. We have tried to find a distinctive niche for our own research, and that niche has been fixed primarily by our own interests and skills. First, in selecting diseases, wars, geographical regions and time periods, we have focused upon the intersection of these variables where quantitative data, capable of being analysed statistically, are available. In the time domain, this means that most of the work reported is post-1850. However, we do use some data for periods prior to the mid-nineteenth century to frame the in-depth analyses. Secondly, the analyses we describe are strongly spatial and locational. We have been concerned to emphasize the locational variable both in describing spatial patterns and in examining the dynamics by which diseases, entrained by war, have moved from one geographical area to another. Our geographical focus has caused us also to examine the war–disease link at different spatial scales, ranging from local conflicts to global conflagrations, to try to identify overarching processes and themes which operate across scale changes. Geography has also meant that we have looked in detail at war and disease in different geographical environments. Finally, our emphasis has been on transmissible or infectious diseases—those which, by nature of their short incubation periods, can be demonstrated to be a direct consequence of a conflict. Thus, although we touch upon such conditions as mental illness and post-conflict syndromes, this forms but a small part of a canvas we paint mainly with contagious diseases.

It is equally important to define what we have not attempted. We have not tried to be inclusive and to cover all major conflicts—apart from any other consideration, space and time would not permit. Rather, we have selected conflicts which act as cameos to illustrate broad principles. Our own competence means that we have not revisited the political or military histories of wars except where it has been necessary to inform our own peculiar geographical slant. As with many areas of history, understanding the political and military context of wars causes active argument among historians, and we would not pretend to make a serious contribution to their debates.

Our research would not have been possible without the unswerving support of a large number of individuals and institutions. Our first and greatest debts are to the Wellcome and Leverhulme Trusts. Without their long-term support, the project could not have been completed. The main body of work reported in this book has been funded by a five-year Leverhulme programme grant entitled Disease in War, 1850–1990: Geographical Patterns, Spread and Demographic Impact. The award of a Philip Leverhulme Prize furnished one of the authors (MSR) with a sabbatical period in which the final manuscript of the book was completed, while the extension of his leave by Nottingham University is gratefully acknowledged.

The Leverhulme Trust also provided additional financial help to fund hand-encoding of data when computer scanning of records failed to cope with the variable and unclear materials being used. These data form part of the record in this book, and they are available electronically from the authors. Accordingly, at Cambridge, we thank Lesley Cliff for undertaking the heavy task of entering up into massive data matrices the individual observations on war and disease from a miscellany of sources. She must have felt, as we often did, that there was no end in sight, and the final accuracy of the data owes much to her skilful inputting and rechecking of material from tables which changed their format in unpredictable ways. Also in Cambridge, Philip Stickler and Owen Tucker in the Drawing Office in the University's Department of Geography and Timothy Cliff at Cliff Cartographics undertook the mammoth task of producing the maps and diagrams. Our especial thanks are due to Philip Stickler, Head of the Cambridge Drawing Office, for undertaking the final assembly of the diagrams himself with both flair and good humour. In Geneva, assistance was provided by two main sections of the World Health Organization. The Global Epidemiological Surveillance section gave us not only a working base but also access to a wealth of regular epidemiological reports. The splendid WHO library allowed us entry to much early epidemiological material from the League of Nations period not readily available elsewhere. Once again, we have to thank Dr John Clements, then at WHO as a senior member of the Global Programme on Vaccines, for his long-term encouragement of our work.

At Divonne-les-Bains, M. Andre Boirét at *La Truite* regularly provided a warm welcome during our working visits to WHO. Despite our wretched French, hand signals normally ensured communication. Coco, the grey Gabonese parrot, has moved from the foyer to the restaurant since our last book, where he has been joined by two companions, while one of us finally forsook nicotine after several evenings mid-meal in the rain looking into a warm restaurant.

As always, personal thanks come last. Complex pressures come, go, and persist over the duration of a project which took over a major part of the lives of both authors for some five years. At critical moments, help arrived from many quarters—families old and new, colleagues and friends. We hope that this book illuminates some of the dark corridors in which the geographies of war epidemics are to be found. We leave that judgement to our critics. But, if we have succeeded, the credit will be more due to the support we have received than the providers would ever allow.

Matthew Smallman-Raynor   Andrew Cliff

Nottingham and Cambridge,
Feast of Saint Sebastian, 2003

CONTENTS

PART III A Regional Pattern of War Epidemics

PART IV Prospects

LIST OF FIGURES AND PLATES

LIST OF TABLES

ACKNOWLEDGEMENTS

The authors and publisher are grateful for permission to reproduce the following material:

By kind permission of Oxford University Press. Coriolanus (Act 4, Scene 5), from "William Shakespeare: The Complete Works", edited by Wells, Stanley & Taylor, Gary (1986) (Prologue, p. xxxiii); and *The Destruction of Sennacherib*, Verse III (4 lines) from "The Complete Poetical Works of Lord Byron" by Byron, George Gordon edited by McGann, Jerome J. (1981) (Ch. 3, p. 123)

Macmillan Publishers, K. Baker, The Faber Book of War Poetry 1996, Wilfred Gibson, *In the Ambulance* (1916) (Ch. 4, p. 175)

R. N. Currey and R. V. Gibson, *Poems from India by Members of the Armed Forces*, 1946, Oxford University Press Bombay 1945 and London 1946. Tara Ali Baig, *Bengal Famine*, 1943 p. 51 (Ch. 5, p. 231)

A. P. Watt Ltd on behalf of the National Trust for Places of Historic Interest or Natural Beauty. Rudyard Kipling, 'Cholera Camp' 1896 (Ch. 9, p. 480) and 'The Spies' March' 1913 (Ch. 12, p. 612)

Constable Press. George Santayana, *Soliloquies in England and Later Soliloquies*, 1922, Soliloquy 25, 'Tipperary' 1924 (Ch. 13, p.689)

Ulm Statarchiv (Plate 1.1)

Réunion des Musées Nationaux Agence photographique (Plate 2.1, Louvre, ref. 94DE15066, and Plate 2.3, Louvre, ref. 85EE1390)

The Wellcome Library, London (Plate 2.2)

Collection Ecole Nationale des Ponts et Chaussées for permission to reproduce 'Napoleon Bonaparte's Russian Campaign (1812–1813)', ref. ENPC Fol 10975 p28 (Plate 2.4)

Edward R. Tufte for permission to reprint 'Napoleon Bonaparte's Russian Campaign (1812-1813)' from *The Visual Display of Quantitative Information*, Graphics Press, Cheshire, CT, 1983 (Plate 2.4)

AP Wide World Photos (Plate 5.1)

BMJ Journals (Plate 5.2)

Library of the College of Physicians of Philadelphia (Plate 7.2C)

Iziko Museums of Cape Town (Plate 8.1)

WHO Collaborating Center for Virus Reference and Research (Plate 9.2)

The American Geographical Society (Plate 9.3)

Medical Department, US Army (Plates 9.1, 11.3, 11.4)

The American Association for the Advancement of Science (Plate 13.1)

Although every effort has been made to trace and contact copyright holders, this has not always been successful. We apologize for any apparent negligence.

PROLOGUE

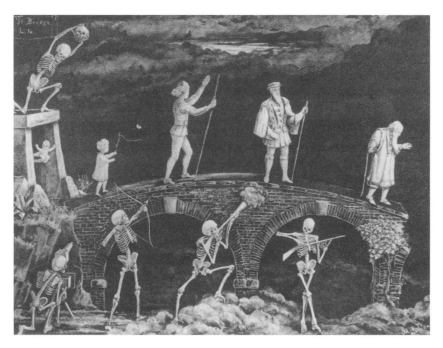

Source: K. S. Pearson (1897). *The Chances of Death and Other Studies in Evolution*. London: Arnold, frontispiece.

1 SERUINGMAN. Let me haue Warre say I, it exceeds peace as farre as day do's night; It's spritely walking, audible, and full of Vent. Peace, is a very Apoplexy, Lethargie, mull'd, deafe, sleepie, insensible, a getter of more bastard Children, then warres a destroyer of men.

William Shakespeare, Coriolanus, iv. v. 1608

PART I

War and Disease

1

Wars and War Epidemics

1.1 Introduction

Disease is a head of the Hydra, War. In his classic book, *The Epidemics of the Middle Ages*, J. F. C. Hecker (1859) paints an apocalyptic picture of the war–disease association. For Hecker, infectious diseases, the 'unfettered powers of nature . . . inscrutable in their dominion, destructive in their effects, stay the course of events, baffle the grandest plans, paralyse the boldest flights of the mind, and when victory seemed within their grasp, have often annihilated embattled hosts with the flaming sword of the angel of death' (Hecker, 1859: 212).

   The theme is developed by August Hirsch who, in the second edition of his *Handbook of Geographical and Historical Pathology* (1883), was repeatedly moved to comment on the manner in which wars fuelled the spread of infectious diseases. Writing of Asiatic cholera in the Baltic provinces and Poland in 1830–1, Hirsch concluded that the 'military operations of the Russo-Polish war contributed materially to its diffusion' (i. 398). Similarly, Hirsch traced one of the last 'considerable' outbreaks of bubonic plague in nineteenth-century Europe to '1828–29, when the Russian and Turkish forces came into collision in Wallachia' (i. 503–4), while the waves of typhus fever that rolled around early-modern Europe were attributed to 'the turmoil of great wars, which . . . shook the whole framework of European society to its foundations' (i. 549).

In much earlier times, Book I of Homer's epic poem the *Iliad*—which may well be based on historical fact—tells of a mysterious epidemic that smote the camp of the Greek Army outside Troy around 1200 BC. According to Homer, the fate of King Agamemnon's legions was sealed thus:

> Say then, what God the fatal strife provoked?
> Jove's and Latona's son; he filled with wrath
> Against the King, with deadly pestilence
> The camp afflicted,—and the people died,—
> For Chryses' sake . . .[1]

Elsewhere, the celebrated works of ancient Greek historians—Herodotus (?484–?425 BC) on the later Assyrian Wars, Thucydides (?460–?395 BC) on the Great Peloponnesian War and Diodorus Siculus (*fl.* first century BC) on the Carthaginian Wars—all attest to the antiquity of the war–disease association. Of ancient Rome, Bruce-Chwatt notes that 'Foreign invaders . . . found that the deadly fevers of the Compagna Romana protected the Eternal City better than any man-made weapons' (cited in Beadle and Hoffman, 1993: 320). Great military leaders—like the minions who stood and fell around them—were not immune to the epidemiological risks of war. Alexander the Great (356–323 BC), it is said, died of one of the most notorious war pestilences (malaria) at the age of 33, before his conquests could be extended into the Indian subcontinent.

Down the ages, war epidemics have decimated the fighting strength of armies, caused the suspension and cancellation of military operations, and have brought havoc to the civil populations of belligerent and non-belligerent states alike (Table 1.1). Factors which have contributed to the spread of war epidemics are well known (Prinzing, 1916; Major, 1940) and include a broad range of social, physical, psychological, and environmental considerations. With war comes the heightened mixing of both military and civil populations, thereby increasing the likelihood of the transmission of infectious disease. The combatants may be drawn from a variety of epidemiological backgrounds,

---

[1] Edward, Earl of Derby (1865). *The Iliad of Homer, Rendered into English Blank Verse by Edward, Earl of Derby*, 2 vols. (5th edn.). London: John Murray, p. 1. For a further consideration of the pestilence that struck the Greek Army during the Trojan War, see: Crawfurd (1914: 4–6); Shrewsbury (1964: 21).

they may be assembled and deployed in disease environments to which they are not acclimatized, and they may carry infections for which the inhabitants of war zones have little or no acquired immunity. For all involved, resistance to infection may be compromised by mental and physical stress, trauma, nutritional deprivation, and the deleterious consequences of rapid exposure to multiple disease agents. Insanitary conditions, enforced population concentration and overcrowding, the destruction of health infrastructure, the interruption or cessation of disease-control programmes, and the collapse of the conventional rules of social behaviour further compound the epidemiological unhealthiness of war.

In this book, we examine the historical occurrence and geographical spread of infectious diseases in association with past wars and war-like events. The disease record is fragmentary. While we summarize what is known of the early history and geography of war epidemics, most of the book is concerned with the 150-year period since 1850 in which the record, particularly the statistical record, is much more complete. Our primary concern is with the great epidemic diseases—cholera, influenza, measles, plague, smallpox, typhoid, and typhus fevers, among others—which, as Table 1.1 indicates, have spread repeatedly with past conflicts. But special attention is also paid to such exotic infections as filariasis, Japanese encephalitis, Q fever, and scrub typhus which have periodically erupted into military consciousness. Sexually transmitted diseases, too, hold a special place in war history and these are considered in the context of both classic (chancroid, gonorrhoea, and syphilis) and newly emerging (HIV/AIDS) diseases.

The analyses to be presented are underpinned by an intrinsically geographical question in the historical association of war and infectious disease: how are the spatial dynamics of epidemics influenced by military operations and the directives of war? To address this question, we draw on a variety of geographical methods and techniques which can contribute to an understanding of the problem. The term *historical geography* is used to indicate our particular concern with archival source materials over a 150-year time period, but we combine this concern with quantitative analyses less frequently associated with historical studies.

In this opening chapter, we set the scene by locating infectious diseases within the broader context of war. We begin in Section 1.2 by looking at definitions and classifications of war. We explore historical trends in the number, type, and geographical location of wars, and we review the mortal impact of past wars upon the populations involved. In Section 1.3, we examine the specific contribution of infectious diseases to morbidity and mortality in military and civil populations on a war footing. Criteria for the selection of certain wars and diseases for especially close study are summarized and the particular choices are defined. In Section 1.4, we review the principal source materials upon which our analyses are based. Finally, in Section 1.5, we outline the structure and chapter arrangement of the book.

Table 1.1. Sample epidemic events associated with war, 500 BC–AD 2000

Year	Conflict	Sample afflicted group and/or location	Disease	Estimated deaths	Source
c.480 BC	Persian Invasion of Greece (480–479 BC)	Persian Army in Greece	Plague or dysentery (?)	>300,000(?)	Zinsser (1935)
430–425 BC	Great Peloponnesian War (431–404 BC)	Athens	Unknown	>100,000(?)	Shrewsbury (1950)
212 BC	Second Punic War (218–202 BC)	Russian Army at Siege of Syracuse	Influenza (?)	?	Crawfurd (1914)
88 BC	Social War (91–88 BC)	Army of Octavius in Rome	?	17,000	Zinsser (1935)
AD 125	Roman Colonial Wars, Africa	Roman Army in Utica	?	up to 30,000	Castiglioni (1947)
251–66	Roman–Gothic War (249–70)	Africa, Europe, and Near East	Measles or smallpox (?)	up to 5,000 per day (Rome)	Castiglioni (1947)
425	Hun Raids on Roman Empire (c.375–454)	Hun Army (advance on Constantinople)	?	? (epidemic forced retreat)	Zinsser (1935)
569 or 571	Elephant War (569 or 571)	Abyssinian Army at Siege of Mecca	Bubonic plague with smallpox (?)	60,000 (?)	Creighton (1965)
638–9	Muslim Conquest of Persia (634–51)	Syrian Army in Amwās	?	25,000 (in 639)	Kohn (1998)
1010 or 1011	Later Viking Raids in England (899–1016)	Danes in Kent	*Dolor viscerum* (dysentery) (?)	?	Creighton (1965)
1148	Second Crusade (1147–9)	Army of Louis VII and civilians at Adalia	Typhoid, dysentery, or bubonic plague (?)	?	Kohn (1998)
1218	Fifth Crusade (1217–21)	Crusader Army at Damietta	Severe scurvy	? (15–20% of army)	Prinzing (1916)
1270	Eighth Crusade (1270)	Crusader Army at Carthage	Dysentery	? ('many deaths')	Crawfurd (1914)
1346	Siege of Kaffa	Tartar Army at Kaffa	Bubonic plague	? ('infinite' numbers)	Derbes (1966)
1485	Wars of the Roses (1455–85)	England	Sweating sickness	? ('most' students at Oxford)	Hunter (1991)
1489–90	War of Granada (1482–92)	Spanish Army in Granada	Typhus fever	? (up to 17,000 prior to 1490)	Zinsser (1935)
1495 ff.	Italian Wars (1494–5)	Continental Europe	Syphilis	?	Prinzing (1916)
1518–20	Wars of Spanish Conquest (1519–46)	Mexico	Smallpox	2–15 million	Hopkins (1983)
1552	Fifth War against Charles V (1552–9)	Army of Charles V at Metz	Typhus fever and dysentery	10,000	Prinzing (1916)
1596–1602	Anglo-Spanish War (1587–1604)	Spain	Bubonic plague	0.5–0.6 million	Kohn (1998)
1632–33	Thirty Years' War (1618–48)	Protestant population, Dresden	Bubonic plague	7,714	Prinzing (1916)
1643	English Civil War (1640–9)	Parliamentary Army at Reading	Typhus fever	? ('great mortality')	Creighton (1965)
1650	Cromwell's Irish Campaign (1649–50)	Garrison at Kilkenny	Bubonic plague	900 (cavalry and foot soldiers)	Creighton (1965)
1689	Irish War (1689–91)	Protestant Army (near Dundalk)	Typhus fever	6,000	Kohn (1998)
1709	Second Northern War (1700–21)	Danzig	Bubonic plague	32,599	Prinzing (1916)
1717	Austro-Turkish War (1716–18)	Austrian troops at Siege of Belgrade	Typhus and dysentery	4,000	Prinzing (1916)

Date	War	Population/Location	Disease	Deaths	Reference
1738	Russo-Austrian War (1735–9)	Russian troops	Bubonic plague	30,000	Prinzing (1916)
1761–2	Seven Years' War	British forces at Siege of Habana	Yellow fever	8,000	Kohn (1998)
1771–2	Russo-Turkish War (1768–72)	Moscow	Bubonic plague	52,300	Alexander (1980)
1781	Comuneros' Uprising in New Granada (1781)	Socorro	Smallpox	6,000	Kohn (1998)
1792–5	War of the First Coalition (1792–7)	Metz	Typhus fever	4,870	Prinzing (1916)
1801–3	Haitian-French War (1801–3)	French Army in Haiti	Yellow fever	22,000	Zinsser (1935)
1808	Peninsular War (1808–14)	Besieged military and civilian population of Saragossa	Typhus fever	72,000	Prinzing (1916)
1809	Walcheren Expedition (1809–10)	British Army on Walcheren Island	Walcheren fever (malaria, typhus, typhoid and/or dysentery)	3,960	McGuffie (1947)
1812–13	Napoleon's Russian Expedition (1812–13)	French soldiers and civilians at Vilna	Typhus fever	55,000	Prinzing (1916)
1831	Polish Insurrection (1830–1)	Warsaw Province	Cholera	13,103	McGrew (1965)
1854–6	Crimean War (1853–6)	British and French Armies, Black Sea	Cholera	c.18,000	Prinzing (1916)
1866	Austro-Prussian War (1866)	Austrian Crownlands	Cholera	165,000	Prinzing (1916)
1870–1	Franco-Prussian War (1870–1)	France and Germany	Smallpox	c.300,000	Prinzing (1916)
1877–8	Russo-Turkish War (1877–8)	Russian Army	Typhoid and typhus fevers	c.33,000	Prinzing (1916)
1898	Spanish–American War (1898)	US Volunteer Army, USA	Typhoid fever	c.1,500	Reed *et al.* (1904)
1902–4	Philippine–American War (1899–1902)	Philippines	Cholera	c.200,000	de Bevoise (1995)
1914–15	World War I (1914–18)	Serbian Soldiers/Austrian POWs, Serbia	Typhus and relapsing fevers	30,000	Soubbotitch (1918)
1917–22	Revolution and Civil War, Russia (1917–21)	Russia	Typhus fever	2.5–3.0 million	Zinsser (19135)
1918–19	World War I (1914–18)	Global pandemic	Influenza	20–40 million	Oxford (2000)
1942–5	World War II (1939–45)	Allied forces in Pacific and SE Asia	Scrub typhus	636	Philip (1948)
1942–3	World War II (1939–42)	Servicemen and civilians, Malta	Poliomyelitis	37	Seddon *et al.* (1945)
1965–75	Vietnam War (1964–73)	Vietnam	Bubonic/pneumonic plague	838 (1966–70)	Velimirovic (1972)
1971	Pakistan Civil War (1971)	East Pakistan refugees in India	Cholera	c.10,000	Kohn (1998)
1980s	Mozambican Civil War (1976–92)	War-displaced persons, Mozambique	HIV/AIDS	?	Palha de Sousa *et al.* (1989)
1984–94	Sudanese Civil War (1956–)	Upper Nile, Southern Sudan	Visceral leishmaniasis	95,000–112,000	Seaman *et al.* (1996)
1984–7	Salvadorian (1977–92) and Nicaraguan (1982–90) Civil Wars	Nicaraguan and Salvadorian refugees in Honduras	Measles	454	Desenclos *et al.* (1990)
1995–7	Burundian Civil War (1993–)	Internally displaced persons	Louse-borne typhus	?	Raoult *et al.* (1998)
1999	Angolan Civil War (1975–)	Luanda and other provinces	Poliomyelitis	c.80	Tangermann *et al.* (2000)

1.2 Wars

The term *war* (stemming from the Old High German *werra*, meaning confusion, discord, or strife) is commonly used to refer to almost any form of sustained opposition or competition between two or more parties. There are wars between the sexes, the races, and the generations; there are economic, industrial, and eco(logical) wars; there are wars against diseases; and there are wars on undesirable manifestations of modern society such as terrorism, drugs, crime, poverty, and want.

In this book, we use the term *war* in a more conventional sense to refer to a particular form of intentional violent conflict between two or more belligerent parties, nations, or states. Even then, the term *war* defies any simple or clear-cut definition. Philosophers, lawyers, and humanitarians have, down the centuries, viewed the essence of war from a broad range of intellectual perspectives— ideological (Grotius), sociological (Cruce), technological (Machiavelli), and psychological (Erasmus). Military thinkers have tended (implicitly or explicitly) to view war as violent conflict between contending groups which, in the first instance, are of sufficiently equal power to render the outcome uncertain. As such, wars are to be distinguished from conflicts between parties of markedly unequal power, including hostilities between 'advanced' versus 'primitive' states (expeditions, explorations, and pacifications), 'large' versus 'small' states (interventions and reprisals), and states versus sub-state 'organizations' (insurrections and rebellions) (Nickerson and Wright, 1962).

1.2.1 Defining Wars

In Book I of his famous treatise *Vom Kriege*, first published in 1832, Karl von Clausewitz conceptualized war as 'nothing but a duel on a larger scale'—'an act of force to compel our enemy to do our will' (Clausewitz, 1976: 75). Notionally, at least, the intrinsic association of war with intentional violence places it in the same broad category as violent crime, prize fights, gladiatorial combats, and reprisals. But war is also a political process for conflict resolution and inter-group relations and, as such, can be classed with mediation, negotiation, conciliation, arbitration, alliance, and entente. Within this dualistic framework of intentional violence and conflict resolution, Table 1.2 samples from Quincy Wright's (1924, 1965) classic series of legal and material definitions of war. Such definitions are not, however, without their detractors. As Richardson (1944: 247) notes: 'The great obstacle to any scientific study of quarrels is contradictory evidence from the opposing sides. Wright's definition of a war involves notions of its "legality" and "political importance" which are always a matter of opinion, and can be permanently controversial.'

Recent Developments

As the nature of armed conflict has evolved during the twentieth century, so new definitions of war have been developed. The increasing recognition of

Table 1.2. Quincy Wright's (1924, 1965) legal and material definitions of war

---

Broad definition of war
'a violent contact of distinct but similar entities' (1965: 8)

Strict definition of war, legal sense
1. 'a condition or period of time in which special rules permitting and regulating violence between governments prevail' (1924: 762)
2. 'a procedure of regulated violence by which disputes between governments are settled' (1924: 762)
3. 'the legal condition which equally permits two or more hostile groups to carry on a conflict by armed force' (1965: 8)

Strict definition of war, material sense
1. 'an act or a series of acts of violence by one government against another' (1924: 762)
2. 'a dispute between governments carried on by violence' (1924: 762)
3. 'a simultaneous conflict of armed forces, popular feelings, jural dogmas, and national cultures so nearly equal [among all the belligerents] as to lead to an extreme intensification of each' (1965: 698)

Source: Wright (1924, 1965).

non-state organizations among the chief combatants has resulted in a shift away from the emphasis of war as an event solely between governments. For example, Shafritz *et al.* (1989: 486) define war as a 'state of violent, armed conflict between organized political entities in their efforts to gain, defend, or add to their national or political sovereignty or power, or to achieve a lesser goal'. More recently, Cioffi-Revilla (1996: 8) has defined war (or a 'war event') as 'an occurrence of purposive and lethal violence among two or more social groups pursuing conflicting political goals that results in fatalities, with at least one belligerent group organized under the command of authoritative leadership'. As Brecke (1999) notes, this latter definition combines sufficient generality to encompass a wide variety of types of violent conflict, and it is also sufficiently focused to exclude such events as gang battles and organized crime vendettas.

1.2.2 Classifying Wars

Although such terms as 'guerrilla', 'civil', 'imperial', and 'low-intensity'—among many others—are commonly used to describe the nature of particular wars, generally accepted and universally applied classifications of war have proved elusive. In a recent review of the literature, Brecke (1999) identified no less than 149 different types or categories of war. Many of the classifications, however, are too broad, too focused, or too simplistic for universal use. For example, within the framework of Marxism-Leninism, a distinction is drawn between *Just Wars* (wars for liberation from foreign control) and *Unjust Wars* (wars to assert imperial control) (Urlanis, 1971: 7–8). An alternative framework draws a distinction between *Absolute Wars* (wars fought for the extermination or unconditional surrender of the enemy) and *Limited Wars* (wars fought for the reparation of injuries, to gain territory, or for recognition of a particular claim) (Nickerson and Wright, 1962: 323). Three further sample classification schemes, utilized by workers in the social and political sciences, are summarized in Table 1.3. As the table indicates, the classifications vary in terms of their core attributes from the qualitative four-category classification of Wright (1965) to the mortality-based classification of Richardson (1960) and the combined typology of Singer and Small (1972).

1.2.3 Historical Trends in Wars

Following Nickerson and Wright (1962: 329), it is convenient to divide the historical sequence of wars into *primitive*, *historic*, and *modern*, with each type of warfare broadly corresponding to major innovations in the fields of communications and weapons. Historic warfare, as differentiated from the primitive (or tribal) warfare of hunter-gatherer societies, emerged around the second millennium BC and was characterized by the use of writing and, typically, the horse. In turn, the development of agriculture, urban civilization, and political organization was associated with a shift in the underpinning motivation for war, away from retribution (typical of primitive wars) to economic gain and political conquest (typical of many historic wars). Modern warfare, emerging with modern civilization around AD 1500, was associated with gunpowder, the propaganda opportunities afforded by the printing press, and, much later, technological developments such as steamboats and steam trains, cars and aircraft, telecommunications, radar, machine guns, and chemical, biological, and nuclear weapons.

TRENDS SINCE ANTIQUITY

If we examine the number of units[2] that were engaged in each of the 2,000 or so sample wars and war-like events listed in Kohn's (1999) *Dictionary of Wars*, we can obtain a broad picture of the geographical distribution of belligerent parties and associated conflicts in the historic and modern categories of warfare, 2000 BC–AD 2000 (Table 1.4). All told, the table identifies over 3,100 engagements, with the number rising steadily down the ages: 372 (historic warfare, antiquity), 786 (historic warfare, Middle Ages), and 1,979 (modern).[3] Geographically, the Old World dominates the record in Table 1.4; entry of the New World awaited European colonization in the modern period and the beginning of a written record for the Americas and Oceania.

---

[2] We use the term 'unit' to refer to belligerent parties down the ages including areas, civilizations, and populations.

[3] The space–time totals in Table 1.4 are based on a count of the individual entries in the Geographical Index to Kohn (1999: 557–94).

Table 1.3. Sample classifications of wars

Type of war	Definition	Examples
Wright's (1965) classification of wars		
Balance of power	War among state members of the modern family of nations	Crimean War (1853–6) World War I (1914–18)
Civil	War within a member state of the modern family of nations	American Civil War (1861–5) Russian Revolution and Civil War (1917–21)
Defensive	War to defend modern civilization against an alien culture	War of Granada (1482–92) Russo-Turkish War (1678–81)
Imperial	War to expand modern civilization at the expense of an alien culture	Conquest of Mexico (1520–1) Zulu War (1879)
Richardson's (1960) magnitude-based classification of wars		
Magnitude 7 ± 0.5	3,162,278–31,622,777 deaths	World War I (1914–18) World War II (1939–45)
Magnitude 6 ± 0.5	316,228–3,162,277 deaths	American Civil War (1861–5) Spanish Civil War (1936–9)
Magnitude 5 ± 0.5	31,623–316,227 deaths	Russo-Turkish War (1828–9) Crimean War (1853–6)
Magnitude 4 ± 0.5	3,163–31,662 deaths	First Burma War (1823–6) Polish Rebellion (1830–1)
Magnitude 3 ± 0.5	317–3,162 deaths	Third Maori War (1863–6) Chinese Revolution (1911–12)
Singer and Small's (1972) classification of international wars		
Interstate	War involving at least one member of interstate system[1] on each side of the conflict, resulting in 1,000 or more battle deaths	Franco-Spanish War (1823) World War II (1939–45)
Extra-systemic (imperial and colonial)	War in which there was a member of the interstate system[1] on only one side of the war, resulting in an average of 1,000 battle deaths per year for system member participants	Cuban Insurrection (1895–8) South African War (1899–1902)

Notes: [1] Interstate system defined variously as: (1) 1816–1919, national entities with independent control over own foreign policy, population of at least 500,000, and diplomatic recognition from Great Britain and France; (2) 1920–65, national entities with independent control over own foreign policy, and either (*a*) membership of the League of Nations or the United Nations or (*b*) population of at least 500,000 and diplomatic recognition from any two major powers.
Sources: Richardson (1960), Wright (1965, app. XX, table 31, p. 641) and Singer and Small (1972, app. A, pp. 381–2).

Table 1.4. Distribution of sample wars and war-like events, by number of
participating units, 2000 BC–AD 2000

Region	Time period			
	Historic Warfare			
	Antiquity (2000 BC–AD 500)	Middle Ages (AD 500–1500)	Modern (AD 1500–2000)	Total
Old World				
Africa	30	15	174	219
Asia	154	180	388	722
Europe	188	591	1,043	1,822
New World				
Americas	0	0	359	359
Oceania	0	0	15	15
Total	372	786	1,979	3,137

Note: Totals are based on counts of the entries in the Geographical Index to Kohn's (1999) *Dictionary of Wars*.
Source: Based on information included in Kohn (1999: 557–94).

TRENDS IN MODERN WARS

We draw on data included in Wright (1965, appendix XX. 636–51) and Brogan
(1992, appendix I. 621–5) to examine trends in wars over the past five centuries.
These two sources provide annual information for 166 types of geographical
area (countries, principalities, cities, and tribal domains): (i) whether the
geographical unit was at war or not, from which the number of wars can be
computed; (ii) the number of states with which each unit was at war; and (iii)
the type of war, as defined by Wright (1965) in Table 1.3.[4]

Aggregate Series

Figure 1.1 plots the annual count of wars (line trace) and participating states
(bar chart) for a global sample of 375 conflicts, 1480–1990. The horizontal
lines mark the median (9) and third quartile (13) of the number of states at war
in each year, while Table 1.5 gives summary details of the sample conflicts. The
bar chart in Figure 1.1 shows that the seventeenth, nineteeth, and twentieth
centuries were particularly warlike. The period of the Thirty Years' War
(1618–48) is especially prominent in the seventeenth century, while the conflicts
of the nineteenth century span the colonial expansion of (and American wars

----

[4] The category 'imperial wars', defined by Wright (1965) as wars to expand modern civilization at the
expense of an alien culture (Table 1.3), poses particular problems in the period since 1945 as new nations
in the developing world lost their colonial status and became independent nations. The former colonial
possessions of the United Kingdom and France in Africa provide examples. We have classified wars
fought to establish independence from colonial status as 'imperial' in this section.

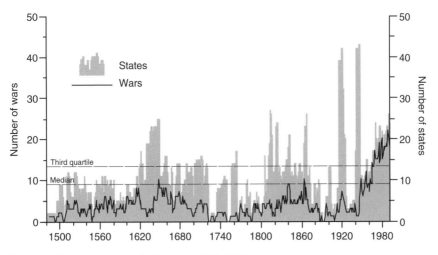

Fig. 1.1. Wars of modern civilization, 1480–1990

Notes: The graph plots the annual count of wars (line trace) and participating states (bar chart) for a global sample of 375 conflicts identified by Wright (1965) and Brogan (1992). The horizontal lines mark the median (9) and third quartile (13) of the number of states at war in each year.

Source: Based on information in Wright (1965, appendix XX, pp. 636–51) and Brogan (1992, appendix I, pp. 621–5).

of independence from) Europe. In the twentieth century, the two world wars rise like spires to claim the dubious distinction of being the largest of the sample conflicts. Finally, a particularly unpleasant feature of the twentieth century is the linearly rising tide of war from a zero base in 1908.

Geographical Theatres

The graphs in Figure 1.2 are annual plots of the percentage proportion of the combatant states in Figure 1.1 that were European (Fig. 1.2A) and non-European (Fig. 1.2B). An ordinary least squares (OLS) polynomial regression line has been fitted to the scattergrams to show the time trends. The trend lines are consistent with a fundamental shift in the geographical location of war from European to non-European theatres after the beginning of the eighteenth century. Initially, this shift reflects the colonial expansion of European powers into other parts of the world and latterly the non-European locations of many civil wars (especially in Africa).[5]

Types of Wars

Figure 1.3 is based on Wright's four-fold classification of wars (Table 1.3) and plots as solid line traces the percentage proportion of war years between 1480

---

[5] The geographical shift in Figure 1.2 may also reflect the European bias of the data set in the period prior to World War II. See e.g. Brecke (1999).

Table 1.5. Summary characteristics of wars, 1480–1990

Characteristic	Time period										Total
	1480–1550	1551–1600	1601–1650	1651–1700	1700–1750	1750–1800	1800–1850	1850–1900	1900–1950	1950–1990	
No. of wars fought	32	31	34	30	18	20	41	48	34	87	375
Type[1]											
Balance of power	18	12	13	14	13	10	17	23	15	4	139
Civil	4	14	14	8	5	5	11	12	11	53	137
Imperial	4	0	3	4	0	5	11	13	6	13	59
Defensive	6	5	4	4	0	0	2	0	0	0	21
Unclassified	0	0	0	0	0	0	0	0	2	17	19
By geographical location											
Predominantly European	28	31	31	26	18	13	15	14	12	4	192
Predominantly extra-European	4	0	3	4	0	7	26	34	22	83	183
No. of states at war	28	19	34	22	20	32	53	53	68	66	—
Average duration of wars	3.8	4.9	7.6	5.2	4.9	3.4	4.2	2.7	3.6	6.3	—

Notes: [1] See Table 1.3 for details of Wright's (1965) classification of wars.
Source: Data from Wright (1965, app. XX, table 45, p. 651 and app. C, pp. 1544–7) and Brogan (1992, app. I, pp. 621–5).

A European states

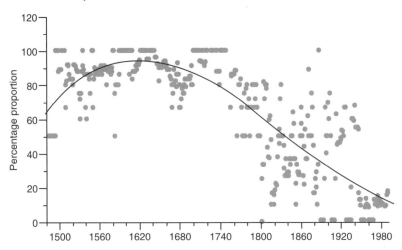

B Non-European states

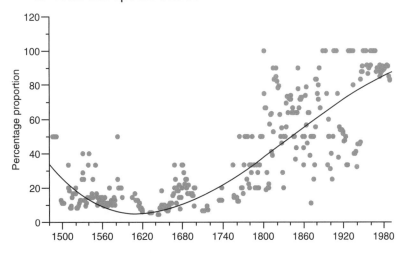

Fig. 1.2. Geographical distribution of states at war, 1480–1990

Notes: For a global sample of 375 conflicts, the graphs plot the annual percentage distribution of warring states by geographical region. (A) European states. (B) Non-European states. Polynomial regression lines depict the temporal trend in each distribution.

Source: Based on information in Wright (1965, appendix XX, pp. 636–51) and Brogan (1992, appendix I, pp. 621–5).

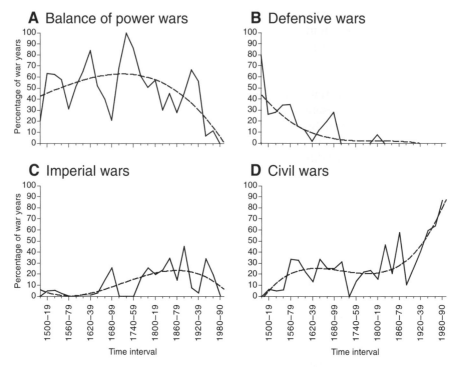

Fig. 1.3. Long-term trends in different types of war, 1480–1990

Notes: The graphs are based on a global sample of 375 conflicts and plot, as solid line traces, the percentage proportion of war years associated with each of four types of war as defined by Wright (1965). Proportions have been computed by 20-year time interval, starting with the period 1480–99. (A) Balance of power wars. (B) Defensive wars. (C) Imperial wars. (D) Civil wars. Polynomial regression lines, plotted as the pecked line traces, depict the temporal trends in each war category. The four types of war are defined in Table 1.3.

Source: Based on information in Wright (1965, appendix XX, pp. 636–51) and Brogan (1992, appendix I, pp. 621–5).

and 1990 associated with balance of power wars (Fig. 1.3A), defensive wars (1.3B), imperial and colonial wars (1.3C), and civil wars (1.3D). To form the graphs, the 500-year period was divided into discrete 20-year windows, with the first window covering the period 1480–99, the second 1500–19, and so on, up to and including the truncated period 1980–90. For each time window, the percentage proportion of war years associated with a given category of conflict was then computed. The resulting values are plotted as the time series in Figure 1.3A–D. As before, OLS polynomial regression lines (pecked line traces) show the temporal trends in each war category.

The graphs in Figure 1.3 show a shift in the dominant types of war over the last five centuries, away from set-piece international conflagrations to civil wars. Figure 1.3A shows that balance of power wars were recorded over the entire observation period. However, despite the repeated occurrence of such wars and their dominance in some epochs (early sixteenth, early-to-mid-seventeenth, eighteenth, late nineteenth, and early twentieth centuries), an underlying downward trend began around 1750. In contrast, Figure 1.3B shows that purely defensive wars had all but ceased by the end of the seventeenth century. Imperial wars (Fig. 1.3C) first appeared on a regular basis in the second half of the seventeenth century, initially associated with the expansion of Holland, Portugal, Spain, and other European states and later, in the twentieth century, with wars for independence from imperial powers. Civil wars (Fig. 1.3D) occurred throughout the 500-year span, but have been a particular feature of the second half of the twentieth century.

1.2.4 Defining Populations: The Geneva Conventions and the Laws of War

Attempts to place war within a legal framework can be traced to antiquity (Corbett, 1962). Classical Roman law contained statutes to limit both the undertaking of war and to moderate the waging of hostilities. Since these early beginnings, an elaborate body of laws relating to war and its conduct has evolved. By the nineteenth century, the prevailing view was to place all belligerents on the same legal footing. The codification of the laws of modern war stem from 1863–4 and the series of meetings in Geneva which established the International Red Cross and the Geneva Conventions. The Geneva Convention of 1864 (explicity concerned with the protection of the wounded and sick in armed forces) inspired the trend towards the international regulation of conflicts and, more recently, the circumstances under which recourse to arms may be made (Corbett, 1962; Mayda, 1962). An overview of major events relating to the development of the international laws of war, 1860–2000, is provided in Table 1.6.

THE 1949 GENEVA CONVENTIONS

While the original Geneva Convention of 1864 was revised and extended in 1906–7 (Conventions I–II) and 1929 (Conventions I–III), Table 1.6 traces the current form of the Conventions to the late 1940s. Following World War II, the International Committee of the Red Cross (ICRC) formulated proposals to adapt and develop international humanitarian law applicable in armed conflicts and, at the XVII International Conference on the Red Cross (Stockholm, 1948), four draft conventions were approved for diplomatic review. The following year, the Diplomatic Conference for the Establishment of the International Conventions for the Protection of Victims of War (Geneva, 1949) undertook a revision of the ICRC draft Conventions, and these were formally approved as the Geneva Conventions on 12 August 1949:

Table 1.6. Some principal events in the development of international laws relating to war and associated populations

Date	Event (including meetings, conventions, protocols, rules, and manuals)
1856	Paris Declaration Respecting Maritime Law
1863	Foundation of the Red Cross
1864	**Geneva Convention** **I. *Wounded and Sick in Armed Forces in the Field***
1868	St Petersburg Declaration Renouncing the Use of Explosive Projectiles
1874	Brussels Conference: Rules of Military Warfare and Draft Code
1880	Institute of International Law: *Manual of the Laws of War on Land*
1899	First Hague Conference on Peace and Disarmament: Conventions, Land War Regulations and Declarations
1906–7	**Geneva Conventions** **I. *Wounded and Sick in Armed Forces in the Field*** **II. *Wounded, Sick, and Shipwrecked Members of the Armed Forces at Sea***
1907	Second Hague Conference: Conventions and Land War Regulations
1909	London Conference: Declaration on the Rules of Naval Warfare
1923	Hague Rules for Aerial Warfare
1925	Geneva Gas Warfare Protocol
1929	**Geneva Conventions** **I. *Wounded and Sick in Armed Forces in the Field*** **II. *Wounded, Sick, and Shipwrecked Members of the Armed Forces at Sea*** **III. *Treatment of Prisoners of War***
1944–5	United Nations Organization established
1945–8	International Military Tribunals (Nuremberg and Tokyo)
1948	Universal Declaration of Human Rights
1949	**Geneva Conventions** **I. *Wounded and Sick in Armed Forces in the Field*** **II. *Wounded, Sick, and Shipwrecked Members of the Armed Forces at Sea*** **III. *Treatment of Prisoners of War*** **IV. *Protection of Civilian Persons in Time of War***
1951	UN Convention Relating to the Status of Refugees
1956	International Committee of the Red Cross: Draft Rules for the Protection of Civilians
1974–7	Geneva Diplomatic Conference for the Reaffirmation and Development of The Law of Armed Conflict
1977	**Geneva Protocols** **I. *Protection of Victims of International Armed Conflicts*** **II. *Protection of Victims of Non-International Armed Conflicts***
1980	UN Convention on Prohibitions or Restrictions on the Use of Certain Conventional Weapons
1994	UN Convention on the Safety of United Nations and Associated Personnel
1997	Ottawa Convention on the Prohibition of the Use, Stockpiling, Production, and Transfer of Anti-Personnel Mines and on their Destruction

Source: Based, in part, on information in Roberts and Guelff (2000).

Convention I: Wounded and Sick in Armed Forces in the Field;
Convention II: Wounded, Sick, and Shipwrecked Members of the Armed Forces at Sea;
Convention III: Treatment of Prisoners of War;
Convention IV: Protection of Civilian Persons in Time of War.

Augmented by the 1977 Geneva Protocols, the Geneva Conventions provide the modern legal framework for the humanitarian operation of war.

Armed Forces

The international legal instruments of war draw a basic distinction between the 'armed forces' and the 'peaceful' (1907 Hague Regulations) or 'civilian' (1949 Geneva Conventions) population. The armed forces, in turn, are viewed as consisting of both combatant and non-combatant personnel (Wright, 1965: 308). As regards definitions of the membership of the armed forces, Table 1.7 reproduces Article 13 of Geneva Conventions I (Armed Forces in the Field) and II (Armed Forces at Sea). By delimiting the persons covered by the Conventions, the article defines the legal units of the armed forces recognized in international law for the sick and wounded. As Table 1.7 indicates, the armed forces of belligerent parties are deemed to include not only regular, militia, and

Table 1.7. Article 13 of the 1949 Geneva Conventions I and II

The present Convention shall apply to the wounded and sick belonging to the following categories:

(1) Members of the armed forces of a Party to the conflict, as well as members of militias or volunteer corps forming part of such armed forces.

(2) Members of other militias and members of other volunteer corps, including those of organized resistance movements, belonging to a Party to the conflict and operating in or outside their own territory, even if this territory is occupied, provided that such militias or volunteer corps, including such organized resistance movements, fulfil the following conditions:
    (a) that of being commanded by a person responsible for his subordinates;
    (b) that of having a fixed distinctive sign recognizable at a distance;
    (c) that of carrying arms openly;
    (d) that of conducting their operations in accordance with the laws and customs of war.

(3) Members of regular armed forces who profess allegiance to a Government or an authority not recognized by the Detaining Power.

(4) Persons who accompany the armed forces without actually being members thereof, such as civil members of military aircraft crews, war correspondents, supply contractors, members of labour units or of services responsible for the welfare of the armed forces, provided that they have received authorization from the armed forces which they accompany.

(5) Members of crews, including masters, pilots and apprentices of the merchant marine and the crews of civil aircraft of the Parties to the conflict, who do not benefit from more favourable treatment under any other provisions in international law.

(6) Inhabitants of a non-occupied territory who, on the approach of the enemy, spontaneously take up arms to resist the invading forces, without having had time to form themselves into regular armed units, provided they carry arms openly and respect the laws and customs of war.

Source: Reproduced from Roberts and Guelff (2000: 202–3).

volunteer corps and their authorized civilian accompaniment but also the crews of merchant ships and civil aircraft and, under certain circumstances, organized resistance movements and spontaneous resistance fighters.

Prisoners of War (POWs)

As Lancaster (1990: 322) notes, the status of 'prisoner of war' (POW) is one of relatively recent times. In the early history of warfare, captives were usually dispatched on the battlefield or taken into slavery. As warfare evolved, however, so too did the treatment of prisoners. In conclusion of the Thirty Years' War (1618–48), the Treaty of Westphalia—which allowed for the release of captives without ransom—is generally held as marking the end of the practice of enslavement of prisoners. By the mid-nineteenth century, most civilized nations had begun to observe a general code of POW treatment, summarized by Francis Lieber during the American Civil War (1861–5). But it was the many POWs involved in the two world wars which prompted the formulation of Convention III (Treatment of Prisoners of War) of the Geneva Conventions. As defined in Article 4, Part I, of the Convention, POWs are 'members of the armed forces of a Party to the conflict' which have 'fallen into the power of the enemy' (sect. A(1)). Subsequent sections of the same article extend this definition to include the enemy detention of, among others: resistance corps; crew members of the merchant marine and civil aircraft; and armed occupants of territories under threat of invasion (sect. A(2)–A(6)); see Roberts and Guelff (2000: 245–6).

CIVIL POPULATIONS

The evolution of international law relating to civilians in wartime is reviewed by Roberts and Guelff (2000: 299–300). While the Hague Conventions of 1899 and 1907 make express reference to civilians (Table 1.6), the first moves to set forth principles for civil populations were made by the ICRC in the wake of World War I. But it was the mass deportations, exterminations, and killings of World War II which finally prompted the formulation of international laws for the protection of civilians in wartime. In a supplement to Convention IV (Protection of Civilian Persons in Time of War) of the Geneva Conventions, Article 50(1) of the 1977 Geneva Protocol I effectively defines a civilian as any person who does not fall into one of the categories of the armed forces in Table 1.7.[6] The same article adds that a civilian population 'comprises all persons who are civilians' (Art. 50(2)), while the 'presence within the civilian population of individuals who do not come within the definition of civilians does not deprive the population of its civilian character' (Art. 50(3)) (Roberts and Guelff, 2000: 448).

---

[6] As Levie (1986: 6) notes, the complex wording of the definition in Article 50(1) of Protocol I simply equates to 'Any person who is not a member of the armed forces is considered to be a civilian'.

WAR-DISPLACED POPULATIONS

Within international law, a complex legal framework has developed around the meaning of the term 'refugee' and the related, but legally distinct, concepts of 'stateless person' and 'internally displaced person'. Prominent legal instruments, including the United Nations (UN) Conventions Relating to the Status of Refugees (1951) and Stateless Persons (1954) are briefly reviewed in Section 5.2, where formal definitions of the various population categories are also provided. Here, we note that war-displaced persons may, in practice, include members of both military and civil populations.

1.2.5 Levels of War-Related Mortality

Although wars occupy an important position in the overall pattern of human mortality, great difficulties are encountered in obtaining accurate information on war-related deaths (Lancaster, 1990). As described in Section 1.4, detailed mortality statistics—for both military and civil populations—only became available from the mid-nineteenth century. Prior to this date, we are largely reliant on broad estimates of the killed and wounded while, even in relatively recent times, the evidence must be treated with caution.

MILITARY POPULATIONS

Prior to the Nineteenth Century

Table 1.8 is based on information included in Sorokin's (1937) *Social and Cultural Dynamics*, Vol. iii and gives, for sample military forces, rounded estimates of mortality arising from wars in the period 500 BC–AD 1800. As the table shows, the latter part of the observation period was associated with a dramatic increase in the estimated number of military deaths, from an annual average of under 1,000 deaths (500 BC–AD 1500) to over 30,000 deaths (AD 1501–1800). All told, almost 11 million died as a consequence of war, with the final three centuries accounting for over 80 per-cent of the estimated toll.

Table 1.8. Estimated war-related mortality in military populations, 500 BC–AD 1800

Period	Estimated Deaths	Average annual number of estimated deaths
500 BC–AD 1500	1,727,000	864
AD 1501–1800	9,112,000	30,373
Total (500 BC–AD 1800)	10,839,000	4,713

Note: Totals are based on sample states and time intervals (Greece, 500–126 BC, AD 1551–1800; Rome, 400 BC–AD 475; Russia, AD 901–1800; France, AD 976–1800; England, AD 1051–1800; Austria-Hungary, AD 1101–1800; Poland and Lithuania, AD 1376–1800; Spain, AD 1476–1800; Italy, AD 1551–1800; Germany, AD 1651–1800).
Source: Based on information in Sorokin (1937, tables 1, 3, 6–14, pp. 293–333, *passim*).

Table 1.9. Global estimates of the average annual
military deaths in wars, by century

Century	Military deaths (per million population per year)
Seventeenth	19.0
Eighteenth	18.8
Nineteenth	10.8
Twentieth	183.2

Source: Data from Garfield and Neugut (1991, table 1, p. 689).

Nineteenth and Twentieth Centuries

The modern era has witnessed a rapid growth in the firepower of belligerent populations. This has been accompanied by a sharp increase in the levels of military mortality associated with wars. So, as Table 1.9 shows, the average annual war-related military death rate (per million of the world's population) varied between 10 and 20 during the seventeenth, eighteenth, and nineteenth centuries. In the twentieth century, the rate spiralled to exceed 183.

Magnitude–duration relationships, I: wars. Figure 1.4A draws on information collated by Singer and Small (1972) and plots the magnitude–duration relationships for 92 sample wars of the nineteenth and twentieth centuries.[7] Magnitude, plotted on the vertical axis of the graph, is the estimated number of military deaths in a given war; duration, plotted on the horizontal axis, is the number of nation-months at war. To assist in the interpretation of Figure 1.4A, the horizontal broken lines mark the first quartile (2,800), median (10,000), and third quartile (33,025) of the number of military deaths in the set of conflicts.

As Figure 1.4A shows, five orders of magnitude separate the smallest wars (~1,000 deaths) from the most lethal conflagrations (~10 million deaths). Generally, magnitude rises with increasing duration. World War I (1914–18), World War II (1939–45), and the Korean War (1950–3) are singled out as wars of exceptional magnitude (>1 million deaths) and duration (>500 nation-months), with the majority of the remainder associated with 1,000–100,000 deaths and 10–100 nation-months of fighting.

Magnitude–duration relationships, II: belligerent states. Figure 1.4B is based on the same data set as Figure 1.4A and plots, for each state engaged in the 92 sample wars, the total number of deaths (magnitude, vertical axis) against the total number of months at war (duration, horizontal axis). In all instances,

---

[7] A further war identified by Singer and Small (Navarino Bay, 1827), included in their original list of 93 wars, has been omitted from the present analysis because of its exceptionally short duration (0.1 months).

A Wars

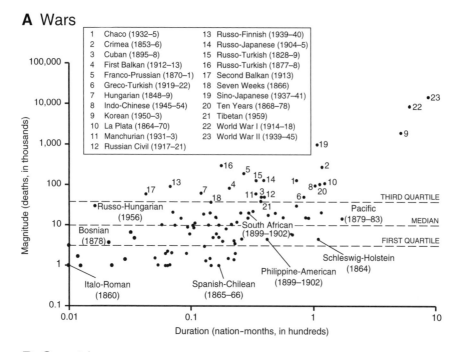

1	Chaco (1932–5)	13	Russo-Finnish (1939–40)
2	Crimea (1853–6)	14	Russo-Japanese (1904–5)
3	Cuban (1895–8)	15	Russo-Turkish (1828–9)
4	First Balkan (1912–13)	16	Russo-Turkish (1877–8)
5	Franco-Prussian (1870–1)	17	Second Balkan (1913)
6	Greco-Turkish (1919–22)	18	Seven Weeks (1866)
7	Hungarian (1848–9)	19	Sino-Japanese (1937–41)
8	Indo-Chinese (1945–54)	20	Ten Years (1868–78)
9	Korean (1950–3)	21	Tibetan (1959)
10	La Plata (1864–70)	22	World War I (1914–18)
11	Manchurian (1931–3)	23	World War II (1939–45)
12	Russian Civil (1917–21)		

B Countries

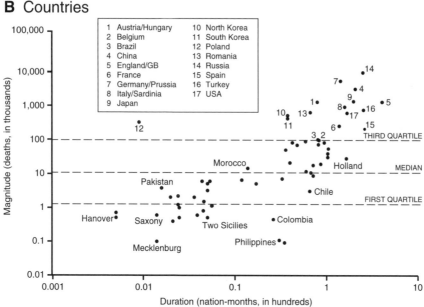

1	Austria/Hungary	10	North Korea
2	Belgium	11	South Korea
3	Brazil	12	Poland
4	China	13	Romania
5	England/GB	14	Russia
6	France	15	Spain
7	Germany/Prussia	16	Turkey
8	Italy/Sardinia	17	USA
9	Japan		

Fig. 1.4. Magnitude–duration relationships for sample wars of the nineteenth and twentieth centuries

Notes: For 92 sample wars defined by Singer and Small (1972), the graphs plot magnitude–duration relationships by (A) war and (B) belligerent country. On both graphs, magnitude is defined as the number of military deaths (all causes); duration is defined in nation-months at war. Horizontal pecked lines mark the first quartile, median, and third quartile of the number of deaths in the respective categories.

magnitude and duration have been computed across the set of wars in which each belligerent was involved. Consistent with Figure 1.4A, Figure 1.4B indicates a general tendency for magnitude to increase with the increasing duration of the hostilities. The graph also marks out those states whose armed forces have, in absolute terms, suffered most in the sample conflicts. States with over 1 million deaths include Russia (9.7 million), Germany/Prussia (5.4 million), China (3.1 million), Japan (1.4 million), Austria-Hungary (1.3 million), and England/Great Britain (1.3 million).

CIVIL POPULATIONS

The involvement of civil populations—either intentionally or unintentionally—has been an enduring feature of war history. In some wars, such as the Thirty Years' War (1618–48), civilians have suffered more than their military counterparts (Bodart, 1916). Historically, civil populations have been particularly affected by direct military action and the hardships of war during the siege of fortified towns and the bombardment of ports. An especially noteworthy feature of the last century has been the stark rise in civilians among the war dead. As Table 1.10 shows, in World War I, an estimated 14–19 per cent of all deaths were among civilians; in World War II the proportion had grown to 48–67 per cent while, for sample wars of the 1980s and 1990s, 75–90 per cent of all deaths are estimated to have occurred in civil populations. These developments are, in large measure, a direct consequence of the low-intensity conflicts of the post-Vietnam era, associated with more sophisticated weaponry and military strategies which have had a more pervasive impact on both the physical and mental well-being of civil populations (Garfield and Neugut, 1997).

Table 1.10. Proportion of war-related deaths estimated to have occurred among civilians, sample wars of the twentieth century

Conflict	Civilians as a proportion of all deaths (%)
World War I (1914–18)	14–19
Spanish Civil War (1936)	50
World War II (1939–45)	48–67
Korean War (1950–3)	34
Vietnam War (1956–75)	48
Sample wars (1980s)	75
Sample wars (1990s)	90

Source: Data from Garfield and Neugut (1997, table 3–4, p. 32 and Figure 3–4, p. 33).

1.3 War Epidemics

In this section, we first define the main causes of war-related morbidity and mortality (Sect. 1.3.1). We then examine the nature of epidemic diseases and their specific contribution to the morbidity and mortality of past wars (Sect. 1.3.2). Finally, we discuss why we have chosen certain wars and epidemic diseases for close study in this book (Sect. 1.3.3).

1.3.1 War-Related Morbidity and Mortality

The human casualties of war—encompassing both military and civil populations—may arise as a result of enemy weapons, by the spread of disease, by privation, physical exhaustion, exposure, accidents, imprisonment, execution, and desertion. Casualties may result from both the direct and indirect effects of military operations, with the latter having the potential to exert an influence on morbidity and mortality for many years after the cessation of active hostilities (Murray *et al.*, 2002).

MILITARY CASUALTIES

For military populations, it is necessary to differentiate between losses in the demographic sense and losses in the military sense (Urlanis, 1971: 21). From a military perspective, losses are usually understood to mean not only the death, but also the disablement (either temporary or permanent), of military personnel. The term *irreplaceable losses* is often used to cover the dead, those taken prisoner, and those otherwise unaccounted for. Irreplaceable losses form a component of those *put out of action*, of which those *discharged from service* (wounded and sick) form the balance. Fatal and non-fatal wounds, injuries, accidents, diseases, and other causes of morbidity and mortality constitute total military losses (see Garfield and Neugut, 1991).

Categories of Mortal Loss

Table 1.11 is based on Urlanis (1971: 28–9) and gives a categorization of mortal losses in mobilized military populations. While all military deaths are classified as direct losses of war, a convenient distinction is made between (A) 'battle losses' and (B) 'non-battle losses'.

(A) Battle losses. As Table 1.11 indicates, battle losses include three major categories of mortality:

  (a) killed on the battlefield (KOB) or, more generally, killed in action (KIA). This category relates to military personnel who died before medical assistance could be given for injuries sustained in active combat;

   (b) died of wounds (DOW) relates to those wounded in action (WIA) and who survived to medical registration, but who later died from their injuries;

   (c) died from poison gas and various diseases directly caused by the enemy. This category relates to deaths arising from purposeful attacks with chemical and biological weapons.

(B) Non-battle losses. As Table 1.11 shows, non-battle losses include deaths from diseases, burns and frostbite sustained under non-battle conditions; deaths from accidents, suicide, and execution; and deaths in captivity.

To the categories of military loss in Table 1.11 can be added *missing* (or *missing, presumed dead*). As Bodart (1916) notes, the 'missing' encompass the dead and wounded who could not be found or identified, prisoners whose fate is unknown, deserters, and dispersed troops.

CIVILIAN CASUALTIES

As noted in Section 1.2, the casualties of war are by no means restricted to military populations. In addition to the mistreatment and/or direct military

Table 1.11. War-related categories of mortality in military and civilian populations

Military Populations	Civil Populations
Direct losses	
(A) Battle losses	(A) Victims of aerial bombing and shelling outside frontline zone
(i) killed on battlefield (KOB)/killed in action (KIA)	(B) Death of civilians in frontline zone from various causes
(ii) died of wounds (DOW) sustained in battle conditions	(C) Victims of terror (including those who died in prisons and concentration camps)
(iii) died from poison gas and various diseases directly caused by the enemy	(D) Losses due to forced transportation of population
(B) Non-battle losses	(E) Deaths of crews and passengers of merchant ships and civil aircraft
(i) died from diseases, burns, frostbite, etc., sustained in non-battle conditions	
(ii) died as a result of accident, suicide, or execution	
(iii) died in captivity from starvation, disease, and other causes	
Indirect losses	
—	War-associated deaths, exclusive of civilian categories (A)–(E) above. Specific causes include deaths arising from: epidemics, starvation, disruption of health-care systems, etc.

Source: Based on Urlanis (1971: 28–9).

targeting of civilians in war zones, armies can spread diseases to civil populations, even in neutral countries. Historically, armies have tended to leave famine behind them, while military forces may impose poor conditions of hygiene on civil populations. The circumstances of civil populations in concentration camps, refugee camps, internment camps, and besieged settlements can be especially severe. Often deprived of food, shelter, clothes, and medical care, such populations may be forced to exist in deplorable conditions.

The right-hand column in Table 1.11 gives a classification of war-related mortality categories for civil populations. As the table shows, direct causes of mortality include deaths arising from aerial bombing and shelling; exposure on the frontline; acts of terror; forced transportation; and enemy attacks on merchant ships and civil aircraft. Indirect losses include all other deaths arising as a consequence of war, including those attributable to disease, starvation, and the disruption of healthcare services. In principle at least, the classification for civil populations in Table 1.11 can be extended to include morbidity as well as mortality.

MEDICINE AND WAR

The development of modern medicine in relation to war is reviewed by Major (1940), Fulton (1953), and Cooter (1993). Some indication of the extent and breadth of medical concern with war and its casualties can be gained from Figures 1.5 and 1.6. The line trace in Figure 1.5 plots the annual number of military- and war-related medical publications over a 200-year period, 1800–2000, as cited in *Index Catalogue of the Library of the Surgeon-General's Office* and *Index Medicus*. The graphs in Figure 1.6 are a subset of Figure 1.5 and plot, using line traces, the annual number of medical publications relating to six war-related topics (air war/air raids, atomic/nuclear war, chemical and biological war, civil defence/protection, refugees, and war crimes), 1900–2000. As a backdrop, the bar charts in Figures 1.5 and 1.6 plot the number of states at war in a given year.

As Figure 1.5 shows, the latter half of the nineteenth century was associated with a rising tide of medical concern with military- and war-related issues which peaked during World War I. Thereafter, a secondary peak during World War II was followed, in the post-war period, by a sustained flow of 300 to 500 citations per year. As regards the shifting nature of the subject matter, Figure 1.6 shows that medical interest in air war/air raids during World War II (Fig. 1.6A) was replaced in subsequent years by concerns over topics such as atomic/nuclear war (Fig. 1.6B), refugees (Fig. 1.6E), and war crimes (Fig. 1.6F). Chemical and biological warfare, which first came to the fore during World War I, continued to occupy a prominent place in the medical literature over the remainder of the twentieth century (Fig. 1.6C), while civil defence/protection declined from a peak in the 1960s (Fig. 1.6D).

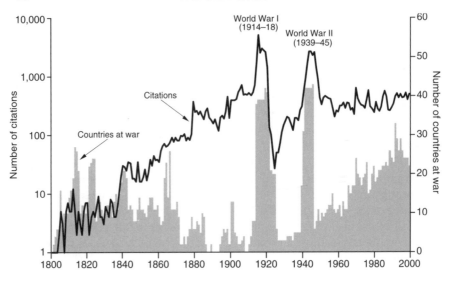

Fig. 1.5. Intensity of medical writing on war, 1800–2000

Notes: The line trace plots the annual count of citations under the headings of Army, Armies, Military Medicine, Naval Medicine, and War as recorded in *Index Catalogue of the Library of the Surgeon-General's Office, United States' Army* and *Index Medicus*. For reference, the bar chart plots the number of countries at war in corresponding years.

1.3.2 Epidemic Diseases and War

Set within the framework of Table 1.11, epidemics of infectious disease have exerted a particularly powerful influence on the (battle/non-battle) military losses and (direct/indirect) civilian losses of past wars. In this subsection, we define the meaning of the terms 'epidemic' and 'epidemic disease', we assess the size of wartime losses arising from epidemic diseases, and we identify the principal infectious diseases that have afflicted military and civil populations in past wars. Finally, we summarize the wartime factors which have promoted the epidemic transmission of the diseases involved.

DEFINING EPIDEMICS AND EPIDEMIC DISEASES

The term *epidemic* comes from two Greek words: *demos* meaning 'people' and *epi* meaning 'upon' or 'close to'. It was used around 500 BC as a title for one

Fig. 1.6. Intensity of medical writing on a sample of six war-related topics, 1900–2000

Notes: On each graph, the line trace plots the annual count of citations as recorded in *Index Medicus*, while the bar chart plots the number of countries at war in corresponding years. (A) Air war/air raids. (B) Atomic/nuclear war. (C) Chemical and biological war. (D) Civil defence/protection. (E) Refugees. (F) War crimes.

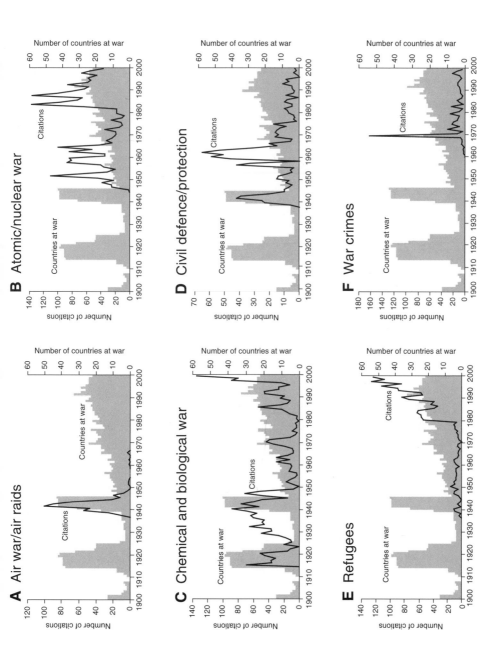

A Air war/air raids

B Atomic/nuclear war

C Chemical and biological war

D Civil defence/protection

E Refugees

F War crimes

major part of the Hippocratic corpus, but the section concerned was mainly a day-to-day account of certain patients and not an application of the word in its modern sense (Risse, 1993: 11). In addition to its wider usage in terms of public attitudes (e.g. Burke's 'epidemick of despair'), the word has been used in the English language in a medical sense since at least 1603 to mean an unusually high incidence of a disease. Here, 'unusually high' is fixed in time, in space and in the persons afflicted as compared with previous experience. Thus the *Oxford English Dictionary* defines an epidemic as: 'a disease prevalent among a people or community at a special time, and produced by some special causes generally not present in the affected locality'. The parallel term, *epizootic*, is used to specify a disease present under similar conditions in a non-human animal community.

In the standard handbook of human communicable diseases, Benenson (1990: 499) defines an epidemic more fully as:

The occurrence in a community or region of cases of an illness (or an outbreak) clearly in excess of expectancy. The number of cases indicating presence of an epidemic will vary according to the infectious agent, size and type of population exposed, previous experience or lack of exposure to the diseases, and time and place of occurrence; epidemicity is thus relative to usual frequency of disease in the same area, among the specified population, at the same season of the year.

Benenson's account goes on to stress that what constitutes an epidemic does not necessarily depend on large numbers of cases or deaths. A single case of a communicable disease long absent from a population, or the first invasion by a disease not previously recognized in that area, requires immediate reporting and epidemiological investigation. Two cases of such a disease associated in time and place are taken to be sufficient evidence of transmission for an epidemic to be declared.

The recognition of an epidemic implies that there is some benchmark against which an 'unusual' concentration of cases or deaths can be measured. In some instances, the benchmark will be zero reported cases but, in others, where the epidemic is a peak rising from a plinth of 'normal' incidence, complex methods of epidemic recognition may be called for (see Fig. 1.7). Cliff *et al.* (1986: 20–2) have reviewed the models used to separate epidemics of influenza from the background incidence of that disease. The term *endemic* is used to describe the usual presence of a disease or infectious agent within a given geographical area. More rarely the term *hyperendemic* is used to describe a persistent intense transmission and *holoendemic* to describe a high level of infection which typically begins early in life and goes on to affect most of the resident population: many tropical areas with endemic malaria may be described as holoendemic (Benenson, 1990: 499).

Types of Epidemics

Epidemics of communicable disease are of two main types. A *propagated* epidemic is one which results from the chain transmission of some infectious

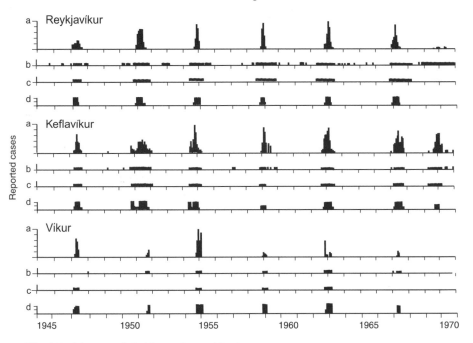

Fig. 1.7. Alternate definitions of an epidemic

Notes: For three Icelandic medical districts, the histograms (charts a) plot the monthly reported cases of measles. Various definitions of an epidemic are attempted in charts b–d. Charts b: Columns are one unit high if cases were reported in a given month. Charts c: Columns are one unit high if the case rate per unit population exceeded a threshold set by the researcher. This crops isolated outlier cases from each epidemic as compared with charts b. Charts d: epidemics are declared if both the case rate (columns one unit high) and the absolute number of cases in a given month exceeded researcher-specified thresholds. Columns are three units high if both criteria were met. This separates out the build-up and fade-out months from the main body of an epidemic.
Source: Cliff *et al.* (1981, fig. 5.10, p. 108).

agent. This may be directly from person to person as in a measles outbreak, or indirectly via an intermediate vector (malaria) or a microparasite. In some cases, indirect transmission may occur via humans (as in louse-borne epidemic typhus fever, or in a mosquito → man → mosquito chain with malaria). In others, the survival of the parasite is independent of man. For example, *Yersinia pestis*, the cause of bubonic plague is continually propagated through rodents, and the infection of man by an infected flea is a sideshow. An example of a propagated epidemic in a war setting is the 1870–1 smallpox epidemic which spread in France and the states of Germany during the Franco-Prussian War (see Sect. 8.3).

The second type of epidemic is a *common-vehicle epidemic* (Maxcy, 1973: 642) which results from the dissemination of a causative agent. In this case, the epidemic may result from a group of people being infected from a common medium (typically water, milk, or food) which has been contaminated by a disease-causing organism. An example of a common-vehicle epidemic in a war setting is the 1898 typhoid epidemic which spread among US Volunteers during the Spanish–American War (see Sect. 7.3).

Routes of Transmission

The major routes of transmission for infectious diseases are listed in Table 1.12. Many disease-causing organisms have several alternate routes, thus enhancing their chances of survival. The sequence of events in successful transmission involves release of the micro-organism from the cell, exit from the body, transport through the environment in a viable form, and appropriate entry into a susceptible host. This may be direct and essentially simple as in the case of the measles virus: the virus is shed from an infected cell and exits the body through exhalation, sneezing, and coughing as an aerosol. If a susceptible host is within range, the virus is inhaled and invades cells in the mucous membranes of the respiratory tract.

By contrast, other contagious diseases spread through a complex chain of contacts in which humans appear only at the end. For example, the transmission of scrub typhus, a rickettsial disease attended in severe cases by haemorrhagic signs and loss of conciousness, depends on the life cycle of a mite (which may bite humans) but also rodents and other zoonotic carriers.

WAR EPIDEMICS

We now move from a consideration of the nature of epidemics and epidemic diseases, to an examination of their occurrence in past wars. We consider military and civil populations in turn.

Military Populations

That epidemic diseases exacted a heavy human toll in many past wars—frequently outstripping battle and battle wounds as the leading causes of death in military populations—is evidenced in Table 1.13. For conflicts of the late eighteenth, nineteenth, and twentieth centuries, the table gives estimates of the number of deaths in sample combatant forces due to (*a*) battle and battle wounds and (*b*) disease. The ratio of deaths from disease to battle, (*b*):(*a*), is also given along with the principal diseases which afflicted the forces.

Table 1.13 shows that, prior to the twentieth century, deaths from diseases regularly exceeded those arising from the bombs and bullets of the enemy. For example, during the French Revolutionary and Napoleonic Wars (1792–1815), the British Army suffered seven or more disease-related deaths for every one battle-related death. Similar statistics are recorded for US forces in the Mexican War (1846–7) and the Spanish–American War (1898) while, across the set of nineteenth-century conflicts in Table 1.13, the aggregate ratio of deaths from disease to battle is approximately 2.5:1. Thereafter, the early years of the twentieth century mark something of a watershed in the epidemiological history of war. Due in part to developments in the firepower of belligerent

Table 1.12. Routes of transmission of infections

Route of exit	Route of transmission	Diseases	Routes of entry
Respiratory	Aerosol	*Chickenpox, diphtheria, influenza, Lassa fever, legionellosis, mumps, pertussis, pneumonia, poliomyelitis, rubella, smallpox, tuberculosis*	? Mouth
	Salivary transfer	*Hepatitis B, mononucleosis, mumps*	Mouth
	Nasal discharges	*Leprosy, smallpox*	? Mouth
	Bite	*Rabies*	Skin
	Mouth: hand or object	*Chickenpox, diphtheria, EBV in children, herpes simplex, pneumonia, smallpox*	Oropharyngeal
Gastrointestinal tract	Stool: hand	*Cholera, cryptosporidiosis, enteroviruses, hepatitis A, poliomyelitis, salmonellosis, shigellosis, typhoid, paratyphoid*	Mouth
	Stool: water, milk	*Cholera, cryptosporidiosis, hepatitis A, tuberculosis*	Mouth
	Stool: ground	*Hookworm disease*	Skin
	Thermometer	*Hepatitis A*	Rectal
Skin	Air	*Poxviruses*	Respiratory
	Skin: skin	*Molluscum cantagiosum, yaws*	Abraded skin
Blood	Mosquitos	*Arboviruses, dengue fever, malaria, yellow fever*	Skin
	Ticks	*Lyme disease, relapsing fever, Rocky Mountain spotted fever, togaviruses (Group B)*	Skin
	Blackflies	*Onchocerciasis*	Skin
	Lice	*Typhus fever*	Skin
	Fleas	*Plague*	Skin
	Blood transfusion	*Hepatitis B, HIV*	Skin
	Injection needles	*Hepatitis B*	Skin
Urine	Rarely transmitted	*CMV, measles, mumps, rubella (congenital)*	Unknown
Genital	Cervix	*Chlamydial infections, gonorrhoeae, herpes simplex, CMV, HIV, syphilis*	Genital
	Semen	*CMV, HIV, syphilis*	Genital
Placental	Vertical to embryo	*CMV, HIV, leprosy, rubella, smallpox, hepatitis B*	Blood

Notes: CMV = cytomegalovirus, EBV = Epstein–Barr virus.
Source: Cliff *et al.* (1998, table 1.1, p. 6), modified from Evans (1982, table 3, p. 10).

Table 1.13. Distribution of deaths by cause in military forces, sample wars (1792–2000)

War	Force	Number of deaths (000s)		Ratio (b):(a)	Major diseases
		Battle and wounds (a)	Disease (b)		
French Revolutionary and Napoleonic Wars (1792–1815)	British Army	25.6	193.9	7.6:1	typhus, dysentery, fevers
Walcheren Expedition (1809–10)	British Army	0.1	4.0	40.0:1	malaria, typhoid, typhus, dysentery
Mexican War (1846–8)	US Army	1.5	11.0	7.3:1	dysentery
Crimean War (1853–6)	Allied Army[1]	24.9	95.1	3.8:1	cholera, typhus, fevers, scurvy
	Russian Army	35.7	37.1	1.0:1	
Italian War (1859)	French Army	5.5	2.0	0.4:1	typhoid, dysentery, malaria
American Civil War (1861–5)	Union Army	91.0–110.0	184.0–224.6	1.7–2.5:1	typhoid, malaria, typhus, dysentery, measles, smallpox
	Confederate Army	72.3	120.0	1.7:1	typhoid
Danish–Prussian War (1864)	Prussian Army	0.7	0.3	0.4:1	
	Danish Army	1.4	0.7	0.5:1	
Austro-Prussian War (1866)	Prussian Army	4.5	6.4	1.4:1	cholera, typhoid fever
	Austrian Army	8.9	19.0	2.1:1	
Franco-Prussian War (1870–1)	German Armies	26.6	14.6	0.5:1	smallpox, dysentery, typhoid, typhus
Russo-Turkish War (1877–8)	Russian Army	34.7	81.1	2.3:1	typhus, typhoid
Cuban and Spanish-American Wars (1895–8)	Cuban forces	5.2	3.4	0.7:1	smallpox, yellow fever, typhoid
	Spanish forces	9.4	53.4	5.7:1	
	US forces	0.7	5.5	7.9:1	
South African (Great Boer) War (1899–1902)	British Army	7.5	14.4	1.9:1	typhoid
Russo-Japanese War (1904–5)	Russian forces	34.0–52.6	9.3–18.8	0.2–0.4:1	typhoid, smallpox, diphtheria, cholera
	Japanese forces	58.9	27.2	0.5:1	
World War I (1914–18)	All forces	8,000.0	3,115.0	0.4:1	various diseases, including typhus, typhoid, cholera, dysentery, malaria, influenza
Revolution and Civil War, Russia (1917–21)	Red Army	308.1	283.1	0.9:1	typhus
World War II (1939–45)	All forces	16,933.0	2,363.0(?)	0.1:1	various diseases
Vietnam War (1956–75)	US forces	45.9	10.0	0.2:1	malaria

Notes: [1] Britain, France, and Sardinia.

states and partly to improvements in military hygiene and disease control, the Russo-Japanese War (1904–5) and World War I (1914–18) signalled the start of an enduring trend in which more soldiers died in battle than in military lazarets (Councell, 1941).

Civil Populations

Writing in the midst of World War I, John Bates Clark (Director of the Division of Economics and History, Carnegie Endowment for International Peace) was moved to comment on the historical importance of war epidemics in civil populations. 'An examination of the facts', Clark observed, 'will indicate that until comparatively recent times, the most serious human cost of war has been not losses in the field, nor even the losses from disease in the armies, but the losses from epidemics disseminated among the civil populations.'[8] It was, Clark noted, 'the war epidemics and their sequelae, rather than direct military losses, that accounted for the deep prostration of Germany after the Thirty Years' War [1618–48]', while such epidemics were also the 'gravest consequence of the Napoleonic Wars [1803–15]'.[9] Further insights into the magnitude of civilian losses associated with wartime epidemics can be gained from Table 1.1. The epidemic of cholera which spread with the Austro-Prussian War (1866) is estimated to have claimed 165,000 lives in the Austrian Crownlands. A few years later, some 300,000 French and German citizens died of smallpox during the Franco-Prussian War (1870–1) and its aftermath while, in the twentieth century, the great epidemic of typhus fever which spread in association with the Russian Revolutions and Civil War (1917–21) resulted in upwards of 2.5 million deaths. Most destructive of all, the 1918–19 pandemic of 'Spanish' influenza—which spread in the closing stages and immediate aftermath of World War I—was associated with an estimated global death toll of 20–40 million or more.

FRIEDRICH PRINZING AND THE 'WAR PESTILENCES'

In his seminal book *Epidemics Resulting from Wars* (1916), the German physician and medical statistician, Friedrich Prinzing (Pl. 1.1), observed how all infectious diseases had the potential to 'spread in consequence of war and develop into epidemics of varying extent' (p. 4). The special term, 'war pestilences', Prinzing reserved for 'those infectious diseases which in the course of centuries have usually followed at the heels of belligerent armies' (p. 4). The war pestilences, according to Prinzing, were six in number: cholera, dsyentery, plague, smallpox, typhoid fever, and (louse-borne) typhus fever.[10] The nature of each disease is summarized in Appendix 1A. Examples of associated

---

[8] Introductory note to Prinzing (1916, p. viii).

[9] Introductory note to Prinzing (1916, p. viii).

[10] To these six diseases, Prinzing added scurvy, the 'etiology of which has not yet been definitively determined' (Prinzing, 1916: 4).

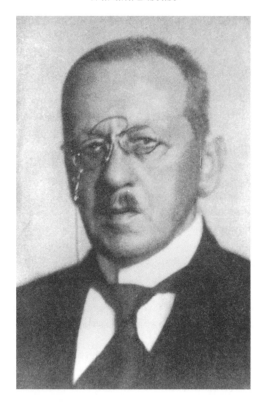

Pl. 1.1. Friedrich Prinzing (1859–1938)

Notes: German physician and medical statistician. After study in Tübingen, Munich, Berlin, and Vienna, Prinzing returned to his home city of Ulm in 1885 where he practised as a physician. In 1916, having already written a handbook of medical statistics (*Handbuch der medizinischen Statistik*, 1906), his book *Epidemics Resulting from Wars* (Oxford: Clarendon Press) was published in association with the Division of Economics and History, Carnegie Endowment for International Peace. Therein, Prinzing identified the principal 'war pestilences' of history as cholera, dysentery, plague, smallpox, typhoid fever, and (louse-borne) typhus fever. To these six infectious diseases, he added scurvy—a malady for which he assumed there to be a specific infective agent.
Source: Hoehn (1937, iv. 379).

epidemics are given in Table 1.1. Here, we provide a thumbnail sketch of the wartime occurrence of each disease.

1. *Cholera*. While diarrhoeal diseases of various aetiologies have been a scourge of military campaigns throughout history (Cook, 2001), the appearance of classic Asiatic cholera as a war pestilence awaited the early nineteenth century and the first pandemic outpourings of *Vibrio cholerae* from South Asia. With epidemic transmission fuelled by insanitary conditions, Table 1.1

shows that cholera spread in association with a long string of nineteenth- and early twentieth-century conflicts, including the Polish Insurrection (1830–1), the Crimean War (1853–6), and the Austro-Prussian War (1866). Cholera claimed the lives of an estimated 200,000 civilians in the immediate aftermath of the Philippine–American War (1899–1902) while, during the Italian occupation of Tripoli (1911), the disease is said to have 'raged' in both the civil population and the occupying forces of the city. Following the introduction of the practice of inoculation, first by the Japanese during the Russo-Japanese War (1904–5) and later by the Greeks during the Balkan Wars (1912–13), cholera activity dropped to low levels in mobilized forces (Prinzing, 1916: 300; Councell, 1941). As Table 1.1 indicates, major epidemics of the disease continued to accompany the movements of war-displaced populations in the twentieth century.

2. *Dysentery*. Fulminating diarrhoeal disease (bloody flux) associated with the dysenteries was a more or less permanent, often crippling, companion of past wars (Patterson, 1993*a*, 1993*b*; Cook, 2001). An epidemic of a disease that may have been dysentery (or plague?) is reputed to have carried away some 300,000 Persian soldiers during the invasion of Greece in 480 BC (Table 1.1) while, in the military camps of later times, Osler notes that dysentery proved 'more fatal . . . than powder and shot' (W. Osler, 1829, cited in Cook, 2001: 95). As far as the historical record allows, dysentery spread widely in the nineteenth century, manifesting as a leading cause of military loss in the Crimean War (1853–6), the American Civil War (1861–5), the Franco-Prussian War (1870–1) and the Sino-Japanese War (1894–5) (Prinzing, 1916; Councell, 1941). In the twentieth century, dysentery was a major source of military loss in parties to the world wars and later the Korean War (Cook, 2001).

3. *Plague*. While many historians have assumed that the ill-defined epidemics of ancient wars were bubonic plague (Lancaster, 1990: 325), confident retrospective diagnoses are often precluded by the ambiguous nature of the clinical evidence (see e.g. Shrewsbury, 1964). By the time that more or less accurate descriptions of epidemics became available, plague—along with louse-borne typhus fever—emerged as one of the most frequently encountered of infectious diseases in wartime (Prinzing, 1916: 328). Bubonic plague was especially prevalent in the Thirty Years' War (1618–48), appearing thereafter in the Second Northern War (1700–21), the Russo-Austrian War (1735–9), the Russo-Turkish War (1768–72), and Napoleon's Egyptian Campaign (1798–1801). The last major war-related epidemic of plague in Europe can be traced to the Russo-Turkish War (1828–9) (Hirsch, 1883, i. 503–4), although the disease continued to spread with wars in other parts of the world (Prinzing, 1916; Councell, 1941).

4. *Smallpox*. While the wartime spread of a disease which may have been smallpox can be traced to antiquity (Table 1.1), the notoriety of smallpox as a war pestilence of early modern times rests with the devastation wrought on the virgin soil populations of the Americas during the Wars of Spanish Conquest

(1519–46). Subsequent conflicts in the Americas, including the French and Indian War (1756–63), the War of American Independence (1775–83), and the Comuneros' Uprising (1781), were all afflicted by the disease while, in Europe, the Franco-Prussian War (1870–1) was associated with a smallpox outbreak of pan-European proportions. However, from the latter part of the nineteenth century, routine vaccination of armed forces generally served to limit the transmission of smallpox in western military campaigns (Prinzing, 1916; Councell, 1941).

5. *Typhoid fever*. Early records of the wartime ocurrence of typhoid fever are scanty, possibly owing to confusion of the disease with such maladies as mucous fevers, bilious fevers, and putrid fevers (Hirsch, 1883). However, by the nineteenth century, there is clear evidence of the epidemic spread of typhoid fever in conflicts such as the American Civil War (1861–5), the Russo-Turkish War (1877–8), the Spanish–American War (1898) and the South African War (1899–1902). Elsewhere, Prinzing (1916) notes that the disease achieved particular prominence during military sieges of fortified settlements, including Torgau (1813), Paris (1870–1), and Port Arthur (1904).

6. *Louse-borne typhus fever*. Louse-borne (epidemic) typhus fever appears to have first manifested as a pestilence of European wars in the latter part of the fifteenth century, spreading widely in the Spanish Army during the War of Granada (1482–92) (Table 1.1). From thereon, observes Prinzing (1916), the disease became the 'Nemesis of belligerent armies' (p. 330), appearing in 'almost every war that was waged between the beginning of the sixteenth century and the middle of the nineteenth century' and acquiring the appellation *war-plague* (p. 328). The notoriety continued into the twentieth century, with major epidemics of typhus fever spreading across Eastern Europe as a consequence of World War I and its aftermath (Zinsser, 1935).

Other Important Diseases

In addition to the major war pestilences, Prinzing (1916: 4) singled out a number of other infectious diseases which, down the ages, were deemed to have played 'an important rôle in many wars'. These diseases included influenza, malaria, measles, louse-borne relapsing fever, and yellow fever (Table 1.1). Although largely overlooked by Prinzing, other workers have highlighted a further malady (tuberculosis) which, among internees in prison and concentration camps, among those working in munitions factories and in other 'dusty' industries, and among the besieged and the famine-afflicted, has repeatedly appeared in times of war (Smallman-Raynor and Cliff, 2003). As described in Section 1.3.3, below, the aforementioned six diseases (influenza, malaria, measles, louse-borne relapsing fever, tuberculosis, and yellow fever), along with the six war pestilences (cholera, dysentery, plague, smallpox, typhoid, and louse-borne typhus fever), form a core set of 12 infectious diseases upon which we base many of the examples in this volume. Again, the nature of each disease is summarized in Appendix 1A.

Factors which contributed to the spread of epidemics in past wars, often exerting an influence beyond the period of active hostilities, are reviewed by Prinzing (1916), Major (1940), and Lancaster (1990: 314–40).

Military Populations

It is possible to isolate a series of factors which, over the centuries, have had a more or less direct influence on the spread of infectious diseases in military populations. As Prinzing (1916: 2–3) explains,

> The causes of the origin and spread of pestilences during a war are clear. Every aggregation of people . . . is necessarily exposed to the danger of pestilence; but this danger is ten times as great in large assemblages of troops during a war. The soldiers are then subjected to all possible kinds of hardship and suffering—lack of food, or food which is inferior and badly cooked, sleeping out in the cold and rain, fatiguing marches, constant excitement, and homesickness—and all those things that greatly lessen their power of resistance.

As regards the geographical sites of war epidemics, the overcrowded and insanitary conditions of military encampments have long been recognized as promoting the spread of infectious diseases—especially 'dirt' diseases such as cholera, dysentery, relapsing fever, typhoid fever, and typhus fever. Again, as Prinzing (1916: 3) observes:

> When large bodies of troops are obliged to remain in one and the same place for a considerable length of time, the additional difficulty presents itself of keeping the locality unpolluted by the excrement of men and animals, and by refuse of all kinds. If an infectious disease reveals its presence in such an aggregation of people, energetic and stringent measures must be adopted . . . to prevent it from spreading. In war times it is often impossible to take the necessary precautions, since the attention of the commanders is directed toward very definite objects, to which all other considerations are subordinate.

The maintenance of a potable water supply, the provision of adequate clothing and shelter, the season of the year, the efficacy of military medical services, and the epidemiological character of the theatre of operations have further served to determine the nature and level of disease activity in the military populations of past wars. Boredom, lack of morale, and/or a fatalistic attitude have also been implicated in the increased risk of exposure to disease agents among deployed personnel while, even in relatively recent conflicts, pressures to meet draft quotas have demanded the enlistment of unseasoned and disease-prone applicants. That military forces have a high level of mobility adds a powerful geographical component to the spread of war epidemics (Prinzing, 1916; Major, 1940; Lancaster, 1990).

Civil Populations

Mass population migration and refugee movements, incarceration in besieged settlements, internment in concentration camps, war-induced nutritional deprivation and famine, the destruction of health infrastructure, and the disruption of disease-control programmes have all served to promote the spread of infectious diseases in the civil populations of past wars. Additional factors have also attained historical prominence. Within theatres of war, military populations have frequently served as a direct source of disease among civilians, while fugitives, prisoners, and demobilized soldiers have often carried infectious diseases beyond the immediate scene of hostilities to the peaceful populations of other lands. Finally, the war-induced disruption of wildlife habitats has occasionally resulted in the appearance and spread of zoonotic diseases in civil populations (see e.g. Prinzing, 1916; Major, 1940; Lancaster, 1990).

1.3.3 Selecting Wars and Diseases

Although we attempt in this book to trace the war–disease association across five millennia of written history, our primary concern is with the 150-year period for which detailed records of war-related morbidity and mortality are available, AD 1850–2000. Even then, a complete and balanced coverage of the approximately 500 recorded wars and war-like engagements to have been fought since the mid-nineteenth century (Kohn, 1999) is not feasible. Consequently, our approach has been to sample from the matrix of wars and diseases, drawing on a small number of examples that illustrate certain key issues and themes. Our selection, which forms the basis of the regional case studies examined in the analytical core of the book, is summarized in Table 1.14. Here, we outline the main criteria which have guided our choice.

1. *Epidemics and war epidemics.* As a fundamental requirement, the epidemic under consideration should be directly or indirectly related in its development to the circumstances of war. In his statistical examination of the demographic impact of wars, for example, Boris Urlanis (1971: 12–13) poses the following question:

If, during a war or immediately after it, an epidemic breaks out claiming thousands, even hundreds of thousands of lives, to what degree should this increased mortality be attributed to war? . . . The question is to what extent can epidemics in war conditions be ascribed to the influence of war and to what extent are they dependent on it?

While the solution to the question can occasionally be found by studying the origins and early course of an epidemic event (Urlanis, 1971), the general problem leads us to restrict our examination to those epidemics for which an

Table 1.14. War epidemics selected for detailed study in this book

War	Epidemic disease	World region (location)	Afflicted population	Principal theme/issue illustrated
Crimean War (1853–6)	Cholera	Europe (Bulgaria, Crimea)	British soldiers	Camp epidemics
American Civil War (1861–5)	Various (including: diarrhoea, dysentery, malaria, measles, scarlet fever, smallpox)	Pan America (United States)	US soldiers	Military mobilization
Franco-Prussian War (1870–1)	Smallpox	Europe (Prussia)	French POWs, Prussian civilians	Camp epidemics
Cuban Insurrection (1895–8)	Enteric fever, smallpox, yellow fever	Pan America (Cuba)	Spanish soldiers and Cuban civilians	Epidemiological integration and war
Spanish–American War (1898)	Typhoid fever	Pan America (United States)	US soldiers	Military mobilization
Philippine–American War (1899–1902)	Cholera	Asia/Far East (Philippines)	Civilians	Post-war epidemic
South African War (1899–1902)	Measles	Africa (South Africa)	Civilians	Population reconcentration
World War I (1914–18)	Various (including: influenza, measles, meningococcal meningitis, mumps, rubella, scarlet fever)	Pan America (United States)	US soldiers	Military mobilization
	Influenza	Oceania (South Pacific Islands)	Troops and civilians	Island epidemics
	Influenza	Europe (England and Wales)	Civilians	Civilian epidemics
	Tuberculosis	Europe (England and Wales)	Civilians	Civilian epidemics
	Typhus fever	Europe (Serbia)	Civilians	Civilian epidemics

Table 1.14. (*cont.*)

War	Epidemic disease	World region (location)	Afflicted population	Principal theme/issue illustrated
World War II (1939–45)	Q fever	Europe (Italy)	US soldiers	Camp epidemics
	Scrub typhus	Asia/Far East (Burma, India)	Allied soldiers	Emerging and re-emerging diseases
	Gonococcal infections, chancroid, syphilis	Africa (Pan-Africa)	US soldiers, Axis POWs	Sexually transmitted diseases
	Dengue, filariasis, malaria, scrub typhus	Oceania (South Pacific Islands)	US forces	Island epidemics
	Various (including: cholera, diphtheria, dysentery, malaria)	Asia/Far East (Burma, Singapore, Thailand)	Allied POWs	POW camps/forced labour
	Poliomyelitis	Europe (Malta)	Civilians	Civilian epidemics
	Diphtheria, poliomyelitis, scarlet fever	Europe (England and Wales)	Civilians (evacuees)	Displaced populations
Korean War (1950–3)	Japanese encephalitis	Asia/Far East (Korea)	UN forces	Emerging and re-emerging diseases
	Korean haemorrhagic fever	Asia/Far East (Korea)	UN forces	Emerging and re-emerging diseases
Vietnam War (1964–73)	Malaria	Asia/Far East (Vietnam)	US forces	Emerging and re-emerging diseases
	Plague	Asia/Far East (Vietnam)	Civilians	Emerging and re-emerging diseases
Ugandan Civil War (1970s)	AIDS	Africa (Uganda)	Civilians	Sexually transmitted diseases
Burundian Civil War (1993)	Louse-borne typhus	Africa (Burundi)	Internally displaced persons	Displaced populations
Rwandan Civil War (1994)	Cholera	Africa (Zaire)	Refugees	Displaced populations

association with the circumstances of war can be clearly established. Thus, particular emphasis is placed upon the spread of diseases in association with specific populations (e.g. soldiers, prisoners of war, war-displaced persons), places (e.g. army camps, concentration camps, refugee camps) and events (e.g. military mobilization, active combat, evacuation) which are closely linked to—indeed, usually contingent upon—the operations of war.

2. *Data availability.* Inevitably, our selection of war epidemics has been conditioned by the availability of the disease records for study (see Sect. 1.4). As we note in Section 1.4.1, the Crimean War (1853–6) was the first major war for which there are official summary data on cause-specific losses during the entire period of hostilities and this marks the earliest war which we examine in statistical detail. The great medical histories of the American Civil War (1861–5), World War I (1914–18), and World War II (1939–45), among other sources, provide further windows of opportunity for the study of infectious diseases in military populations. But such sources take us only so far and, for civil populations, we are largely reliant upon the availability of relevant information gathered through the registration systems of civil health and medical services. As described in Section 1.4.3, such systems may be subject to partial or complete disruption during periods of active hostilities, thereby limiting the availability of reliable data.

3. *Themes and regions.* Special prominence is given in this book to a series of repeating themes linking war and infectious disease. These themes, which are played out in Part III (Chs. 6–12), include:

(i) *Theme 1*: *military mobilization* which, at the outset of wars, has usually provided a fertile breeding ground for epidemics among unseasoned recruits;

(ii) *Theme 2*: *camp epidemics*, historically associated with the unhealthful conditions of army field camps, prisoner of war camps, and other forms of temporary and makeshift military settlement systems;

(iii) *Theme 3*: *emerging and re-emerging diseases*, reflecting the long-established role of war as a facilitating factor in the appearance of apparently 'new' infections, and the reappearance of classical infections, in human populations;

(iv) *Theme 4*: *sexually transmitted diseases (STDs)*, highlighting one of the great scourges of past military forces and the wars in which they were deployed;

(v) *Theme 5*: *island epidemics*, marking the particular epidemiological interest which attaches to islands as environments for the wartime transmission of infectious diseases.

Although each of the five themes could be examined in a number of geographical theatres, we have taken the great world regions of Pan America (Theme 1), Europe (Theme 2), Asia/Far East (Theme 3), Africa (Theme 4), and Oceania (Theme 5) as the spatial framework for our thematic analysis. Within this framework, conflicts have been selected to ensure a regional balance in the global coverage of wars and diseases.

4. *Infectious diseases.* While many infectious diseases have the potential to spread as a consequence of war, the 12 infectious diseases identified in Appendix 1A (cholera, dysentery, influenza, malaria, measles, plague, relapsing fever, smallpox, tuberculosis, typhoid fever, typhus fever, and yellow fever) form the core set from which we draw most of our examples. However, steadfastly limiting our consideration to these diseases would preclude a discussion of other major diseases and disease groups which have served as central actors in modern wars. Consequently, we have sampled broadly from the war–disease record, augmenting the core set of 12 diseases with infectious conditions such as meningococcal meningitis, Japanese encephalitis, Korean haemorrhagic fever, poliomyelitis, Q fever, scrub typhus, and a range of sexually transmitted diseases (chancroid, gonococcal infections, HIV/AIDS, and syphilis).

5. *Historical significance of wars.* Finally, in choosing wars for close study, we have been acutely aware of the wide historical gulf which separates the many minor skirmishes from the few mighty conflagrations which have served as pivot points in world history (Richardson, 1960). Although any judgement on historical significance is inherently subjective, our choice of wars has been guided by a broad concern for some of the more noteworthy conflicts of modern military and political history. Thus our selection includes wars such as the Crimean War (1853–6), the American Civil War (1861–5), the Franco-Prussian War (1870–1), the World Wars (1914–18 and 1939–45), and the Korean War (1950–3)—wars which, in the context of Figure 1.4, were of large magnitude (>100,000 military deaths) and, with notable exceptions, long duration (>100 nation-months). But, to these great clashes, we add a series of somewhat less prominent conflicts, with each selected on the basis of the particular insights it offers into the historical geography of war epidemics.

Applying the foregoing criteria, we arrive at the set of war epidemics in Table 1.14. These war epidemics form the basis of the main regional case studies examined in subsequent sections of the book.

1.4 Epidemiological Data Sources

Meaningful insights into the geographical occurrence and spread of war epidemics are contingent upon the availability of accurate and precise data. While details of the data sources upon which we draw are given at relevant points in the book, it seemed useful in this opening chapter to provide a general overview of the sources we have used. A selection of such source materials is illustrated in Plate 1.2. Our consideration begins with a review of local and national data sources for military and civil populations (Sect. 1.4.1) before turning to the publications of international agencies such as the Health Organization of the League of Nations, the World Health Organization, and the International Committee of the Red Cross (Sect. 1.4.2). We conclude with an overview of the potential limitations of infectious disease statistics in wartime (Sect. 1.4.3).

1.4.1 Local and National Sources

MILITARY POPULATIONS

It is convenient to divide data on morbidity and mortality in military populations into official and semi-official sources. Official sources embrace a diverse set of military accounts, dispatches, lists, memoranda, unpublished and published inquiries, reports, and official histories relating to the sick and dead of the armed forces in past wars. Semi-official sources, often written by (ex-)members of official organizations, generally based on official materials and sometimes prepared with the assistance of the organizations involved, embrace publications which have been issued in the capacity of individual authors (see Urlanis, 1971).

Official Data Sources

In his historical review of official data sources for the assessment of war-related losses in military populations, Urlanis (1971: 38–9) divides the Medieval and Modern eras into four broad periods.

(i) *Middle Ages (c.500) to the Thirty Years' War (1618–48)*. While fragmentary data exist on the killed and wounded in some of the most important battles, there is no reliable documentary evidence on wartime losses during this period.

(ii) *Thirty Years' War (1618–48) to the War of the Spanish Succession (1701–13)*. The first war dispatches appeared during this period, permitting insights into losses sustained in battles of various magnitudes.

(iii) *War of the Spanish Succession (1701–13) to the mid-nineteenth century.* For wars in this period, a wide variety of records, dispatches, reports, and accounts are available for battles and, in some instances, entire campaigns. The sources permit estimates of the strength of military forces along with counts of the number of sick, wounded, killed, and taken prisoner. As evidenced in Chapter 2, records have been preserved for campaigns such as the Continental Army's Canadian Campaign (1775–6), Napoleon's Egyptian Campaign (1798–1801), Sir John Moore's Corunna Campaign (1808–9), and the British Expedition to Walcheren (1809–10). By the 1820s, major causes of morbidity and mortality were being routinely recorded for the US Army, with general returns for US forces in the Mexican War (1846–7) appearing in the consolidated *Statistical Report* for 1839–55 (US Army, 1856: 605–24; Pl. 1.2A).

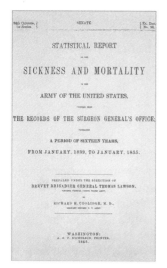

A

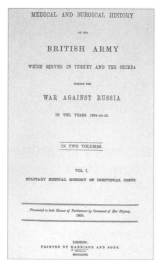

B

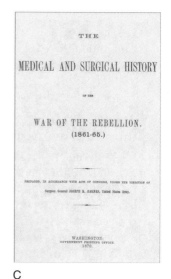

C

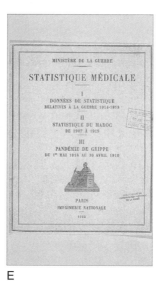

D

E

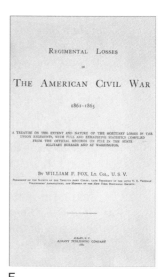

F

Pl. 1.2. Sample statistical sources for the study of war epidemics

Notes: (A) The US Army's consolidated *Statistical Report* for 1839–55, including general returns for the Mexican War of 1846–7. (B) The British Army's *Medical and Surgical History of the British Army which Served in Turkey and the Crimea*, published in 1858. (C) The US Army's *The Medical and Surgical History of the War of the Rebellion (1861–65)*, published between 1870 and 1888. (D) The US Army's *Report on the Origin and Spread of Typhoid Fever in US Military Camps During the Spanish War of 1898*, published in 1904. (E) The French Ministère de la Guerre's *Statistique Médicale*, published with a statistical summary for the 1914–18 War and the 1918–19 'Spanish' influenza pandemic. (F) William F. Fox's *Regimental Losses in the American Civil War, 1861–1865: A Treatise*, published in 1889.

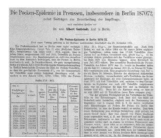

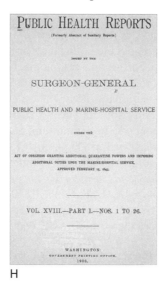

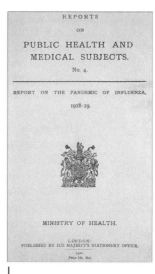

G H I

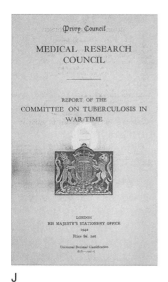

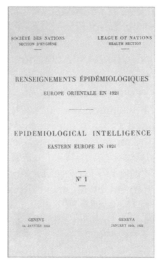

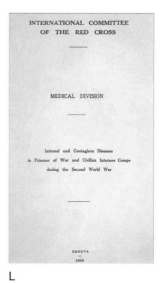

J K L

Pl. 1.2. (*cont.*)

(G) Albert Guttstadt's (1873) 'Die Pocken-Epidemie in Preussen', summarizing the spread of smallpox among French POWs in Prussia during the Franco-Prussian War (1870–1). (H) The US *Public Health Reports*, containing regular reports on epidemic activity in Cuba during the insurrection against Spain (1895–8) and on cholera in the Philippines in the closing stages and aftermath of the Philippine–American War (1899–1902). (I) *Report on the Pandemic of Influenza, 1918–19*, prepared by the British Ministry of Health and published in 1920. (J) The British Medical Research Council's *Report of the Committee on Tuberculosis in War-Time*, published in 1942. (K) Edition No. 1 of *Epidemiological Intelligence*, prepared by the Health Section of the League of Nations and published in January 1922. (L) Summary report on *Internal and Contagious Diseases in Prisoner of War and Civilian Internee Camps during the Second World War*, prepared by the Medical Division of the International Committee of the Red Cross (ICRC) and published in 1950.

(iv) *Mid-nineteenth century to twentieth century.* In this period, which coincides with the development of national and international systems of
health surveillance, detailed official reports of military losses are available not only for battles and campaigns but also for entire wars. The
Crimean War (1853–6) was one of the first major conflicts for which
there are official summary data, with a detailed classification of morbidity and mortality for the various divisions and regiments of the
British Army appearing in the monumental *Medical and Surgical History of the British Army* in 1858 (Army Medical Department, 1858; Pl.
1.2B). Likewise, military losses in the American Civil War were recorded in *The Medical and Surgical History of the War of the Rebellion
(1861–65)* (Surgeon-General's Office, 1870–88; Pl. 1.2C). To such general sources can be added the official reports of specific epidemic events
in mobilized forces including the US War Department's *Report on the
Origin and Spread of Typhoid Fever in US Military Camps during the
Spanish War of 1898* (Reed *et al.*, 1904; Pl. 1.2D) and the French Ministère de la Guerre's *Pandémie de Grippe du 1ᵉʳ Mai 1918 au 30 Avril 1919*
(Ministère de la Guerre, 1922; Pl. 1.2E). Among other types of official
data source, the several multi-volume medical histories of the world
wars, exemplified by the publications of Britain (Macpherson *et al.*,
1922–3; MacNalty, 1952–72) and the United States (Lynch *et al.*,
1923–9; Hoff, 1955–69) are especially noteworthy.

Semi-Official Data Sources

In addition to official data sources, semi-official sources provide information
on military losses sustained as a consequence of the wartime spread of infectious diseases. Among the more prominent examples, William F. Fox's *Regimental Losses in the American Civil War, 1861–1865: A Treatise* (1889) draws
on official documents of the US General Government and the State Militia
Bureaus to provide a regiment-by-regiment digest of cause-specific losses in
the Union Army, 1861–5 (Fox, 1889; Pl. 1.2F). Likewise, Albert Guttstadt's
extended article 'Die Pocken-Epidemie in Preussen' (1873), published by the
Prussian Statistical Office (Berlin), contains valuable summary information on
the geographical occurrence of smallpox in French POWs during the Franco-
Prussian War (1870–1) (Guttstadt, 1873; Pl. 1.2G). Much more recently, Frank
A. Reister's *Medical Statistics in World War II* (1976)—prepared with the
assistance of the erstwhile US Army Medical Statistics Agency—provides
monthly estimates of US Army admissions and deaths for 68 categories of
infectious/parasitic disease in eight theatres of operations, 1942–5.

CIVIL POPULATIONS

Prior to the mid-nineteenth century, few detailed records exist of the killing
or wounding of civilians or of their morbidity and mortality from infectious

diseases in wartime. So, while parish and land tax records—among other sources—provide early 'windows' on war-related losses in civil populations (Lancaster, 1990: 314; see Ch. 2), the analyses in this book are largely dependent on the development of civil systems of public health and disease surveillance from the mid-nineteenth century (Fig. 1.8). The sources on which we draw embrace a series of different types of statistical publication, ranging from national disease surveillance reports such as the US *Public Health Reports* (Pl. 1.2H) to consolidated accounts of major epidemic events (Pl. 1.2I) and the special wartime reports of councils, committees, and boards of inquiry (Pl. 1.2J).

1.4.2 International Sources

HEALTH ORGANIZATION OF THE LEAGUE OF NATIONS

The systematic international recording of information about morbidity and mortality from disease begins with the Health Organization of the League of Nations,[11] established in the aftermath of World War I (Health Organization, League of Nations, 1931). Prompted by the devastating epidemics of typhus fever, relapsing fever and cholera that spread across Eastern Europe with the population upheavals of the Russian Civil War (1918–21), the Russo-Polish War (1919–20), and the Greco-Turkish War (1921–2), a provisional Health Committee of the League was formed in Geneva. The first meeting of the Committee took place in August 1921 to consider 'the question of organising means of more rapid interchange of epidemiological information' (Health Section, League of Nations, 1922: 3). To meet this need, a series of publications—including the key surveillance report *Epidemiological Intelligence* (Pl. 1.2K)—were instituted. Details of the content of *Epidemiological Intelligence* and related publications (including: *Annual Epidemiological Report*; *Monthly Epidemiological Report*; *Weekly Epidemiological Record*; and *Bulletin of the Health Organization*) are provided elsewhere (Cliff *et al.*, 1998: 389–93). Here, we note that *Epidemiological Intelligence* and its successors are the main source of published international data on mortality in the period between the world wars.

WORLD HEALTH ORGANIZATION

The remit of the Health Organization of the League of Nations was transferred to the newly established World Health Organization (WHO) in the aftermath of World War II. Details of WHO statistical publications relevant to this book are given in Cliff *et al.* (1998: 393–5) and include *Annual Epidemiological*

---

[11] The Health Organization of the League of Nations consisted of a Health Committee, an Advisory Council, and the Health Section, the latter operating as an executive organ and forming an integral part of the League Secretariat (Health Organization, League of Nations, 1931: 4).

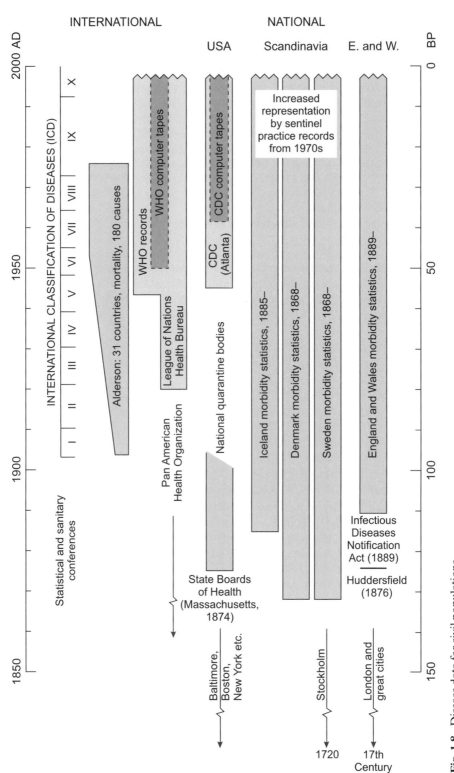

Fig. 1.8. Disease data for civil populations

Note: Time span of archival epidemiological records, 1850–2000.
Source: Cliff *et al.* (1998, fig. 1.7, p. 34).

and Vital Statistics (later renamed *World Health Statistics Annual*), *Weekly Epidemiological Record*, and *Epidemiological Information Bulletin*. To these printed sources can be added the on-line data bank files of morbidity (*c*.1950–80) and mortality (*c*.1950–) in WHO member states (see World Health Organization, 1976, i, pp. v–vi, 784–8).

OTHER INTERNATIONAL SOURCES

To complement the Health Organization of the League of Nations/WHO epidemiological data, we also draw on several other international sources.

International Committee of the Red Cross

The origins of the Red Cross movement can be traced to the opening year of the Italian War of Independence (1859–61) and the efforts of Jean Henri Dunant to provide assistance to the 40,000 dead and dying on the battlefield of Solferino (Willemin and Heacock, 1984). Several years later, in 1863, Dunant established the International Committee for Relief to Military Personnel— forerunner of the International Committee of the Red Cross (ICRC) and insti-gator of the 1864 Geneva Convention (Sect. 1.2.4). Since that time, the ICRC has acted as guardian of the principles of humanitarian law in times of war; a remit which, through the operation of ICRC delegates, has allowed the collec-tion of epidemiological information of outstanding interest, as illustrated by the ICRC Medical Division's report on *Internal and Contagious Diseases in Prisoner of War and Civilian Internee Camps during the Second World War* (ICRC, 1950; see Pl. 1.2L).

Other Organizations

In addition to the international organizations already mentioned, use is made in this book of the published and unpublished statistics and surveillance ma-terials of other official bodies, including the UN High Commission for Refugees (UNHCR) and the UN Relief and Works Agency for Palestinian Refugees in the Near East (UNRWA).

1.4.3 Data Limitations

The geographical analysis of infectious diseases in wartime is confronted by an insidious problem in epidemiological studies: the quality of the data available for examination. As Urlanis (1971: 37) explains:

War-time conditions are little conducive to the provision of complete statistical data. In areas captured by the enemy every current recording of the natural movement of the population is frequently brought to a halt. As for data on war losses, they too are often incomplete and fragmentary owing to the very nature of military operations. Moreover, in a number of instances army leaders give false information on losses, seeking to minimise their own and exaggerate enemy casualties. Napoleon at one time remarked: 'it's as false as a war bulletin'.

MILITARY POPULATIONS

Detailed insights into the limitations of disease statistics in mobilized forces can be gained from summary war reports of the type described in Section 1.4.1. For example, with reference to the cholera epidemic that struck the British Army during the Crimean War (1853–6), the Army Medical Department (1858, i) observes how many regimental surgeons had little or no previous experience of classic Asiatic cholera. In some regiments, diagnoses were purposely limited to the most severe and unambiguous cases of the disease (p. 180), while the reporting of milder cases as diarrhoea, dysentery, and 'English' cholera—among a raft of conditions—must be strongly suspected (pp. 138, 432). In some instances, the progression of cholera was so rapid that there was insufficient time to change any initial (mis)diagnoses (p. 172) while, in yet other instances, pressures on time and hospital resources dictated against the admission (and, hence, the hospital-based reporting) of anything other than the most desperately ill cholera patients (p. 453). Similar circumstances are reported to have prevailed in other nineteenth century wars for which detailed records are available (Woodward, 1863; Reed *et al.*, 1904). In the twentieth century, the limitations of British medical statistics for World War II are attributed by Mellor (1972, p. xiii) to 'the loss of documents in transit owing to enemy action, fast-moving warfare leaving little time for medical recording and the inexperience of some Service Medical Officers'.

CIVIL POPULATIONS

The destruction of public health infrastructure, the redeployment, transfer, or elimination of health resources and personnel, the collapse of communications systems, the lack of diagnostic capabilities, censorship, and propaganda all conspire to limit the availability and reliability of civil disease statistics in wartime. By way of example, the testimony of medical staff attached to the United Nations Relief and Rehabilitation Administration (UNRRA), operating in Europe in the immediate aftermath of World War II, highlights the limitations of statistics for one infectious disease (tuberculosis) in a modern theatre of war:

When we went into the liberated countries, in our innocence we asked for figures to show the tuberculosis death-rates during the war years . . . In some countries, public health records were lost or destroyed; in a couple of Polish cities, wartime records were preserved only through the grim tenacity of a few doctors who could foresee their use . . . the unreliability of many statistics was apparent when one examined their source . . . In examining pre-war figures we were convinced that the desire to please a dictator who took a benevolent interest in tuberculosis may well have made rather steeper a decline in the death-rates. Figures of incidence were quoted . . . but it was soon apparent that they could be of no value. (Daniels, 1947: 202–3)

According to the same source, the mortality records for Yugoslavia 'everywhere were destroyed', no records were available for Greece, while, for the Nazi concentration and extermination camps, information was largely dependent on post-war autopsies conducted on the dead of such places as Belsen and Dachau (Daniels, 1947). But the experience of occupied Europe in World War II provides just one example and, in the latter half of the twentieth century, high- and low-intensity conflicts in Vietnam (Allukian and Atwood, 1997), Cambodia (Heng and Key, 1995), Lebanon (Armenian, 1989), Nicaragua (Siegel *et al.*, 1985), and the former Yugoslavia (Toole *et al.*, 1993), among many other countries, have been associated with the acute or chronic disruption of surveillance for infectious diseases.

1.5 Organization of the Book

The structure of the book is laid out in Figure 1.9. The opening two chapters, constituting Part I: War and Disease, provide the foundation for the main part of the volume. Following on from the present chapter, Chapter 2 surveys the early history of the war–disease association from ancient times to the brink of the statistical period (1500 BC–AD 1850).

The main part of the book, concerned with the 140-year period from 1850, is split into two parts. Part II: *Temporal Trends* provides a longitudinal time-based analysis of infectious disease activity in three different war-afflicted populations: civilians (Chapter 3), military (Chapter 4), and the war-displaced (Chapter 5). In Part III: *A Regional Pattern of War Epidemics*, the treatment switches from the longitudinal analysis of Part II to a series of regional–thematic case studies. As a prelude, Chapter 6 illustrates the range of geographical techniques which may be used to follow the time–space tracks of war epidemics. Subsequent chapters are organized by the great world regions and examine the themes of military mobilization (Pan America, Chapter 7), camp epidemics (Europe, Chapter 8), emerging and re-emerging diseases (Asia and the Far East, Chapter 9), sexually transmitted diseases (Africa, Chapter 10), and island epidemics (Oceania, Chapter 11). Chapter 12 concludes the regional–thematic survey by illustrating further prominent themes (concentration camps, epidemiological integration and war, forced labour, and civilian epidemics) which, either because of their subject-matter or because of their geographical location, were beyond the immediate scope of the foregoing chapters.

In the concluding Part IV: *Prospects*, Chapter 13 examines the disease consequences of wars and war-like events in the years since 1990. Looking forwards, the chapter also isolates a series of war-related issues which—given the balance of probabilities—are likely to be of continuing epidemiological significance in the twenty-first century. Finally, for the disease events analysed in the present volume, Appendix 1B provides a list of electronic data sets which may be obtained from the authors.

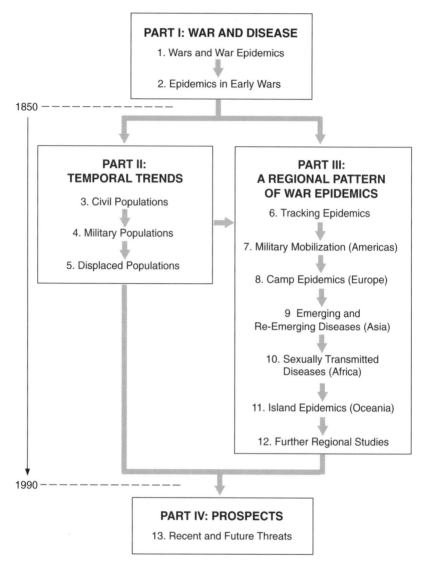

Fig. 1.9. Organization of book

Note: Schematic diagram of sequence of topics covered in this volume.

Appendix 1A

Disease Descriptions (Section 1.3.2)

This appendix provides brief profiles of the 12 sample infectious diseases (cholera, dysentery, influenza, malaria, measles, plague, louse-borne relapsing fever, smallpox,

tuberculosis, typhoid/enteric fever, louse-borne typhus fever, and yellow fever) identified in Section 1.3.2 as having a close historical connection with war. Detailed accounts
of the aetiology, epidemiology, history, and clinical course of the diseases included in
this appendix can be found in relevant standard works including Benenson (1990),
Kiple (1993), Evans and Kaslow (1997), Evans and Brachman (1998), and Mandell
et al. (2000). For reference, Table 1.A1 summarizes the current geographical distribu-
tion/occurrence of each sample disease; alpha-numeric International Classification of
Diseases (ICD-10) codes are indicated.

1. Cholera

Classic Asiatic cholera (ICD-10 A00) is a severe, often rapidly fatal, diarrhoeal disease
produced by the bacterium *Vibrio cholerae*. Transmission of the bacterium usually
occurs via the ingestion of faecally contaminated water and, less commonly, food. As
regards its clinical course, an incubation period of two to five days is usually followed by
the sudden onset of diarrhoea and vomiting, giving rise to massive fluid loss and dehydration. Consequent symptoms include cramps, a reduction in body temperature and
blood pressure leading to shock and, ultimately, death within a few hours or days of
symptom onset. Mortality is typically witnessed in 40 to 60 per cent of untreated cases
(Speck, 1993; Seas and Gotuzzo, 2000).

2. Dysentery

Dysentery is a potentially severe diarrhoeal disease arising from infection of the
intestines with bacteria or amoeba. Bacillary dysentery (ICD-10 A03), or shigellosis, is

Table 1.A1. Geographical distribution/occurrence of sample diseases

Disease[1]	Geographical distribution/occurrence
Cholera (A00)	Global in pandemics
Dysentery, bacillary (A03) and amoebic (A06)	Global
Influenza (J10–11)	Global in pandemics, epidemics, and local outbreaks
Malaria (B50–54)	Currently widespread in tropics and subtropics, with resurgence in the late twentieth century
Measles (B05)	Global, with interruption of indigenous transmission in some countries (United States)
Plague (A20)	Persistent wildlife foci in Africa, South and Southeast Asia, South America, and the western United States
Relapsing fever (louse-borne) (A68.0)	Parts of Central, East, and North Africa, Asia, and South America
Smallpox (B03)	Globally eradicated by 1979
Tuberculosis (A15–19)	Global
Typhoid (A01.0)/enteric fever (A01.1–01.4)	Global
Typhus fever (louse-borne) (A75)	Endemic in parts of Africa, Central and South America, Eastern Europe, and Asia
Yellow fever (A95)	Tropical areas of Africa and South America

Note: [1] Alpha-numeric ICD-10 codes are given in parentheses.

caused by infection with bacteria of the *Shigella* genus while amoebic dysentery (ICD-10 A06), or amoebiasis, is caused by infection with the parasitic protozoan *Entamoeba histolytica*. For both bacillary and amoebic forms of the disease, the route of transmission is faecal–oral, with contaminated water and food serving as important sources for epidemic outbreaks. Direct infection may occur in overcrowded and/or insanitary environments. As regards the clinical course of dysentery, differences are apparent in the bacillary and amoebic forms of the disease:

(i) *Bacillary dysentery.* A typical incubation period of two to three days (range one to ten days) is commonly followed by the abrupt onset of fever, diarrhoea, and, frequently, vomiting, cramps, and tenesmus. Stools may be watery and, in severe cases, may contain blood, mucus, and pus. The duration of disease ranges from a few days to two to three weeks, with the severity of attack linked to such factors as age, pre-existing nutritional state, size of infecting dose, and the infecting serotype. Severe disease is most commonly associated with *Shigella dysenteriae 1* (Patterson, 1993*a*; Keusch and Bennish, 1998).

(ii) *Amoebic dysentery.* A variable incubation period of days to years (typically, two to four weeks) gives way to insidious onset of disease. Symptoms may vary in severity, from mild diarrhoea and abdominal discomfort to fulminating disease with fever, chills, and semi-formed bloodstained or mucoid stools. Duration of disease may range from a few days to weeks, with remission followed by relapse. Complications may include intestinal perforation and peritonitis, while dissemination by the bloodstream may result in potentially lethal abscesses of the liver and, less commonly, the lung or brain (Patterson, 1993*b*).

3. Influenza

Influenza (ICD-10 J10–11) is a highly contagious respiratory disease caused by influenza A, B, and C viruses. Epidemic events are restricted to influenza A and B viruses, while pandemic events are associated with the genetically unstable A virus. In human populations, the predominant route of virus transmission is via exposure to droplet emissions from the respiratory tract. Clinically, a short incubation period (typically one to three days) is followed by the sudden onset of sore throat, cough, headache, fever, generalized muscle pain, lassitude, and prostration. In mild cases, symptoms may subside in one to two weeks, although lethargy and depression may persist for three to four weeks. Secondary complications, with potentially fatal outcome, involve the organs of the lower respiratory tract, the cardiovascular system, and the central nervous system (Kilbourne, 1987; Glezen and Couch, 1997).

4. Malaria

Malaria (ICD-10 B50–54) is an infection produced in man by several species of protozoan parasites which are members of a single genus, *Plasmodium*. The parasites (*P. vivax, P. falciparum, P. malariae*, and *P. ovale*) are transmitted naturally from human to human by the bite of an infected female anopheline mosquito. The symptoms produced include alternate bouts of chill, followed by high fever, sweating, and prostration. The time intervals between these episodes (paroxysms) are a function of the precise species of the parasite involved. Malaria due to *P. falciparum* presents the most serious form of the disease, with case fatality rates in excess of 10 per cent for non-immune adults. With the exception of the young and those with concurrent disease, malaria due to other

Plasmodium spp. is not generally considered to be life threatening (Dunn, 1993; Krogstad, 2000).

5. Measles

Measles (ICD-10 B05) is a highly communicable viral disease. The predominant route of virus transmission is by droplet spread or direct contact with the nasal and throat secretions of infected persons. The incubation period is of the order of ten days (range one to two weeks). Clinically, measles is characterized by a prodromal fever, conjunctivitis, coryza, cough, Koplik spots on the buccal mucosa, and a red blotchy rash. Complications may result from viral replication or bacterial superinfection, and include otitis media, pneumonia, diarrhoea, and encephalitis. Measles is presently a more severe disease in developing countries, especially among very young and malnourished children, in whom it may be associated with haemorrhagic rash, protein-losing enteropathy, mouth sores, dehydration, diarrhoea, blindness, and severe skin infections; the case fatality rate may be 5 to 10 per cent or more (Kim-Farley, 1993; Black, 1997).

6. Plague

Plague (ICD-10 A20) is a zoonosis caused by the bacillus *Yersinia pestis.* The natural vertebrate reservoir of *Y. pestis* is wild rodents (especially ground squirrels). The disease in humans occurs as a result (i) of intrusion into the zoonotic (sylvatic) cycle, or (ii) by the entry of sylvatic rodents or their infected fleas into human habitats. The most frequent source of exposure resulting in human disease worldwide has been the bite of infected fleas (especially *Xenopsylla cheopis*, the oriental rat flea). Plague occurs in two major forms. Bubonic plague is caused by the bite of an infected flea and manifests as a painful swelling of the lymph glands ('buboes'). Bacteraemia and septicaemia often follow, as may secondary pneumonia. Primary pneumonic plague (contracted through exposure to the airborne exhalations of patients with primary pneumonic plague or the secondary pneumonia of bubonic plague) manifests as severe malaise, frequent cough with mucoid sputum, severe chest pains, and rapidly increasing respiratory distress. The incubation period is usually one to seven days (bubonic plague) and one to four days (primary pneumonic plague). Untreated bubonic plague has a case fatality rate of 50 to 60 per cent; untreated primary pneumonic plague is almost invariably fatal (Carmichael, 1993a; Butler, 2000).

7. Relapsing Fever (Louse-Borne)

Louse-borne relapsing fever (ICD-10 A68.0) is a systemic disease caused by the parasitic spirochete *Borrelia recurrentis.* Human beings are the only reservoir of the causative agent. The disease is transmitted from person to person by the human body louse, *Pediculus humanus.* The body louse is infected by feeding on the blood of a patient, with onwards transmission to other human beings via the crushing of infective lice over bite wounds and skin abrasions. The disease flourishes in circumstances favourable to the multiplication and passage of the body louse, especially cold, over-crowded, and insanitary living conditions. Clinically, an incubation period of five to eight days gives way to the abrupt onset of fever, headache, body pains, and, commonly, jaundice. Relapses occur in approximately 50 per cent of cases. The total duration of the disease is of the order of two weeks. The fatality rate is usually less than 10 per cent in untreated cases, but may exceed 50 per cent in war- and famine-associated epidemics (Felsenfeld, 1971; Hardy, 1993).

8. Smallpox

Although eradicated globally by 1979, smallpox (ICD-10 B03) was historically a severe and often fatal viral disease. Transmission was through direct contact with the oropharyngeal secretions of an infected person and, less commonly, by contact with the clothing or bedding of a smallpox patient. The disease took a characteristic clinical course. An incubation period of about 12 days was followed by the abrupt onset of fever, headache, and muscle pain. After two to five days, a papular rash appeared on the face, palms, soles, and other parts of the body. Soon thereafter, the pimples of the rash turned to pustules, eventually to form scabs which fell off three to four weeks after onset. In addition to extreme scarring, possible sequelae included blindness and male infertility. Death as a result of toxaemia and massive haemorrhaging occurred in up to 30 per cent of untreated cases (Fenner *et al.*, 1988; Benenson, 1997).

9. Tuberculosis

Tuberculosis (ICD-10 A15–19) is a potentially severe disease caused by a bacterial complex, including *Mycobacterium tuberculosis* primarily from humans, and *M. bovis* primarily from cattle. The principal route of human to human transmission is via exposure to bacilli in the airborne exhalations of infected individuals. The initial infection usually goes unnoticed. Lesions at the site of lodgement of the organism commonly heal, leaving no residual changes except occasional pulmonary or tracheobronchial lymph node calcifications. Approximately 95 per cent of those initially infected enter this latent phase from which there is lifelong risk of reactivation. In approximately 5 per cent of cases, the initial infection progresses directly to *pulmonary tuberculosis* or, by lymphohaematogenous dissemination of bacilli, to pulmonary, miliary, meningeal, or other extra-pulmonary involvement. Serious outcome of the initial infection is more frequent in infants, adolescents, and young adults. *Extra-pulmonary* tuberculosis is much less common than the pulmonary form. It may affect any organ or tissue and includes tuberculous meningitis, acute haematogenous (miliary) tuberculosis, and involvement of lymph nodes, pleura, pericardium, kidneys, bones and joints, larynx, skin, intestines, peritoneum, and eyes. *Progressive* pulmonary tuberculosis arises from exogenous reinfection or endogenous reactivation of a latent focus remaining from the initial infection. If untreated, about half the patients will die within a two-year period (Johnston, 1993; Comstock and O'Brien, 1998).

10. Typhoid/Enteric Fever

Enteric fever is a generalized term to cover typhoid (ICD-10 A01.0) and paratyphoid fevers (ICD-10 A01.1–A01.4); both are infections of the bowel and are produced by the bacteria *Salmonella typhi* (typhoid) and *Salmonella paratyphi* (paratyphoid). Transmission of the bacteria occurs via the ingestion of faecally contaminated food, water, and other fluids; the disease flourishes in insanitary conditions, particularly areas with inadequate sewerage systems and a lack of potable water. Other routes of transmission include contaminated dust, flies, and other insects. For typhoid fever, a typical incubation period of eight to 14 days is followed by the onset of a sustained fever with headache, abdominal distension, non-productive cough, and 'rose spot' rash on the trunk, constipation, and, more commonly, diarrhoea. Mortality due to profound toxaemia, circulatory failure, intestinal perforation, haemorrhage, or inter-current pneumonia is typically witnessed in 10 to 20 per cent of untreated cases. Paratyphoid fever presents a similar clinical picture but tends to take a much milder course (LeBaron and Taylor, 1993; Levine, 1998).

11. Typhus Fever (Louse-Borne)

Louse-borne (classical epidemic) typhus fever (ICD-10 A75) is an acute febrile disease caused by infection with *Rickettsia prowazekii*. The disease is transmitted from person to person by the human body louse, *Pediculus humanus*. The body louse is infected by feeding on the blood of a febrile typhus patient, with onwards transmission to other human beings via the exposure of wounds and skin abrasions to the faeces of infected lice. Human infection may also result through the inhalation of dust containing rickettsiae. The disease flourishes in circumstances favourable to the multiplication and passage of the body louse, especially cold, overcrowded, and insanitary living conditions. As regards the clinical course of louse-borne typhus, an incubation period of one to two weeks gives way to the abrupt onset of headache, malaise, unremitting fever, prostration, and, in severe cases, progressive neurological symptoms. A characteristic rash, becoming widespread and petechial, appears on the trunk after about five days. The disease usually resolves in death or recovery in the third week. Fatality rates may reach 40 per cent or more in untreated cases (Harden, 1993; Saah, 2000*a*).

12. Yellow Fever

Yellow fever (ICD-10 A95) is a severe, sometimes fatal, viral disease of the tropics. Within a human population, person-to-person spread of the virus occurs via a mosquito vector (*Aëdes aegypti*). As the flight range of *Aëdes aegypti* is short (of the order of 100 metres), long-distance spread is dependent upon (i) the relocation of infected people to spark a new human–mosquito–human cycle and/or (ii) the transportation of infected mosquitos. As regards the clinical course of the disease, an incubation period of three to six days is usually followed by fever, chills, headache, nausea, and muscular aches. For the majority of patients, remission and recovery follows two to three days after symptom onset. But, for some patients, the remission is short-lived and gives way to a severe clinical course that frequently results in death after seven to ten days. In yet other patients, especially children, the disease may take a very mild, or even sub-clinical, path (Cooper and Kiple, 1993; Shope and Meegan, 1997).

Appendix 1B
Electronic Data Sets (Section 1.5)

In producing this book, a large number of epidemiological and demographic data sources have been accessed. The data contained in many of these sources have been digitally encoded as PC EXCEL spreadsheets, especially if they were either temporally or geographically referenced. This appendix summarizes the data that have been encoded. The data are freely available from the authors. We ask that the source of the data and, in particular, the Leverhulme Trust Programme Grant which met the cost of the work, is acknowledged. Suggested references are: M. R. Smallman-Raynor and A. D. Cliff (2004), *War Epidemics: An Historical Geography of Infectious Diseases in Military Conflict and Civil Strife, 1850–2000* (Oxford: Oxford University Press); Leverhulme Trust Programme Grant F/753/D, Disease in War, 1850–1990: Geographical Patterns, Spread and Demographic Impact.

1. United States Army (1839–1859)

Description of data: Quarterly counts of cases and deaths, by disease category and major geographical division (1839–59).

Sources of data: (1) US Army (1856). *Statistical Report on the Sickness and Mortality in the Army of the United States, Compiled from the Records of the Surgeon General's Office; Embracing a Period of Sixteen Years, from January, 1839, to January, 1855.* Washington; (2) US Army (1860). *Statistical Report on the Sickness and Mortality in the Army of the United States, Compiled from the Records of the Surgeon General's Office; Embracing a Period of Five Years, from 1855–60.* Washington.

2. Crimean War (1853–1856)

Description of data: Cholera admissions and deaths in the British Army of the East, by month and regiment (April 1854–June 1856).

Source: Army Medical Department (1858). *The Medical and Surgical History of the British Army which Served in Turkey and the Crimea during the War against Russia in the Years 1854–55–56*, I and II. London: Harrison and Sons.

3. Colonial Armies (1859–1913)

Description of data: Army deaths per 1,000 mean strength, British, French, and Netherlands armies at home and in Algeria, West Indies, India–Madras, and the Netherland Indies in five- to ten-year blocks, 1859–1913.

Source: Curtin, P. D. (1989). *Death by Migration: Europe's Encounter with the Tropical World in the Nineteenth Century*. Cambridge: Cambridge University Press, app., pp. 162–222.

4. American Civil War (1861–1865)

Description of data: Monthly cases/case rates, mortality/mortality rates from all recorded infections and battle wounds, 1861–6, for Black soldiers and officers, White soldiers and officers and by geographical army divisions.

Source: Surgeon-General's Office (1870–88). *The Medical and Surgical History of the War of the Rebellion. (1861–65)*. Washington: Government Printing Office.

5. Cuban Insurrection (1895–1898)

Description of data: Monthly counts of deaths from enteric fever, smallpox, and yellow fever in seven Cuban towns and cities, 1887–1902.

Source: US Marine Hospital Service, *Public Health Reports* (1895–8). Washington: Government Printing Office.

6. Spanish–American War (1898)

Description of data: Typhoid fever cases and deaths in the US Volunteer Army, by week and regiment (May 1898–Feb. 1899).

Source: Reed, W., Vaughan, V. C., and Shakespeare, E. O. (1904). *Report on the Origin and Spread of Typhoid Fever in US Military Camps during the Spanish War of 1898*, I and II. Washington: Government Printing Office.

7. Philippine–American War (1899–1902)

Description of data: Weekly counts of cholera cases and deaths in the civilian population of the Philippine Islands, by province and island (Mar. 1902–Mar. 1904).

Source: US *Public Health Reports* (1902–4). Washington: Government Printing Office.

8. World War I (1914–1918)

Data Set 1: French Army (1914–1918)

Description of data: French army deaths from various infectious diseases by theatre of operation, 1914–18.

Source: Ministère de la Guerre (1922). *Données de Statistique Relatives à la Guerre 1914–1918*. Paris: Imprimerie Nationale.

Data Set 2: England and Wales (1911–1920)

Description of data: Registrar General's *Weekly Returns* for infectious diseases and other causes for 76 great towns and nationally, 1910–20. Weekly mortality from nine infectious diseases, violence, inquests, deaths in public institutions. Total births, deaths, and population.

Source: Registrar General (1911–21). *Weekly Return of Births and Deaths*. London: HMSO.

Data Set 3: England and Wales, Influenza (1918–1919)

Description of data: Weekly counts of influenza deaths in London and the county boroughs of England and Wales, June 1918–April 1919. Daily count of influenza admissions to the First Eastern General Hospital, Cambridge, June 1918–March 1919.

Source: Local Government Board (1919). *Forty-Eighth Annual Report of the Local Government Board, 1918–1919: Supplement Containing the Report of the Medical Department for 1918–19*. London: HMSO, 24–7. Copeman, S. M. (1920). 'Report on incidence of influenza in the University and Borough of Cambridge and in the Friends' School, Saffron Waldon'. In: Ministry of Health, *Report on the Pandemic of Influenza, 1918–19*. Reports on Public Health and Medical Subjects, No. 4. London: HMSO, app. I, 388–444.

9. Russia (1823–1924)

Description of data: Cases and case rates for nine infectious diseases, Russia, annually, 1900–20 (cholera and typhoid, 1823–1920); monthly, 1900–24 for five infectious diseases for Russia and 45 cities and districts in European Russia; reported cases for six infectious diseases, monthly, January–November 1921, for 45 cities and districts in European Russia, prison, rail, waterway populations.

Source: League of Nations Health Committee (1922–4). *Epidemiological Intelligence* (E.I.1–6). Geneva: League of Nations.

10. World War II (1939–1945)

Data Set 1: US Army, 1942–1945

Description of data: Monthly counts of admissions and deaths for 68 categories of infectious and parasitic disease, by theatre of operations (1942–5).

Source: Reister, F. A. (ed.) (1976). *Medical Statistics in World War II.* Washington: Government Printing Office.

Data Set 2: England and Wales, 1933–1951

Description of data: Quarterly counts of diphtheria, poliomyelitis, and scarlet fever cases in counties of eastern and southern England, covering World War II evacuation and reception areas.

Source: Registrar General (1933–52). *Weekly Return of Births and Deaths.* London: HMSO; Registrar General (1933–52). *Quarterly Return of Births, Deaths and Marriages.* London: HMSO.

11. Palestinian Refugees (1960–1987)

Description of data: Annual morbidity for 30 infectious diseases by UNRWA field of operation (Jordan, West Bank, Gaza, Lebanon, Syria).

Source: UNRWA (unpublished).

12. US Military Applicants (1985–1989)

Description of data: HIV-1 reports by ethnic group and sex among civilian applicants for military service, by state and standard metropolitan statistical area.

Source: CDC (1990). *Prevalence of HIV-1 Antibody in Civilian Applicants for Military Service, October 1985–December 1989*. Selected tables prepared by the Division of HIV/AIDS. Atlanta: Centers for Disease Control and Prevention.

13. Backcloth Disease Data: 33 Countries (1887–1975) and World Cities (1913–1938)

Data Set 1: World Countries, 1901–1975

Description of data: Quinquennial standardized mortality ratios for 33 countries on all causes and 60 conditions.

Source: Alderson, M. (1981). *International Mortality Statistics*. London: Macmillan.

Data Set 2: 30 World Cities, 1913–1921

Description of data: Weekly data, 1913–21 inclusive, giving number of reported cases for 30 cities from around the world for all causes, diphtheria, measles, scarlet fever, tuberculosis, typhoid fever, and whooping cough. Cities are: Alexandria (Egyptians), Alexandria (foreigners), Amsterdam, Berlin, Bombay, Brussels, Budapest, Cairo (Egyptians), Cairo (foreigners), Calcutta, Chicago, Christiana, Cologne, Copenhagen, Frankfurt, Hamburg, Leipzig, Madras, Moscow, Munich, New York, Paris, Philadelphia, Prague, Rio de Janeiro, St Petersburg, Stockholm, Trieste, Venice, Vienna.

Source: Registrar General (1911–21). *Weekly Return of Births and Deaths*. London: HMSO.

Data Set 3: 115 World Cities, 1925–1938

Description of data: Tuberculosis cases, 1925–35 (quarterly) and 1925–38 (annually).

Source: League of Nations Health Committee (1925–41). *Epidemiological Intelligence*; *Annual Epidemiological Report and Corrected Statistics of Notifiable Diseases*; *Epidemiological Report*. Geneva: League of Nations.

14. Modern wars (1614–1913)

Description of data: Estimated losses of life in modern wars, Austria–Hungary and France (1614–1913).

Source: Bodart, G. (1916). *Losses of Life in Modern Wars: Austria–Hungary; France*. Oxford: Clarendon Press.

2

Epidemics in Early Wars

Whip! thro' both camps, halloo! it ran,
Nor uninfected left a man . . .
Hence soon thro' Italy it flew
Veiled for a while from mórtal view,
When suddenly in various modes,
It shone display'd in shankers, nodes,
Swell'd groins, and pricking shins, and headaches
And a long long long string of dread aches . . .
From thence with every sail unfurl'd
It traversed almost all the world . . .
Until at length this Stygian fury
Worked its foul way to our blest Drury,
Where still Lord Paramount it reigns,
Pregnant with sharp nocturnal pains

Andrew Tripe, 'The Smallpox, A Poem' (1748) [1]

---

[1] Cited in Creighton (1965, i. 432 n. 2).

2.1 Introduction

While our selection of the time period, AD 1850–1990, for the analytical work we undertake in Chapters 3 to 12 is conditioned by the availability of consolidated morbidity and mortality data for both military and civil populations from the middle of the nineteenth century, this time-window gives only the most recent outlook upon an association between war and disease which can be traced back to the great struggles of ancient times (see Table 1.1). So in the present chapter, in so far as the historical record allows, we review the early history of war epidemics. Our narrative follows a temporal sequence. We consider in turn evidence from antiquity (1500 BC–AD 500) (Sect. 2.2), the Middle Ages (AD 500–1500) (Sect. 2.3), and the modern period (AD 1500–1850) (Sect. 2.4–2.6).

To obtain a picture of the geographical distribution of belligerent parties and associated conflicts, 1500 BC–AD 1850, Table 2.1 is based on a subset of the information included in Table 1.4 and gives the number of units[2] engaged in each of the *c.*2,000 wars and war-like events listed by Kohn (1999). All told, Table 2.1 identifies 2,267 engagements, with the number rising from 365 (antiquity), to 786 (Middle Ages) and 1,116 (modern). As noted in Section 1.2.3, the Old World and Europe especially dominate the geographical record; entry of the New World awaited European colonization in the modern period and the beginning of a written record for the Americas and Oceania.

As a marker of recorded conflicts, Table 2.1 defines the broad geographical limits to an historical review of war-related epidemics. A review of all the wars that underpin the tabulation is outside the compass of this book. As noted in Section 1.4, relevant information is simply not available for the majority of early wars while, even for relatively recent conflicts, the nature of the disease(s) that beset military and civil populations continues to defy confident retrospective diagnosis. Inevitably, language barriers offer a further limit to our coverage. But within these constraints it is possible to sample from the available evidence and to obtain some idea of the magnitude and scope of war epidemics prior to AD 1850. In so doing, we lay particular emphasis on the occurrence of the major war pestilences listed in Section 1.3.2 (cholera, dysentery, plague, smallpox, and typhoid and typhus fevers) in European and American theatres.

---

[2] Here, we use the term 'unit' in a general sense to refer to belligerent parties down the ages, including areas, civilizations, and populations.

Table 2.1. Distribution of sample wars and war-like events, by number of participating states/areas, 1500 BC–AD 1850

Region	Time period			Total
	Antiquity (1500 BC–AD 500)	Middle Ages (AD 500–1500)	Modern (AD 1500–1850)	
Old World				
Africa	28	15	40	83
Asia	149	180	204	533
Europe	188	591	710	1,489
New World				
Americas	0	0	157	157
Oceania	0	0	5	5
Total	365	786	1,116	2,267

Source: Based on information included in Kohn (1999: 557–94).

For other theatres, especially those of Sub-Saharan Africa and Asia, the available evidence is largely restricted to a small number of conflicts in which European forces were directly involved.

One complication of the present review is the variation in the names and time brackets frequently allotted to early wars. As a general rule, our coverage of conflicts in the modern period adopts the nomenclature and dates given in the second edition of Quincy Wright's *A Study of War* (Wright, 1965, tables 31–42, pp. 640–7). For earlier periods, we tend to follow Kohn (1999).

2.2 Antiquity (1500 BC–AD 500)

It is generally held that many of the ancient epidemics recorded from the second millennium BC were related to warfare, mass migrations, and the consequent breakdown of public health (Adamson, 1980; Wiseman, 1986). Table 2.2 lists a sample of such epidemics, along with summary information on the possible nature of the associated disease and the principal afflicted populations. See also Figure 2.1A.

The prophets and compilers of the Old Testament frequently portrayed the Lord's wrath in terms of apocalyptic visitations of war, famine, and disease.[3] For example, Joshua's account of the sacking of Jericho in the fourteenth century BC (Josh. 6) has been attributed by Hulse (1971) in part to contamination of the city's main water supply (Elisha's Well) with the agent of urino-genital

---

[3] See e.g. Ezekiel 5: 17 and Leviticus 26: 25.

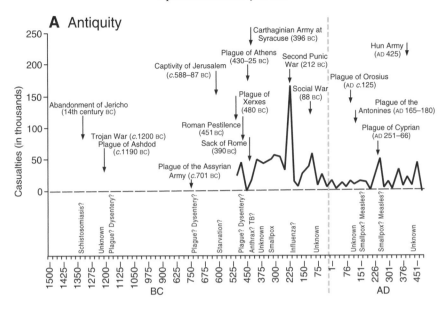

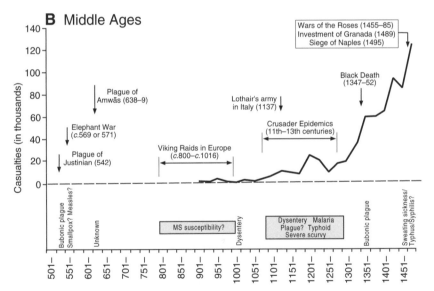

Fig. 2.1. Wars and war epidemics, 1500 BC–AD 1850

Notes: Graphs identify major wars and phases of war, and associated diseases, examined in the present chapter. (A) Antiquity (1500 BC–AD 500). (B) Middle Ages (AD 501–1500). (C) Modern (AD 1501–1850). For reference, the line trace on each graph is based on information in Sorokin (1937) and plots the estimated total number of military casualties by 25-year period for sample states and time periods: Ancient Greece (500–126 BC); Ancient Rome (400 BC–AD 475); Russia (AD 901–1850); France (AD 975–1850); England (AD 1051–1850); Austria and Hungary (AD 1101–1850); Poland and Lithuania (AD 1376–1800); Spain (AD 1476–1850); Greece (AD 1551–1850); Italy (AD 1551–1850); Germany (AD 1651–1850).

Source: Casualty data from Sorokin (1937, tables 1, 3, 6, 7, 8, 9, 10, 11, 12, 13, 14, pp. 293, 301, 306–7, 311, 315, 319, 322, 325, 328, 331, 333).

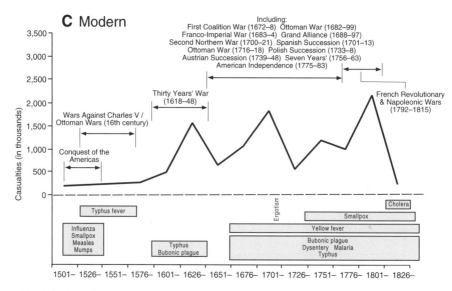

Fig. 2.1. (*cont.*)

schistosomiasis (*Schistosoma haematobium*). In a similar vein, the Plague of Ashdod (I Sam. 5) which afflicted the Philistines at Ashdod during the Hebrew–Philistine War, *c.*1190 BC (Pl. 2.1) has been interpreted as bubonic plague (Simpson, 1905; Wilson and Miles, 1946; Rendle Short, 1955; Hirst, 1953) or bacillary dysentery (Shrewsbury, 1964).

The intersection of war and disease also appears in the writings of the Greeks. As noted in the introduction to Chapter 1, Book 1 of Homer's epic poem, the *Iliad*, tells of a mysterious epidemic that smote the Greek Army outside Troy during the Trojan War (*c.*1200 BC); see Crawfurd (1914) and Shrewsbury (1964). In later times historians such as Herodotus, Thucydides, and Diodorus Siculus provide classical accounts of the devastation wrought by war pestilences. During the Persian Invasion of Greece (480–479 BC) Herodotus describes an epidemic (λοιμός) which attacked the 800,000-strong Persian Army under Xerxes in 480 BC. With failing supplies and with under-nourishment lowering the resistance of the army, λοιμός (possibly, plague and/or dysentery) spread widely in the Persian ranks, reputedly claiming many tens of thousands of lives and forcing the Persian retreat from Thessalia (Zinsser, 1935: 154).

The Peloponnesian War (431–404 BC) and the Plague of Athens

One of the great war epidemics of classical times was the Plague of Athens, described by Thucydides (460?–395? BC) in Book 2 of his celebrated *History of the Peloponnesian War* (431–404 BC). See Figure 2.2.

Table 2.2. Sample war epidemics in Antiquity, 1500 BC–AD 500

Year	War	Epidemic/disease	Afflicted population/area
Biblical References			
c.1190 BC	Hebrew–Philistine War (c.1190 BC)	Plague of Ashdod (Bubonic plague? Dysentery?)	Philistines at Ashdod, Gath, and Ekron
c.701 BC	(Later) Assyrian Wars (c.746–609 BC)	Plague of the Assyrian Army (Bubonic plague? Dysentery?)	Assyrian Army at Jerusalem or Pelusium
c.588–587 BC	Babylonian Expedition and Captivity of Jerusalem (589–538 BC)	Starvation (accompanied by disease?)	Jerusalem
Ancient Greece			
c.1200 BC	Trojan War (c.1200 BC)	Literary reference to undetermined disease	Greek Army outside Troy
480 BC	Persian Invasion of Greece (480–479 BC)	Plague of Xerxes (Bubonic plague? Dysentery?)	Persian Army
430–425 BC	Great Peloponnesian War (431–404 BC)	Plague of Athens	Athens and Southern Greece
396 BC	Carthaginian Wars (409–367 BC)	Smallpox?	Carthaginian Army at Syracuse
Rome and Roman Empire			
451 BC	(Planned) Aequian attack on Rome (451 BC)	Roman Pestilence of 451 BC (Anthrax? Tuberculosis?)	Romans and Aequians
390 BC	Celtic Sack of Rome (390 BC)	?	Gaul Army besieging Rome
212 BC	Second Punic War (218–212 BC)	Influenza?	Carthaginian, Roman, and Sicilian Armies at Syracuse
88 BC	Social War (91–88 BC)	?	Army of Octavius at Rome
AD c.125	Roman defence of African colonies	Plague of Orosius	Roman Army at Utica
AD 165–180	Roman Eastern War (AD 162–5)	Plague of the Antonines/Galen (Smallpox? Measles?)	Roman Empire (and beyond)
AD 251–266	Roman–Gothic Wars (AD 249–68)	Plague of Cyprian (Smallpox? Measles?)	Roman Empire (and beyond)
AD 425	Hun Raids on Roman Empire (AD 375–454)	?	Hun Army advancing on Constantinople

Sources: Based on information in Castiglioni (1947), Crawfurd (1914), Kohn (1998), Major (1940), Prinzing (1916), Shrewsbury (1950, 1964), Wiseman (1986), and Zinsser (1935).

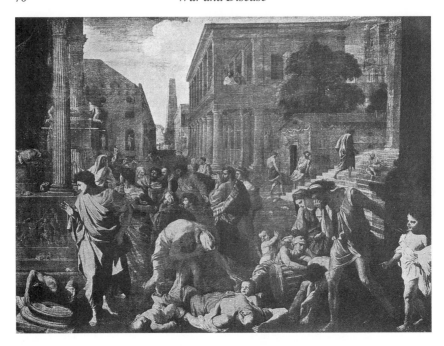

Pl. 2.1. *La Peste d'Asdod dit les Philistins frappés de la Peste*

Notes: Outbreak of an infectious disease among the Philistines at Ashdod, *c.*1190 BC. As described in the *Old Testament* (I Sam. 5: 6–12), the epidemic struck the Philistine Army following the capture of the Ark of the Covenant from the Hebrews. On the arrival of the Ark at Ashdod, 'the Lord laid a heavy hand upon the people of Ashdod; he threw them into distress and plagued them with tumours, and their territory swarmed with rats [or mice]. There was death and destruction all through the city' (I Sam. 5: 6). Opinion is divided as to the nature of the disease, although the biblical description is suggestive of either bubonic plague or bacillary dysentery.
Source: Original painting (canvas, 148 × 198 cm) by Nicolas Poussin (1594–1665) (Louvre, Photo © RMN).

The disease is said to have begun south of Egypt in Aethiopia; thence it descended into Egypt and Libya, and after spreading over the greater part of the Persian empire, suddenly fell upon Athens. It first attacked the inhabitants of Piraeus . . . It afterwards reached the upper city, and then the mortality became far greater. (Thucydides, 2. 48, transl. Jowett, 1900, p. 135)

The 200,000 or so refugees that had fled the Athenian countryside for the relative safety of the city appeared to have suffered most. 'For, having no houses of their own, but inhabiting in the height of summer stifling huts', Thucydides noted, 'the mortality among them was dreadful, and they perished in wild disorder. The dead lay as they had died, one upon another, while others hardly alive wallowed in the streets and crawled about every fountain craving for water' (Thucydides, 2. 52, trans. Jowett, 1900: 138–9).

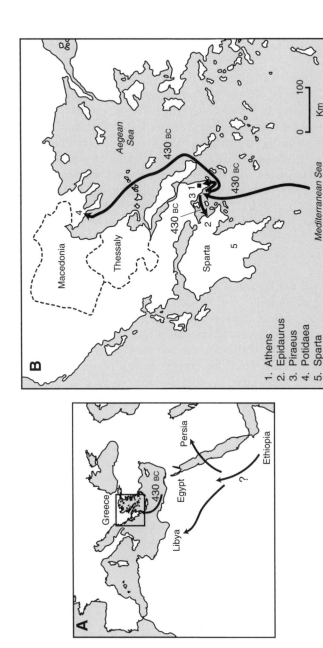

Fig. 2.2. Spread of the Plague of Athens (430–425 BC)

Notes: Vectors show the documented routes of disease transmission in the period up to 430 BC. According to the celebrated account of Thucydides, the epidemic began 'south of Egypt in Aethiopia; thence it descended into Egypt and Libya, and after spreading over the greater part of the Persian empire, suddenly fell upon Athens. It first attacked the inhabitants of Piraeus . . . It afterwards reached the upper city, and then the mortality became far greater' (Thucydides, *Peloponnesian War*, Book 2, ch. 54, trans. Jowett, 1900: 140). The epidemic appeared in Athens during the invasion of Attica by the Peloponnesian (Spartan) Army in the summer of 430 BC. Thereafter, the disease followed Athenian military excursions to Portidaea and Epidaurus. Having spread in Athens as two waves, the epidemic was finally extinguished in the winter of 426–425 BC.

From Athens, military operations served to spread the pestilence to other parts of Greece. In the summer of 430 BC, the disease followed the Athenian troops who were sent as reinforcements in the blockade of Potidaea. Elsewhere, Plutarch (AD 46?–120?) records that a second Athenian expedition—to Epidaurus—suffered a similar fate in the summer of 430 BC (see Major, 1940: 15).

All told, the initial outbreak of the plague is said to have lasted for some two years, abating in the summer of 428 BC. Thereafter, the disease lingered on in southern Greece, recrudescing in the early winter of 427–426 BC. By the following winter, the epidemic was finally spent (Thucydides, 2. 87, trans. Jowett, 1900: 246–7). Exactly how costly the epidemic was in terms of human lives is not known. Pericles, the Athenian strategus, was one of many notables to succumb during the first wave of the visitation, while the second wave is said to have claimed the lives of 4,400 hoplites, 300 horsemen, and an unknown number of 'common people' (Thucydides, 2. 87, trans. Jowett, 1900: 246–7). More generally, the Athenian mortality rate is estimated to have been of the order of 25 per cent (Carmichael, 1993*b*) in a population that, at a maximum in 430 BC, had been swelled by refugees from 100,000 to 300–400,000 (Morens and Littman, 1992).

Identifying the cause of the Plague of Athens has given rise to a lively academic debate. Most recently Olson *et al.* (1996) have speculatively added Ebola fever to an already existing list of 30 or so contending diseases ranging from typhus fever, smallpox, typhoid fever, and bubonic plague through to measles and influenza. Others have argued that the disease may have been 'antique plague' or some other malady which no longer occurs (Prinzing, 1916; Holladay, 1986). The latter suggestion is not implausible. As we note in later sections, the history of war is studded with examples of epidemic diseases which we can no longer trace.

Like Greece, Rome also occasionally found its military aspirations, as did Rome's aggressors, thwarted by infectious diseases; see Table 2.2 and the writings of classical historians such as Livy (59 BC–AD 17) and Dionysius of Halicarnassus (*fl. c.*20 BC). At one level the geographical location of Rome—protected as it was by malaria and the other 'deadly fevers' of the Campagna di Romana—posed a severe epidemiological threat to any would-be invader of the city (Beadle and Hoffman, 1993: 320). At another level the size, mobility, and geographical extent of the Imperial Roman military machine occasionally served as an efficient mechanism in the spatial spread of epidemic (sometimes, pandemic) events.

While Table 2.2 traces the war–disease record for Rome and the Roman Empire back to at least 451 BC when the so-called 'Roman Pestilence' of that year forced the Aequians to forgo a planned attack on the Eternal City, the available evidence suggests that war epidemics were relatively geographically contained in the pre-Christian era. In the early Christian era, events changed for the worse when military operations associated with the maintenance and control of the Roman Empire fuelled two of the major pandemics of early European history: the Plague of the Antonines (AD 165–80) and the Plague of Cyprian (AD 251–66).

The Roman Eastern War and the Plague of the Antonines (AD 165–80)

The origins and course of the Plague of the Antonines (sometimes referred to as the Plague of Galen from the medical description of the disease given in Galen's *Methodus Medendi*) is summarized by Major (1940: 17–21). Descriptions of symptoms suggest smallpox, possibly spreading in a virgin soil population, but others have viewed the disease as typhus fever, measles, a form of 'antique plague', or a mixture of diseases (see e.g. Crawfurd, 1914: 72; Prinzing, 1916: 12). Whatever the exact nature of the epidemic, its effects were severe and wide-ranging. The disease was first carried to Rome by returning soldiers where the subsequent spread within the civil population is said to have resulted in tens of thousands of victims. From Rome the disease spread throughout the rest of Italy resulting in large-scale depopulation. North of Italy, the plague advanced as far as the Rhine while, to the west, it is said to have reached the shores of the Atlantic. All told, the epidemic continued for some 15 years until AD 180, during which time it claimed the lives of two Roman Emperors: Lucius Verus (d. AD 169) and his co-regent, Marcus Aurelius Antoninus (d. AD 180). Some nine years after the death of Marcus Aurelius, Rome is said to have been revisited by the disease, when up to 2,000 citizens a day are believed to have perished (Major, 1940; Kohn, 1998).

The Roman–Gothic Wars and the Plague of Cyprian (AD 251–66)

The Plague of Cyprian (AD 251–66) gravely affected the entire Mediterranean Basin during the period of instability associated with the Roman–Gothic Wars (AD 249–68). The epidemic spread throughout much of North Africa, the Near East, and Europe. At its height, it is documented to have claimed 5,000 victims a day in Rome. The pestilence devastated the Roman legions. It disrupted supply lines and the means of revenue collection, thereby contributing further to the military and political instability of the Empire. As described by Saint Cyprian, the Bishop of Carthage, symptoms of the disease included reddened eyes, an inflamed throat, vomiting, and diarrhoea, with loss of senses (hearing and sight) in survivors. The disease may have been measles or smallpox; bubonic plague has largely been ruled out as contemporary accounts fail to mention swellings (Castiglioni, 1947; McNeill, 1976; Kohn, 1998).

2.3 The Middle Ages (AD 500–1500)

We use the term 'Middle Ages' in a loose sense to mark the 1,000 years or so between the downfall of the classical Roman Empire and the ascendancy of the Renaissance in politics and society. Figure 2.1B summarizes the war–disease interface over the millennium. In this section we outline the main associations.

2.3.1 Before the Holy Crusades

BUBONIC PLAGUE AND BYZANTINE WARS: PLAGUE OF
JUSTINIAN (AD 542)

As Carmichael (1993a) notes, the sixth century AD is generally recognized as marking the first of three great cycles of human bubonic plague. An eyewitness account of the emergence and initial spread of the first cycle and its particular coincidence with Byzantine military operations during Emperor Justinian's wars with the Goths and the Persians is provided by the Byzantine historian, Procopius (AD c.500–?), in Book 2 of his *History of the Wars*. Unlike many earlier references to 'plague', where the term is used in a general sense, Procopius leaves little doubt as to the nature of the disease under consideration: the disease, he says, was characterized by 'a bubonic swelling . . .; and this took place not only in the particular part of the body which is called "boubon" ["groin"] . . . but also inside the armpit, and in some cases also beside the ears, and at different points on the thighs' (Procopius, 2. 22, trans. Dewing, 1914: 457, 459).

According to Procopius, the disease first came to light among the Egyptians at Pelusium in 541. As for the spread of the disease from this putative origin,

it divided and moved in one direction towards Alexandria and the rest of Aegypt, and in the other direction it came to Palestine on the borders of Aegypt; and from there it spread over the whole world . . . And this disease always took its start from the coast, and from there went up to the interior. (Procopius, 2. 22, trans. Dewing, 1914: 455)

The plague reached Byzantium in the spring of 542 where, during the height of the four-month visitation, 'the tale of the dead reached five thousand each day, and again it even came to ten thousand and still more than that' (Procopius, 2. 23, trans. Dewing, 1914: 465).

It seems reasonable to infer that the epidemic spread outwards from Byzantium with the movements of soldiers who were deployed in operations against the Italian Goths to the west and the Persians to the east (see Kohn, 1998). We learn from Procopius that plague 'fell . . . upon the land of the Persians and visited all the other barbarians besides' (Procopius 2. 23, trans. Dewing, 1914: 473). The same source (2. 24) cites the appearance of the disease among the former peoples both as a precipitating factor in Persian efforts to treat for peace in 543 and as an immediate spur for the Roman Byzantine forces to invade Persarmenia. More generally, Russell (1972) suggests that the epidemic resulted in a contraction of the European–Mediterranean population by some 25 per cent. With later recrudescences, the epidemic caused a regional population decline of some 50 to 60 per cent in the period to 570 and it has been viewed as a major contributor to the political and military decline of the classical Mediterranean civilizations.

LATER WARS AND WAR-LIKE EVENTS

Wars in Arabia, Persia, and Syria

Epidemiological details of the many wars involving the peoples of Arabia, Persia, and Syria during the later sixth to eleventh centuries are largely unrecorded. Legend has it that an epidemic of smallpox (possibly measles?) decimated the Abyssinian Army at Mecca during the Elephant War (*c*.569 or 571) with some 60,000 Abyssinian soldiers failing to return home. A disease that could have been smallpox or measles also appeared among Greek troops who were returning from Mecca at about this time (Creighton, 1965; Kohn, 1998). Later, during the Byzantine–Muslim War (633–42), the so-called 'Plague of Amwās' spread as two waves of infection (638 and 639), the second striking the Syrian Army at Amwās with considerable ferocity. The disease, which spread onwards to Egypt and Persia, is reputed to have claimed the lives of 25,000 Arab soldiers, including the Syrian military commander Abu 'Ubaydah (Dols, 1977; Kohn, 1998).

Europe: The Viking Raids

The Viking Raids on Europe extended over two centuries (*c*.800 to *c*.1016) and were typified by swift incursions, sieges, and sackings by Scandinavian raiding parties especially in the British Isles, France, the Low Countries, Germany, Italy, Russia, and Spain. Nothwithstanding the broad temporal and geographical extent of the incursions, the historical record provides very little evidence of the spread of disease in direct association with such war-like events.

However, Poser (1994, 1995) postulates a much longer-term epidemiological legacy. Noting that, today, the highest prevalences of multiple sclerosis (MS) are to be found in Scandinavia and the countries settled by the Norseman and their descendants, Poser suggests that peoples of Viking descent may have a particular genetic susceptibility to MS (cf. Cliff *et al.*, 2000: 355–8). If correct, the Viking Raids, coupled with the engagement of Vikings and their progeny in such geographically disparate factions as the Byzantine, Mongol, and Crusader Armies, may have played a critical role in the geographical dissemination of susceptibility to multiple sclerosis during the Middle Ages (Poser, 1994, 1995).

2.3.2 The Era of the Holy Crusades

The Holy Crusades (1095–1291) encompassed a series of eight major (and many more minor) military campaigns organized by western European Christendom to recover the Holy Land from the Muslims (Runciman, 1951–5). Variously viewed as either holy wars or penitentiary pilgrimages to Christ's

Holy Sepulchre, the Crusades marked not only an upsurge in Christian revival but also an epoch of European social upheaval and change. The dissolution of feudalism, the development of modern urban settlement systems, the growth of scholasticism, the emergence of west European colonization, the establishment of trade networks, and developments in warfare can all be traced to the era of the Holy Crusades (for general overviews, see: Le Goff, 1988; Heer, 1998).

Table 2.3 provides a summary overview of the principal epidemic events to afflict the Christian armies during the crusades. While many of the campaigns were associated with major outbreaks of disease, variously in North Africa and the Near East, opinion is often divided as to the nature of the disease(s) concerned. During the First Crusade (1095–9), for example, an unidentified disease appeared in the largely French army at Antioch, northern Syria, in the summer of 1098. Chroniclers relate how, at the height of the epidemic, 40 or more corpses were buried each day (Kohn, 1998: 69), while a 1,500-strong German contingent is reputed to have been 'almost completely anihilated' on its arrival in the city (Prinzing, 1916: 13). The epidemic continued into 1099, apparently spreading with the movements of the various army factions and serving to delay the crusaders' advance on Jerusalem. The nature of the disease that appeared at Antioch is uncertain, but malaria, scurvy, and typhoid fever have all been posited (Prinzing, 1916; Kohn, 1998).

Later expeditions were to fare little better. During the Second Crusade (1147–9), many thousands of pilgrims are reputed to have died when the army

Table 2.3. Epidemic events during the Crusades, AD 1095–1291

Crusade	Epidemic events
First (AD 1095–9)	Crusader Army at Antioch (AD 1098–9), possibly malaria, typhoid, or scurvy.
Second (AD 1147–9)	Army of Louis VII at Attalia (AD 1148), possibly bubonic plague, dysentery, or typhoid.
Third (AD 1189–92)	Crusader Army besieging Acre (AD 1189–91), possibly scurvy and other diseases; Crusader Army besieging Antioch (AD 1190), disease unknown.
Fifth (AD 1217–21)	Crusader Army besieging Damietta (AD 1218–19), possibly severe scurvy.
Seventh (AD 1248–54)	Crusader Army at Al Mansurah (AD 1250), 'army sickness' (scurvy?).
Eighth (AD 1270–2)[1]	Crusader Army at Carthage, possibly dysentery.

Note: [1] Fighting continued as part of the Crusader–Turkish Wars until 1291.
Sources: Based on information in Prinzing (1916), Major (1940), and Kohn (1998).

of Emperor Louis VII was beset by an epidemic (possibly of bubonic plague, dysentery, or typhoid fever) at Attalia in 1148. Likewise, during the Third Crusade (1189–92), diseases—which may have included severe scurvy—appeared among the besieging Christian armies at Acre in 1189–91 and Antioch in 1190 (Prinzing, 1916; Kohn, 1998).

Scorbutic Diseases in the Later Crusades

In the thirteenth century, chroniclers leave us in little doubt as to the occurrence of scorbutic diseases among the Christian armies. During the Fifth Crusade (1217–21), a disease—which was almost certainly a severe form of scurvy—broke out among the Christian forces as they besieged Damietta in the winter of 1218–19 (Jaques de Vitry, cited in Major, 1940: 29). One-sixth of the pilgrims are estimated to have succumbed (Prinzing, 1916: 14). The besieged of Damietta, too, suffered from severe scurvy, ophthalmia, and other diseases. When the city finally capitulated in November 1219, less than 10 per cent of the original population of 80,000 is estimated to have survived (Wilken, 1826, cited in Prinzing, 1916: 15).

Severe scurvy, possibly complicated by typhoid fever and other infectious diseases, reappeared during the Seventh Crusade (1248–52), this time in the Christian camp at Al Mansurah, on the road to Cairo. The disease, which first appeared in February 1250, persisted until Easter 1250, forcing a Christian retreat to Damietta and, ultimately, resulting in the collapse of the Seventh Crusade (Major, 1940: 31).

An Old Plague: Leprosy in Medieval Europe

As Prinzing (1916) notes, the apparent upsurge of one of the ancient infectious diseases of the Holy Land—leprosy—in medieval Europe has frequently been attributed to the Crusades. While there is ample evidence to suggest that crusaders did contract the disease in the Holy Land (Ell, 1996), a direct link to the rapid expansion in the number of lazar houses in Europe during the era of the crusades is unclear (Prinzing, 1916). On the one hand, there is some uncertainty regarding the nature and diagnosis of 'leprosy' in Europe at this time (Watts, 1997) while, on the other hand, the Crusades represented just one form of contact between Europe and the Middle East (Ell, 1996). As Ell (1996: 185) concludes, 'It is tempting to connect the rise of leprosy in Europe with the crusades, but there had been many peaceful contacts between Western Europe and the Middle East. Whatever the crusades may have contributed in terms of the incidence of leprosy must have been a matter of degree rather than as a primary cause.'

Other European Evidence: The Holy Roman Empire

The forces of the Holy Roman Empire were repeatedly beset by epidemics during their various expeditions to Italy. In 1137, for example, Lothair's army was attacked by an unknown infectious disease whilst in Italy (Prinzing, 1916).

Later, during the Wars of the Lombard League (1167–83), the army of Frederick Barbarossa was struck by an epidemic in August 1167 shortly after the capture of Rome. The epidemic almost annihilated the German army, forcing Barbarossa to withdraw into northern Italy. Opinion is divided as to the nature of the disease, although bubonic plague (Prinzing, 1916), typhus fever (Zinsser, 1935), and malaria (Kohn, 1998) have been suggested. Finally, Prinzing (1916) notes that a fatal epidemic disease appeared in the army of Henry VI just as it had laid siege to Naples in the winter of 1190–1.

2.3.3 After the Crusades

THE BLACK DEATH AND WAR

In terms of its grip on the public imagination, the Black Death probably remains the most visible symbol of the power and influence of epidemic disease. In 1346, Europe, Northern Africa, and the Levant (the westward parts of the Middle East) had a population of the order of magnitude of 100 million (McEvedy, 1988). Within a decade, nearly a quarter of them had died and the population rise that had marked the evolution of medieval society had come to an abrupt end. The cause of what was known as the Great Dying or the Great Pestilence (it was only later that the term 'Black Death' emerged) was the agent of human plague (*Yersinia pestis*) which, a full eight centuries after its first pandemic cycle in the human population (Plague of Justinian; see Sect. 2.3.1), again spread across the Eurasian land mass. The disease is thought to have emerged among marmots, large rodents native in central Asia, and to have been introduced by fur traders moving along the Silk Road from Astrakhan and Saray. The subsequent spread to Kaffa, Constantinople, Egypt, Sicily, and Genoa (all infected by 1347) is shown in Figure 2.3. As the time-contours on the map show, most of Europe was affected before the epidemic finally subsided in 1352.

The geographical progress of the Black Death was intimately associated with war and war-like events. From its putative origin in central Asia, the disease was carried to Persia by the forces of Malik Ashraf, who returned to Baghdad in 1347 after an attack on Tabriz (bordering Azerbaijan) where plague was present. Ashraf's troops laid siege to the town of Shaykh Hasan Buzurg, near Baghdad, but had to abort the siege when plague appeared in the army (Kohn, 1998). As for the westwards diffusion plotted in Figure 2.3, the

---

Fig. 2.3. Spread of the Black Death, 1347–1352

Notes: Vectors show the main routeways by which bubonic plague diffused from Central Asia, via the Ukrainian city of Kaffa, to the Mediterranean and Northern Europe. The Mongol–Italian conflict of the mid-1340s, centred on the Genoan occupation of Kaffa, facilitated the spread of the disease from the Black Sea to the Mediterranean ports of Genoa, Venice, and elsewhere.
Source: Cliff *et al.* (1998, fig. 1.3, p. 15), reproduced from Brock (1990, fig. 1, p. 5).

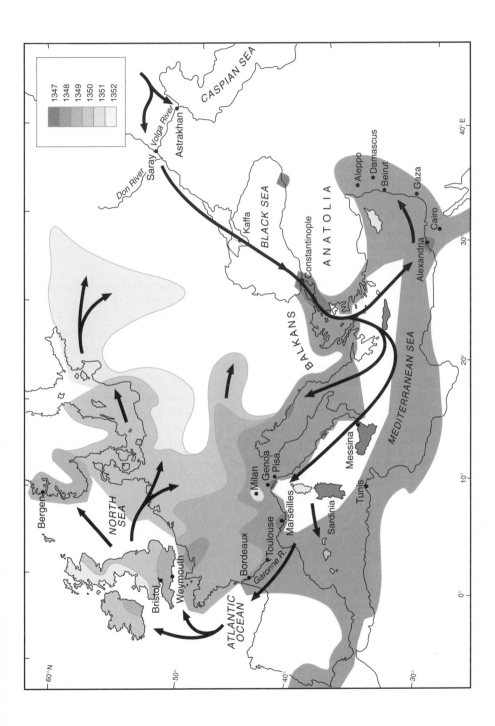

Tartar siege of the Genoese-occupied Crimean city of Kaffa was to prove a pivotal event in the onwards spread of plague to Europe. In 1346, during the third year of the Siege of Kaffa, the besieging Tartar forces experienced a sudden outbreak of plague. According to one eyewitness account,

Infinite numbers of Tartars and Saracens suddenly fell dead of an inexplicable disease . . . and behold the disease invading all the army of the Tartars . . . every day . . . thousands were killed . . . arrows having been hurled from Heaven to oppress the pride of the Tartars . . . who at once showed signs in their bodies . . . the humours coagulated in the groins, they developed a subsequent putrid fever and died, all council and aid of doctors failing. (de Mussis, cited in Derbes, 1966: 60)

In an early reference to biological warfare, the same source tells how the Tartars attempted to take advantage of their misfortune:

the Tartars, fatigued by such a plague and pestiferous disease, stupefied and amazed, observing themselves dying without hope of health ordered cadavers placed on their hurling machines and thrown into the city of Caffa [*sic*], so that by means of these intolerable passengers the defenders died widely. (ibid.)

Whatever the exact source of plague within the besieged stronghold, either via the hurling machines of the Tartars or as part of a natural cycle of sylvatic and urban rats and their fleas (see Christopher *et al.*, 1997), the disease forced the Italian capitulation and abandonment of the city. From Kaffa, the fleeing refugees—with plague victims among them—carried the disease to Constantinople, Genoa, Venice, and other Mediterranean ports, with onwards spread to the whole of southern, central, and northern Europe; see Figure 2.3. The appearance of plague, in turn, brought the nascent Hundred Years' War (1337–1453) to a halt; a truce between England and France was renewed no less than three times between 1347 and 1351 (Kohn, 1998).

EMERGENT DISEASES AND EUROPEAN WARS IN THE LATE MIDDLE AGES

English Sweating Sickness and the Wars of the Roses

In the mid-summer of 1485—just as the English Wars of the Roses (1455–85) were about to reach their conclusion at Bosworth Field—a previously unknown, and rapidly fatal, infection began to extend across England. As described by T. Forrestier in 1490, the disease had an acute onset with 'a sudden great sweating and stinking with redness of the face and of all the body' (Forrestier, 1490, cited in Hunter, 1991: 303)—symptoms from which the name 'English sweating sickness' was derived. Other manifestations included fever, headache, lethargy, pulmonary involvement, and delirium. The course of the disease was generally swift, often with fatal outcome (probably due to dehydration, circulatory shock, and electrolyte loss) within a day of clinical onset; for those that did not succumb, there was usually complete recovery in one to two weeks (Hecker, 1859).

Exactly where the sweating sickness originated, and what (if any) connection it had with the closing stages of the Wars of the Roses, has been an ongoing source of scholarly contention. According to the account of Polydore Vergil, written some 50 years after the event, the disease first showed itself when the (largely French) mercenary army of Henry VII landed at Milford Haven, South Wales, on 1 August 1485. While the general impression of a northern French origin with Henry's army is consistent with the appearance of a similar disease (the 'Picardy sweat') in Flanders some two centuries later, the historical evidence for an introduction with Henry's forces is equivocal (Wylie and Collier, 1981; Hunter, 1991). First, as Wylie and Collier (1981) note, archival records provide no evidence of the occurrence of the disease, either among Henry's army or the Welsh people, during the 21-day march from Milford Haven to Bosworth Field. Secondly, available evidence suggests that the disease was present in Yorkshire and northern England more generally in the months preceding the arrival of Henry (Wylie and Collier, 1981). Wylie and Collier (1981) propose that the disease originated with trade links between the Yorkshire–Lincolnshire seaports and Russia–Scandinavia.

Whatever the source of English sweating sickness, the population flux which accompanied Henry's victory at Bosworth Field almost certainly contributed to the dissemination of the disease. The sickness showed itself in London on 19 September when, Creighton (1965, i. 266) notes, the city must have been 'unusually full of people' in the build-up to Henry's coronation. The disease remained in the capital for five weeks, claiming the lives of at least two mayors and six aldermen (Hecker, 1859) and causing 'more devastation . . . than the sword, which had been ruling for thirty years in a fearful civil war' (B. M. Lersch, 1896, cited in Prinzing, 1916: 18). Elsewhere, many scholars are said to have succumbed at Oxford while, by the end of 1485, the disease is believed to have reached across the kingdom (Hecker, 1859; Creighton, 1965).

The English sweating sickness of 1485 appears to have been an entirely novel disease; it spread in epidemic form on just four subsequent occasions (1508, 1517, 1528, and 1551), before apparently disappearing from the epidemiological scene. The exact nature of the disease is uncertain (Wylie and Collier, 1981; Hunter, 1991; Thwaites *et al.*, 1997; Taviner *et al.*, 1998; Carlson and Hammond, 1999). Medieval and early-modern observers appear to have distinguished it from influenza, malaria, plague, and typhus fever (Thwaites *et al.*, 1997). Wylie and Collier (1981) dismiss the possibility of a bacterial aetiology, and suggest that the disease was probably caused by an arbovirus. Hunter (1991) favours an enterovirus, while Thwaites *et al.* (1997) and Taviner *et al.* (1998) postulate a viral agent with a marked pulmonary component and a rodent reservoir. In a further contribution to the debate, Carlson and Hammond (1999) contend that the epidemiological and clinical profile corresponds to one of the haemorrhagic fevers, of which only Crimean Congo haemorrhagic fever had the potential to establish itself in enzootic form in England during the medieval period.

Venereal Syphilis and the Italian Wars

The apparent epidemic ascendancy of venereal syphilis in late-fifteenth-century Europe and its reputed association with the wars of that time holds a particularly controversial place in disease history. As Arrizabalaga (1993: 1028) notes, medical historiographers of the past have usually identified modern-day venereal syphilis with *morbus gallicus* (var. *mal franzoso, mala napoletana*), a severe and commonly fatal venereal disease that first erupted in Europe in the 1490s. The apparently sudden appearance of *morbus gallicus* and its temporal association with the return of Columbus from the Americas has prompted some scholars to argue for a New World origin for venereal syphilis. Opponents of this view, on the other hand, contend that the disease existed in the Old World long before the discovery of the Americas. The evidence, however, remains equivocal; see Guerra (1978) and Wood (1978).

Whether *morbus gallicus*—when viewed as the conceptual forerunner of venereal syphilis—originated in the New World or not, all available evidence suggests that its epidemic dissemination in Europe was closely associated with the Italian War of Charles VIII (1494–5). Details are sketchy, but it is generally held that the disease began to spread widely in the French mercenary army of Charles in early 1495, coincident with its entry into the city of Naples (Prinzing, 1916; Creighton, 1965).[4] At about the same time, medical evidence points to the occurrence of the same malady among the Venetian and Milanese troops that had gathered at Novara while, in 1496, the German troops aligned against France under Maximilian I were also afflicted by the disease (Creighton, 1965).

Seeded in the forces of France, German, and Italy in this manner, the subsequent disbanding of the various armies was to result in the dissemination of *morbus gallicus* across much of Europe. According to H. Häser, 'Those who had most to do with the further dissemination . . . were the Albanian and Roumanian estradiots serving in the Venetian army . . . and also the German and Swiss *Landsknechte* [mercenary foot soldiers] returning from Italy' (H. Häser, 1882, cited in Prinzing, 1916: 17). Certainly it appears that the disbanded *Landsknechte* had carried the disease to French and German towns, including Metz, Nördlingen, and Strasbourg by the end of 1495 (Prinzing, 1916), with the disease appearing later in Greece and Holland (1496), the British Isles (1497), and Hungary, Poland, and Russia (1499) (Kohn, 1998).

---

[4] The source of the disease among the French army in Naples is entirely uncertain. According to Garrison (1917), syphilis is supposed to have been communicated to the French soldiers by the Spanish occupants of the city. The latter, in turn, contracted the disease from sailors who had returned from the New World with Christopher Columbus. As noted by Creighton (1965, i. 433), however, there is some evidence that the disease may have been present in France before the war with Italy, and that the French forces may have conveyed the disease to Liguria. In summarizing the conflicting evidence, Creighton (1965, i. 433) observes: 'we have a theory of a Spanish origin, of a French origin, and also perhaps of a native Italian origin—all agreeing that Italy during the state of war from 1494 to 1496 was the theatre of its first ravages on the great scale, and the source from which the disease was brought to all the countries of Europe by the returning soldiery'.

2.4 The Old World, I: European Theatres (AD 1500–1850)

The principal links between war and infectious diseases over the period are summarized in Figure 2.1C.

2.4.1 Before the Thirty Years' War

THE EPIDEMIC ASCENDANCY OF WAR TYPHUS

The late fifteenth and sixteenth centuries are identified by disease historians such as Hecker (1859), Hirsch (1883), and Zinsser (1935) as signalling the appearance of the first great epidemic waves of a disease that, over the next 450 years, would spread repeatedly with the wars of modern Europe: typhus fever. The exact origins of epidemic typhus in Europe are unknown (Hirsch, 1883), although some connection with the Orient—and particularly with successive conflicts with the Ottoman Turks—is generally suspected (see Zinsser, 1935: 265–70). In this context, the earliest documentary evidence of typhus fever as a pestilence of European wars can be traced back to the Castilian investment of Granada during the Spanish Christian–Muslim War (1481–92). According to the Spanish historian, Joaquin Villalba, a typhus-like disease ('malignant spotted fever') first appeared among the Castilian troops in 1489, having originated with Spanish soldiers from Cyprus—a place where the fever was said to be prevalent. As Villalba explains, 'In Cyprus, these soldiers fought with the Venetians against the Turks, and thence they carried the seeds of the disease not only to the Spaniards, but also to the Saracens' (Joaquin Villalba, cited in Zinsser, 1935: 243). From the Castilian camps in Granada, the disease spread onwards to the army of Don Fernando the Catholic, such that:

when the [Spanish] army was reviewed at the beginning of the year 1490, the generals noticed that 20,000 men were missing from the rolls, and of these 3,000 had been killed by the Moors and 17,000 had died of disease, not a few of them succumbing to the severe cold—a kind of death which . . . was very miserable. (Joaquin Villalba, cited in Zinsser, 1935: 243)

After the war in Granada, typhus fever spread to Italy and France, and then northwards, forming the first of a series of epidemic waves that diffused with the great European struggles of the time.

War Typhus in the Sixteenth Century

In his seminal biography of typhus fever, *Rats, Lice and History*, Hans Zinsser (Pl. 2.2) identifies two groups of conflicts—each extending over a number decades—which facilitated the dissemination of epidemic typhus in sixteenth-century Europe: the wars against the Holy Roman Emperor, Charles V, and the Ottoman Wars in Hungary (Zinsser, 1935). We consider each group of conflicts in turn.

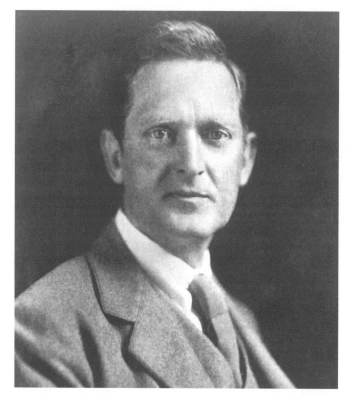

Pl. 2.2. Hans Zinsser (1878–1940)

Notes: US bacteriologist and biographer of typhus fever. Professor Zinsser had first witnessed the tragic consequences of epidemic typhus during his work with the Red Cross Typhus Commission in Serbia during World War I (see Sect. 12.5.2). Having co-authored *Typhus Fever with Particular Reference to the Serbian Epidemic* (Cambridge, Mass.: Harvard University Press, 1920), his interest in the disease was further stimulated when, in 1923, he was posted to Russia as sanitary commissioner for the Health Section of the League of Nations. In 1935, his famed book *Rats, Lice and History* postulated a link between the historical emergence of typhus fever in fifteenth- and sixteenth-century Europe and the Ottoman wars of the time.
Source: The Wellcome Library, London.

Wars against Charles V. The antecedents of the second major wave of typhus fever in Europe can be traced to the French siege of Naples during the Second War against Charles V (1526–9). A 30,000-strong French force had laid siege to Naples and the ensconsed Imperial Roman Army at the beginning of May 1528. At first, mild and non-specific camp diseases (diarrhoeas and fevers) went largely unnoticed in the siege camp, and it was only when the strategy to cut the city's water supply had backfired—resulting in the flooding of the French siege plain—that illness became more general in the French forces. Beginning in mid-July, the French Army experienced a period of great mortality which, by the end of August, had resulted in the deaths of up to 25,000 soldiers and forced the lifting of the siege. The principal cause of the mortality is thought to have been typhus fever; a disease that is reputed to have been widely distributed in Italy and which, by most acccounts, was carried to Germany and elsewhere after the end of the siege (Hecker, 1859; Prinzing, 1916; Zinsser, 1935).

Almost a quarter of a century later, during the Fifth War against Charles V (1552–9), Prinzing (1916) records how a 'great pestilence' (probably typhus and dysentery) forced Charles V to lift the allied (German–Italian–Spanish) siege of Metz on New Year's Day 1553. By that time, the combined effects of disease, disablement, and desertion had reduced the *c.* 80,000-strong siege army by one-third of its original strength. The besieged, too, suffered from typhus fever, with the disease continuing to spread in the razed environs of Metz in the summer of 1553 (Prinzing, 1916; Zinsser, 1935).

Ottoman Wars in Hungary. Although the weight of evidence suggests that typhus fever spread widely during the early wars against Charles V, Zinsser (1935) contends that the epidemic emergence of the disease in Europe was contingent on the contemporaneous conflicts of the Ottoman Turks in Hungary:

> . . . we are inclined to believe that the Hungarian wars and their consequences created the circumstances which gave typhus the opportunity of passing from man to man by lice in uninterrupted cycles, short-circuiting the rat–flea phase and adapting the parasitism firmly as a man–louse–man transmission in the form we now know as the 'classical European type' or 'virus humanise'. (Zinsser, 1935: 270)

The earliest reliable evidence of typhus fever in Hungary can be traced to 1542 when the disease (referred to by chroniclers as '*Pestartige braüne*') ravaged the German army of Joachim, Margrave of Brandenburg, claiming the lives of some 30,000 soldiers. Whether the disease had been introduced by the Turks or some other party, or whether it was already present in Hungary, is unknown. By all accounts, however, the Germans suffered a great deal more than the Hungarians, suggesting that some degree of herd immunity had been established in Hungary before the Germans had arrived (Prinzing, 1916; Zinsser, 1935).

In direct consequence of the Ottoman War of 1565–9, typhus fever (having now acquired the label *morbus Hungaricus* or 'Hungarian disease') spread widely in Hungary during 1566. The epidemic continued until 1568 and, according to Hirsch (1883) and Prinzing (1916), extended to Austria, Belgium, Bohemia, Germany, Holland, Italy, Spain, and beyond. 'Ever since that time,' observes Zinsser (1935: 270), 'typhus has remained endemic in Hungary, the Balkan States, and the adjoining territories of Poland and Russia. These are still, at the present day, the "home stations" from which modern European epidemics take origin.'

2.4.2 The Thirty Years' War

In terms of its human costs, the Thirty Years' War (1618–48) ranks as one of the most destructive conflicts in European history. Cast as a religious war between European factions of Protestantism and Roman Catholicism, but also fuelled by the political tensions of a modernizing continent, Germany and the Holy Roman Empire provided the soil for the marches, counter-marches, and clashes of armies aligned with some 25 warring states.[5] The Imperial campaigns under Tilly, Wallenstein, and Spinola, the Protestant campaigns under Mansfield, Gustavus Adolphus, and Christian IV of Denmark and, later in the war, the Swedish campaigns under Banér, Torstensson, and Wrangel, all contributed to a field of destruction that extended from Hungary in the east to the Franco-German border in the west, and from the Baltic Sea in the north to the border with the Swiss Confederation in the south; see Figure 2.4 for locations. Punitive killings, the razing of crops, land, and property, mass population displacement, famine, and a long series of lethal epidemics in both military and civilian populations all contributed to the devastation. Such was the severity that, during the course of the war, the population of Germany is estimated to have fallen by 50 per cent or more, to 8 to 9 millions (Prinzing, 1916). In some places, such as Mecklenburg, Württemberg, and western Bavaria, the population loss may have exceeded two-thirds (see Fig. 2.5) while, in Bohemia, it is said that little more than 6,000 (of an original 35,000) villages were left standing at the end of the conflict (Prinzing, 1916; Lancaster, 1990).

THE WAR PESTILENCES

Epidemics, often in association with famine, followed closely on the movements of the various mercenary armies such that Europe became 'a spot map of constant . . . outbreaks of every conceivable disease' (Zinsser, 1935: 272–3). The nature of the disease(s) at a given time and place, however, is not always apparent. Disease historians are largely reliant on the evidence of contemporary chroniclers and these frequently fail to provide sufficient information for accurate retrospective diagnosis. On the basis of fragmentary evidence, Prinzing (1916) draws a broad epidemiological division between the earlier phase of the war (1618–30) when typhus fever spread as the principal disease in both military and civil populations, and the later phase (1630–48) when bubonic plague gained ascendancy. While some have opposed this simple division, contending that bubonic plague was also present in the early period (Zinsser, 1935: 274), there is little doubt as to the prominence of bubonic plague and typhus fever, along with dysentery, as the major pestilences of the Thirty Years' War (Hirsch, 1883). To these diseases, the chroniclers add scurvy and, in the latter stages of the conflict, smallpox (Prinzing, 1916), while the occurrence of diph-

---

[5] For English-language overviews of the origins and course of the Thirty Years' War, see Wedgwood (1938), Steinberg (1966), Pagès (1970), Polišenský (1971), and Parker (1984).

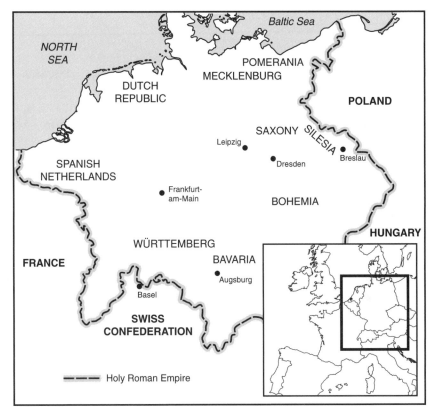

Fig. 2.4. Location map of Germany and the Holy Roman Empire at the outbreak of the Thirty Years' War (1618–1648)

theria, scarlet fever, and typhoid fever, among other conditions, may be surmised (Zinsser, 1935).

EPIDEMIC PATTERNS

The first major epidemic event associated with the Thirty Years' War can be traced to the initial focus of the conflict—Bohemia. In the early part of 1620, typhus fever appeared among the invading forces of Tilly and the Catholic League. The outbreak is said to have claimed the lives of some 20,000 soldiers, with the survivors carrying the disease on to the civil populations of Bavaria and Württemberg in the following year (Prinzing, 1916); see Figure 2.4 for locations. During the remainder of the war, the primary geographical centre of disease activity tracked the shifting locus of military operations: first in the south and west of Germany (1620–5); and then in the north and east (1625–30); down the central spine (1630–5); again in the north (1635–40);

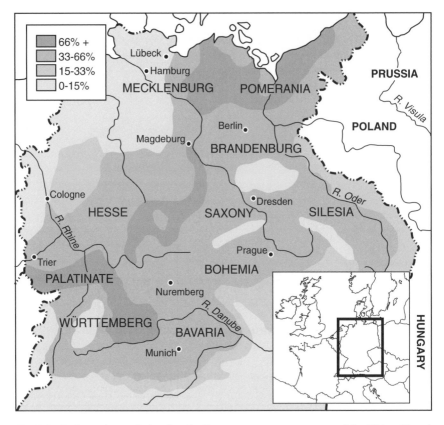

Fig. 2.5. Estimated population loss in Germany as a consequence of the Thirty Years' War, 1618–1648

Source: Redrawn from Pennington (1989, map 4, p. 587).

and, finally, with the breakdown of centralized warfare, the entire country (1640–8).

Patterns in Time

In his review of disease in the Thirty Years' War, Friedrich Prinzing (1916: 28–72) documents some 450 local epidemic outbreaks in the civil settlement system of Germany, 1622–39. The annual distribution of Prinzing's sample series of outbreaks, formed to the year of epidemic onset, is plotted as the bar chart in Figure 2.6. For reference, the periods associated with the constituent conflicts of the Thirty Years' War have been indicated on the chart. As Figure 2.6 shows, the outbreak distribution is bimodal with a primary peak of activity in the years 1625–6 (>50 outbreaks per annum) coinciding with the onset of the Danish and Swedish–Prussian conflicts. Thereafter, the number of documented outbreaks fell to low levels in the years 1627–9 (<10 outbreaks per

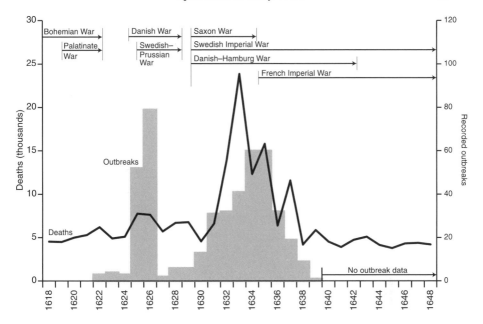

Fig. 2.6. Temporal distribution of epidemic outbreaks in Germany during the Thirty Years' War, 1618–1648

Notes: The bar chart plots the annual count of local epidemic events as documented by Prinzing (1916) for the civil settlement system of Germany, 1622–39. The line trace plots the aggregate number of deaths recorded in sample cities of Germany (Augsburg, Breslau, Dresden, Frankfurt-am-Main, Leipzig) and the Swiss Confederation (Basel), 1618–48.

Source: Based on information in Prinzing (1916: 28–78).

annum) before increasing steadily to a secondary peak with the Saxon, Danish–Hamburg, Swedish, and French Imperial conflicts in 1634–5 (>50 outbreaks per annum).

Patterns in Space

Unfortunately demographic and epidemiological information on which to judge the duration and severity of many of the outbreaks charted in Figure 2.6 is unavailable. Consequently, we limit our spatial consideration to six sample towns and cities of Germany (Augsburg, Breslau, Dresden, Frankfurt-am-Main, and Leipzig) and the neighbouring Swiss Confederation (Basel) for which unbroken records of annual mortality, 1618–48, are available from Prinzing (1916: 78). The locations of the settlements are given in Figure 2.4. The corresponding series of annual mortality are plotted as the line traces in Figure 2.7. To assist in the interpretation of Figure 2.7, the charts have been grouped by broad geographical location:

1. Figures 2.7A–C (Dresden, Leipzig, and Breslau): northern and eastern Germany;

Table 2.4. Epidemic outbreaks in sample cities of Germany and the Swiss Confederation during the Thirty Years' War, 1618–1648

Settlement[1]	Epidemic period	Disease	Deaths	
			All causes[2]	Excess[3]
Northern/eastern Germany				
Dresden (13,000[5])	1626	typhus fever	740	340
	1632–5	bubonic plague	7,714	6,100
	1637	*plague*[4]	1,897	1,500
	1639	?[4]	1,845	1,400
	1643	?[4]	1,041	600
Leipzig (14,500[5])	1626	typhus fever	1,268	800
	1631–3	*plague*[4]	5,988	4,700
	1636–7	*plague*[4]	5,447	4,600
	1642–3	?[4]	2,114	1,200
Breslau	1625	typhus fever	3,000	1,800
	1633	*plague*[4]	13,231	12,000
Southern/western Germany and Swiss Confederation				
Augsburg (*c.* 80,000[6])	1626–8	?[4]	8,454	4,400
	1632–5	?[4]	17,756	12,300
Frankfurt–am–Main	1622	typhus fever	1,785	1,200
	1625	?[4]	1,871	1,200
	1632	?[4]	2,900	2,100
	1634–7	various[4]	15,908	15,300
Basel	1629	*pestilence*[4]	2,656	2,100
	1634	*pestilence*[4]	2,115	1,600

Notes: [1] Estimated population size in parentheses. [2] Deaths recorded in epidemic years among citizens. [3] Estimated as reported deaths in excess of expectation (expectation is based on reported mortality in the year 1618). [4] Specific disease(s) not stated; the term *plague* is used in a loose sense. Writing of Saxony (including the cities of Dresden and Leipzig) in the period from 1630, Prinzing (1916: 41) notes that 'We may safely assume that bubonic plague was the most common disease, although both typhus fever and dysentery were of frequent occurrence'. [5] Population estimate for 1626. [6] Population estimate for 1624.
Source: Based on information in Prinzing (1916: 28–78).

2. Figures 2.7D–F (Augsburg, Frankfurt-am-Main, and Basel): southern and western Germany and the Swiss Confederation.

For reference, the bar charts on each graph have been formed in the manner described for Figure 2.6 and plot the annual distribution of sample disease outbreaks recorded by Prinzing (1916) for northern and eastern sectors[6] (Figs. 2.7A–C) and southern and western sectors[7] (Figs. 2.7D–F) of Germany. Finally, Table 2.4 provides summary details of the major epidemic events recorded for each of the sample cities. The aggregate annual mortality count for the six cities is plotted as the line trace in Figure 2.6.

[6] Including Brandenburg, Lusatia, Mecklenburg, Pomerania, Saxony, Schleswig-Holstein, and Thuringia.
[7] Including Alsace, Baden, Bavaria, Hesse, Lorraine, Palatinate, Upper/Middle Rhine, and Württemberg.

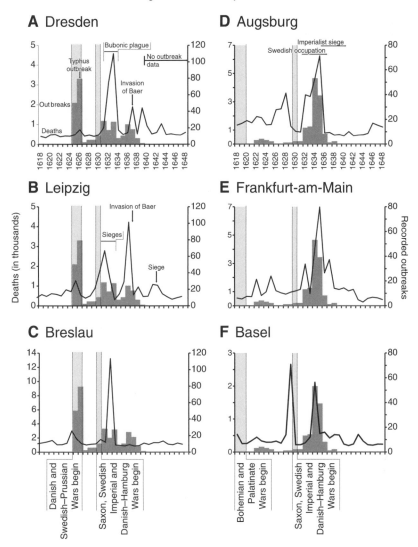

Fig. 2.7. Mortality in the Thirty Years' War, 1618–1648

Notes: Mortality in sample towns and cities of Germany and the Swiss Confederation during the Thirty Years' War, 1618–48. Charts A–C: settlements of northern/eastern Germany (Dresden, Leipzig, and Breslau). Charts D–F: settlements of southern/western Germany and the Swiss Confederation (Augsburg, Frankfurt-am-Main, and Basel). The line traces plot the annual mortality count for each settlement, while the bar charts plot the annual distribution of sample outbreaks of disease in northern/eastern Germany (A–C) and southern/western Germany (D–F) as documented by Prinzing (1916). See Fig. 2.4 for location of settlements.

Source: Based on information in Prinzing (1916: 28–78).

Although Figure 2.6 clearly identifies the period to 1635 as the main period of heightened mortality across the six sample cities, the city-level graphs in Figure 2.7 show highly complex patterns of localized mortality.

Northern and Eastern Germany (Figures 2.7A–C). All told, the sample locations recorded 11 epidemic events (Table 2.4), with each event manifesting as a clearly defined peak in mortality (Figs. 2.7A–C). While typhus fever spread to all three settlements in 1625/6, associated with a more general epidemic which had been sparked by Wallenstein's early incursions into the region, Table 2.4 and Figure 2.7 indicate that the major mortality crises awaited the 1630s. The repeated sieges of Leipzig in 1631, 1632, and 1633 were associated with the high-level spread of a disease which may have been bubonic plague. At about the same time, bubonic plague spread widely in Dresden, while Wallenstein's invasion of Silesia in 1633 was associated with a major epidemic in Breslau. Although Breslau escaped further epidemics of any consequence, the long series of Swedish military campaigns, variously under Banér, Torstensson, Wrangel, and others, were associated with subsequent epidemics in Dresden and/or Leipzig during 1636–7, 1639, and finally 1642–3 (Fig. 2.7 and Table 2.4).

Southern and Western Germany and the Swiss Confederation (Figures 2.7D–F). The sample mortality series in Figures 2.7D–F follow the same broad pattern as Figures 2.7A–C, but with more pronounced evidence of epidemic activity in the period prior to the 1630s. So, as Table 2.4 indicates, epidemics spread in Frankfurt-am-Main in 1622 and 1625, Augsburg in 1626–8, and Basel in 1629. But for Augsburg and Frankfurt-am-Main, these early events were eclipsed by major epidemics associated with Swedish occupation and related sieges in the mid-1630s. Finally, given the geographical proximity of Switzerland, it seems reasonable to infer that the 1634 epidemic in Basel was connected to events in southern and western Germany (see Prinzing, 1916: 73–4).

INTERNATIONAL DIFFUSION

As intimated by the evidence for Basel, the epidemiological effects of the Thirty Years' War were by no means contained within the borders of Germany; the cross-border movements of armies, fugitives, and others all contributed to the international diffusion of disease. In Holland, for example, the presence of Mansfield's ailing troops prompted an epidemic of typhus fever which spread throughout the upper tiers of the civilian settlement system in 1623–4. In France, severe outbreaks of typhus fever and bubonic plague occurred in Paris, Lyons, Marseilles, and Toulouse, among many other towns and cities, during 1628–33 while, at about the same time, German or French troops are believed to have sparked major epidemics of bubonic plague and typhus fever in Italy (Prinzing, 1916; Zinsser, 1935).

2.4.3 The English Civil War

Unlike many earlier civil and dynastic wars in England, the epidemiological overspill from the ongoing Thirty Years' War beset both military and civil populations during the English Civil War (1640–9). In the spring and summer of 1643, typhus fever spread among the Royalist and Parliamentary forces in Berkshire (Reading) and Oxfordshire (Oxford), while the local civil populations were also severely afflicted by the disease. Whether the epidemic became more generally widespread in England is uncertain, although Creighton (1965, i. 522) records that 29 county registers (of 88 examined) revealed a 'sickly death rate' in that year.

While typhus fever reappeared in 1644, this time in association with military activities around the Devon market town of Tiverton, it was bubonic plague that now began to spread widely in consequence of the war. At the Royalist stronghold of Banbury, Oxfordshire, an epidemic of plague began in March 1644; it continued throughout the period of the Parliamentary siege of the town (July–Oct. 1644) and claimed 161 lives. Likewise, at Newcastle-upon-Tyne, the Royalist surrender of Tynemouth Castle—where plague had been smouldering for much of October 1644—resulted in the dissemination of the disease to surrounding settlements, including Gateshead and Sunderland. Thereafter, war-related outbreaks of plague occurred in towns and cities across England, including Bristol (1645), Leeds (1645), Oxford (1645), Lichfield (1645–6), Newark-on-Trent (1646), Totnes (1646–7) and Chester (1647); see Creighton (1965, i. 557–62).

2.4.4 Wars 1650–1792

Space does not permit a detailed examination of the many European conflicts and their associated epidemics in the 150 years or so between the close of the Thirty Years' War (1648) and the onset of the French Revolutionary and Napoleonic Wars (1792). In this section, therefore, we focus on sample wars to illustrate general epidemiological themes from the period. By way of background, our consideration begins with a brief overview of major war epidemics and associated trends, 1650–1792. We then turn to one of the great war epidemics of the period—the epidemic of bubonic plague that spread in Russia during the Russo-Turkish War (1768–72)—to illustrate how an exotic disease agent can be swept back from a military front into the civil population of a belligerent nation. Finally, for a century-long time-window to 1725, we examine the role of war as a factor in the periodic demographic crises of a single continental locality: the Basse–Meuse region of Belgium and the Netherlands.

OVERVIEW

Table 2.5 provides summary information on major war epidemics in European theatres, 1650–1792. When read in conjunction with the evidence for earlier time periods (Sects. 2.4.1–2.4.3), the most prominent feature of the table is the continuing importance ascribed to typhus fever in the modern epoch—a feature that lasted into the Napoleonic period and beyond (Sects. 2.4.5 and 2.4.6). According to Hirsch (1883, i. 551), the typhus 'took a new start' in Germany after the outbreak of the First Coalition War against Louis XIV (1672–8) and, during the wars of the next 100 years, spread repeatedly in the military and civil populations of central and northern Europe. Among the other diseases listed in Table 2.5, the Second Northern War (1700–21) and more particularly the Campaign of Charles XII of Sweden contributed materially to the diffusion of the last major epidemic of bubonic plague in central Europe (1701–13; see Eckert, 2000). Thereafter, the spread of plague as a pestilence of European conflicts was geographically restricted to the vicinity of the Balkan Peninsula, Hungary, Transylvania, European Russia, and the Ottoman–Turkish principalities of southeastern Europe.

THE SPREAD OF BUBONIC PLAGUE IN THE RUSSO-TURKISH WAR, 1770–1772

The final entry in Table 2.5—the Russo-Turkish War (1768–74)—provided the foundations for one of the great epidemics of bubonic plague in Imperial Russia. From an apparent origin with Russian forces in the Black Sea territories of the Ottoman Empire in early 1770, *Yersinia pestis* was swept back along the lines of communication into Russia where, during the next several years, the disease claimed upwards of 120,000 lives. The course of the epidemic and its particular association with the Russo-Turkish War has been examined by Prinzing (1916) and Alexander (1980) and we draw upon their accounts here.

Diffusion Patterns

The vectors in Figure 2.8 are based on the time-ordered sequence of appearance of bubonic plague in sample settlements of Moldavia, Poland, and Russia and trace the implied route by which the disease spread to, and within, Russia during the year 1770. As described by Alexander (1980), the exact source of the disease in the region is unknown, although an importation into the Ottoman territories of Bulgaria and Moldavia (possibly with Turkish military drafts in the late 1760s) is generally suspected. Indeed, plague may have contributed to the widespread sickness that forced the Turkish Army to abandon Moldavia in September 1769, while the Russian occupation of the same place in the winter of 1769–70 may have brought the latter army into contact with the plague bacterium (Prinzing, 1916; Alexander, 1980).

Some of the first recognized cases of bubonic plague in Russian troops can be traced to the Moldavian town of Jassy—where part of the Russian Army had wintered—in mid-March 1770. In subsequent days and weeks, plague (possibly in association with typhus fever) spread among both the soldiery and the townsfolk such that, by mid-May, half the population of Jassy is said to

Table 2.5. Sample war epidemics in military and civilian populations, European theatres (1650–1792)

War	Disease	Notes	Source
First Coalition War against Louis XIV (1672–8)	Typhus fever	Epidemic in Germany	Hirsch (1883)
Ottoman War (1682–99)	Typhus fever	Epidemic in Hungary and Germany	Hirsch (1883), Prinzing (1916)
Franco-Imperial War (1683–4)	Typhus fever	Epidemic in Germany	Hirsch (1883)
War of the Grand Alliance (1688–97)	Typhus fever	Conveyed by Bavarian troops to southern Germany	Prinzing (1916)
Irish War (1689–91)	Typhus fever and dysentery	Epidemic among soldiers and civilians during the siege of Londonderry (1689)	Kohn (1998)
Second Northern War (1700–21)	Bubonic plague	Epidemic dissemination with the Campaign of Charles XII of Sweden, across Eastern Europe, northwestern Germany, Denmark, and Sweden	Prinzing (1916)
War of the Spanish Succession (1701–13)	Typhus fever	Epidemic in civilian and military populations at Augsburg (1702–5) Epidemic on British troopships off Iberia (1706–7)	Prinzing (1916), Cantlie (1974)
Ottoman War (1716–18)	Typhus fever, dysentery, and bubonic plague	Siege of Belgrade (1717): epidemics of typhus fever and dysentery among Austrian troops, bubonic plague epidemic among Turkish troops	Prinzing (1916)
War of Polish Succession (1733–8)	Typhus fever	Prevalent over Eastern and Central Europe in the period to 1744, having first appeared among Polish troops in 1734	Hirsch (1883), Prinzing (1916)

Table 2.5. (*cont.*)

War	Disease	Notes	Source
Russo–Turkish War (1736–9)	Bubonic plague	Epidemic in Ukraine, Hungary, and Transylvania	Hirsch (1883), Prinzing (1916)
War of Austrian Succession (1739–48)	Typhus fever	Epidemics in southern Germany and Prague, 1742; epidemic on board English transports, 1748	Prinzing (1916), Creighton (1965)
	Dysentery	Epidemic among English forces in Germany, 1743	Creighton (1965)
First Silesian War (1740–2)	Typhus fever	Epidemic in Bohemia	Hirsch (1883)
Russo–Swedish War (1740–3)	Dysentery, typhus fever, and relapsing fever	Epidemic in Sweden, especially in the southwest of the country	Kohn (1998)
Jacobite Rebellion (1745–6)	Typhus fever (?)	Epidemic among English forces returning from the Low Countries, 1745	Creighton (1965)
Seven Years' War (1756–63)	Typhus fever	Epidemic in Germany (1757–61), eastern France (1760–1), and Spain (1764 ff.)	Hirsch (1883), Prinzing (1916)
Russo–Turkish War (1768–74)	Bubonic plague	Epidemic in Moldavia, Wallachia, Transylvania, and European Russia	Alexander (1980)

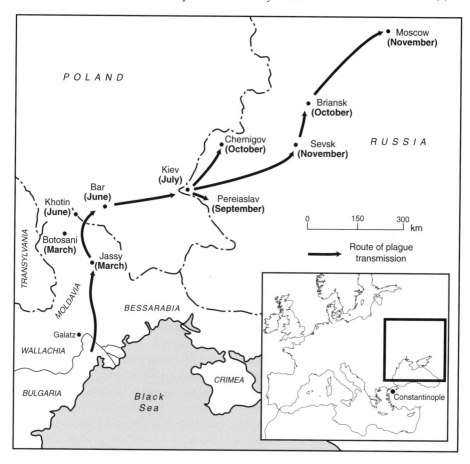

Fig. 2.8. Spread of bubonic plague during the Russo-Turkish War (1768–1774)

Notes: Vectors depict the implied direction of transmission of bubonic plague to Moscow during the Russian campaign of 1770. The month of first appearance of bubonic plague in sample settlements is indicated for reference.

Source: Based on information in Prinzing (1916) and Alexander (1980).

have been either sick or dead. Variously fuelled by interactions associated with the Russian Army supply system, the movements of travellers, refugees, troops, and prisoners, as well as the ordinary civil commerce of the Danubian provinces and their northern neighbours, Figure 2.8 traces a northwards spread of plague from Jassy. The disease is reputed to have reached the civil population of Botosani by late March, the Russian military field hospital at Khotin by mid-June, and, over the border in southeastern Poland, the town of Bar (site of a Russian supply depot) by late June. In addition, to the west of the diffusion route plotted in Figure 2.8, plague also spread with Moldavian and Wallachian fugitives along the Transylvanian border (Prinzing, 1916; Alexander, 1980).

Quarantine

In recognition of the plague threat from Poland, orders to protect the southwestern frontier of Russia were issued in late August 1770. The orders came too late. With cross-border movements buoyed by the spring campaign, Figure 2.8 indicates that bubonic plague had entered the Russian city of Kiev in July. From Kiev, the disease spread eastwards and northwards, carried by soldiers, fugitives, and others along the main overland route to Moscow. Despite efforts to halt the advance of the disease on the latter place (cordons were established in October, and strengthened in November), bubonic plague reached the city of Moscow by the end of 1770 (Alexander, 1980). From here, the disease spread onwards to the whole of central Russia in the months and years that followed.

Plague in Moscow

Course of the epidemic. The epidemic of bubonic plague in Moscow was to prove especially severe. Cases of a suspicious disease that may have been bubonic plague had begun to appear among attendants at the city's General Infantry Hospital as early as mid-November 1770. However, the main epidemic phase in the city awaited the following summer and autumn. To illustrate the course of the epidemic, Figure 2.9 plots the daily count of deaths from all causes (solid line trace) and the corresponding count of deaths in government quarantines (broken line trace) for Moscow, July–December 1771. From relatively low overall levels of mortality in early July (<50 deaths per day), the solid line trace grows steeply in August,[8] to a peak of mortality (>900 deaths per day) at about the time of the social disturbances associated with the Moscow 'Plague Riot' (15–16 Sept.). Thereafter overall mortality began a gradual decline to December. By January 1772, plague had all but disappeared from the city.

Impact. In reviewing the demographic and economic impact of the 1770–2 plague epidemic in Moscow, Alexander (1980: 257) estimates the number of plague deaths at about 52,300 in a population of some 250,000 to 300,000. Demographic recovery from the period of crisis mortality was relatively rapid; in the two decades that spanned the epidemic, 1762–82, the male population of Moscow province grew from less than 400,000 to more than 440,000. Nevertheless, the short-term population loss had severe economic ramifications for the city. The reduced labour pool, the enforced closure of businesses,

---

[8] According to Alexander (1980: 167), the sharp spike of mortality on 2 August (Fig. 2.8, solid line trace) is assumed to be an inflated statistic, possibly associated with batch reporting or an error in transcription.

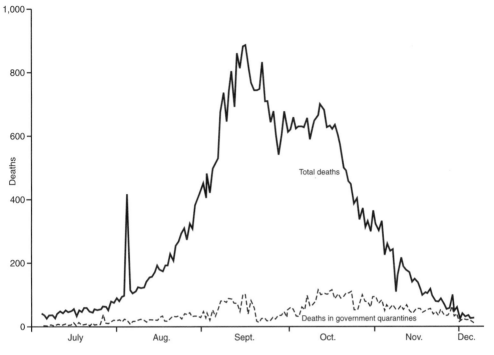

Fig. 2.9. Daily count of deaths in Moscow during the bubonic plague epidemic, July–December 1771

Source: Redrawn from Alexander (1980, graphs 2–4, pp. 161, 185, 224).

the resulting loss of revenue, and, not least, depleted liquid and fixed capital, all contributed to a sharp (if temporary) downturn in the municipality's economic prosperity (see Alexander, 1980: 265–71).

LOCAL DEMOGRAPHIC CRISES IN CONTINENTAL WARS: LONGITUDINAL EVIDENCE

Our consideration of local demographic crises and war in continental Europe draws on Gutmann's (1977) longitudinal study of the Basse–Meuse region of Belgium and the Netherlands, 1628–1725. The location of the study site, positioned between the cities of Maastricht (Netherlands) and Liège (Belgium), is plotted in Figure 2.10. During the period under examination, the immediate vicinity of the Basse–Meuse was subject to repeated wars and war-like events:

(i) the Dutch occupation of Maastricht (1632–8) during the Thirty Years' War (1618–48);

(ii) the French conquest of Maastricht (1673) during the Franco-Dutch War (1672–9);

(iii) the French attack on Liège (1691) during the War of the Grand Alliance (1689–98);

(iv) campaigns in the Spanish Netherlands during the first phase (1701–6) of the War of the Spanish Succession (1701–13).

Although the Thirty Years' War lies strictly outside the time bracket of the present section, the crisis events in the years prior to 1650 provide a benchmark against which to judge subsequent patterns. Accordingly, information for the pre-1650 period has been retained in the following analysis.

Time Series

The graphs in Figure 2.10 plot as bar charts the annual count of civil deaths (Fig. 2.10A) and baptisms (Fig. 2.10B) in sample parishes of the Basse–Meuse, 1628–1725. The line traces superimposed on the bar charts provide an annual index of the corresponding demographic parameter. In each instance, the index has been scaled to 1 (=average annual deaths/baptisms in the set of sample parishes); values above 1 mark years in which deaths/baptisms exceeded the annual average. For reference, the intervals associated with major wars are marked by the vertical pecked lines.

Civil deaths (Figure 2.10A). The line trace in Figure 2.10A plots a steep rise in civil deaths (annual index values >1.0) during the first three conflicts, underscoring the association between war and the periodic civil mortality crises in the Basse–Meuse. According to Gutmann (1977: 113), the principal causes of death during these crises were recorded by the local priests as *contagion*, dysentery, and *peste*, from which we can infer the occurrence of epidemic pulmonary and gastrointestinal diseases, along with plague. The two highest peaks in the deaths index, in 1676 (Franco-Dutch War) and 1694 (War of the Grand Alliance), coincide with 'combination crises': war (and associated disease), aggravated by bad weather and harvest failure (1694). In contrast, the marginally lesser peak for 1634 (Thirty Years' War) was associated with war alone (Gutmann, 1977). Finally, Figure 2.10A indicates that the somewhat less dire War of Spanish Succession had little discernible impact on local mortality.

Fig. 2.10. Demographic impact of war on the civil population of sample parishes of the Basse–Meuse region, Belgium, 1620–1730

Notes: Bar charts plot the annual count of deaths (A) and baptisms (B) in sample parishes, while line traces plot an index of the respective demographic parameters. The indices have been scaled to 1 (=average annual number of deaths/baptisms) for the sample units; index values above 1 (marked by the horizontal line) denote years of above-average deaths/baptisms. Graph A is based on the parishes of Cheratte, Dalhem, Haccourt, and Hermalle-sous-Argenteau (1620–59) and Cheratte, Dalhem, Hermalle-sous-Argenteau, Herstal, and Wandre (1660–1730). Graph B is based on the parishes of Dalhem, Hermalle-sous-Argenteau, Herstal, Heure-le-Romain, Vivegnis, and Wandre. The location of the study area is indicated on the inset map.

Source: data from Gutmann (1977, tables 2 and 3, pp. 109–10 and table 4, p. 116).

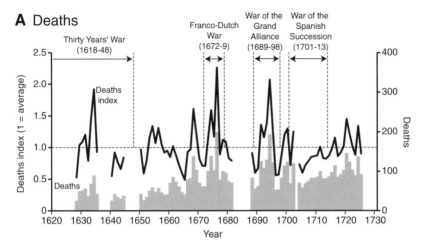

A Deaths

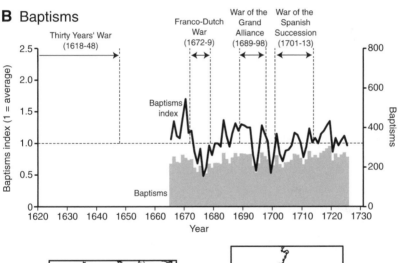

B Baptisms

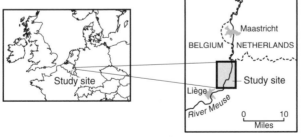

Baptisms (Figure 2.10B). Notwithstanding the highly truncated nature of the data series, it is apparent from the line trace in Figure 2.10B that wars of the seventeenth and early eighteenth centuries were associated with a marked reduction in baptisms (index values <1.0) and, by inference, the level of child-bearing in the Basse–Meuse. Moreover, comparison with Figure 2.10A reveals that two of the three years with the lowest numbers of baptisms (the war years of 1676 and 1694) coincided with the years of peak civil mortality. Given the observed sensitivity of baptisms to food supply in the region at this time, Gutmann (1977: 118–19) contends that war—through a breakdown in food supply chains—served as an indirect limiting factor on births.

2.4.5 French Revolutionary and Napoleonic Wars

Beginning with the French National Assembly's declaration of war on Emperor Francis II of Austria on 20 April 1792, and extending until the final defeat of Napoleon Bonaparte at Waterloo on 18 June 1815, continental Europe was overtaken by more than two decades of near-continuous warfare. At one time or another, all major European powers were involved in the fighting, with the scene of hostilities shifting back and forth across the continental mainland and beyond. Conventionally, the constituent wars—of which Wright (1965) lists 13 in total—are divided into the Revolutionary (1792–1802) and Napoleonic (1803–15) periods, and we adopt this basic division in the present section.

While the Revolutionary and Napoleonic Wars were associated with the spread of a range of diseases, typhus fever again held the epidemiological sway in both military and civil populations (Hirsch, 1883, i. 554).

FRENCH REVOLUTIONARY WARS (1792–1802)

War of the First Coalition (1792–7)

Severe epidemics of infectious disease showed themselves from the very outset of hostilities. As early as August 1792, the Prussian advance on northeastern France was marred by the appearance of dysentery and typhus fever, with onwards spread of the latter disease to the local inhabitants of Ardennes, Meurthe, Meuse, and Moselle and, subsequently, the pursuing French Army (Prinzing, 1916; Kohn, 1998). During the next two years, 1793–4, French prisoners of war (POWs) sparked epidemics of typhus fever in the civil settlement system of central and southern Germany (cf. Sect. 8.3), extending from the Rhine to the Black Forest, Bavaria and eastwards, and along the upper reaches of the Danube (Prinzing, 1916: 93–5). Elsewhere, in northern Italy, the French siege of Mantua (1796–7) was accompanied by virulent outbreaks of malaria and later typhus fever and dysentery; by the time Mantua had capitulated on 3 February 1797, the city's dead probably numbered 20,000 (Prinzing, 1916: 304–6).

Bubonic Plague and Napoleon's Egyptian Expedition (1798–1801)

Napoleon's designs on Egypt, the Levant, and, ultimately, British India were severely hampered by repeated outbreaks of bubonic plague and endemic ophthalmia (trachoma), in the French expeditionary forces (Major, 1940; Kohn, 1998). Plague first appeared in epidemic form among French units in the Egyptian settlements of Aboukir, Alexandria, Damietta, and Rosetta towards the end of 1798 (Kohn, 1998) and continued to beset the forces in Egypt during the following year. The French troops sent on to Syria fared even worse: plague decimated the occupying French troops in Jaffa (Tel Aviv) soon after the conquest of the city in March 1799 (Pl. 2.3). Thereafter, plague continued to strike the Gallic line with a major outbreak of the disease, eventually forcing the French capitulation of Cairo in 1801 (Major 1940; Kohn 1998). Although the total French loss to bubonic plague is not known, Bodart (1916: 110) estimates that some 17,000 of the original 42,000-strong French force were killed, drowned, died of disease, or otherwise lost during the expedition to Egypt.

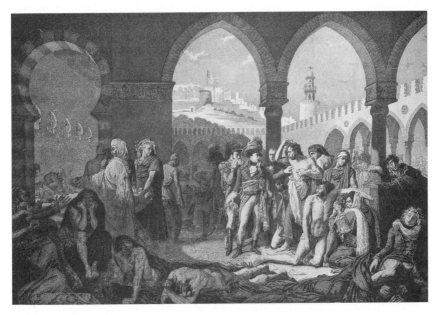

Pl. 2.3. *Les Pestiférés de Jaffa*

Notes: Soon after Napoleon Bonaparte's conquest of Jaffa (Tel Aviv) in March 1799, the occupying French Army fell victim to an epidemic of bubonic plague. In an effort to allay the fears of the soldiers, Bonaparte engaged personally in the care of plague patients; the celebrated painting *Les Pestiférés de Jaffa* portrays Bonaparte touching a plague victim.
Source: Original painting (canvas, 523 × 715 cm) by Antoine-Jean Gros (1771–1835) (Louvre, Photo © RMN).

If the French were to suffer at the hands of plague in Egypt and surrounding lands, so too did the defending forces of Turkey and Britain. To assist the Mameluke, Turkish, and Arab opposition, a British expeditionary force had landed in Egypt in early March 1801. With Alexandria blockaded and preparations for an advance on Cairo under way, plague began to attack the British troops on the Egyptian coast. Between April and June 1801, 380 plague cases and 173 deaths were recorded in the British home contingent at Aboukir and Rosetta. Alexandria fell on 26 August and, soon thereafter, the British troops began to re-embark. Plague, however, appeared in the hospital of the Connaught Rangers at Rosetta on 14 September. Isolation was enforced, but cases continued throughout October (Kempthorne, 1930).

THE NAPOLEONIC WARS AND RELATED EXPEDITIONS (1803–1815)

Before the Peninsular War

Typhus fever spread widely with the War of the Third Coalition (1805) and the Franco-Prussian War (1806–7). In 1805, hostilities between France and Austria gave rise to the dissemination of the disease across Moravia, Bohemia, Upper and Lower Austria, Galicia and Hungary, and, via the transportation of POWs, southern Germany and France. Prisoners again brought typhus fever to parts of southern Germany (Baden) and France (Aube and Yonne) in 1806–7, while the same disease—possibly mixed with typhoid fever—broke out in the Prussian cities of Danzig and Königsberg, among other locations, during the latter half of the Franco-Prussian War (Prinzing, 1916).

The Peninsular War (1808–1814)

Howard (1991) provides epidemiological details of the British Army's disastrous retreat to Corunna during Sir John Moore's Campaign of 1808–9. Moore's advance into northern Spain had begun towards the end of October 1808 but, with the allied Spanish forces repeatedly routed by the French and with the 25,000-strong British force under pressure from the advancing French Army, Moore ordered a British retreat to Corunna on 25 December. In the mid-winter, in harsh terrain and with mounting disarray in the ranks, the 300-mile trek to Corunna was to result in the loss of several thousand British troops. Approximately 3,000 men died of exposure, typhus fever, dysentery, and other causes on the march between Astorga and Villafranca. By the time of the Battle of Corunna, on 16 January 1809, a further 4,035 troops were listed as sick. Some impression of the nature of the illnesses can be gained from Tables 2.6 and 2.7. Here, Table 2.6 gives the distribution of the sick aboard one transport (Transport no. 309, *Alfred*) at Corunna on 18 January 1809 at about the time of embarkation for England, while Table 2.7 summarizes the sick return from receiving hospitals at Portsmouth and vicinity, 24 January–24 July 1809. The tables highlight the prominence of dysentery and fever (predominantly, typhus) as causes of morbidity and mortality among the troops

(Howard, 1991); see also Creighton (1965, ii. 166). All told, British losses during the Corunna Campaign amounted to 5,998, of which 2,189 were taken prisoner by the French and 3,809 perished in battle, on the roadside, or in hospital (Howard, 1991).

The French Army, too, suffered greatly from disease during the course of the Peninsular War. Prinzing (1916: 101) places Napoleon's losses at 400,000 dead, with disease accounting for 75 per cent of the mortality. At the same time, the constant movement of Spanish prisoners gave rise to the wider dissemination of typhus in the civil settlement system of France. The town of Dax, near the French border with Spain, was one of the first settlements to experience the ravages of the disease. Thereafter, and despite efforts to segregrate Spanish

Table 2.6. Distribution of sick on board Transport no. 309 (*Alfred*) at Corunna, 18 January 1809

Condition	No. of men
Dysentery	68
Fever	56
Wounded	36
Convalescent	77
'Trifling' complaints	20
Total	257

Source: Howard (1991, table 1, p. 300).

Table 2.7. Return of the sick of the army from Spain and Portugal received into hospitals in Portsmouth and vicinity from 24 January to 24 July 1809

Disease	Admitted	Discharged	Died
Febris (Continuous)	824	717	107
Febris (Intermitt.)	11	11	
Ophthalmia	5	5	
Pneumonia	81	61	20
Rheumatismus	13	13	
Catarrhus	11	11	
Dysenteria	1,053	801	252
Hydrops	4	4	
Icterus	4	4	
Variola	1	1	
Lues venerea	6	6	
Puniti	1	1	
Vulnera and ulcers	413	373	26
Total	2,427	2,008	405

Source: Howard (1991, table 2, p. 301).

POWs and the French civil populaton, prisoners carried typhus fever to Limoges, Guéret, Châteauroux, Issoudun, Moulin, Nevers, and other interior locations (Prinzing, 1916: 103).

Another Emergent Disease: Walcheren Fever

According to Howard (1991: 301), the Walcheren Expedition (1809–10) constituted 'one of the greatest medical disasters ever to befall the [British] army'. The expedition and its medical consequences are reviewed by McGuffie (1947), Feibel (1968), and Howard (1999). In July 1809, a British expeditionary force of 40,000—one of the largest expeditionary forces yet assembled by Britain— set sail from Kent for the island of Walcheren in the Scheldt Estuary, Holland. The aim of the mission: to strike a blow at French naval activity in Antwerp, to cripple enemy resources at the mouth of the Scheldt, and to render the river unnavigable for ships of war (McGuffie, 1947). But before these aims could be achieved, the expeditionary force was overtaken by a virulent and lethal epidemic.

The first cases of so-called 'Walcheren' or 'Flushing' fever appeared in the British expeditionary force during August 1809. By 3 September, some 8,000 troops were in hospital, with the number rising to 9,000 in late October. Houses, churches, and warehouses were converted into makeshift lazarets while, back in England, hospitals were overwhelmed by the sudden influx of returning patients. Such was the extent of the epidemic that, by the end of the expedition in February 1810, 40 per cent of the force had contracted the disease, 3,960 officers and men had died, while around 11,000 were to be registered among the longer-term sick (McGuffie, 1947; Howard, 1999).

The exact nature of Walcheren fever is not known. Clinically, the disease followed a relapsing course and this has been interpreted by some as evidence of malaria. Howard (1999), however, contends that malaria alone would not account for the severe and rapidly fatal nature of the disease. Walcheren fever, he suggests, was a combination of malaria, along with typhus fever, typhoid fever, and dysentery, manifesting in a physically compromised military population.

Napoleon's Russian Expedition (1812–1813)

The origins and course of Napoleon's disastrous Russian Expedition, and the particular role of disease as a cause and consequence of the campaign's collapse, have been outlined elsewhere (see e.g. Prinzing, 1916; Major, 1940; Tarlé, 1942; Austin, 1993). Spurred by Russia's renunciation of the economic blockade of Britain under the Continental System, but further aggravated by French interests in Poland, Sweden, and the Balkan Peninsula, Napoleon's 450,000-strong *Grande Armée* began to move on Russia in late June 1812. The subsequent disintegration of the army, from its point of assembly on the River Nieman (modern-day Latvia), along the line of the *c*.1,000 km march to Moscow, and back again, is portrayed in Charles Minard's classic map of 1861 (see Pl. 2.4). As the map shows, by the time Napoleon entered Moscow in mid-September, the army had been whittled down to about 100,000 men. Only 10,000 returned across the Nieman in the winter of 1812–13. Exposure, fatigue, starvation, battle, and desertion all contributed to the dramatic loss. At the forefront of the disaster, however, were two of the great camp diseases: dysentery and typhus fever.

Disease had appeared in the *Grande Armée* soon after the initial crossing of the Nieman. By the beginning of August, Prinzing (1916) notes that some 80,000 men were suffering from dysentery while, at about the same time, typhus fever also made an appearance—albeit at a relatively low level—in the ranks. After the battle of Smolensk (14–18 Aug.), typhus fever and other diseases (including diarrhoea, gastric fever, and dysentery) became more widespread in the army. Typhus, at least, accompanied the troops into Moscow where, during the period of Russian occupation (14 Sept.–19 Oct.), it manifested as the most common ailment among the men.

The epidemiological dimensions of Napoleon's wintertime retreat from Moscow are reviewed by Prinzing (1916: 116–19). Here, we note that the

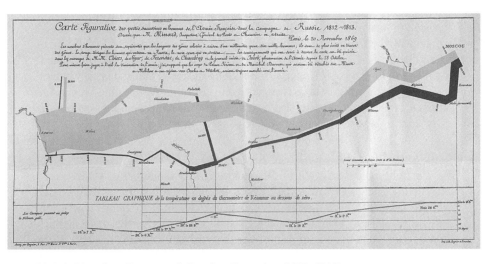

Pl. 2.4. Napoleon Bonaparte's Russian Campaign (1812–1813)

Notes: Charles Joseph Minard's (1781–1870) graphical portrayal of the losses incurred by the French Army during the Russian Campaign of 1812–13. Starting from the left of the map, the upper band depicts the reducing size of the French Army as it marched from the Polish border (422,000 men) to Moscow (100,000 men); the lower, dark, band depicts the losses incurred during the retreat to the Polish border (10,000 men). The map was drawn in 1861.
Source: Collection Ecole Nationale des Ponts et Chaussées, ref. ENPC Fol 10975 p. 28.

withdrawal was associated with the high-level spread of typhus fever in the retreating army, the pursuing Russian forces, and in the civil populations of surrounding lands. Typhus broke out in the city of Vilna during December 1812 following the abandonment of some 30,000 sick soldiers from Napoleon's army. By this time, the disease had become more generally widespread in the region of the Baltic Sea, attacking both St Petersburg and the hospitals and garrison at Riga. Once across the Niemen, the remnants of the *Grande Armée* scattered, with the consequent dispersal of typhus fever across much of Germany. Settlements of Prussia (including Gumbinnen, Insterburg, Königsberg, Konitz, and Tilsit) and the free city of Danzig, whose French and allied defenders had come under Russian siege in January 1813, were among the first to suffer. From thereon, the disease appeared at increasingly distant locations in Brandenburg and Saxony, Silesia, Bohemia, Bavaria, Württemberg, Switzerland, and elsewhere (Prinzing, 1916).

War of Liberation (1813–1814)

The epidemic transmission of typhus fever in Central Europe was rekindled by the war of 1813–1814. Fresh outbreaks of the disease first appeared with Napoleon's advance into Saxony in the summer of 1813. Thereafter, the foci of epidemic activity tracked the movements of troops, prisoners, and fugitives in southern, western, and northern Germany and, as the French retreat progressed, northeastern France and the *départements* to the south and east of Paris in the winter of 1813–14 (Prinzing, 1916). While equivalent figures for France are unavailable, Prinzing (1916: 163) estimates that approximately 10 per cent of the German population of *c*.20 million was infected with typhus fever during 1813–14 resulting in some 200,000 to 300,000 deaths. In accounting for such high levels of infection, Prinzing observes that the largely urban-based system of military lazarets operated in Germany by both the French and Russian armies almost certainly contributed to the widespread dissemination of typhus in the civil settlement system of the country.

NAPOLEONIC WARS: OVERALL MORTALITY ESTIMATES

For the fighting forces, Bodart (1916) places the total number of deaths in the Napoleonic armies at 1 million, of which 400,000 were lost to battle and battle wounds and 600,000 to disease, along with exhaustion, accidents, starvation, and other causes. Assuming a similar combined loss in the other armies, Bodart concludes, 'it will not be far from the truth to assert that the wars of the First French Empire cost Europe about 2,000,000 men killed, besides an equal number wounded of whom perhaps fifteen or twenty per cent were disabled for life' (Bodart, 1916: 133). Equivalent estimates for civil populations are unavailable but, on the basis of Prinzing's (1916: 163) appraisal of typhus in Germany during 1813–14 alone, losses due to disease may be assumed to run into many hundreds of thousands.

2.4.6 After the Napoleonic Wars

The conflicts that followed in the wake of the Napoelonic Wars were associated with the epidemic transmission of many of the long-established war pestilences. Typhus fever in the Spanish Civil War of 1821–3 (Hirsch, 1883), malaria in the Greek Revolt of 1821–30 (Kohn, 1998), and bubonic plague in the Russo-Turkish War of 1828–9 (Hirsch, 1883; Prinzing, 1916) all attest to the continuing importance of these diseases in the years to 1850. At the same time, however, a new and rapidly lethal disease emerged on the European war scene: Asiatic cholera. From an apparent hearth in South Asia, the first pandemic outpouring of cholera (1817–23) had stopped short of the European continent (Cliff and Haggett, 1988; Patterson, 1994). However, subsequent pandemics of the disease in 1826–36 and 1840–55 reached into Europe and spread with the wars of those times (Hirsch, 1883).

PANDEMIC CHOLERA IN EUROPEAN WARS:
THE POLISH INSURRECTION

The outbreak of the Polish Insurrection (1830–1) was temporally coincident with the first significant penentration of cholera into the European continent. Cholera had swept westwards across Central Asia in the latter years of the 1820s reaching the heart of European Russia by September 1830 (Patterson, 1994). Two months later, and with the disease now poised along the Russian frontier with Poland (McGrew, 1965), Warsaw revolted against her Russian overlords. Hirsch (1883, i. 398) contends that the subsequent Russian military offensive 'contributed materially' to the diffusion of cholera in Poland. McGrew (1965: 100), on the other hand, cites evidence to suggest that cholera had begun to spread in Poland 'well before the Russian campaign to suppress the revolution took form'. Whatever the exact role of Russian military operations in the primary diffusion of the disease, the Russian Army was the first to suffer heavy casualties. At the height of the epidemic, in 1831, the monthly count of cholera cases in Russian military hospitals—both in Poland and Russia—grew from less than 700 (March) to over 8,700 (April), with 2,800 cholera deaths in the latter month alone. The Polish Army, too, suffered greatly from the disease while, from May, cholera also began to spread widely in the civil population of Poland; by the following September, the province of Warsaw had recorded no less than 22,700 cases of cholera with 13,100 fatalities (McGrew, 1965).

From Poland, cholera spread onwards for central Europe during 1831–2. Nothwithstanding the intensification of Prussian frontier regulations, cholera crossed the border from Poland in the mid-summer of 1831 with the subsequent appearance of the disease in many German provinces in the weeks and months that followed (see Hirsch, 1883, i. 398–9 for further details).

2.5 The Old World, II: European Engagements in Africa and Asia (AD 1700–1850)

2.5.1 European Wars with Persia

Kohn (1998) reviews evidence for the epidemic occurrence of disease associated with the European–Persian conflicts of the eighteenth and nineteenth centuries. During the first year of the Russo-Persian War (1722–3), an outbreak of ergotism[9] resulted in the death of many thousands of Russian troops in the Volga region of southern Russia, thereby forcing the abandonment of the planned campaign in Persia. Five years later, in 1727, the Volga region of Russia was again struck by disease: this time, bubonic plague, whose appearance was a direct result of Russian military incursions into Persia. The earliest recorded cases of the disease occurred in July, August, and September 1727, among Russian soldiers newly returned from Persia to the Volga port city of Astrakhan. Sporadic cases of plague occurred throughout the winter of 1727–8, to be followed by an explosive epidemic among the civil population of Astrakhan in the spring and early summer of 1728. Finally, a century on, Kohn (1998) notes that the operations of the Turko-Persian War (1821–3) contributed to the spread of the first great cholera pandemic (1817–23) across Persia with onwards transmission to the Caucasus in the north and Syria in the east.

2.5.2 British Forces in Africa and Asia, 1800–1850

Evidence for the spread of infectious disease among British forces engaged in Africa and Asia, 1800–50, is reviewed by Sir Neil Cantlie (1974, i. 454–93). We draw on his account here.

AFRICA

On the Gold Coast of West Africa (present-day Ghana), the bush warfare that characterized the First Ashanti War (1824–6) was associated with major outbreaks of fever and dysentery among the British troops, while smallpox spread widely among the native African population. In 1825, an experiment was undertaken by the British Army; 108 fresh young recruits from Chatham, apparently free of the excesses of the older soldiers, were stationed on the Isles of Los, a location of reputedly 'salubrious aspect' and free from the 'miasmal exhalations' of the mainland. Between June 1825 and December 1826, however, 48 (44.4%) of the recruits had died, 21 (19.4%) were invalided, and 29 (26.9%) were declared unfit as a consequence of fever. All told, there were 1,298

---

[9] A severe, potentially lethal, disease of the central nervous system caused by the ingestion of grains infected with the fungus *Claviceps purpurea*.

deaths among the 1,658 Europeans sent out to the Royal African Corps in the period 1822–30. From 1830, the War Office ceased the practice of sending European soldiers to West Africa and, thereafter, the West Coast of Africa was garrisoned by the West India Regiment (Cantlie, 1974, i. 459–62).

ASIA AND THE FAR EAST

The dire epidemiological experiences of British forces in the Far East during the first half of the nineteenth century are salutary. For example, during the First Anglo-Burmese War (1824–6), European regiments of the British Army were so decimated by disease that, within 11 months of landing in Rangoon, nearly 50 per cent of the European contingent had died. The chief causes of death were amoebic dysentery and related complications (hepatitis and liver abcesses) with malaria, scurvy, and, later, cholera adding to the health problems of the expedition. All told, annual hospital admissions for the British Army during the war amounted to 3,540 per 1,000. The original British regiments counted 1,215 disease-related deaths in a total strength of 2,716, with only 96 deaths attributable to battle and battle wounds (Cantlie, 1974, i. 454–9).

Cholera spread in epidemic form among the British forces stationed at Baug, southern Afghanistan, during the First Afghan War (1838–42) while, at about the same time, the First Opium War (1839–42) was to underscore the unhealthful nature of Hong Kong and the entire Chinese coast. An initial Indian–British expedition to the mouth of the Yangtse-Kiang River was so marred by malaria, dysentery, and diarrhoea that, in a period of six months, the combined force of 2,500 men had registered 3,239 hospital admissions and 445 deaths. The remnants of the force were subsequently transferred to Canton where, with reinforcements, the city was taken in May 1841. At nearby Hong Kong, which formed the new operational base of the army, malaria and dysentery again spread widely; within a short period, some two-thirds of the force had been admitted to hospital. Later, in 1842, 2,700 men were dispatched from Hong Kong to capture the cities of Amoy, Chin-hai, and Ningpo. Malaria proved the major problem in these operations; at Amoy, some 50 per cent of the troops perished on account of the lack of quinine. Between July and October 1842, HMS *Minden*, positioned off the mouth of the Yangtse-Kiang, received 107 cases of Asiatic cholera and 1,313 cases of dysentery (Cantlie, 1974, i. 477–81).

2.6 War Epidemics in the New World (AD 1500–1850)

2.6.1 The Conquest of the Americas

'The most sensational military conquests in all history', observed Alfred Crosby (1967: 321), 'are probably those of the Spanish conquistadores over the

Aztec and Incan empires.' With armies of just a few hundred men, but aided
by wave upon wave of Old World infections for which the native American
Indians lacked acquired immunity, Hernán Cortés and Francisco Pizarro succeeded in the overthrow of entire civilizations. Some of the epidemics spread
with the conquistadores, some ahead of them but, with the drastic population
loss that ensued, all facilitated the Spanish conquest (see e.g. Cook, 1981, 1998;
A. W. Crosby, 1986; Ramenofsky, 1987; Stannard, 1992). As such, the Spanish
conquest of the Americas illustrates—in dramatic fashion—one recurring
feature of the war–disease association: the role of conflict in the introduction,
and high-level spread, of infectious diseases in non-immune (virgin soil)
populations.

For various geographical divisions, Table 2.8 summarizes the principal disease events during the century or so after European contact in 1492. As the
upper section of the table shows, the early years (1492–1517) were accompanied by the spread of influenza, fevers, and ill-defined maladies among the
native inhabitants of the Caribbean island of Hispaniola and later the Isthmus
of Panama (see Fig. 2.11 for locations). For Hispaniola, these outbreaks were
sufficient to reduce the native population to just a few thousand by 1520 (Cook,
1998). From 1518, however, the great 'eruptive fevers' of the Old World
(measles, plague, smallpox, and typhus, among others) began to sweep across
the Caribbean Basin, Central and Southern America, claiming tens of millions
of lives and stripping away the native civilizations. As the lower section of Table
2.8 shows, major pandemics of smallpox (1518–28) and measles (1531–4) were
the first to appear, and these coincided with the initial conquests of Cortés in
Mexico and Pizarro in Peru.

The First Pandemic: Smallpox (1518–1528)

Figure 2.11A charts the routes by which the smallpox pandemic of 1518–28
spread in the Americas. The earliest reference to the disease in European
sources can be traced to Hispaniola on 10 January 1519. On that date, the local
friars reported that an epidemic of the disease, which probably began in the
previous month, had carried away almost one-third of the native population.
The source of the infection on Hispaniola is entirely unknown, although an
importation from Spain is generally suspected. The disease appeared in nearby
Puerto Rico by 21 January and, soon thereafter, all islands of the Greater
Antilles (Crosby, 1967; Cook, 1998).

As regards the circumstances surrounding the spread of smallpox to
Mexico, the biographer of Cortés, Francisco López de Gómara, tells how the
disease appeared at Cempoala, in the vicinity of Veracruz, in early March 1520.
The disease was carried there by the expedition of Pánfilo de Navárez which
had been dispatched by the governor of Cuba to bring Hernán Cortés to justice
(Cook, 1998). According to López de Gómara: 'among the men of Narváez
there was a Negro sick with smallpox, and he infected the household in
Cempoala where he was quartered; and it spread from one Indian to another,

Table 2.8. Early disease occurrences (1493–1517) and major pandemic events (1518–1600) in the Americas to 1600

Date	Caribbean and Mesoamerica	Date	Andean America
Early disease occurrences, 1492–1517			
1493–8	Influenza, sickness (Hispaniola)		
1498	'Epidemic' syphilis? (Hispaniola)		
1500	Sickness, fevers (Hispaniola)		
1502	Illnesses general, fevers (Hispaniola)		
1507	Illnesses general		
1514–17	Influenza (Isthmus of Panama)		
Major pandemic events, 1518–1600			
1518–21	Smallpox	1524–8	Smallpox
1531–4	Measles	1531–3	Measles
1545	Pneumonic plague, typhus	1546	Pneumonic plague, typhus
1550	Mumps		
1559–63	Measles, mumps, influenza, diphtheria	1557–62	Measles, influenza, smallpox
1576–80	Typhus, smallpox, measles, mumps	1585–91	Typhus, smallpox, measles
1595	Measles	1597	Measles

Source: Based on Cook (1998, table 1.2, p. 58 and table 3.2, p. 132).

and they, being so numerous and eating and sleeping together, quickly infected the whole country' (Francisco López de Gómara, cited in Cook 1998: 65). By June 1520, smallpox had reached the Aztec capital, Tenochtitlán, where it spread widely in the days and weeks that followed Cortés's forced retreat from the city. By mid-August, however, and with up to half the inhabitants of Tenochtitlán having died of smallpox, Cortés was able to recapture the city and lay claim to the lands of the former empire (Crosby, 1967; Cook, 1998).

As regards Andean America, Figure 2.11A shows that smallpox spread well ahead of Pizarro's conquest of the Inca in early 1530s. The disease arrived among the Inca in the mid-1520s, lasted until at least 1527, and claimed the life of the Incan ruler, Huayna Capac, along with his wife, brother, sister, uncle, and his legitmate son and heir, Ninan Cuyoche (Dobyns, 1963). Facilitated by a vastly reduced population, a ruptured power structure, and an ongoing dynastic struggle that served to split the remnants of the Incan empire, Pizarro took the Incan capital, Cuzco, in the latter months of 1533 (Crosby, 1967).

The Second Pandemic: Measles (1531–1534)

It is highly probable that measles reached the tropical New World soon after the arrival of the first European settlers. Outbreaks may have occurred during the early years of the sixteenth century, although the disease is difficult to identify accurately in the records of the eruptive diseases described by the

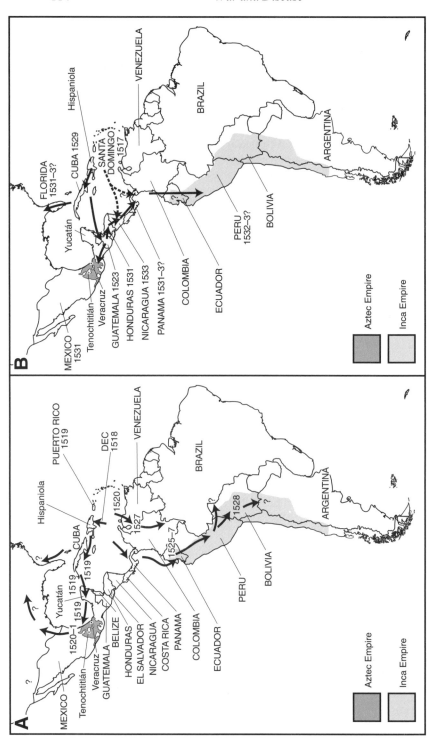

Fig. 2.11. Epidemic transmission and the Spanish conquest of the Americas

Notes: Vectors trace the diffusion of the smallpox epidemic of 1518–28 (map A) and the measles epidemic of 1531–4 (map B). The geographical extent of the Aztec and Inca civilizations at about the time of European contact is indicated for reference.

Source: Redrawn from Cook (1998, map 2.1, pp. 74–5) and Cliff *et al.* (1993, fig. 3.6, p. 62).

chroniclers of the period. McNeill (1976: 208) cites the views of Aristides A. Moll that there were probably epidemics of measles as early as 1517 in Hispaniola. Measles may have struck Guatemala in 1519–23, and the disease is recorded in Cuba in 1529 (Marks and Beatty, 1976). These outbreaks, however, were to pale against the measles pandemic of 1531–4.

Figure 2.11B traces the routes by which measles spread in the Americas during the pandemic of 1531–4. Measles was introduced into the Caribbean in 1531, probably having been imported from the Spanish mainland. From this entry point, the disease spread onwards to Mexico, Nicaragua, and Panama in the following months and years. Whether the disease extended south of Panama is open to conjecture (Dobyns, 1963: 499).

Later Sixteenth-Century Epidemics

Of the subsequent epidemics listed in the lower section of Table 2.8, Dobyns (1963) speculates that the appearance and spread of typhus fever in Andean America during the latter half of the 1580s may well have been directly associated with war-like events. During the course of Sir Francis Drake's raids on Spanish possessions in 1585–6, his 2,300-strong force fell victim to a typhus fever-like disease. The illness first appeared on the sea voyage between Cape Verde and Hispaniola and had probably been contracted at the former place. Notwithstanding the heavy death toll on board ship, Drake took Santo Domingo (Hispaniola) by force, before capturing Cartagena (Colombia) in mid-January 1586. While the illness so weakened Drake's expedition that he was compelled to return to England, the imputed introduction of typhus fever to Cartagena would accord with the known history of a virulent disease that spread southwards from the city subsequently to infect Quito, Lima, Cuzco, and Chile (Dobyns, 1963).

Demographic Impact of Disease

Two factors enhanced the impact of the sixteenth-century visitations of disease on the Amerindian population. First, relatively trifling endemic infections of the Old World became death-dealing epidemics among New World populations that were wholly lacking in acquired resistance. Secondly, the Spaniards were nearly immune to the terrible diseases that raged so mercilessly among the Indians. They had almost always been exposed in childhood and so developed immunity to subsequent attacks.

Estimates of Amerindian population loss are, at best, sketchy. For central Mexico, Crosby (1967) suggests that the Aztec population fell from 25 million on the eve of conquest to 16.8 million a decade later. It seems reasonable to infer that much of this decrease was directly or indirectly associated with the smallpox pandemic of 1518–28. Elsewhere in Mesoamerica, Table 2.9 provides high and low estimates of the Maya population of Yucatán, Guatemala, for the period 1520–1600 (see Fig. 2.11 for location). While the population estimates for 1520 vary widely, the overall message of the table is clear: by the end of the observation period, the Maya population had collapsed to just 10 to 20 per cent of its initial level (Lovell, 1992).

2.6.2 Later Wars in the Americas

CARIBBEAN AND CIRCUM-CARIBBEAN THEATRES

The Anglo-Spanish War (1655–1659)

As Creighton (1965, i. 633–43) notes, the English assault on the Spanish Antilles in 1655 was beset by infectious disease. The opening gambit—the English advance on Santo Domingo (Hispaniola) in April 1655—was accompanied by a severe outbreak of dysentery such that, when the English force re-embarked on 3 May, some 1,700 men had been lost to battle and disease. The subsequent assault on Jamaica was to fare even worse. A 7,000-strong English force had landed on the island on 10 May but, with rations in short supply and with dysentery still present in the ranks, the condition of the troops rapidly declined. By 13 June, Venables placed the English sick at 'about 2000', adding that 'Our men die daily' (Venables, 13 June 1665, cited in Creighton, 1965, i. 638). When reinforcements reached Jamaica on 1 October, the commander of the fresh contingent, Robert Sedgwick, found the original force to be in a piteous state. The newcomers, too, soon began to sicken and it is estimated that some 50 soldiers died each week in the period 5 November 1665 to 24 January 1656 (Creighton, 1965, i. 640).

As for the diseases that contributed to the high mortality among the English forces in Jamaica, Charles Creighton has speculated on the possible role of yellow fever in addition to dysentery in the latter months of 1655 (Creighton, 1965, i. 643).

Yellow Fever in Later Wars

While the contribution of yellow fever to morbidity and mortality in the Anglo-Spanish War (1655–9) is unclear, the latter decades of the seventeenth century were to witness the emergence of the disease as a major epidemiologic-

Table 2.9. Guatemala, Central America: estimates of Maya depopulation, 1520–1600

Year (approximate)	Low estimate	High estimate
1520	300,000	2,000,000
1550	121,000	428,000
1575	75,000	148,000
1600	64,000	195,000

Source: Lovell (1992, table 2.2, p. 58).

al threat to European fighting forces in the region. The nature of yellow fever is described in Appendix 1A but, for raw recruits from temperate European latitudes, the disease—a tropical arthropod-borne viral disease for which they lacked any prior exposure or immunity—was to prove devastating. By way of illustration, Table 2.10 gives the estimated levels of mortality associated with sample epidemics of yellow fever among European forces on active service in the Caribbean Basin, 1680–1810. With estimated mortality ranging up to 80 per cent of strength, the table highlights a critical facet of the war–disease relationship: the potentially dire consequences of deploying troops in epidemiological environments to which they are not acclimatized (see Curtin, 1989; Earle, 1996).

NORTH AMERICAN WARS

Smallpox in the French and Indian War (1756–1763): Biological Warfare

The contending British and French forces, along with their allies among the native Indian tribes, were beset by severe epidemics of smallpox during the French and Indian War of 1756–63. Initially manifesting as a southerly extension of the Quebec smallpox epidemic of 1755–7, the disease had appeared in the British-held Forts William Henry and Edward, upstate New York, soon after the beginning of the conflict. Fort William Henry was taken by an 8,000-strong combined French and Indian force in mid-summer 1757, with the onwards dissemination of smallpox both to the native Indian contingent and the French captors of the British forces (Hopkins, 1983; Kohn, 1998).

Subsequent events have earned the French and Indian War some notoriety as a possible early example of biological warfare (see Sect. 13.4). Details are given by Christopher *et al.* (1997). During the course of the conflict, Sir Jeffrey Amherst, Commander of the British forces, is reputed to have promoted the tactical use of smallpox against Indians hostile to the British forces. The plan is said to have been executed when, on 24 June 1763, Captain Ecuyer, a subordinate of Amherst, supplied native Indians with blankets and a handkerchief from the smallpox hospital at the British-held Fort Pitt. Perhaps coincidental with this event, an epidemic of smallpox subsequently spread among the native Indians of the Ohio River valley; see Christopher *et al.* (1997).

Smallpox in the War of American Independence (1775–1783): Vaccination

The Canadian Campaign (1775–1776). As described by Cash (1976), the American forces under General Richard Montgomery and Colonel Benedict Arnold were to suffer a major epidemic of smallpox during the expedition to Canada in 1775–6. While the forces had been severely weakened by starvation and disease (including dysentery, diarrhoea, and rheumatism) on the advance to Canada, smallpox did not appear in the army until the units had come together outside Quebec City in late 1775. The newly established military hospital in the convent at St Roche, a suburb of Quebec, provided the first evidence

Table 2.10. Estimated mortality associated with epidemic outbreaks of yellow fever in sample forces and wars, Caribbean Basin, 1680–1810

War	Force	Estimated strength[1]	Epidemic		Estimated yellow fever deaths[2]
			Year	Location	
War of the Grand Alliance (1688–97)	British	?	1691	Barbados	3,100 (?)
War of Jenkin's Ear (1739–41)	British	12,000	1741	Cartagena (Colombia)	8,400 (70)
Seven Years' War (1756–63)	British	15,000	1762	Habana (Cuba)	8,000 (53)
Haitian Revolt (1802–3)	French	c.50,000	1802–3	Haiti	40,000 (80)

Notes: [1] At time and location of epidemic. [2] Estimated mortality, expressed as a percentage proportion of strength, in parentheses.
Source: Data from Cantlie (1974) and Kohn (1998).

of the disease. On 19 December 1775, three of the hospital's in-patients were diagnosed with smallpox, while two further cases presented on the following day. Thereafter, smallpox began to spread through the lines of the Continental Army.

After the failed attempt to take Quebec on New Year's Day 1776, and with the original leadership either dead (Montgomery) or ailing (Arnold), the incidence of smallpox began to spiral in the American forces. On 12 February, the number of smallpox cases was documented at 50. By the start of May, and with the disease having now taken on a more virulent character, the number of smallpox cases had risen to 800. The situation was to get even worse so that, by the termination of the Canadian Campaign in July 1776, no less than 5,000 Continental troops—representing about 50 per cent of all those engaged—had either died or deserted from the army (Cash, 1976).

As Bayne-Jones (1968) observes, the smallpox epidemic of 1775–6 not only operated as a central factor in the failure of the Canadian Campaign. It also served to reduce the number of available troops while, at the same time, discouraging further recruitment into the Continental Army. In response, on 6 January 1777, the Commander-in-Chief, General Washington, wrote to the Physician in Charge of the Army, William Shippen, Jr., with the following:

Finding the small pox to be spreading much and fearing that no precaution can prevent it from running thro' the whole of our Army, I have determined that the Troops shall be inoculated. This Expedient may be attended with some inconveniences and some disadvantages, but yet I trust, in its consequences will have the most happy effects. (General Washington, 1777, cited in Bayne-Jones, 1968: 52)

Washington's inoculation policy worked well and, although the army was thereafter never entirely free of smallpox, the disease did not spread in the epidemic form of 1775–6. Indeed, it is generally agreed that inoculation policy contributed materially to the winning of the war (Bayne-Jones, 1968).

Overall mortality in the Continental Army. An estimated 70,000 soldiers died in the Continental Army during the period 1775–81. Of these, some 7,000 deaths were battle-related, while most of the remainder were attributable to disease. Assuming the average annual strength of the army to have been 50,000, battle injuries and disease accounted for an annual death rate of 20 and 180 per 1,000 strength, respectively. In addition to smallpox, the principal disease-related causes of death included hospital fever (typhus) and dysentery, along with measles, meningitis, and pneumonia (Bayne-Jones, 1968).

2.7 Conclusion

Drawing on a small sample of a vast historical literature, this chapter has traced the intersection of war and infectious disease from the earliest accounts of classical scholars to the brink of the modern statistical period. Our primary focus has been on the great conflicts of the ages, and the diseases that repeatedly spread in both military and civil populations. Geographically, our coverage has been conditioned by the pattern of recorded wars and the associated level of epidemiological information over a 3,350-year sweep from 1500 BC.

For Europe and neighbouring lands, we have been able to trace a broad epidemiological sequence of war pestilences from the earliest possible manifestations of dysentery in the pre-Christian period, through the certain epidemic appearance of bubonic plague (sixth century AD), to typhus fever (sixteenth century) and cholera (nineteenth century). Elsewhere, in the Americas, the European military conquests of the early sixteenth century were materially aided by wave upon wave of Old World diseases (smallpox, measles, and typhus fever, among others) which, spreading in a virgin soil, ravaged the native Indian populations. By the following century, another disease (yellow fever) had emerged as a severe epidemiological threat to those unacclimatized European forces that ventured into the Caribbean Basin.

Only on relatively rare occasions do we find sufficient epidemiological information to plot the geographical spread of war epidemics in the period prior to the mid-nineteenth century. Where such information is available, an intimate epidemiological association is usually found to exist between military and civil populations. As evidenced by the diffusion of bubonic plague during the Russo-Turkish War of 1770–2 (Sect. 2.4.4), the geographical progress of the disease from Turkish–Ottoman territories into European Russia was fuelled by the intersection of military and civilian activities. Here, the wintering of soldiers alongside civilians in villages and towns, the flight of civilian refugees, movements along military supply lines, and regular patterns of commerce, among other factors, all contributed to the spatial diffusion of the disease. Such interactions at the interface of military, civil, and war-displaced populations serve to underscore the complexity of war epidemics, and it is to epidemiological time trends in these three populations that we turn in the next three chapters.

PART II

Temporal Trends

3

Mortality and Morbidity in Modern Wars, I: Civil Populations

> For the Angel of Death spread his wings on the blast,
> And breathed in the face of the foe as he pass'd;
> And the eyes of the sleepers wax'd deadly and chill,
> And their hearts but once heaved, and for ever grew still!
>
> Lord Byron, 'The Destruction of Sennacherib' (verse 3, 1815)

3.1 Introduction

In this chapter, we examine the time trends that have occurred in the causes of morbidity and mortality in civil populations over the last century and a half.

Particular attention is paid to the period since 1900 when international comparative data become readily available. We begin with two case studies—of Australia, and England and Wales—to establish the main trends affecting the advanced economies over this period. Next, using data collected by Alderson (1981), we extend our analysis to 31 countries to give global coverage. We look first at the statistical evidence of change. It is shown that mortality and morbidity from all causes have declined. Since 1850, it is the infectious diseases which have witnessed the most spectacular falls in their contribution to total mortality and morbidity. Within the general decline, however, sharp upturns in both mortality and morbidity from infectious diseases occur during times of war. In the second half of the chapter, we examine some of the factors which lie behind the declines. Notwithstanding the general falls, in recent years there has been a revolution of interest in infectious diseases arising from a sharp resurgence of both old and new diseases. The former include drug-resistant strains of tuberculosis and the latter HIV (human immunodeficiency virus). The disease setting is also evolving with environmental change and increased human interaction. And so the chapter is concluded with an assessment of the potential significance of infectious diseases in the present century in times of peace and war.

3.2 Twentieth-Century Trends in Mortality: Australia and England and Wales

3.2.1 Australia

THE DATA

In Australia, notifiable diseases data are collected by states and territories under their public health legislation; collection has taken place on a regular basis since 1917. The legislation has required medical practitioners and some other classes of people to notify health authorities of the number of cases recorded of certain communicable and other diseases. The resulting data were published in the *Medical Journal of Australia* from 1917 to 1922, *Health*, 1924 to 1939, and in the *Commonwealth Year Book* since 1945. Additionally, the Commonwealth Department of Health and its successors have published an annual compilation of notifiable diseases data in the Department's *Annual Report*.

Since 1917, a total of 157 different rubrics have been used at various times to collect notifiable diseases data. Several of these rubrics are no longer recognized as independent nosological entities, while others represent stages in the evolution of diagnostic techniques to identify the same diseases. The task of pulling the data into a consistent body of statistics covering the time span from 1917 to the present has been undertaken by Hall (1993), and it is his annual data, 1917–91, on reported cases and case rates for 89 communicable diseases and other conditions that are analysed in this section. The diseases are listed in Hall, and cover a wide spectrum of infections ranging, for example, from quarantine diseases like plague and yellow fever, respiratory infections like influenza and measles, parasitic diseases, haemorrhagic fevers, through to HIV.

As with all surveillance data, Hall attaches the usual 'health warnings' to the figures. For example, the proportion of cases notified is not known with certainty for any disease and may vary over time, between diseases and between jurisdictions. This may affect secular trends. Not all disease categories have been uniformly notifiable in all states and territories. Intra-state variation has been ignored by Hall in the calculation of rates of notification; denominator populations were defined as being the whole of the state or territory. Frequently diseases were notifiable only in endemic or epidemic areas. Overestimates of the rate of notification of some diseases will follow from this. The sensitivity of the surveillance systems varies from disease to disease. For example, for malaria and tuberculosis, proactive surveillance may give a better indication of the epidemiology of these diseases in Australia than for diseases like measles where passive reporting is the norm. But, subject to the uncertainties described, Hall's data represent best estimates of Australian rates of notifiable diseases.

The time series published by Hall are very complete. Data are missing for the years 1941, 1943, and 1952 and do not appear to have been published. Data for the Northern Territory for 1942 to 1946 were suppressed. For some diseases, some states or territories are missing in an irregular manner scattered through the 75-year data run. Case rates (per 100,000 population) were calculated using population estimates from the Australian Bureau of Statistics for each state and territory at mid-year for the years 1917 to 1991. Crude rates, rather than rates standardized for age and sex, are analysed here.

MORBIDITY TRENDS

Over the 75 years from 1917 to 1991 a total of 2,200,194 notifications was received by Australia's routine disease notification system. The peak number in any one year was 120,023 in 1919 when 89,941 cases of influenza were reported. Figure 3.1A plots as line traces the annual notified case rate per 100,000 population for each of the 89 diseases in Hall's data set. A logarithmic scale has been used. The heavy lines mark the maximum case rate and the three quartiles recorded each year across the 89 diseases. No attempt has been made to pick out individual diseases. The broad trends are clear. Bearing in mind the logarithmic scale used for the vertical axis, case rates from the infections have declined exponentially over the 75-year period. Up to the beginning of World War II, the band of rates is effectively horizontal, with a slight hint of an increasing range to the encompassing envelope through the 1930s. After 1945, the steady fall in case rates that has persisted through to the present day set in,

although there is some evidence for a levelling out in the speed of fall after
c.1970. From *c*.1950, the range of rates also declined as compared with
1917–39.

To aid comparison between the rates for different diseases over time, Figure
3.1B replots from Figure 3.1A the line traces for the maximum case rate and the
three quartiles as index numbers (1917 = 100). Again, a logarithmic scale has
been used for the vertical axis. In contrast to Figure 3.1A, the use of index numbers has enabled us to illustrate the time series for the minimum annual rates by
avoiding a plotting problem that arises when showing the raw data on a log
scale—namely many years with zero or near zero rates. Like Figure 3.1A, Figure 3.1B shows the sharp fall in rates after 1945. The time series for minimum
rates emphasizes this decline by reflecting how very low are the rates for many
infectious diseases at the end of the twentieth century.

Figure 3.2 emphasizes the morbidity trends shown in Figure 3.1 by plotting
as index numbers on an annual basis the mean, standard deviation, and the
coefficient of variation of the notified rates. In each year of the time series,
these summary statistics have been calculated across the rates for the 89
diseases. We define CV as

$$CV = 100(s/\bar{x}),\qquad\qquad\qquad(3.1)$$

where $\bar{x}$ and s are the arithmetic mean and standard deviation respectively of
the 89 rates in each year. The coefficient is large where there is great variation in
relation to the mean, and small when the variation is relatively small. Because
the three time series are in different units, they have been converted to index
numbers (1917 = 100) to aid comparisons; a log scale has again been used for
the vertical axis.

While the coefficient of variation remained effectively constant over the
entire period, Figure 3.2 makes clear (i) the roughly constant or slightly rising
level (mean) and variation (standard deviation) of rates between 1917 and
1940; (ii) the shift to a lower level and degree of variability after 1945; (iii) the
sharpest decline in rates and variability in the immediate post-World War II
period from 1946 to 1951.

3.2.2 England and Wales: Trends in Mortality since 1841

THE DATA

The data upon which the discussion in this section is based appear in *The
Health of Adult Britain 1841–1994*, prepared in association with the Office for
National Statistics (Charlton and Murphy, 1997).

Any attempt to examine long-term trends in mortality must confront a number of difficulties. Over the 150-year period considered in this book, there have
been changes in the way causes of death have been recorded, as well as improvements in the accuracy of diagnosis and reporting. The manner in which dis-

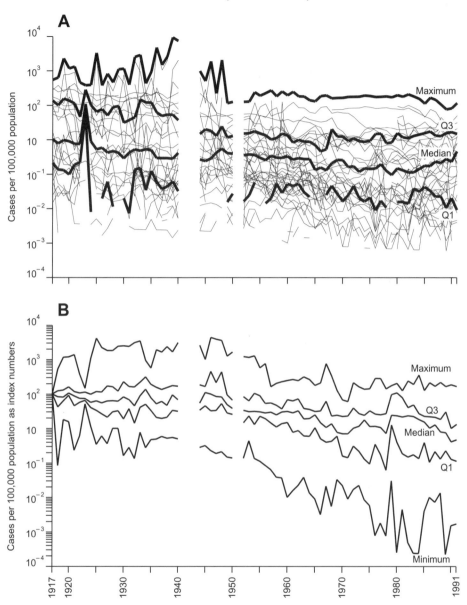

Fig. 3.1. Australia, 1917–1991: annual morbidity rates from 89 infectious diseases

Notes: (A) The line traces plot the notified number of cases per 100,000 population at the national level. The heavy lines give the maximum rate and the three quartiles (Q1, median, and Q3) calculated on an annual basis across the 89 diseases. A log scale has been used for the vertical axis. (B) Maximum and minimum rates and three quartiles replotted as index numbers (1917 = 100). *Source*: Data from Hall (1993).

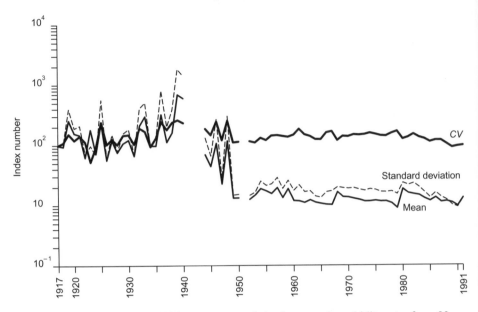

Fig. 3.2. Australia, 1917–1991: summary statistics for annual morbidity rates from 89 infectious diseases

Notes: Mean, standard deviation, and coefficient of variation (*CV*) of rates plotted as index numbers (1917 = 100). The statistics have been calculated annually across the notified rates for the 89 diseases.

Source: Data from Hall (1993).

eases are described and classified has also varied. These issues are discussed in Cliff *et al.* (1998: 26–34). To circumvent some of these difficulties, the Office for National Statistics (ONS) data cover trends for the periods 1841–1910 and 1911–92 separately. For the earlier period, they rely on the tables produced by Logan (1950). For the latter period, they have matched cause data to the International Classification of Diseases (ICD) chapters used in the ninth revision of the ICD and to past and present coding practices of the ONS.

MORTALITY TRENDS

In the period 1848–72 the main causes of death (in order) were: infectious, respiratory, nervous, digestive, and circulatory diseases. Infectious diseases accounted for one death in every three, and a third of these deaths were due to respiratory tuberculosis. Cancers formed only a small proportion of all deaths, but their rates increased more than threefold for men and twofold for women by 1901–10. During the twentieth century the decline of infectious disease mortality has been the most important cause of increased life expectancy. Infectious diseases now only account for around 0.5 per cent of all deaths. The decline in respiratory disease mortality was second in importance. There have also been major declines in death rates from digestive, genito-urinary, and nervous system diseases. Figure 3.3A shows these changes since 1911 by plotting on an annual basis for males aged 15–74, the death rate per million population

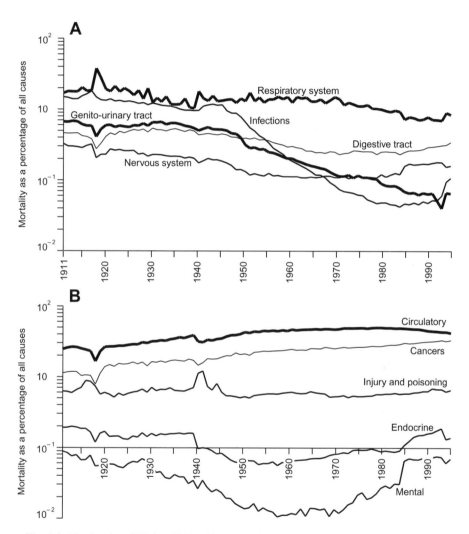

Fig. 3.3. England and Wales, 1911–1994: annual mortality rates for males aged 15–74 per million population

Notes: The death rates have been plotted as a percentage of the rate for all causes, and they have been age-standardized to the populations of Europe. (A) Infections, diseases of the digestive, nervous, and respiratory system, and of the genito-urinary tract. (B) Cancers, circulatory, endocrine, and mental diseases, injury and poisoning.

Source: Redrawn from Charlton and Murphy (1997, fig. 4.3, p. 37).

as a percentage of the rate for all causes. The death rates have been age-standardized to the populations of Europe. Bearing in mind the logarithmic scale used for the vertical axis, the fall in deaths from infectious diseases has been especially dramatic.

To set against these falls, there have been increases in mortality from circulatory diseases and cancers, especially in men. The number of deaths from diseases of the circulatory system increased from 83,000 in 1911 (16% of all deaths) to 293,000 in 1971 (52% of deaths), falling to 255,000 by 1992 (46% of all deaths). Most of these deaths (57%) are due to ischaemic heart disease, but 26 per cent are due to stroke. The increase in mortality has been more marked in men than in women. The number of deaths from cancer rose from 37,700 in 1911 to 146,000 by 1992 (from 7 to 26% of all deaths, respectively). Currently the most common sites recorded on death certificates are: lung (23%); colon and rectum (11%); female breast (9%); prostate (6%); and stomach (6%). Although diseases of the circulatory system and neoplasms now account for most male deaths below age 65 (72% of male deaths), they account for only half of the years of life lost below age 65. Figure 3.3B plots deaths from these classes of diseases on the same basis as Figure 3.3A. The gently rising trends for cancers and circulatory diseases over most of the period are evident.

Increasingly important as causes of death among the young are suicides and accidents. In 1992, 36 per cent of the 17,300 deaths resulting from injury and poisoning were due to suicide, 24 per cent to motor vehicle accidents, 20 per cent to accidental falls, 4 per cent to accidental poisoning, 3 per cent to fires, and 2 per cent each to homicides and drownings. For men these constituted 5.3 per cent of all deaths, for women 3.9. Among the under-65s, accidents and suicides accounted for only 3 per cent of deaths but 19 per cent of years of life lost for males because these deaths occur at younger ages. Some of these features are evident in Figure 3.3B. Mortality from mental disorders was roughly constant until *c*.1930. It then fell steadily until *c*.1970 and has risen sharply since then.

The line trace for injury and poisoning is of especial interest in the context of the link between war and disease. There are sharp local peaks during both the world wars. This link is returned to at an international scale in the next section.

3.3 Twentieth-Century Trends in Mortality: International Patterns

To give a measure of uniformity to our discussion, we have used the monumental collection of mortality data assembled by Alderson (1981) in his *International Mortality Statistics*. These cover 31 countries (listed in Table 3.1) for each of the 15 quinquennial periods from 1901–5 to 1971–5 inclusive. European countries dominate the list, but there is at least one country from each of

Table 3.1. International mortality trends, 1901–1975: list of countries studied by Alderson (1981)

Country	WHO region	Country	WHO region
Australia	Western Pacific	Netherlands	Europe
Austria	Europe	New Zealand	Western Pacific
Belgium	Europe	Norway	Europe
Bulgaria	Europe	Poland	Europe
Canada	America	Portugal	Europe
Chile	America	Romania	Europe
Czechoslovakia	Europe	Spain	Europe
Denmark	Europe	Sweden	Europe
Eire	Europe	Switzerland	Europe
Finland	Europe	Turkey	Europe
France	Europe	UK—England and Wales	Europe
Greece	Europe	UK—Northern Ireland	Europe
Hungary	Europe	UK—Scotland	Europe
Iceland	Europe	USA	America
Italy	Europe	Yugoslavia	Europe
Japan	Western Pacific		

the other main world regions used by the World Health Organization (WHO) for surveillance purposes. Because Alderson's data pre-date the ready availability of computers, they have been little used, yet they provide the only readily available source data that allow inter-country and inter-disease trends to be studied over a 75-year time span.

In assembling his data, Alderson was mindful of the tensions between geographical coverage, data validity, the need to obtain long time series, and problems of alignment of disease definitions between the various revisions of the ICD list. A winnowing process which involved application of these considerations led ultimately to Alderson's selection of countries and causes of death. For our purposes in this book, studying the impact of war upon patterns of disease in the general population as well as among the military, we have selected a subset of 53 causes from Alderson's list of 178; we have, however, analysed all 31 countries.

The subset of causes chosen appears in Table 3.2. The list is dominated by sicknesses for which an element of transmission is probable over the likely duration of conflicts (from a few days in the case of the Six-Day War between Israel and Egypt in 1967 to years for major international conflicts). Patterns of transmissible diseases are likely to be profoundly affected by the population flux that accompanies war. We have not considered causes of mortality which are unlikely to be strongly linked to war. These include, for example, malignant neoplasms and various heart and circulatory disorders. But in the 'non-transmissible' category, we have included a number of conditions likely to be greatly affected by war. Examples are suicides, homicides, and mental illness.

Table 3.2. International mortality trends, 1901–1975: list of causes of death studied by Alderson (1981)

Mortality cause	Mortality cause
Anthrax	Respiratory diseases—all forms
Broncho-pneumonia	Rheumatic fever
Cholera	Scarlet fever
Diphtheria	Septicaemia
Dysentery	Skin diseases
Gastroenteritis	Smallpox
Genito-urinary system—all diseases	Syphilis—all forms
Gonococcal infection	Syphilis—all other
Homicide and war injury	Syphilis—central nervous system
Homicide, suicide, and war injury	Syphilis—general paralysis of the insane
Infections—all forms	Syphilis—tabes dorsalis
Influenza	Tetanus
Malaria	Tuberculosis—alimentary
Measles	Tuberculosis—all forms
Meningococcal infections	Tuberculosis—all other forms
Meningitis—non-meningococcal	Tuberculosis—bones and joints
Mental illness—all forms	Tuberculosis—meninges and central nervous system
Nephritis, acute	Tuberculosis—non-respiratory
Nephritis, chronic	Tuberculosis—respiratory system
Nephritis and nephrosis	Typhoid
Paratyphoid	Typhoid and paratyphoid
Plague	Typhus and other rickettsial diseases
Pleurisy	Venereal disease
Pneumonia—all forms	War injury
Pneumonia—lobar	Whooping cough
Pneumonia—primary	Yellow fever
Poliomyelitis	

3.3.1 Data Standardization

To allow for the variable demographic composition of each of the countries, Alderson employed mortality and age-structure data for each country at each period to compute a Standardized Mortality Ratio (*SMR*) by the indirect method for the various causes of death in males, females, and for all persons.[1] The various ways in which *SMR*s may be calculated are summarized in Benjamin (1968, ch. 6). The basic idea behind *SMR*s is, however, straightforward. If a country has a relatively 'old' population (as, for example, in western economies) there may be an excess of deaths from diseases of age simply because the country concerned has an undue proportion of older people. In these circumstances, the conventional mortality rate will not reflect the true

---

[1] Except, of course, for gender-specific diseases like breast and testicular cancer where only the data relevant to the appropriate gender are given.

risk of death from such causes. By the same token, countries with high birth rates and young populations may have excess deaths from certain diseases that especially afflict the young.

Thus mortality from many diseases is not independent of either the geographical environment or of the age–sex composition of the population at any moment in time. Without standardizing for this effect, inter-area and inter-disease comparisons of the impact of different sicknesses over long time periods are restricted, especially if the demographic composition of the population changes very much. *SMR*s allow for these effects by referencing each country's mortality to the mortality expected in a 'standard' population, generating a ratio with the standard population in the denominator. A ratio greater than 1 (or some multiple of this) denotes an excess of deaths from a given cause as compared with the standard population.

3.3.2 Time Trends in Mortality

Given the inevitably uneven nature of international mortality data we opted, notwithstanding Alderson's meticulous approach, to base our analysis upon robust statistics of the time series behaviour of the *SMR*s. Accordingly, for each cause, the first, second (i.e. the median), and third quartiles of the *SMR*s in each quinquennium were calculated across the 31 countries. This yielded three time series of quartile values for each of the 53 causes. Next, the 53 time series of medians were subjected to a complete linkage cluster analysis to classify the causes in terms of their median *SMR* time series behaviour between 1901 and 1975. The dendrogram is plotted in Figure 3.4. Five well-defined groups are picked out; for the discussion below, group 3 is subdivided into groups 3 and 3A. The median time series for the causes which comprise each group is plotted in Figure 3.5.

We begin our discussion of the dendrogram with class 3 which contains the specifically war-related causes of death (war injuries, and homicides and suicides occurring in war). Into this class also fall the great quarantine diseases—typhus, smallpox, yellow fever, plague, cholera, typhoid, and paratyphoid—as well as the classic war-related infection of poliomyelitis and one sexually transmitted disease. The median *SMR* curves for the causes of mortality in classes 3 and 3A illustrated in Figure 3.5 reflect the association of these diseases with war. Substantial upturns in mortality are seen in the quinquennia spanning the two world wars for group 3A (the quarantine diseases), while the line trace for group 3 as a whole has marked 'shoulders' in the same quinquennia; these stand out against a steady decline in deaths from these causes over the course of this century.

The causes of mortality in the other groups of Figure 3.5 share one common feature with group 3 (and with the earlier results for Australia and England and Wales; cf. Figs. 3.1–3.3)—the loglinear decline over the 75-year period considered by Alderson. In much reduced form, they also show slight rises during the

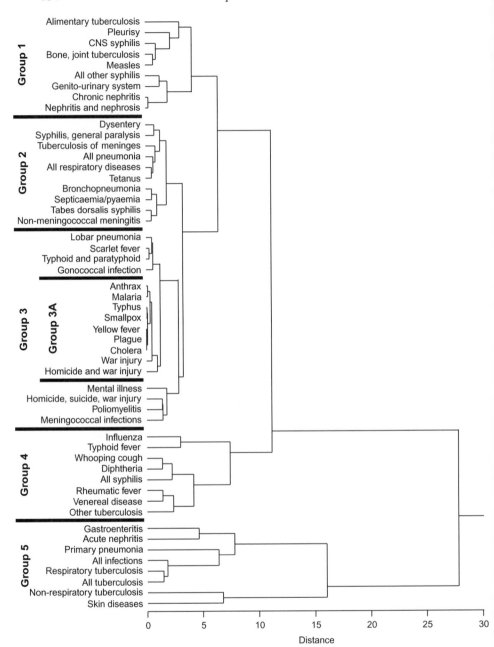

Fig. 3.4. Classification of 53 causes of death in terms of their time-series behaviour, 1901–1975

Note: For each cause, the input data consisted of the median standardized mortality ratio in each quinquennium across the 31 countries listed in Table 3.1.

Source: Data from Alderson (1981).

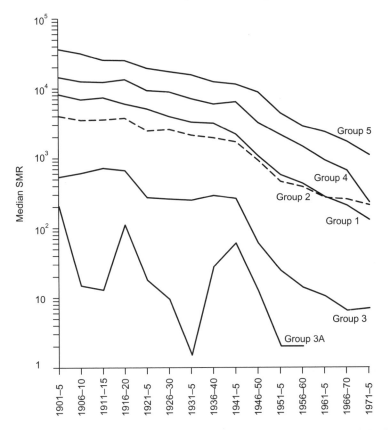

Fig. 3.5. Time series of median standardized mortality ratios for the causes of death in each group of Fig. 3.4

world wars, although this is small compared with the group 3 causes. To identify quinquennia with excess mortality from a particular group of causes more precisely, the model

$$\log(SMR_t) = \beta_0 + \beta_1 t \tag{3.2}$$

was fitted to the time series plotted in Figure 3.5. Here, SMR_t is the median standardized mortality ratio in the tth quinquennium plotted in Figure 3.5. The regression results are summarized in Table 3.3 while, for each of the groups, Figure 3.6 plots the time series of residuals from equation (3.2).

The uniformly good fits of the loglinear model to the time series is confirmed by the values for R^2 given in Table 3.3. Despite this, the residual plots show a number of interesting features:

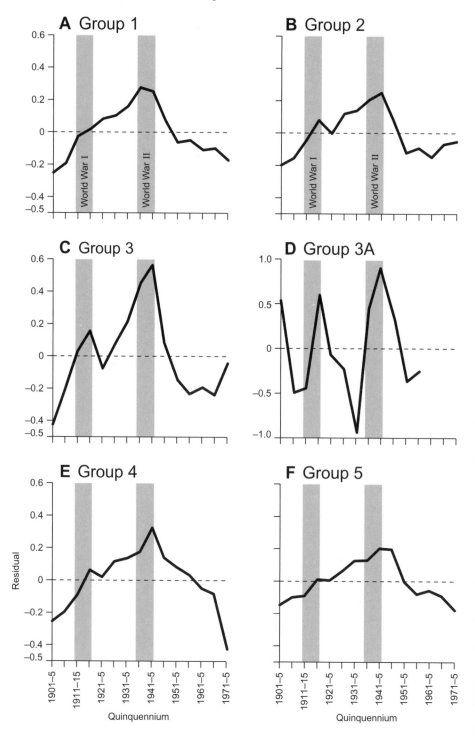

Table 3.3. International mortality trends, 1901–1975: results from loglinear model fitted to time series of the median *SMR*s for causes of mortality in groups 1–5 of the dendrogram shown in Fig. 3.4

Mortality group	$\hat{\beta}_0$	$\hat{\beta}_1$	(t)	R^2
1	52.4	−0.0269	(−13.77)	0.94
2	39.6	−0.0204	(−11.98)	0.92
3	61.9	−0.0325	(−9.82)	0.88
3A	41.0	−0.0222	(−2.30)	0.35
4	45.7	−0.0233	(−9.95)	0.88
5	42.4	−0.0214	(−14.26)	0.94

1. Causes in groups 2, 3, and 4 have local maxima in World War I (quinquennium 1916–20).
2. All plots peak during World War II, generally in the quinqunnium 1941–5.
3. With the exception of group 3A, the general time trend of the residual plots is quadratic, with above average mortality from these causes between 1916 and 1950.
4. For the diseases in group 3A, Figure 3.6D emphasizes the excess mortality from these causes during the two world wars. The fundamentally different time series behaviour of these diseases is also show by the comparatively low value for R^2 in Table 3.3.

3.3.3 Deaths from All Causes

To provide a context for assessing trends in mortality for each of the groups of causes used above, it is useful to subject deaths from all causes based upon the Alderson *SMR* data to the same analysis as for the medians of the five classes. The general decline in mortality is shown in Figure 3.7A for the 15 quinquennial periods from 1901–5 to 1971–5. This graph plots the median *SMR* value for the 31 countries as a heavy line, while the shaded area forms an envelope delimiting the range of values from the highest to the lowest *SMR* in each five-year time period.

Compared with a median *SMR* of 30,000 in the first quinquennium of the century (1901–5), the figure had fallen nearly threefold to a value of 12,400 by

◄───

Fig. 3.6. Quinquennia with excess mortality from different causes, 1901–1975

Notes: Time-series plots of residuals from a loglinear trend model fitted to time series of median standardized mortality ratios of disease groups 1 to 5 in Fig. 3.4. Quinquennia corresponding to World Wars I and II are highlighted.

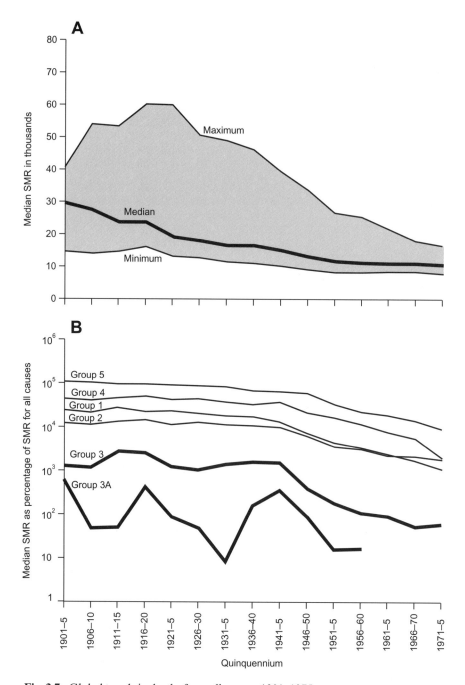

Fig. 3.7. Global trends in deaths from all causes, 1901–1975

Notes: (A) Median value (heavy line) of standardized mortality ratios (*SMRs*) for males in 31 countries. The shaded area forms an envelope which delimits the range of values from the highest to lowest *SMR* in each five-year time period. (B) Comparison of the median *SMRs* for causes in groups 1 to 5 as a percentage of the median *SMR* for deaths from all causes.
Source: Based on data in Alderson (1981, table 24, p. 161).

the last quinquennium (1971–5). For the median, the decline was fairly constant and gentle over the period. For some countries, the experience was different. As the upper edge of the shaded envelope indicates, the effect of World War I was to push the maximum *SMR* in each quinquennium to a high level, from which it declined in a similar steady fashion to the 31-country median over the period of the Depression and World War II. It was only after 1945 that the outlier *SMR*s converged rapidly on the 31-country median. Although, as we would expect, in comparative terms the fall in *SMR*s for deaths from all causes is much less striking than that for any of the five dendrogram classes, the same steady decline over the 75-year period covered by Alderson's data is apparent.

Figure 3.7B shows the median *SMR*s for the causes in groups 1 to 5 against all causes by plotting them as the ratio

$$100 \text{ (median } SMR \text{ for class } i/\text{median } SMR \text{ for all causes)}. \qquad (3.3)$$

The graph highlights the increased contribution of the quarantine and other war-related causes of death (dendrogram class 3) to total deaths during the two world wars. By comparison, there is no significant increase for the causes in dendrogram groups 1, 2, 4, and 5.

The post-World War II decline is illustrated further in Figure 3.8 using World Health Organization data. This graph plots the age-standardized death rate between 1950 and 1989 by five-year periods for 12 of the countries recorded by Alderson for which particularly good mortality records exist: Australia, Belgium, Denmark, England and Wales, Italy, Japan, the Netherlands, Norway, Portugal, Sweden, Switzerland, and the United States. This reduced set retains the global coverage of the 31 countries considered by Alderson by omitting mainly European countries from the full set. The heavy line plots the median, while the shaded envelope delimits the maximum and minimum value in each quinquennium. For the 12 countries, the death rate from all causes stood at 905 per 100,000 population in 1950 and, by 1990, this had been reduced by one-third to 611.

3.3.4 Geographical Patterns of Decline

A detailed analysis of the geographically disaggregated patterns of decline in deaths from all causes over the course of this century would be a massive undertaking and take us well outside the scope of this book. For the period to mid-century, the topic has been discussed in a number of major studies (e.g. Erhardt and Berlin, 1974; Preston, 1976; and Wrigley, 1969), and the reader should consult these sources for detailed accounts. But, for the war-related diseases in groups 3 and 3A, we can isolate some of the broad trends in Alderson's data.

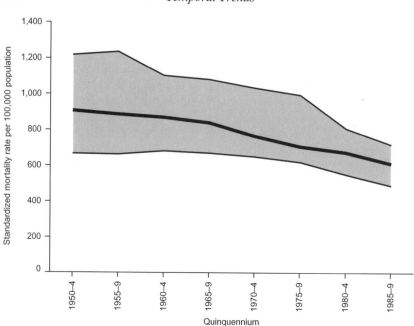

Fig. 3.8. Trends in deaths from all causes in the developed world, 1950–1989

Note: Median value and ranges for World Health Organization age standardized death rate per 100,000 population.

Source: Cliff *et al.* (1998, Fig. 7.11, p. 340).

THE WAR DISEASES

To illustrate the geographical variation in the impact of the group 3 diseases in times of war, Alderson's data were re-examined on a country-by-country basis. In each quinquennium, and for each of his 31 nations, the maximum *SMR* across the diseases in each of the classes was calculated. For those countries with reasonably complete time series, Figure 3.9 plots the resulting graphs. The data for each graph have been standardized by their ranges prior to plotting. This standardization permits easy comparison between graphs by making 1 the maximum value on any chart; it also emphasizes the quinquennia with the larger *SMR*s.

For many countries, sharp peaks of mortality can be seen in one or both of the quinquennia spanning the two world wars (shaded black on the plots). The graph for Spain is especially interesting, peaking sharply between 1936 and 1941, rather than in the next five-year period. The quinquennium, 1936–41, spans the Spanish Civil War which affected Spain more dramatically than the world war. Some countries in Figure 3.9 show no marked peak of *SMR* in either of the world wars. These were either outside the main theatres of war in

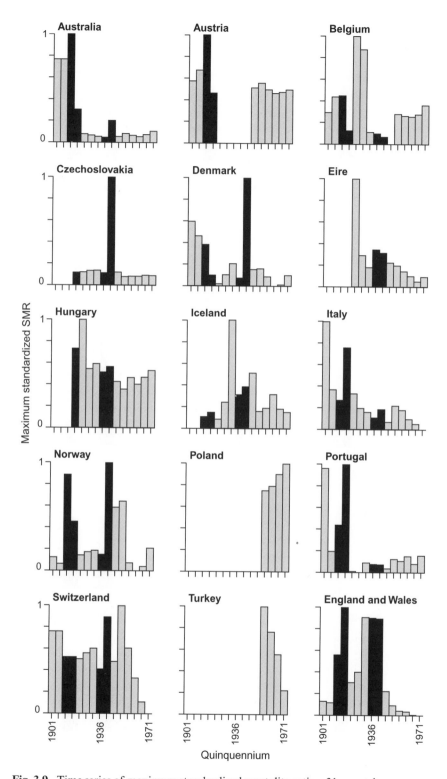

Fig. 3.9. Time series of maximum standardized mortality ratios: 31 countries

Notes: For each country, the maxima have been calculated across the causes of mortality for the group 3 diseases of Fig. 3.4, and the resulting time series has been standardized by its range prior to plotting. The quinquennia spanning the world wars are shaded black.

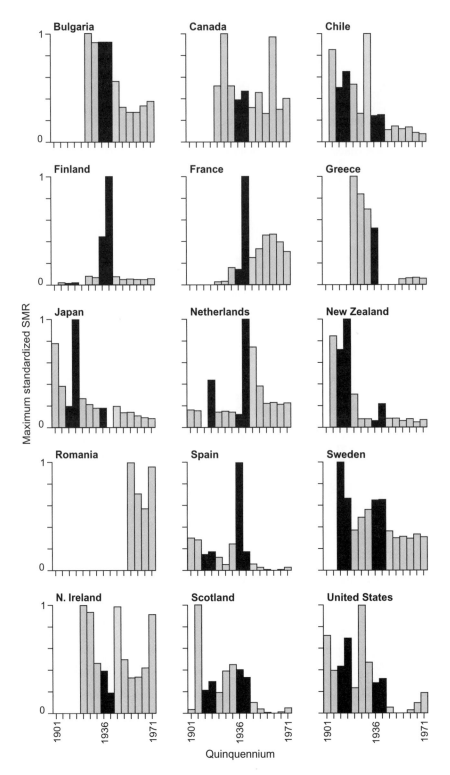

Fig. 3.9. (*cont.*)

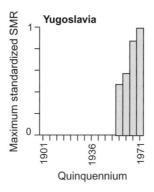

Fig. 3.9. (*cont.*)

the global conflicts (United States, Canada, Australia, New Zealand) or were neutral (Switzerland).

3.4 The Causes of Epidemic Disease Decline

3.4.1 *Explaining Mortality Change*

The fact that we can demonstrate clearly that (i) mortality and morbidity from diseases, especially those which are transmissible, have steadily declined over the last 150 years (albeit in a cyclic, loglinear manner rather than in a simple linear fashion), (ii) considerable variations exist between countries in the rate of decline, (iii) infectious diseases have enhanced significance during war, and (iv) mortality from cancers and heart disease has increased steadily since 1850, throws little light on why these declines and variations have occurred. We look briefly at the debate over the reasons for change, drawing upon Cliff *et al.* (1998: 134–8).

Few topics cause as much controversy amongst economic historians, demographers, and historians of medicine as the causes of the long mortality decline which has affected western Europe over the last three centuries. As we have seen, so far as the available demographic data indicate, the facts of decline are not in dispute, at least in the round. But, outside the broad picture, the detail of the ways in which particular age cohorts or sexes were affected remains an area for active research and argument. Wrigley and Schofield's (1989) monumental *Population History of England, 1541–1871* confirms the extent to which the specific demographic parameters of decline still remain to be unravelled. And, what is true for England, with one of the best recorded and most pored-over demographic histories, is likely to be all the more true for most countries around the world.

In an introduction to *The Decline of Mortality* (Schofield *et al.*, 1991), the Cambridge demographer, Roger Schofield, succinctly summarizes the historical development of mortality in Europe in the following terms:

Pre-decline patterns typical of most *Ancien Régime* societies were characterized by high overall levels, punctuated by periodic bouts with epidemics caused by infectious disease (plague, smallpox, typhus, etc.). During the eighteenth century, and chiefly thanks to ever more efficient government intervention, the incidence of crisis mortality diminished drastically in most of Europe. It was the 'stabilisation of mortality' as Michael Flinn (1974) called it, and was essential to the subsequent spurt in European growth rates. With the reduction of epidemics, endemic infectious diseases became relatively more important and gains in life expectancy slowed considerably. It was not until the latter part of the nineteenth century that mortality once again declined sharply in most areas of Europe. Child mortality and, somewhat later, infant mortality were responsible for much of this decline, though gains in life expectancy affected all age groups. Mortality improvement was due mostly to the decline in diseases such as diarrhoea and tuberculosis. The third period of mortality decline began after World War II, spread throughout the world, and seems inextricably, though not exclusively, linked to the discovery and use of sulpha drugs and antibiotics. (Schofield *et al.*, 1991: 1)

A useful review of the mortality changes both within and outside Europe is provided by Kunitz (1986).

But, if the facts are slowly becoming clearer, the causes which lie behind the observed decline remain a hotbed of controversy. The range of the debate suggests that any understanding of precisely what happened, both when and where, remains tenuous. In general terms there are six main hypotheses, each with a penumbra of minor variations that lie outside our immediate concern. We term them 'hypotheses' here because most remain speculative and the opportunity for testing them as models remains limited. The complex interactions among the factors underpinning the hypotheses are summarized in Figure 3.10.

1. *Crisis hypotheses.* These suggest that the background level of mortality in so-called 'normal' years remained roughly constant over long periods of time. Long-term decline in mortality is then attributed to a reduction in the number of 'epidemic years' which are characterized by a flare-up of excess mortality. The concept is discussed at length by Landers (1993: 14–22). As he notes, an implication of the crisis hypothesis is that mortality crises had an essential character of their own, that they were qualitatively distinct from the background mortality characterizing 'normal' years, and that they stemmed from some external shock. Mortality crises have been correlated with environmental triggers (leading to poor harvests, for example), epidemics of infectious disease, and military crises brought on by war. Equally, there must be instances when aspects of all three combined to create a mortality crisis. Further, as Flinn (1981: 53) has pointed out, 'whatever the basic cause of a crisis, epidemic disease generally took over, so that mortality crises of all kinds very commonly appear as great increases in the number of deaths from infectious diseases'.

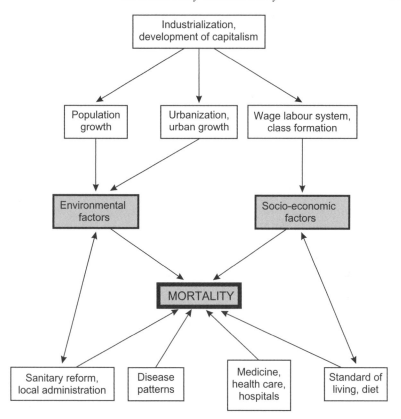

Fig. 3.10. Schematic model of factors affecting levels of mortality
Source: Cliff *et al.* (1998, fig. 4.1, p. 136), from Woods and Woodward (1984, fig. 1.1, p. 21).

Schofield and Reher (1991, p. 3) link the early phase of the mortality transition over a period stretching from the latter part of the seventeenth century to the beginning of the nineteenth to the decline, or even disappearance, of crisis mortality caused by epidemics of plague which had all but disappeared from the continent by the early part of the eighteenth century.

2. *Urbanization hypotheses.* To the contemporary mid-Victorian urban observer such as Charles Dickens or Émile Zola, the living conditions in crowded and filthy cities were seen as a major obstacle to any mortality decline. As Schofield and Reher (1991: 14) observe: 'Towns had always been characterized by higher mortality rates due mainly to greater population densities which facilitated infection and filth; and during the nineteenth century increasing proportions of the population were living in those urban centres'. In *An Atlas of Victorian Mortality*, Woods and Shelton (1997) use Registrar General's records for 614 small districts in England and Wales to test the hypothesis that

urbanization had a profound influence on national mortality because an increasing proportion of the population of England and Wales became concentrated in a relatively small number of urban districts. Generally speaking, the rural districts were the healthy ones, where mortality was at its lowest compared with the urban areas, but not all the groups or causes of death considered in the atlas showed clear urban–rural differentials. In infancy, diarrhoea and dysentery, and, in old age, diseases of the lung were especially important in establishing and maintaining the urban–rural mortality differential. In early childhood, Woods and Shelton found that the infectious diseases displayed the most sensitivity to differences in population density, with measles and scarlet fever exhibiting a pronounced mortality gradient between town and country. But the maps show a complex pattern. That for scarlet fever mortality in the 1860s picks out some of the largest urban centres and it is these places that benefited most from the lower mortality at the end of the century. But, unlike measles, there are many counter-examples, especially at mid-century, of relatively high mortality in more rural areas. The maps also emphasize the uncertainty concerning the extent to which pulmonary tuberculosis was principally an urban disease, throw doubts on whether urban areas fostered tuberculosis, and challenge the prevailing nineteenth-century explanation that rural life afforded some protection against the disease.

3. *Economic and nutritional hypotheses.* Thomas McKeown (1976) in *The Modern Rise of Population* argued forcefully that the fall in mortality was mainly due to improved nutrition, linked to increased levels of economic development. His arguments were largely based on British data for deaths classified by age and certified cause from 1837 onwards. He observed that diseases spread by airborne micro-organisms (especially tuberculosis) had accounted for most of the decline in mortality during the nineteenth and the twentieth centuries. From this observation he went on to argue that, since tuberculosis and some of the other airborne diseases like measles, were largely unaffected by advances in public health until well into the twentieth century, exposure to them could not have been limited during that part of the mortality transition prior to significant medical intervention. His conclusion—that therefore resistance to them must have grown on account of the improved nutritional status of the population—has been widely criticized. Wrigley and Schofield (1989: 224–48) have demonstrated that the role McKeown attributed to mortality decline in eighteenth-century population change is inaccurate: changes in fertility trends were the key to population growth rates. Szreter (1988) has also shown that social intervention played a much larger part in mortality decline in the period from 1850 to 1914 than McKeown would allow.

4. *Public health and sanitation hypotheses.* Expanding on Szreter's critique of McKeown, this explanation stresses the key role of the state in organizing public defence against disease, providing basic health facilities, and informing the population of advances in health care. A leading advocate of this view is Preston (1976) who, in his *Mortality Patterns in National Populations with Spe-*

cial Reference to Recorded Causes of Death, used twentieth-century national data to demonstrate that income, nutrition, and other indicators of the standard of living cannot have been responsible for more than 25 per cent of the rise in life expectancy. Public-health technology is left as the most important residual explanation for declining mortality. Such ideas have been supported by evidence from the developing world since 1950 where mortality has been reduced drastically despite few improvements in the standard of living.

5. *Medical hypotheses*. As Schofield and Reher (1991: 14) point out, the role of medicine and medical science in the decline of mortality has been belittled by McKeown and many other scholars. Medical advances could not be credited with the decline in mortality since, with the exception of smallpox and diphtheria, most other diseases (whooping cough, measles, scarlet fever) were declining long before effective chemotherapy or other scientific techniques became available. Before the discovery of antibiotics and sulpha drugs during the middle part of the present century, physicians had almost no effective weapons with which to combat disease and infection directly. By and large, hospitals were places noted for the spread of contagion rather than centres of cure. But, as with the other hypotheses, evidence is building up to suggest that the role of the physician may be more important than McKeown's arguments would suggest (see, for example, Kunitz, 1991).

6. *Environmental hypotheses*. A few studies have explored the links between climatic variation in determining both long- and short-term fluctuations of mortality in Europe. For example, Galloway (1985, 1986) has associated warmer summers or colder winters with higher-than-average mortality especially among very young children. In the same vein, Caselli (1991) has observed that infant, and especially child, mortality patterns in Europe suggest that, in areas with hot, dry summers, there may be deleterious consequences for food and water purity. Such regions display anomalously high child mortality levels from diarrhoea and other intestinal diseases when compared with other parts of the continent.

3.4.2 *The Continuing Debate on Mortality Decline*

The lively debate on the causes of the overall mortality decline did not stop with data at the end of the nineteenth century. As the discussion in the previous section indicated, the views over the 'long decline' have drawn on demographic information which spans from the start of the eighteenth century through to the end of the twentieth. So the rumbling battle on the role of nutrition that followed McKeown's thesis on *The Modern Rise of Population* (1976) has seen a number of studies which have questioned the arguments by using twentieth-century data: Vallin and Meslé's (1988) study, *Les Causes de Décès en France de 1925 à 1978* is a case in point. Like many recent studies, this eschews a grand central theory and sees mortality decline as the end-product of a complex bundle of factors which interact in different time periods and different demographic regions. This continuing shift towards such models of cautious complexity led Schofield and Reher (1991: 7) to comment: 'there may have been multiple paths to mortality transition which have yet to be unearthed by scholars'.

But there are two areas in which debates using twentieth-century data (and still more the data of the next century) may have advantages over those from earlier periods. First, more is now known about the changing nature of disease itself. The best example is that of influenza where the recognition that the influenza A virus was subject to both major shifts and minor drifts (Cliff *et al.*, 1986) is a major explanation for mortality changes. The 1918–19 pandemic (with its estimated 20–40 million or more deaths worldwide) and the lesser pandemics of Asian, Hong Kong, and 'Red' flu in more recent decades each illustrate the direct effect of disease change on mortality, as do the minor 'drift' changes which boost winter mortality on a regular two- or three-year cycle. This contasts with earlier periods when hypothesized changes in the virulence of diseases are more speculative. For example, Lancaster (1990: 115) conjectures that the decline in mortality from scarlet fever from the nineteeth century may be attributable to the existence of scarlet fever strains operating in earlier centuries which are no longer in circulation '. . . for no other explanation [of the decline] has ever been given'. In the absence of direct virological or bacteriological knowledge, changes in virulence remains a potentially powerful explanation of last resort.

A second difference in studying the present century is (*a*) the dramatic increase in medical knowledge and (*b*) its consequent effect on prevention and treatment. The links between (*a*) and (*b*) are shown in Table 3.4 which summarizes some of the major advances in medical treatment and prevention in so far as they affect six of the great killing infectious diseases.

3.4.3 Treatment versus Prevention

Nature of the Hypotheses

The enhanced role of medical technology in the present century allows some light to be thrown on the relative roles of treatment and prevention in disease reduction.

1. The *treatment hypothesis* states that mortality decline arises from improvements in the treatment of patients who are unfortunate enough to succumb to a particular disease, so preventing them from dying from the disease. Thus we should expect the improved treatment of a disease to be marked by a reduction in the number of cases which become deaths. This may be assessed by computing a (scaled) case–fatality ratio: here we use the reported number of deaths per 1,000 reported cases. A time-series plot of this case–fatality ratio should have a declining trend under the treatment hypothesis.

2. The *prevention hypothesis* states that mortality decline arises from those conditions which prevent cases of the disease arising in the first place; a decline

Table 3.4. Some major twentieth-century microbiological advances with implications for six marker diseases (diphtheria, enteric fever, measles, scarlet fever, tuberculosis, and whooping cough)

Date(s)	Event	Discoverer and/or Developer	Disease implications
1906–21	BCG Vaccine	Calmette, Guerin	Method for immunizing children against tuberculosis
1907	Scarlet fever serum	Moser Garbritchewsky	Serum from horses immunized with cultures of streptococci for scarlet fever immunization
1908	Tuberculin tests	Mantoux	Diagnostic tests for recognizing tuberculosis
1914–18	Anti-typhoid vaccine	Wight and Semple	Successful deployment of anti-typhoid vaccine first developed in 1897
1918	Antibodies in measles convalescents	Nicolle	Sero-prevention and sero-attenuation in measles
1923	Toxoid for immunization	Glenny and Hopkins	Use of toxoid for human immunization against diphtheria
1924	Test for scarlet fever	Dick and Dick	Dick test to determine susceptibility of a subject to scarlet fever
1928	Penicillin	Fleming	Treatment of diphtheria and scarlet fever
1933	Whooping cough vaccine	Madsen	Trials in Faroe Islands of whooping cough vaccine: only slight influence on prevalence but decreased severity of attack
1943	Streptomycin	Waksman	Antibiotic treatment of tuberculosis
1944	Human immune serum globulin	Cohn	Measles
1948	Chloramphenicol		Antibiotic for typhoid fever treatment; resistant strains since early 1970 caused switch to other antibiotics
1952	Isoniazid	Robitzek and Selikoff	Treatment of tuberculosis
1954	Measles virus	Enders and Peebles	Isolation of measles virus
1955	Cycloserine		Treatment of tuberculosis
1963	Measles vaccine licensed	Enders, Katz, and Milanovic	Licensing of attenuated live virus produced by Enders and colleagues in 1958

Source: Cliff *et al.* (1998, table 7.3, pp. 346–7).

in mortality automatically follows. The preventive conditions may include both medical factors (e.g. vaccination) and non-medical (e.g. reduced virulence, improved social conditions, diet, knowledge). Successful prevention of cases of a disease should be reflected in a decline in the number of reported cases per unit of population. We capture this here by studying the number of reported cases per 100,000 population.

We now consider how the importance of these two classes of factors—treatment and prevention—in accounting for mortality decline may be assessed. We take the indices defined above and apply them to two case studies: (i) changes in measles mortality in a single country (the United States, 1960–88) and (ii) changes in mortality from four diseases (diphtheria, measles, scarlet fever, and whooping cough) in four developed countries (Australia, Ireland, Japan, and the United States) between 1930 and 1990.

Case Study I: Measles in the United States, 1960–1988

To provide a benchmark for testing the two hypotheses, we have graphed in Figure 3.11 the annual crude mortality rate for measles alongside the case–fatality ratio (a measure of the treatment hypothesis) and incidence (a measure

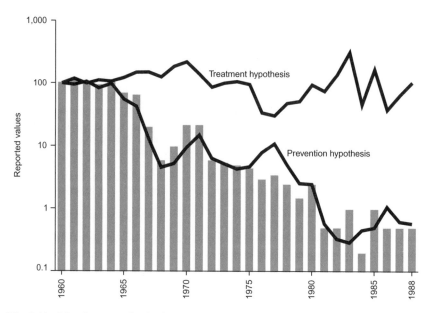

Fig. 3.11. Measles mortality in the United States, 1960–1988

Notes: Time trends in indices of the treatment and prevention hypotheses (line traces) benchmarked against the crude reported death rate (histogram). For plotting purposes, the series have been expressed as index numbers (1960 = 100).
Source: Cliff *et al.* (1998, fig. 7.15, p. 351).

of the prevention hypothesis). Because the three time series are in radically different units, they have been converted to index numbers (1960 = 100), and a log scale has been used for the vertical axis. The implication of the log scale is that deaths from measles per unit of population (bar graph) fell exponentially over the period, and this trend is followed faithfully by the line trace for cases per 100,000 population (prevention hypothesis). In contrast, the time series for deaths per 1,000 cases (treatment hypothesis) oscillates about a constant mean over the period. We conclude that there is prima facie evidence to suggest that the prevention of cases of measles in the population achieved more than treatment of actual cases in contributing to the decline of measles mortality in the United States over this period.

Case Study II: Diphtheria, Measles, Scarlet Fever and Whooping Cough in Four Developed Countries, 1930–1990

To extend our evaluation of the treatment and prevention hypotheses as possible explanations of twentieth-century trends in mortality, we took yearly data from WHO's *World Health Statististics Annual* (and its precursors) for the period 1930–90 on reported deaths, cases, and total populations for four countries (Australia, Ireland, Japan, and United States) and for four of our marker diseases—diphtheria, measles, scarlet fever, and whooping cough. The choice of countries and the absence of enteric fever and tuberculosis were dictated solely by data availability. As described earlier in this section, the raw data were used to construct annual time series for prevention, treatment, and crude deaths for each disease and country.

To check for possible time changes in the relative importance of treatment and prevention over the 60-year period, each time series was divided into a series of ten-year windows (1930–9; 1940–9; 1950–9; 1960–9; 1970–9; 1980–9). For each window, disease, and country, we computed the simple Pearson correlation coefficient between (i) deaths per million population and deaths per 1,000 cases (treatment), and (ii) deaths per million population and cases per 100,000 population (prevention); this yielded potentially 144 correlation coefficients for study. We regarded ten-year windows as the absolute minimum size for which it was reasonable to calculate correlations. We would have preferred bigger windows but, even at this size, randomly occurring missing observations meant that in practice our potential 144 coefficients were reduced to only 26 with a full complement of data and these we used for further work.

Given the way the analysis has been structured, a positive influence of either prevention or treatment upon death rates will yield a positive correlation coefficient. Figure 3.12 plots the results obtained. The correlations defined in the previous paragraph were used as x (treatment) and y (prevention) coordinates to plot each time window/disease/country observation in Figure 3.12A; the disease information associated with each point has been retained. Figures 3.12B and 3.12C have been derived from Figure 3.12A. In Figure 3.12B, the average coordinate position of each time window irrespective of disease and country is

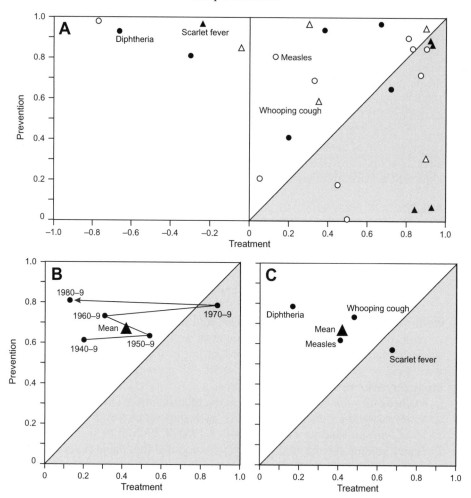

Fig. 3.12. Time changes in mortality from four diseases (diphtheria, measles, scarlet fever, and whooping cough), 1930–1990, attributable to prevention and treatment

Notes: (A) Scattergram of diseases on measures of prevention and treatment irrespective of time window and geographical location. (B) Average prevention/treatment position by time periods. (C) Average prevention/treatment position by disease. Shaded regions mark chart areas in which the treatment hypothesis is more important than the prevention hypothesis.
Source: Cliff *et al.* (1998, fig. 7.16, p. 352).

recorded, along with the grand mean over all 26 observations. In Figure 3.12C, the average coordinate position of each disease, ignoring time window and country is plotted, along with the grand mean. The 45° line marks equality between the treatment and prevention hypotheses. Below the line (shaded), treatment is more important than prevention and vice versa.

Figure 3.12B shows that it was only in the decade 1970–9 that treatment was more important than prevention, and then only by a small margin. The vectors linking the points show that, over this 60-year period, the evidence in favour of the prevention rather than the treatment hypothesis systematically strengthened. Figure 3.12C indicates that this was true for three of the four diseases studied. The exception was scarlet fever and, given the period studied here, Lancaster's work (1990: 114-15) suggests why (cf. earlier in this section): 'The decline in death rates from scarlet fever has occurred in many countries; it cannot be ascribed to progress in medical science, with the possible exception of the improvement about 1940 that may have been partly due to the use of the sulphonamide drugs.'

Summary

We recognize the provisional nature of our attempt to assess the relative importance of prevention as opposed to treatment (or, as Lancaster describes it, 'progess in medical science') in accounting for post-1930 trends in mortality decline. In particular, our analysis suffers from sample-size limitations in terms of countries and time periods. But the preliminary evidence is consistent: prevention has been better than cure in reducing mortality, a truism that has increased in force over the course of the century.

3.4.4 Impact of War

We noted in Section 3.3 that, within the long-term decline in mortality from infectious diseases, the traditional killers rapidly returned to cause excess mortality in times of war. Taking Europe as an example, Alderson (1981: 13–42) identifies four dimensions to war-induced mortality:

(*a*) the identification of the military who are killed (primarily fit males aged 15 to 40);

(*b*) the number of civilians killed (of much greater and major importance in World War II than in World War I);

(*c*) the forced migration that occurs during and after a war;

(*d*) major alterations in national boundaries (particularly marked after World War I which resulted in the delineation of new countries).

While the assocation of disease with refugee populations is explored fully in Chapter 5, Figure 3.13 gives some idea of the potential impact of (*c*) and (*d*) on the spread of disease. The map shows the complex mass population movements that took place in Europe between 1944 and 1951 as a result of the new political regimes and boundaries that emerged in the aftermath of World War II. Large numbers of ethnic Germans moved into West Germany from Poland, Czechoslovakia, and Hungary. With other refugees, these totalled some 8 million by 1950. Ogden (1984: 37) quotes an estimate of 25 million as the number of people who moved during and after World War II. Lest these figures be

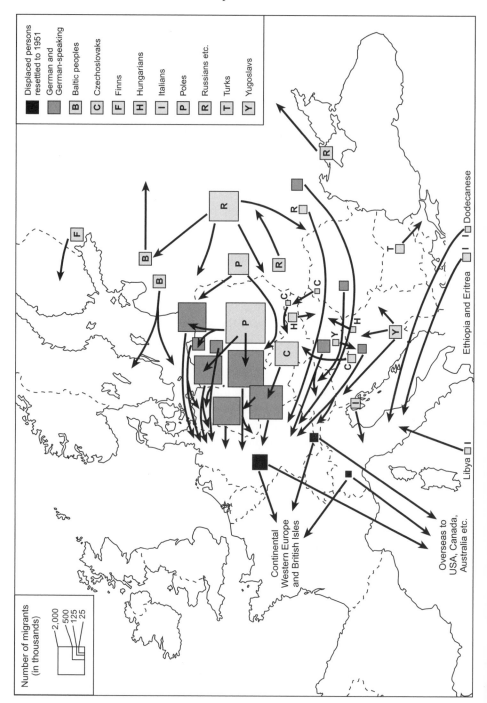

thought wholly exceptional, other wars of the twentieth century caused similar massive population fluxes: World War I led to a movement of nearly 8 million people, while a somewhat smaller move (3 million) accompanied the Spanish Civil War.

3.5 The Changing Disease Environment

In looking at the changing picture of disease in civil populations since 1850, it is important to look also at the factors which are shaping the geographical patterns of all diseases, both old and emerging, at the start of the new millennium. This section is based upon Cliff *et al.* (1998: 7–12).

3.5.1 The Demographic Impact of Diseases

Despite decades of research and data collection, establishing the precise impact of diseases, especially the infectious, at the world level remains difficult. Here we take our figures from the World Health Organization's (WHO) *World Health Report 1995* (World Health Organization, 1995a), although we recognize that the figures given there can be little more than rough estimates.

INTERNATIONAL ESTIMATES

There are several ways in which an estimate may be made. One approach to measuring the demographic impact of diseases is through the deaths they cause—the mortality approach. Despite the long-term decline in the importance of infectious diseases as causes of mortality, Table 3.5 shows that infectious diseases still occupy half of the top ten places as global killers. Taken together, infectious diseases and parasites take 16.4 million lives a year, ahead of heart disease which kills 9.7 million. Table 3.5 also shows that another way to measure disease is through disease incidence—the number of new cases of a disease each year. Again, the table illustrates the still-dominant position of infectious diseases (but note that the figures here are in 100,000s compared to 1,000s for deaths). Diarrhoea in children under 5 accounts for 1.8 billion

---

Fig. 3.13. Migrations in Europe, 1944–1951

Notes: The aftermath of war and new political regimes and boundaries provoked complex population movements. Particularly marked is the movement into West Germany of ethnic Germans from Poland, Czechoslovakia, and Hungary, and of many other refugees who totalled some 8 million by 1950.
Source: Ogden (1984, fig. 3.1, p.36).

Table 3.5. Communicable diseases as part of the global health situation (1993 estimates)

Rank	Deaths Disease/condition	Deaths no. (thousands)	Incidence Disease/condition	Cases no. (hundred thousands)
1	Ischaemic heart diseases	4,283	Diarrhoea under age 5, including dysentery[2]	18,210
2	Acute lower respiratory infections under age 5[1]	4,110	Acute lower respiratory infections under age 5[2]	2,483
3	Cerebrovascular disease	3,854	Occupational injuries due to accidents	1,200
4	Diarrhoea under age 5, including dysentery	3,010	Chlamydial infections (sexually transmitted)	970
5	Chronic obstructive pulmonary diseases	2,888	Trichomoniasis	940
6	Tuberculosis	2,709	Gonococcal infections	780
7	Malaria	2,000	Occupational diseases	690
8	Falls, fires, drowning, etc.	1,810	Measles	452
9	Measles	1,160	Whooping cough	431
10	Other heart diseases	1,133	Genital warts	320

Notes: [1] Estimates for some diseases may contain cases that have also been included elsewhere; for example, estimates for acute lower respiratory infections and diarrhoea include those associated with measles, pertussis, malaria, and HIV. [2] Estimates refer to number of episodes.
Source: Cliff *et al.* (1998, table 1.2, p. 8), from World Health Organization (1995*a*, table 1, p. 3).

episodes a year (and claims the lives of 3 million children). Acute lower respiratory conditions in children, sexually transmitted diseases, measles, and whooping cough remain major problems.

Another way of measuring the disease burden is in terms of prevalence—the total number of people with a given condition—or the burden of disability that a disease causes. Global figures are hard to find and we know all too little about some major infectious diseases. Notwithstanding the long-term decline in mortality and morbidity from communicable diseases, such fragments of information as we have at the world scale underscore their continuing importance: for example, schistosomiasis has a prevalence of some 200 million cases on a worldwide scale, while 10 million are permanently disabled by paralytic poliomyelitis.

NATIONAL ESTIMATES

An alternative approach to estimating the size of the disease burden is to use figures for a single country. For the United States, the Centers for Disease Control and Prevention (CDC) believe that 83 per cent of all deaths from infections occur outside the 'classic' ICD disease codes 1 to 113: infections and infection-related deaths are important contributors to circulatory, respiratory, and gastrointestinal disease, to infant mortality and morbidity, and to arthritis. Infections complicate a wide range of injuries and have been found to cause malignancies in humans (Bennett *et al.*, 1987).

It is thus difficult to obtain a clear statistical picture of the real role of infectious diseases in causing mortality and morbidity. For this reason, the Carter Center Health Policy Project reworked the available statistics for the United States and compared these with CDC Survey Data to provide a revised estimate of the effects of infectious diseases on morbidity and mortality. They concluded that 740 million symptomatic infections occur annually in the United States, causing 200,000 deaths per year. Such infections resulted in more than $17 billion annually in direct costs, not including costs of deaths, lost wages and productivity, and other indirect costs. About 63,000 deaths are currently prevented annually and a further 80,000 deaths could be prevented by using current or soon-to-be available interventions.

Figure 3.14 summarizes the Carter Center findings. This plots on logarithmic scales the number of deaths and number of cases for the main infectious diseases. Note that only diseases causing more than ten deaths or more than 1,000 cases per year are shown. The largest number of deaths (32,000) are caused by pneumoccocal bacteria, followed by nosocomial deaths in acute (26,400) and chronic care (24,700). In terms of morbidity, the largest number

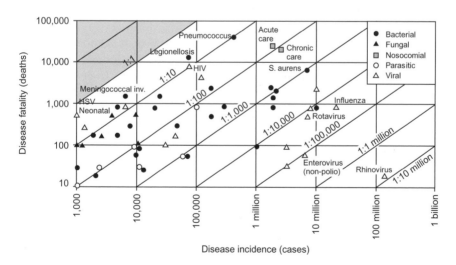

Fig. 3.14. Annual mortality and morbidity from major infectious and parasitic diseases in the United States in the mid-1980s

Notes: Note that both disease fatality and disease incidence are plotted on logarithmic scales. The diagonal lines represent the fatality-case ratio.

Source: Drawn from data in Bennett *et al.* (1987: 102–10; table 1, pp. 104–7).

of cases are generated by the rhinovirus (125 million) that causes the common cold, followed by another group of viruses, influenza (20 million).

The figure illustrates only the leading 56 of the 117 specific infections considered in the Carter Center study. Although those not shown have fewer than ten deaths per year or fewer than 1,000 cases, they include many diseases which rank highly on the 'dread' factor. For example, amoebic meningoencephalitis was recorded only four times in the United States in the year studied, but each resulted in death: rabies killed all ten of those infected, while half of the 100 cases infected with the cryptosporidiosis parasite died. The case-to-fatality ratio is marked by the diagonal lines in Figure 3.14 for the more frequently occurring diseases. Those on or above the 1:10 diagonal include HIV, legionellosis, meningococcal invasions, and neonatal HSV.

3.5.2 *The Increasing Range of Communicable Diseases*

In 1917, the American Public Health Association published the first edition of its pioneer handbook on *Control of Communicable Diseases in Man* (Benensen, 1990). It listed control measures for 38 communicable diseases, all those then officially reported in the United States. Since 1917, the number listed has expanded steadily, so that the fifteenth edition of the handbook details some 280 different diseases. Examples of some of these emerging diseases are given later in Table 9.1.

One of the disease groups that has shown the sharpest increase is that of the arboviruses (*ar*thropod-*bo*rne viruses). In 1930, only six viruses were known to be maintained in cycles between animal hosts and arthropod vectors like mosquitoes, gnats, and ticks. Only one of these, yellow fever, was known to cause disease in humans, although the other five caused epizootics and major economic loss in domestic animals (e.g. African swine fever). Over the last 60 years, the number of arboviruses recognized has leapt from six to 504 worldwide (Lederberg *et al.*, 1992). One-quarter of these are associated with viral diseases. North America alone now has around 90 different arboviruses and these include a few consistently associated with human disease: Colorado tick fever, California encephalitis, and dengue fever.

Most of the 'new' viruses discovered have probably existed for centuries, escaping detection because they existed in remote or medically little-studied populations or because they produced disease symptoms not previously identified as being due to infectious agents. As with Marburg disease, they are recognized when they impinge on middle-latitude rather than tropical populations. Improvements in viral detection technology and in particular the invention of the polymerase chain reaction (PMR) method have opened up new frontiers in biology and medicine. It seems likely that the disease list will expand as links between previously unnoticed slow viral infections and chronic conditions (these include neurological problems and cancers) are unravelled.

3.5.3 Environmental Change and Disease Control

Diseases spread in a specific historical and geographical context. In the twenty-first century, the environmental context within which disease control is set is evolving at a faster rate than at any time in human history. Again, some of the geographical changes that have disease implications are summarized later in Table 9.1. We illustrate here the impact of four factors: (1) demographic growth and migration of the host population, (2) the collapse of geographical space, (3) global land-use changes, and (4) global warming.

RAPID GROWTH AND RELOCATION OF THE HUMAN POPULATION

Whatever the rate of past disease emergence, there are reasons to consider the present time as one of special significance for the human host population. Figure 3.15A shows the historical pattern of growth in the human population from 1750, with a forward projection to 2100. Three aspects of this change call for comment. First, the rapid acceleration in growth is very recent. In the past few decades, the world's population has more than doubled, from 2.5 billion in 1950 to 5 billion in 1988. On the United Nations' 'medium-growth' assumptions, this total is expected to reach 6.3 billion by the end of the twentieth century and 8.5 billion by the year 2025 (Sadik, 1991). Although that rate of growth is now decelerating (its peak was at 2.1% p.a. in the quinquennium from 1965 to 1970) the multiplier of resource use per capita continues to increase, with evident environmental implications.

Secondly, a geographical redistribution of world population is accompanying this growth. For example, it is expected that some 94 per cent of population growth over the next 20 years will occur in the developing countries. Figure 3.15B illustrates the present geographical distribution of population, with its marked concentration in northern mid-latitudes. Present and future growth will shift the balance of world population towards the tropics and low latitudes. As a result of this shift, Haggett (1991) has estimated that the average temperature experienced by the global population will rise by around +1°C, from 17°C to 18°C. Figure 3.15B also shows that this latitudinal shift in the concentration of population will place more people than at any time in the world's previous history in areas of high microbiological diversity, potentially exposing a greater share of the world's population to conventional tropical diseases.

Thirdly, the world's growing population is increasingly concentrated in cities. In 1800, less than 2 per cent of the world's population lived in urban communities. By 1970, this had risen to one-third and, by the start of the present millennium, the fraction is estimated to have reached one-half. Along with the increasing proportion of urban population, the number of large cities and their average density has also increased. On United Nations' estimates, the number of cities with a million or more inhabitants increased from 200 in 1985 to 425 by the end of the twentieth century. At that date there were estimated to be 25 cities with populations in excess of 11 million.

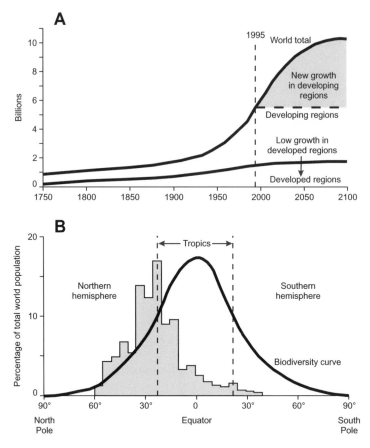

Fig. 3.15. Global population growth

Notes: (A) Course of global population growth for the period from 1750 and projected forward to 2100. (B) Geographical distribution of population distribution (histogram) in terms of 5-degree latitudinal bands north and south of the equator. The biodiversity curve is approximate and does not make allowances for the global distribution of humidity.
Source: Cliff *et al.* (1998, fig. 7.17, p. 355), from Haggett (1995).

    The disease implications of urbanization are complex (Williams, 1989). Positive effects from improved sanitation or better access to health-care facilities have to be set against the negative effects from increased risk of disease contacts through crowding and pollution. Crompton and Savioli (1993) have shown that where rural–urban migration in developing countries results in peri-urban shanty settlements, high rates of intestinal parasitic infections (notably amoebiasis, giardiasis, ascariasis, and trichuriasis) can result. Each are common intestinal infections caused by protozoan parasites or helminths transferred from human to human by the faecal–oral route. They pose an increasing health burden as the share of urban population in developing countries rises towards one-half of all population. In a long-term historical context, Haggett (1992) has indicated that the aggregation of human populations into high-density urban 'islands' has had important effects in providing the host reservoirs necessary to maintain infection chains for many diseases. The implications of urbanization for measles have been discussed by Cliff *et al.* (1993: 7, 47–8) and, for a wide range of other infectious diseases, by Fine (1993).

THE COLLAPSE OF GEOGRAPHICAL SPACE

The second main environmental change has come from the collapse (in terms of both time and cost) of geographical space, and the increased spatial mobility of the human population which has accompanied this collapse. We look first at the evidence for such change and then at its disease implications.

1. *Changes in travel patterns.* The manner in which travel patterns have changed for the host population over recent generations has been illustrated in an interesting way by the distinguished epidemiologist, D. J. Bradley. Bradley (1988) has compared the travel patterns of his great-grandfather, his grandfather, his father, and himself. The life-time travel track of his great-grandfather around a village in Northamptonshire could be contained within a square of only 40 km side. His grandfather's map was still limited to southern England, but it now ranged as far as London and could easily be contained within a square of 400 km side. If we compare these maps with those of Bradley's father (who travelled widely in Europe) and Bradley's own sphere of travel, which is worldwide, then the enclosing square has to be widened to sides of 4,000 km and 40,000 km respectively. In broad terms, the spatial range of travel has increased tenfold in each generation, so that Bradley's own range is one thousand times wider than that of his great-grandfather.

Against this individual cameo, we can set some general statistical trends from recent years. One indicator of the dramatic increase in spatial mobility is shown in Figure 3.16. This plots for France over a 200-year period the average number of kilometres travelled daily both by transport mode and by all modes. Since the vertical scale is logarithmic the graph shows that, despite changes in the mode used, average travel has increased exponentially, a trend broken only by the two world wars. Over the whole period, mobility has increased by more than 1,000. The precise rates of flux or travel of population both within and between countries are difficult to catch in official statistics. But most available evidence suggests that the flux over the last few decades has increased at an accelerating rate. While the world population growth rate since the middle of this century has been running at between 1.5 and 2.5 per cent per annum, the growth in international movements of passengers across national boundaries has been between 7.5 and 10 per cent per annum. One striking example is provided by Australia: over the last four decades its resident population has

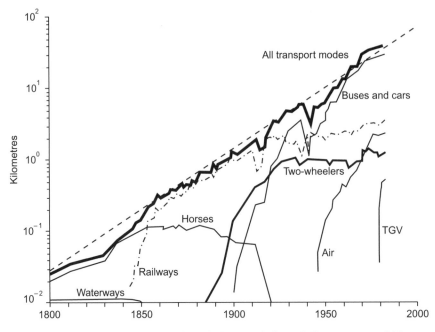

Fig. 3.16. Increased spatial mobility of the population of France over a 200-year period, 1800–2000

Notes: Curves give the average kilometres travelled daily by mode. Note that the vertical scale is logarithmic so that increases in average travel distance increase exponentially over time.
Source: Cliff *et al.* (1998, fig. 7.18, p. 358) and Haggett (1994, fig. 7.4, p. 101), based on data in Grubler and Nakicenovic (1991).

doubled, while the movement of people across its international boundaries (i.e. into and out of Australia) has increased nearly one hundred fold.

2. *Disease implications of increased travel.* The implications of increased travel are twofold: short-term and long-term. First, an immediate and important effect is the exposure of the travelling public to a range of diseases not encountered in their home country. The relative risks met in tropical areas by travellers coming from western countries (data mainly from North America and Western Europe) have been estimated by the World Health Organization (1995*b*: 56) and are illustrated in Figure 3.17. These suggest a spectrum of risks from unspecified 'traveller's diarrhoea' (a high risk of 20%) to paralytic poliomyelitis (a very low risk of less than 0.001%). Another way in which international aircraft from the tropics can cause the spread of disease to a non-indigenous area is seen in the occasional outbreaks of tropical diseases around mid-latitude airports. Typical are the malaria cases that appeared within 2 km of a Swiss airport, Geneva–Cointrin, in the summer of 1989 (Bouvier *et al.*, 1990). Cases occurred in late summer when high temperatures allowed the in-

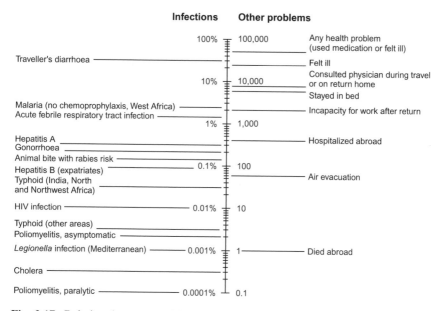

Fig. 3.17. Relative threats posed by communicable diseases to travellers in tropical areas

Note: The scale is logarithmic.
Source: Redrawn from World Health Organization (1995*b*, fig. 7.1, p. 56).

flight survival of infected *anopheles* mosquitoes that had been inadvertently introduced into the aircraft while at an airport in a malarious area. The infected mosquitoes escaped when the aircraft landed at Geneva to cause malaria cases among several local residents, none of whom had visited a malarious country.

A second short-term factor with modern aircraft is their increasing size. Bradley (1988) postulates a hypothetical situation in which a person in the travelling population is assumed to have a chance of 1 in 10,000 of being in the infectious stage of a given communicable disease. With a 200-seat aircraft, the probability of having an infected passenger on board (x) is 0.02 and the number of potential contacts (y) is 199. If we assume homogeneous mixing, this gives a combined risk factor (xy) of 3.98. If we double the aircraft size to 400 passengers, then the corresponding figures are $x = 0.04$, $y = 399$, and $xy = 15.96$. In other words, *ceteris paribus*, doubling the aircraft size increases the risk from the flight fourfold. Thus the new generation of wide-bodied jets presents fresh possibilities for disease spread, not only through their flying range and their speed, but also from their size.

On a longer time-scale, increased travel brings some possible long-term genetic effects. With more travel and longer-range migration, there is an enhanced probability of partnerships being formed and reproduction arising from unions between individuals from formerly distant populations. As Khlat and Khoury (1991) have shown, this can bring advantages from the viewpoint of some diseases. For example, the probability of occurrence of conditions such as cystic fibrosis or spinal muscular atrophy is reduced; the risk of these is somewhat higher in children of consanguineous unions. Conversely, inherited disorders such as sickle cell anaemia may become more widely dispersed.

CHANGING GLOBAL LAND USE

The combination of population growth and technological change has given mankind the capacity to alter environments in ways which are unprecedented in human history. We illustrate the disease implications of three such changes.

1. *Agricultural colonization.* Accelerated world population growth has put pressure on food supplies in tropical areas and has led to the colonization of new environments in the search for expanded food production. Venezuelan haemorrhagic fever is a severe and often fatal zoonotic virus disease only recently identified in the Guanarito area in central Venezuela. Cases were not found in the cities but were confined to rural inhabitants of the area who were largely engaged in farming or cattle ranching. Major outbreaks in 1989 and again in 1990–1 had fatality rates of around one-quarter. First diagnosed as due to dengue haemorrhagic fever, the disease is now known to be due to a separate virus, named the Guaranito virus, which is associated with rodent reservoirs.

Guaranito appears to be one of a family of arenaviruses known to cause haemorrhagic fevers in humans. They include the Junin and Machupo viruses, the cause of haemorrhagic fever outbreaks in Argentina and Bolivia. In each case, transfer appears to be from a wild rodent host (*Akodon azarae* and *Calomys musculinus* in Argentina and *C. callosus* in Bolivia); the main risk of transfer occurs during the corn-harvesting season. Similar seasonal risks from epidemics of haemorrhagic fevers are associated with the family of Hantaan viruses in China which appear to be spread to humans during the rice harvest. Field mice, rats, and bank voles are involved in fever transmission in different parts of the world (see Sect. 9.4.2).

2. *Deforestation and reforestation.* Changes in the global forest cover also appear to be linked to disease changes. The deforestation of the tropical rain forests has been spatially complex, with a fern-like pattern of new logging roads being driven into the forests to abstract the highest-quality timber. New settlers following the logging roads into Amazonia encountered heavy malarial infections. This is partly because the land-use changes have greatly increased the forest-edge environments suitable for certain mosquito species.

Disease changes can also result from an opposite process in which abandoned farmland reverts to woodland. The classic case is the emergence of Lyme disease, caused by the spirochetal bacterium *Borrelia burgorferi* (Schmid,

1985). Lyme disease is now the most common vector-borne disease in the United States, but retrospective studies suggest it was not reported there until 1962 in the Cape Cod area of New England. The link between Lyme disease and 'Lyme arthritis' was not established until the 1970s, when an endemic focus was recognized around Old Lyme in south-central Connecticut. The critical land-use change which precipitated the emergence or re-emergence of the disease appears to have been the abandonment of farmland fields to woodland growth. The new woodland proved an ideal habitat for deer populations, the definitive host for certain Ixodes ticks which spread the bacterium through bites. The complex seasonal cycle of the vectors, which involves the ticks, the deer, the white-footed mouse (the reservoir for the pathogen), and human visitors using the forest, illustrates how sensitive is the ecological balance in which disease and environment is held. Epidemic Lyme disease is now a growing problem in Europe, fuelled by reversion of farmland to woodland (partly due to EU set-aside land policies), deer proliferation, and increased recreational use of forested areas. Lyme disease has now been reported from most temperate parts of the world in both northern and southern hemispheres.

3. *Water control and irrigation.* Until recently, Rift Valley fever was primarily a disease of sheep and cattle. It was confined to Africa south of the Sahara, with periodic outbreaks in East Africa, South Africa, and, in the mid-1970s, the Sudan. The first major outbreak as a human disease occurred in Egypt in 1977 when there were 200,000 cases and 600 deaths; the deaths were usually associated with acute haemorrhagic fever and hepatitis.

The Egyptian epidemic has been provisionally linked to the construction of the Aswan Dam on the Nile. Completed in 1970, the dam created an 800,000-hectare water body and stabilized water tables so that its surface water provided breeding sites for mosquitoes. Whether the mosquito population provided a corridor that allowed the virus to enter Egypt from the southern Sudan has yet to be proved. But the possibility led to concern for the epidemiological implications of other dam-building schemes in the African tropics. Completion of the Diama dam on the Senegal River in 1987 was followed by a severe outbreak of Rift Valley fever upstream of the new dam. Over 1,200 cases and 244 deaths resulted. But, in contrast to Egypt, immunological studies demonstrated that Rift Valley fever was already endemic in people and livestock in a wide area of the Senegal River basin. Ecological changes favouring the vector and associated with dam building seem to be implicated in allowing both (i) invasion of the virus into a previously virgin population and (ii) severe flare-ups in a population with low-level endemicity.

GLOBAL WARMING

Of the many global scenarios for disease and the environment in the early part of the twenty-first century, it is the health implications of global warming that has caught the attention of governments and press worldwide. There have already been major studies of this issue in at least three countries: the United States (Smith and Tirpak, 1989), Australia (Ewan *et al.*, 1990), and the United Kingdom (Bannister, 1991). The World Health Organization also has a committee looking at the topic.

It has been postulated that a number of health effects will follow from a worldwide increase in average temperature from global warming. For infectious diseases, the main effects relate to changes in the geographical range of pathogens, vectors, and reservoirs. So far, few attempts have been made to compute the relative burden of morbidity and mortality that would be yielded by these effects. Any such calculation would also need to offset losses against gains that might accrue (e.g. reductions in hypothermia against increases in hyperthermia).

The magnitude and spatial manifestations of global warming are still speculative. One of the main conclusions of the report of the Intergovernmental Panel on Climate Change (IPCC) in 1990 was how far research still had to go before reliable estimates of global warming could be made. But some rough orders of magnitude can be computed from the estimates of the different models that have been used. In global terms, warming appears to range from '. . . a predicted rise from 1990 to the year 2030 of 0.7°C to 1.5°C with a best estimate of 1.1°C' (Intergovernmental Panel on Climatic Change, 1990).

We can obtain some idea of the implications of the predicted shift for local mean temperatures with reference to the United Kingdom. Current differences between the coldest (Aberdeen, latitude 57.10°N.) and warmest (Portsmouth, latitude 50.48°N.) of its major cities is 2.4°C; this is well beyond the postulated IPCC warming effect by the year 2030. Climate is a much more complex matter than average temperature, but—if the global warming models carry over to the UK—then, by 2030, Edinburgh might have temperatures something like those of the English Midlands and London something like those of the Loire valley in central France. If we accept the much higher estimate of +4.8°C warming over 80 years, this brings London into the temperature bands of southern France and northern Spain. Provided that these projections are sensible, something might be gained by comparative studies of disease incidence within the UK and adjacent EU countries, and disease incidence in warmer climates that match those predicted for the UK.

The biological diversity of viruses and bacteria is partly temperature dependent, and it is much greater in lower than higher latitudes (see Fig. 3.15). Conditions of higher temperature would favour the expansion of malarious areas, not just for the more adaptable *Plasmodium vivax* but also for *P. falciparum*. Rising temperatures might also allow the expansion of the endemic areas of other diseases of human importance: these include, for example, leishmaniasis and arboviral infections such as dengue and yellow fever. Higher temperatures also favour the rapid replication of food-poisoning organisms. Warmer climates might also encourage the number of people going barefoot in poorer countries, thereby increasing exposure to hookworms, schistosomes, and Guinea worm infections. But not all effects would be negative. Warmer external air temperatures might reduce the degree of indoor crowding and lower the transmission of influenza, pneumonias, and 'winter' colds.

While modest rises in average temperatures are the central and most probable of any greenhouse effects, they are likely to be accompanied by three other main changes: (*a*) sea level rises of up to a metre: (*b*) increased seasonality in rainfall, thus reducing the level of water available for summer use; and (*c*) storm frequency increases (Henderson-Sellars and Blong, 1989).

3.6 Controlling Epidemic Spread

Efforts to prevent the spatial spread of communicable diseases lie deep in human history. While archaeological evidence from Peru to China provides evidence only of disease control by extensive civil engineering works (to supply safe water and to dispose of human and animal wastes) later historical accounts show increasing concerns about imported diseases. By the thirteenth century, most Italian cities were posting gatemen to identify potential sources of infection from visitors to the city. Venice, with its widespread trading links with the Levant and the Oriental lands beyond, pioneered the idea of quarantine. Its tiny Dalmatian colony, Ragusa (now Dubrovnik) saw the first recorded attempt, in 1377, to place a moratorium on travel and trade. Originally a 30-day waiting period (a *trentino*), it was widely adopted by port cities as a defence against the plague and was later extended to 40 days (a *quarantino*), the familiar quarantine period (Carmichael, 1993*c*: 198).

The steps by which the early Venetian quarantine measures were extended to become the International Quarantine Regulations of today have been outlined elsewhere (Roemer, 1993). Highlights included the earliest sanitary conference at Venice in 1576, the first International Sanitary Conference convened in Paris in 1851, and the formation of key international control bodies: the Pan American Sanitary Bureau (1902), the International Office of Public Hygiene (1907), the Health Section of the League of Nations (1922), and the World Health Organization (1946). For the medieval world, the main threat came from imported plague but, by the nineteenth century, it was concern about cholera and yellow fever that drove the need for regulations. Smallpox, louse-born typhus, and relapsing fever were not added to the international list of regulated diseases until 1922.

In this section, we examine the prime achievement of international public health in the twentieth century—the global eradication of smallpox—and ask how far this provides a model for the eradication of other communicable diseases. In conclusion, we note briefly some of the problems which are likely to affect disease control in the next few decades.

3.6.1 Global Control Programmes

When the epidemiological history of the twentieth century comes to be written, the outstanding success that historians will be able to record is the global eradication of smallpox. The complex story which culminated in the last recorded natural case in October 1977 (there were to be two subsequent laboratory deaths) has been superbly told and in massive detail by Fenner *et al.* (1988). The success has inevitably raised questions as to whether other infectious diseases, measles among them, can also be eradicated. We look briefly at the smallpox eradication programme and compare its success with the prospects for poliomyelitis.

THE GLOBAL ERADICATION OF SMALLPOX

Although the WHO has from time to time conducted major campaigns against infectious disease (notably malaria and yaws) only one disease—smallpox—has so far been globally eradicated. The practical reality of devising, coordinating, and financing a field programme involving more than 30 national governments, as well as some of the world's most complex cultures and demanding environments proved to be of heroic proportions. Until the mid-1960s, control of smallpox was based primarily upon mass vaccination to break the chain of transmission between infected and susceptible individuals by eliminating susceptible hosts. Although this approach had driven the disease from the developed world, the less developed world remained a reservoir area. Thus between 1962 and 1966, some 500 million people in India were vaccinated, but the disease continued to spread. Between 5 to 10 per cent of the population always escaped the vaccination drives, concentrated especially in the vulnerable under-15 age group. Nevertheless, the susceptibility of the virus to concerted action had been demonstrated and led to critical decisions at the Nineteenth World Health Assembly in 1966.

This Assembly embarked upon a ten-year global smallpox eradication programme which was launched in 1967. It started with mass vaccination, but rapidly recognized the importance of selective control. Contacts of smallpox cases were traced and vaccinated, as well as the other individuals in those locations where the cases occurred. The success of the four-phase programme (*preparatory*, *attack*, *consolidation*, and *maintenance*) may be judged from the maps and graph in Figure 3.18. By 1970, retreat was in progress in Africa. By 1973, the disease had been eliminated in Latin America and the Philippines; a few strongholds remained in Africa, but most of the Indian subcontinent remained infected. Despite a major flare-up of the disease in 1973 and 1974, the hunt by WHO for cases and case contacts continued. By 1976 the disease had been eradicated in Southeast Asia and only a part of East Africa remained to be cleared. The world's last recorded smallpox case was a 23-year-old man of Merka town, Somalia, on 26 October 1977. After a two-year period during which no other cases (other than laboratory accidents) were recorded, WHO

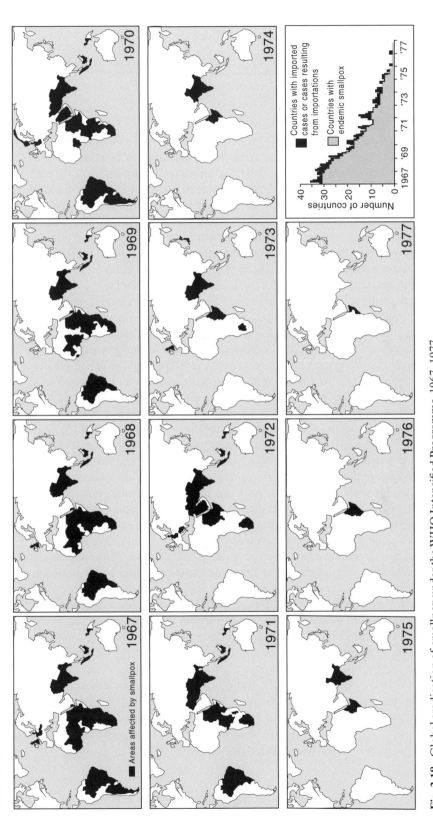

Fig. 3.18. Global eradication of smallpox under the WHO Intensified Programme, 1967–1977

Note: Countries with smallpox cases for the year in question marked in black.

Source: Cliff *et al.* (1998, fig. 7.25, p. 374), redrawn from Fenner *et al.* (1988, fig. 10.4 and pls. 10.42–10.51, pp. 516–37 *passim*).

formally announced at the end of 1979 that the global eradication of smallpox was complete.

THE POLIOMYELITIS ELIMINATION CAMPAIGN

The dramatic success of the WHO smallpox programme has inevitably raised the prospect and hope that other virus-borne diseases can be eradicated. In 1974, WHO established its Expanded Programme of Immunization (EPI) with the objective of greatly reducing the incidence of six other crippling diseases: diphtheria, measles, neonatal tetanus, pertussis, poliomyelitis, and tuberculosis (Pl. 3.1). Two further diseases (hepatitis B and yellow fever) were later added. As we have seen, these diseases are among the traditional killers of civil populations in times of peace and war. With the exception of yellow fever, Table 3.6 summarizes some of the characteristics of the diseases and indicates in the final two columns the continental variation in vaccination levels achieved to date for two areas of the world, Africa and Europe. Very high levels are being reached in Europe holding out the prospect of elimination of some diseases from these regions. Indeed, some countries, like Finland, are already free of measles.

Comprehensive reviews of the impact of such vaccination programmes upon world health appear in Cutts and Smith (1994) and in the WHO's *Immunization Policy* (Global Programme for Vaccines and Immunization, World Health Organization, 1995). An important consideration is how far smallpox is a useful control model for other communicable diseases. For, whatever the huge difficulties in practice, in principle smallpox was well suited (perhaps uniquely well suited) to global eradication: Fenner (1986) has summarized the special characteristics of smallpox which allowed global eradication. Fenner also recognized that the biological features of smallpox, while a necessary precondition for global eradication, were not in themselves sufficient to ensure success. For example, Fenner has demonstrated that the disease was economically significant in the West. Quite apart from the disease and death from smallpox itself, the cost of vaccination, plus that of maintaining quarantine barriers, is calculated to have been about $US1,000 million per annum in the last years of the virus's existence in the wild. These costs disappear completely if, and only if, *global* eradication is achieved.

Eleven years after the close of its successful smallpox campaign, the Forty-first World Health Assembly, meeting in Geneva in 1988, committed WHO to the global eradication of a second disease, poliomyelitis. Like smallpox, this target involves not only eliminating the disease, but totally eradicating the causative virus. The goal was made possible by 40 years of research and vaccine development since Enders, Weller, and Robbins succeeded in growing poliovirus in cell culture. The licensing of the Salk inactivated (1955) and Sabin attenuated live vaccine (1961) was reinforced by the early success of the countries of the Pan American Health Organization which had agreed in 1985 to eradicate the wild poliovirus from the Americas.

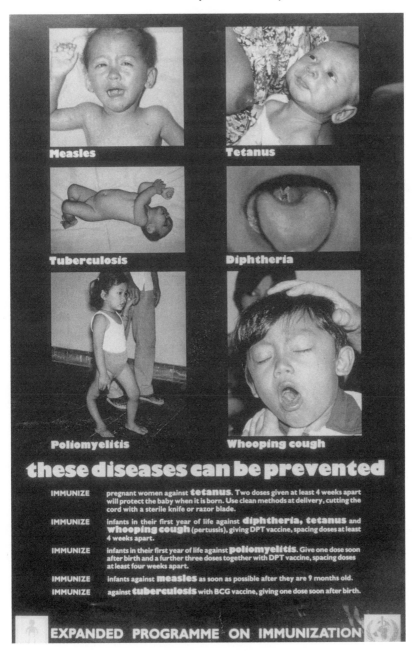

Pl. 3.1. The Expanded Programme on Immunization

Note: One of several posters produced by WHO to publicize its immunization campaign.
Source: Cliff *et al.* (1998, pl. 7.1, p. 377), courtesy of Dr John Clements, Expanded Programme of Immunization, World Health Organization, Geneva.

Table 3.6. Target diseases in the WHO Expanded Programme on Immunization

Disease	Infectious agent	Reservoir	Spread	Nature of vaccine	Form of vaccine (Doses)	Immunization coverage (%) Africa	Immunization coverage (%) Europe
Diphtheria	Toxin-producing bacterium (*C. diphtheriae*)	Humans	Close contact respiratory or cutaneous	Toxoid	Fluid (1)	50.0	86.0
Hepatitis B	Virus	Humans	Perinatal; child–child; blood; sexual spread	HBsAg	Fluid (3)	0.2	12.0
Measles	Virus	Humans	Close respiratory contact and aerosolized droplets	Attenuated live virus	Freeze-dried (1)	49.0	78.0
Pertussis	Bacterium (*B. pertussis*)	Humans	Close respiratory contact	Killed whole cell pertussis bacterium	Fluid (3)	50.0	86.0
Poliomyelitis	Virus (serotypes 1, 2, and 3)	Humans	Faecal–oral; close respiratory contact	Attenuated live viruses of 3 types	Fluid (4)	50.0	92.0
Tetanus (neonatal)	Toxin-producing bacterium (*Cl. tetani*)	Animal intestines; soil	Spores enter body through wounds, umbilical cord	Toxoid	Fluid (3)	35.0	N/A
Tuberculosis	*Mycobacterium tuberculosis*	Humans	Airborne droplet nuclei from sputum positive person	Attenuated *M. Bovis*	Freeze-dried (1)	68.0	81.0
Yellow fever	Virus	Humans; monkeys	Mosquito-borne	Attenuated live virus	Freeze-dried (1)	6.0	N/A

Note: Immunization coverage at March 1994. Africa excludes South Africa.
Source: Based on data in Global Programme for Vaccines and Immunization, World Health Organization (1995, tables 1–3, pp. 2–5).

The level of global success to the year 2000 is mapped in Figure 3.19. Figure 3.19A shades those countries in which wild poliovirus transmission was recorded in 1988, at the outset of the global eradication initiative, while Figure 3.19B shows the equivalent information for 2000. Figure 3.19 indicates that, by 2000, poliomyelitis had retreated from vast tracts of the globe. The WHO Americas Region was certified poliomyelitis free in 1994, to be followed by the Western Pacific Region in 2000 and, subsequently, the European Region in 2002. Elsewhere, however, tropical Africa and South Asia remained major zones of wild poliovirus transmission.

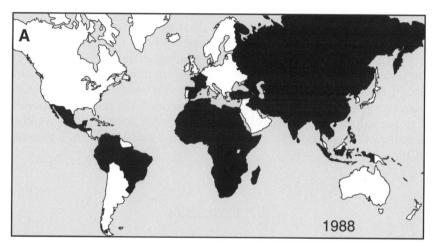

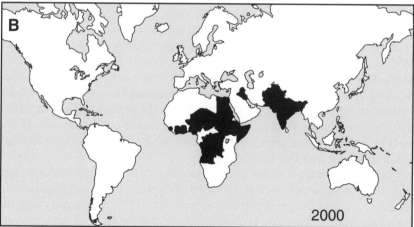

Fig. 3.19. Progress towards global poliomyelitis eradication, 1988–2000

Note: Shading has been used for those countries of the world in which wild poliovirus transmission was reported during (A) 1988 and (B) 2000.
Source: Redrawn from World Health Organization (2001, fig. 2, p. 9).

WHO has warned against complacency. Declining polio incidence mostly reflects individual protection from immunization, and not wild virus eradication, for although surveillance is improving, less than 15 per cent of cases are being officially reported. The global strategy has five components: (*a*) high immunization coverage with oral polio vaccine, (*b*) sensitive disease surveillance detecting all suspected cases of poliomyelitis, (*c*) national or subnational immunization days, (*d*) rapid, expertly managed outbreak response when suspected cases are detected, and (*e*) 'mopping-up' immunization in selected high-risk areas where wild virus transmission may persist.

The major cost of eradicating poliomyelitis will be borne by the endemic countries themselves but donor country support will be required for vaccine, laboratories, personnel, and research. Of these, the most urgent need is for vaccine: although each dose of oral vaccine currently costs only 7 US cents, over 2 billlion doses will be required per year for routine and mass immunization. In the longer run, the economic benefits of disease eradication far exceed the cost. Since its own last case in 1977, the United States has saved its total contribution once every 26 days. If present progress is maintained, the global initiative will start to pay for itself by the year 1998, and will produce savings of half a billion dollars by the year 2000. These savings will increase to US$3 billion annually by the year 2015.

3.7 Conclusion

In this chapter, we have examined trends in mortality and morbidity in the general population over the 150-year period since 1850. Infectious diseases were the most significant causes of mortality in the nineteenth century. In the developed world, these diseases have declined exponentially in significance since 1900 as the onslaught of improved treatments and vaccination has grown apace. As a consequence, although they are far from eradicated, they have been replaced by cancer, heart, and circulatory disorders as the main causes of death in these countries. In the developing countries, the picture is different. Infectious diseases remain of central importance as causes of death, although the story here is also one of retreat in the face of the World Health Organization's Expanded Programme of Immunization.

The historical impact of war upon disease in civil populations appears clear. With the breakdown of normal standards of hygiene, the frequent collapse of medical care, and the mass population movements that accompany war, the great infections of history—typhus, smallpox, yellow fever, plague, cholera, typhoid, and paratyphoid fever—along with sicknesses like measles and poliomyelitis, which are in abeyance and are strictly controlled in peacetime—rapidly re-establish themselves as major killers.

4

Mortality and Morbidity in Modern Wars, II: Military Populations

Two rows of cabbages,
Two of curly-greens,
Two rows of early peas,
Two of kidney-beans.

That's what he keeps muttering,
Making such a song,
Keeping other chaps awake
The whole night long.

Wilfred Gibson, 'In the Ambulance' (1916)

4.1 Introduction

In the previous chapter, we looked at the main trends in morbidity and mortality in civil populations since 1850. In this chapter our focus shifts to the military. An invaluable recent source of information on this topic is Lancaster

(1990: 314–40) who gives a disease-by-disease account of morbidity and mortality among soldiers from the seventeenth century. Until the twentieth century, soldiers were lucky to survive military medicine. Basic treatments included the cauterizing of wounds and the removal of limbs to prevent gangrene. The biggest early advances in military medicine came when doctors started to wash their hands. The role of Florence Nightingale in transforming the military hospitals during the Crimean War (1853–6), and her broader role in improving the welfare of the British Army, is legendary. Yet, notwithstanding the gigantic losses directly attributable to battle, up to World War I, most deaths in war among soldiers were caused by epidemic diseases like dysentery, enteric fever, cholera, typhus, plague, and simple infections like measles—the traditional killers encountered in civil populations. And, as with civil populations, the real advances in controlling these infections came with the development of antibiotics and vaccination after 1945.

In this chapter, we begin by looking at mortality trends in a number of theatres of war between 1859 and 1914 using data from Curtin (1989). As a specific illustration of the role of one simple infectious disease, measles, as a cause of mortality in military camps during this period, we take the American Civil War (1861–5). By the end of World War I in 1918, the role of many infectious diseases as causes of military mortality and morbidity had changed from lethal to nuisance value. This shift is shown through an examination of the role of measles in World War I.

After 1945, the use of antibiotics and the generalized availability of vaccination against most of the common infectious diseases ensured that the historic infectious diseases waned in their impact on military populations just as they did in civil populations. Again we use measles and the American army as examples to show these declining effects. But, from 1979, a new infection emerged to threaten the human population, namely the human immunodeficiency virus (HIV), the causative agent of AIDS. One principal mechanism of spread for HIV is unprotected heterosexual and homosexual intercourse between infected and susceptible individuals. As a sexually transmitted disease, the military and war have played a special role in the propagation of the disease. This theme is studied in detail in Chapter 10. Here, we examine HIV in the US Army, 1985–9.

4.2 Mortality and Morbidity, 1850–1914

In his book, *Death by Migration*, Curtin (1989) uses the remarkable records kept by certain European governments on the health of their armies to determine the main trends in mortality, causes of death, and the excess mortality that arose when European armies were sent overseas into epidemiological environments which differed from those they experienced at home. In this section, some of Curtin's data is reworked to show his principal findings for the period from 1850 to the outbreak of World War I.

Curtin (1989, p. xvi) notes that, by the early twentieth century, military medical data covered scores of overseas territories and several European and North American armies. His data focus principally upon the British and French armies in Europe and three colonial settings, the British West Indies, Algeria, and the Madras Presidency of British India; some Dutch data are also included. Curtin chose the British West Indies to represent the New World humid tropics. Algeria represents a Mediterranean climate epidemiologically different from Europe. South India is an example of monsoon Asia.

4.2.1 Mortality Trends

Figure 4.1A plots the annual death rate per 1,000 enlisted men, 1859–1914, for armies in Great Britain, France, and the Netherlands, and for armies from these nations stationed in India and the West Indies (Great Britain), Algeria (France), and the Netherlands Indies (Netherlands). A logarithmic scale has been used for the vertical axis. As we saw in Sections 3.2 and 3.3 for civil populations, Figure 4.1A shows that death rates among the military fell exponentially over this period as well. Additionally, Figure 4.1A plots the annual interquartile range for death rates calculated across the seven geographical locations. The negative gradient implies that the degree of variability from one area to another also declined over the 50 years.

Although all areas experienced a fall in rates and variability, Figure 4.1A suggests that rates and variability were similar and lower in Europe than in other parts of the world. The inset chart, Figure 4.1B, illustrates this by plotting the median rate each year for (i) the three European armies and (ii) the four armies posted overseas. Figure 4.1B also shows the annual interquartile range on the same basis as the medians. The explanation for these differences is straightforward. Men from European armies posted to tropical and subtropical regions were subjected to a disease environment not encountered in their homeland. The lack of immunity to the ensuing infections resulted in excess mortality or, as Curtin puts it, the cost of posting overseas.

Figure 4.1C explores this excess mortality in more detail by plotting on an annual basis the ratio

$$R_O/R_E. \tag{4.1}$$

Here R_O is the death rate in an army in a non-European location and R_E is the rate for the corresponding army based in Europe. The median ratio, 1859–1914, calculated from equation (4.1) was 2.7 (India), 2.0 (West Indies), 1.8 (Algeria), and 4.6 (Netherlands Indies). Figure 4.1C shows that, over the period, the variability in the rates from one location to another diminished so that, by 1914, the ratio had stabilized to a median value of 2.0. As part of this stabilization, extremely high ratios of around 10 found in the 1860s disappeared.

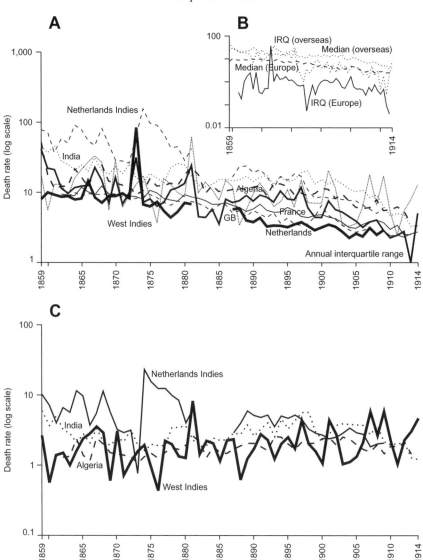

Fig. 4.1. Time trends in mortality rates for armies in seven geographical locations, 1859–1914

Notes: (A) Death rates per 1,000 enlisted men (log scale) in the armies of Great Britain, France, and the Netherlands, and in the armies of these nations posted in the West Indies, India, Algeria, and the Netherland Indies. The annual interquartile range is also shown. (B) Annual median rate and interquartile range (IRQ) for European and overseas armies. (C) Annual death rate in each of the overseas armies as a ratio of the death rate in the corresponding army in Europe (Great Britain for the West Indies and India; France for Algeria; Netherlands for Netherlands Indies).
Source: Data assembled from Curtin (1989, tables A31–A37, pp. 194–202).

The trends illustrated in Figure 4.1 are echoed in many other locations. Figure 4.2 uses nested bars to show the mortality rate of European troops at home (Britain, France, Netherlands, Germany, and America) and abroad (all other locations) in 1817–38 (Fig. 4.2A) and 1909–13 (Fig. 4.2B). They reveal the general decline in rates between the two dates, and the much higher rates experienced by European and American troops posted abroad than in their homelands.

4.2.2 Causes of Death

To maximize the data available for analysis, we use figures from Curtin that relate to hospital admission rates as well as to mortality.

Using stacked bar graphs, Figures 4.3A–E plot the percentage of admissions (deaths for France and Algeria) attributed (i) to disease (light shading) and (ii) to other causes (dark shading) in six time blocks between 1859–67 and 1909–13. The graphs show the dominance of disease compared with other causes in hospital admissions/deaths over the 50-year period, irrespectively of time and location. Figure 4.3F uses line traces to show the change in admissions/deaths attributable to diseases and other causes over the period. For each location, it plots the ratio

$$100(R_6 - R_i)/R_i \tag{4.2}$$

where R_i is the rate in the *i*th time period. The lines show negative changes for admissions/deaths from diseases and for all causes irrespective of location. In contrast, causes other than disease showed negative changes in only two of the five locations (United Kingdom and India). These patterns are consistent with Figure 4.1. Admissions/deaths from causes other than disease generally gained at the expense of those from disease over the period but, at the same time, the negative change is consistent with the long-term decline in mortality experienced in both civil and military populations.

As regards the causes of death among the diseases, Curtin (1989: 94) summarizes the position during this period as follows:

Differences among the three overseas territories are to be expected. Men died of malaria in Algeria and the Caribbean—but much less so in India. They died of yellow fever in the West Indies and nowhere else. They died far more often of cholera and gastrointestinal infections in Madras than anywhere else, and the death rates from tuberculosis everywhere overseas were less than half those in either European [UK and France] sample.

To illustrate these differences, Figure 4.4 shows hospital admission rates for different groups of diseases between 1859 and 1914. The groups have been generated from Curtin's data using the British army's disease classification of 1859–68, but modified to enable the main time trends for certain diseases to be shown more clearly. The classification is described in Curtin (1989: 12–13).

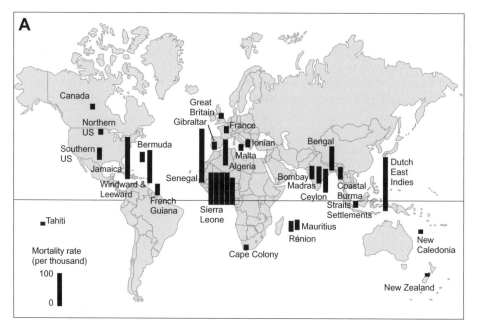

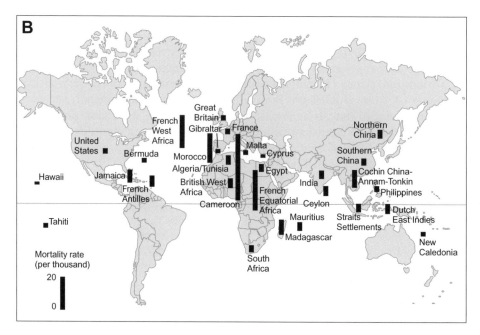

Fig. 4.2. Mortality rates (per 1,000 enlisted men) of troops at home (Britain, France, Netherlands, Germany, and America) and abroad (all other locations), 1817–1838 (map A) and 1909–1913 (map B)

Source: Based on Curtin (1989, maps 1.1 and 1.2, pp. 11, 19).

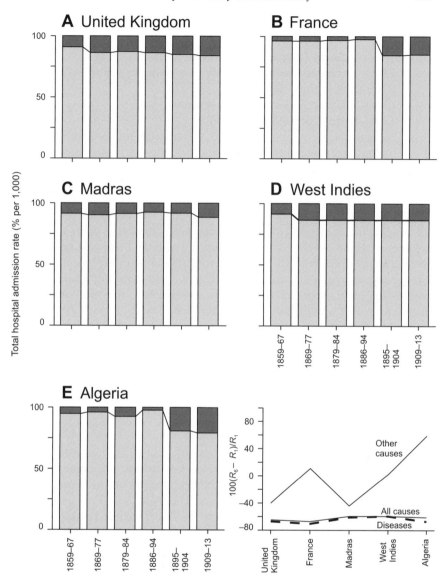

Fig. 4.3. Time trends in causes of death for armies in five geographical locations, 1859–1914

Notes: The stacked bar chart shows the percentage of the total hospital admission rate (graphs A, C, D) or mortality (graphs B, E) per 1,000 mean strength attributed to (i) disease (light shading) and (ii) all other causes (dark shading). The latter includes battle injuries, accidents, homicides, suicides, and punishment. (A) United Kingdom. (B) France. (C) Madras, India. (D) West Indies. (E) Algeria. (F) Change in rates, defined in equation (4.2), between the 1860s and 1914 for all causes, disease, and causes other than disease.

Source: Data from Curtin (1989, tables A3–A30, pp. 167–93).

For our purposes, we note the critical diseases in each group as far as sickness in armies is concerned:

- (*a*) *Venereal disease.* Syphilis, gonorrhea, etc.
- (*b*) *Fevers.* Includes smallpox, chickenpox, malaria, yellow fever, black-water fever, typhus, measles.
- (*c*) *Constitutional diseases.* Includes tuberculosis.
- (*d*) *Local diseases.* Includes pneumonias.
- (*e*) *Nervous diseases.* Including apoplexy and delerium tremens. Separated out here in an attempt to capture sicknesses due to combat fatigue ('shell shock').
- (*f*) *Dysentery.* Including diarrhoea, enteritis, and cholera.

United Kingdom

To benchmark the impact of non-European environments upon European soldiers, we begin our discussion of Figure 4.4 with the United Kingdom. For the British army in Great Britain, the dominant groups among hospital admissions were venereal and local diseases. Curtin comments with measurement caveats (p. 156), 'Venereal disease was, nevertheless, the most important single cause of hospitalization in most nineteeth-century armies—at home or overseas'. The local diseases included pneumonia which was the principal killer among diseases of the respiratory system. But there is a striking downwards trend in rates for both these disease groups over the 50-year period. Among the constitutional diseases, tuberculosis was the main reaper. This was also on a falling trend. The water-borne diseases—dysentery, cholera, etc.— made a steady contribution to mortality.

India

Curtin (1989: 17–18) remarks that monsoon Asia is an epidemiologically diverse region. The graphs for India (Fig. 4.4B) show clear differences as compared with the UK. The contrasts are most marked for the constitutional diseases, fevers, and dysentery and cholera. These are the disease groups that bring home Curtin's 'death by migration'. The fevers included malaria as well as typhoid. Dysentery and cholera are self-explanatory, while tuberculosis of the lungs was the chief cause of mortality among the constitutional diseases. Over time, however, both the dysentery/cholera and constitutional groups fell steadily in terms of hospital admission rates.

West Indies

Curtin (1989: 18) notes that the main culprit causing excess mortality among European arrivals was yellow fever and (p. 69) 'In the nineteeth-century Caribbean . . . yellow fever struck somewhere nearly every year'. It had a very high case–fatality rate but provided the survivors with permanent immunity. The impact of yellow fever is clearly seen in Figure 4.4C. Like the UK, venereal disease and the local group were also strongly in evidence.

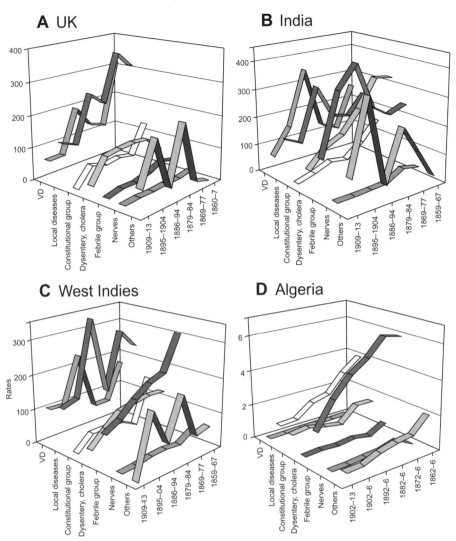

Fig. 4.4. Time trends in causes of deaths by types of disease, 1859–1914

Notes: (A) United Kingdom. (B) India. (C) West Indies. (D) Algeria. The diseases in each class broadly follow the British disease classification of 1859–68 defined in Curtin (1989: 12–13). Principal diseases are listed in the text.

Source: Data from Curtin (1989, tables A3–A30, pp. 167–93).

Algeria

Climatically, the southern shore of the Mediterranean is much like the north shore in Italy and southern France, and the epidemic environment was not radically different in many regards. Venereal diseases and fevers (malaria was a persistent problem) were the dominant groups among hospital admissions over the period, but both experienced strong declining trends.

4.2.3 Changes, 1850–1914

Curtin's work yields three principal conclusions.

1. Infectious diseases rather than battle were the main cause of morbidity and mortality among soldiers during this period.
2. As in civil populations, morbidity and mortality from infectious diseases generally declined over the 50 years.
3. Venereal disease was a persistent problem.

In the next section, we consider the impact of one infectious disease, measles, during the American Civil War as a type example of the effect such diseases could have upon military operations in the second half of the nineteenth century.

4.3 Measles in the American Civil War

Our account is based upon Cliff *et al.* (1993: 101–7). The American Civil War started on 12 April 1861 with Southern shelling of Fort Sumter (South Carolina) and ended four years later on 9 April 1865 with the Southern surrender at Appomattox Court House (Virginia). No one knows precisely how many men served on both sides, but 2.4 million is a commonly agreed figure. Of these, 1.5 million served in the Union Army (out of a Northern population of 22 million) and 0.9 million in the Confederate army (out of a Southern population of 9 million, including 3.5 million slaves).

4.3.1 War and Disease

In terms of human casualties, the Civil War cost more lives than any other American war. Inevitably, attention has focused on the great battlefields (Fig. 4.5). At Gettysburg, the largest of the battles, there were 40,000 casualties in three days. But it was not necessary to be fighting to lose men. Steiner (1977, p. xvii) describes the plight of General McClellan who, while the fate of his army was being discussed, was losing the equivalent of a regiment per day from disease in his idle army on the Peninsula after the Seven Days battles. During the entire Civil War, only 204,000 troops were thought to have been killed on the battlefields; twice as many (another 419,000) died of disease (Fig. 4.5, inset). Sanitary conditions in the hospitals, camps, and prisoner-of-war camps were shocking by modern standards. For example, at Andersonville in southwest Georgia, as many as 30,000 Northern prisoners were enclosed in a log stockade of only 16.5 acres. The disease consequences are

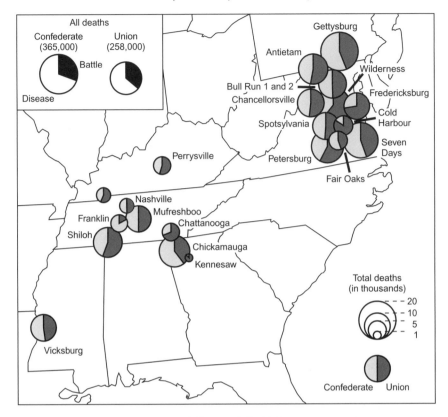

Fig. 4.5. Deaths in the American Civil War, 1861–1865

Notes: (Map) Location of the 23 largest battles, with deaths plotted as circles proportional to the estimated losses. Exact figures are impossible to gain and those charted represent a compromise between conflicting data. (Inset) Overall deaths in the Union and Confederate armies with the proportions due to disease given.
Source: Cliff *et al.* (1993, fig. 5.3, p. 102).

summarized in Table 4.1, while Table 4.2 shows that conditions were no better in the North.

The fact that diseases were recorded alongside conflict data arises from their importance at this time (Pl. 4.1). As a cause of death, disease was twice as common as combat; in the prison camps, Tables 4.1 and 4.2 indicate the situation was even worse. As a cause of non-fatal disability, disease was about six times greater than non-fatal wounds. Although comparative civilian illness data for the United States are not available for a long period, records of illness (admission to sick report) among the active-duty personnel of the Army are available back to 1819, and those for the Navy back to 1865. The US Army's *Annual Reports of the Surgeon General on Medical Statistics* and the US Navy's

Table 4.1. Deaths of Northern troops held as prisoners in Andersonville, 1864

Cause of death	Deaths	Annual rate per 1,000
Typhoid fever, typhus fever	199	20.5
Malaria	119	12.2
Smallpox, measles, scarlet fever, erysipelas	80	8.2
Diarrhoea, dysentery	4,529	465.6
Scurvy	999	102.8
Bronchitis	90	9.2
Inflammation of the lungs and pleurisy	266	27.4
Other diseases	844	86.7
Wounds and uncertain maladies	586	60.2
Total	7,712	792.8

Source: Lancaster (1990, table 33.11.2, p. 323).

Table 4.2. Deaths of Southern troops held in prisons of the Northern states

Cause of death	Deaths	Annual rate per 1,000
Typhoid fever, typhus fever	1,109	13.6
Malaria	1,026	12.6
Smallpox, measles, scarlet fever, erysipelas	3,453	42.3
Diarrhoea, dysentery	5,965	73.0
Scurvy	351	4.3
Bronchitis	133	1.6
Inflammation of the lungs and pleurisy	5,042	61.7
Other diseases	1,729	21.3
Wounds and uncertain maladies	252	0.3
Total	19,060	230.7

Source: Lancaster (1990, table 33.11.3, p. 324).

Annual Reports of the Surgeon General on Medical Statistics provide useful sources for measles incidence, especially during the Civil War period. The definitive source of summary casualty statistics for the latter conflict is *The Medical and Surgical History of the War of the Rebellion* (1861–65) (Surgeon-General's Office, 1870–88) (see Sect. 7.2).

4.3.2 High Measles Mortality and Morbidity

Measles was a particularly troublesome disease to the combatants. Thus, Steiner (1977: 84) writes:

An account of camp measles in the Civil War sounds improbable today, but in reality its importance can hardly be exaggerated. It was axiomatic that army measles, like army

REPORT OF SICK AND WOUNDED.

Station : .... *Month :* .... , 186 .

		TAKEN ON SICK REPORT DURING THE MONTH. *(Cases remaining from last month are not to be entered, except in the Summary.)*			
Classes of Diseases.	Orders of Diseases.	TABULAR LIST OF DISEASES.	Cases from other Hospitals.	All other Cases.	All Deaths.
CLASS I.—ZYMOTICI. (Zymotic Diseases.)	ORDER 1.—MIASMATIC DISEASES.	Typhoid fever..............................			
		Typhus fever..............................			
		Typho-malarial fever..........			
		Yellow fever..............................			
		Remittent fever			
		Intermittent fever. { Quotidian ..... Tertian........ Quartan........ Congestive....			
		Diarrhœa............. { Acute.......... Chronic........			
		Dysentery............ { Acute.......... Chronic........			
		Epidemic cholera........................			
		Erysipelas..............................			
		Hospital gangrene.......			
		Pyæmia..............................			
		Smallpox			
		Varioloid..............................			
		Measles			
		Scarlet fever..............................			
		Diphtheria..............................			
		Mumps..............................			
		Epidemic catarrh			
		Other diseases of this order............			
		Carry forward			

Pl. 4.1. Civil War epidemiological records

Note: Extract from the standard report form *Report of Sick & Wounded* as used by the Union army during the Civil War.
Source: Cliff *et al.* (1993, pl. 5.1, p. 103), from Woodward (1964, app., p. 333).

itch, never got well . . . The mortality was relatively high both in camp measles and its complications, and both left many sequels . . . The direct mortality could be 5 per cent and the complications over 20 per cent.

Joseph Janvier Woodward (Pl. 4.2), Assistant Surgeon-General during the Civil War, provides a classic description of camp measles in his *Outlines of the Chief Camp Diseases of the United States Armies*. His original account was published in 1863, and then republished in 1964 (Woodward, 1964). In this section, we draw upon Woodward's original text to give the full flavour of both

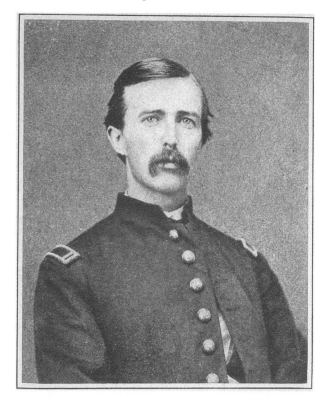

Pl. 4.2. Joseph Janvier Woodward (1833–1884)

Notes: US Army medical officer who served with the Army of the Potomac in the early years of the American Civil War (1861–5). Assigned to the US Surgeon General's Office in 1862, Woodward's treatise on camp epidemics in the Civil War appeared under the title *Outlines of the Chief Camp Diseases of the United States Armies* in 1863. Woodward later contributed to the production of the monumental *Medical and Surgical History of the War of the Rebellion*.
Source: Cliff *et al.* (1993, pl. 5.2, p. 104), from Thompson (1911: 233).

the importance of measles, and contemporary North American beliefs regarding its treatment, prevention, and aetiology, during the American Civil War.

Woodward begins his observations on camp measles by describing it as '. . . one of the most characteristic diseases of the present war . . . from which few of the new regiments escaped' (Woodward, 1964: 267). He continues by stressing the weaknesses of numerical evidence regarding the occurrence of camp measles:

The official returns to the Surgeon-General's office for the first year of the war [1861–2] greatly underestimate the prevalence of this disorder, and this especially because a large number of regiments suffered from disease while still in the camps of instruction in their respective States, prior to being mustered into the service of the United States. In this case no reports of the number taken sick were forwarded to the Surgeon-General's office. Even after the new regiments were mustered into the service of the United States, however, it was generally some months before the regimental surgeons learned regularity in making the reports of sick and wounded required by regulations, and it was precisely during this early period, for which so often no reports were made, that measles most frequently occurred. (ibid. 267)

Despite fragmentary data, Woodward placed the number of reported measles cases during the first year of the war at 21,676, with 551 fatalities (Woodward, 1964: 267). At this date, the short-term impact of measles on the strength of a regiment could be dramatic.

Frequently from one-third to one-half of the effective strength was attacked [by measles] . . . The duration of the epidemic in a regiment was usually from one to two months, and the patients continued to suffer from its sequelae for a still longer period . . . No part of the army escaped. The new levies on the Pacific slope suffered as well as the great armies of the central basin and the Atlantic coast. (ibid. 268–9)

Although camp measles tended to make its appearance in the early months of the history of each regiment and, as a consequence, measles prevailed most actively during the autumn, winter, and spring of 1861–2 (ibid.), measles continued unabated throughout the war. The main record of measles mortality and morbidity is given in the *Medical and Surgical History*. In this, 76,318 examples of measles in Union soldiers were tabulated and the deaths therefrom totalled 5,177. The mortality rates were different as between White and Coloured troops; 6.3 per cent among the former, but 10.9 per cent among the latter. Steiner (1977: 85) stresses that this difference reflected the general position for the whole country but in a more extreme form. According to the US mortality tables for 1860, the relative mortality was 119 in the Negro and 100 in Whites (Steiner, 1977: 85).

Brooks (1966: 120) notes that measles was but one of the fevers to plague the troops of both sides in the combat.

There were also the much-dreaded *eruptive* fevers—smallpox, measles, scarlet fever, and erysipelas—epidemics of which at times wrought more havoc than the Springfields and Napoleons . . . Sometimes an entire regiment or brigade would be hit, with thousands of desperately sick men chattering with chills or burning with fever. Among the Confederates held prisoner in the North, eruptive fevers were the third ranking cause of death. (ibid. 120)

These infections proved even more deadly among the Union Negro soldiers; they experienced a mortality rate nearly six times greater than their White colleagues.

RURAL–URBAN RECRUITING FIELDS

Ordinarily, these 'eruptive fevers' were infections of childhood, but not necessarily so among those coming from remote rural areas away from the viruses and streptococci of the cities. As Brooks (1966: 120) argues, not having had these infections as a child, and without the protection of vaccination, the farm boy proved a fertile field for microbial multiplication. As a consequence, regiments made up of rural troops were especially hard hit (see Sect. 7.2). Training programmes were so thoroughly disrupted by measles epidemics that companies, battalions, and even whole regiments were disbanded temporarily and the men sent home. Cunningham (1958: 188) notes that over 8,000 cases of measles were reported in the Army of the Potomac during the months of July, August, and September 1861; one out of every seven men in this command contracted the disease. In a camp near Raleigh, North Carolina, 4,000 cases of measles developed among 10,000 troops, and hospitals in the cities as well as those in the field were filled with men suffering from this sickness. When Samuel H. Stout took charge of the Gordon Hospital in Nashville, for example, he found 650 patients, most of whom had measles. And the sick who filled the Overton Hospital in Memphis early in 1862 were mostly victims of measles and exposure.

While measles struck its most devastating blows in the first part of the war, the disease never subsided completely; thus 2,207 cases were reported by the Virginia general hospitals from 1 October 1862 to 31 January 1864 (ibid. 188).

MEASLES IN THE SIXTY-FIFTH REGIMENT

One regiment may be selected for special study because of its exceptionally bad health record: it stands first in deaths from disease among the approximately 2,000 Union regiments. Yet it was never in combat and, during its three years of service, it was always assigned to guard and garrison duty. The regiment was recruited in Missouri in the winter of 1863–4, and it was discontinued in January 1867 by the discharge of the survivors.

A typical Civil War regiment originally contained only about 1,000 men, but the Sixty-Fifth had, at one time or another, 1,707 enlisted men and 62 commissioned officers. No less than 772 of these died of disease or camp injuries. On first inspection, measles was not a major cause of these deaths: only 21 were directly attributed to the disease, and all came in the first four months of service. Attack rates were, however, massive throughout the war, and deaths from the sequelae of measles, rather than measles itself, commonplace. The first case was recorded at Benton Barracks shortly after Christmas 1863, and an epidemic with 400 cases was recorded. Bearing in mind normal incubation periods for measles (around 7–14 days), it is apparent that these recruits had been infected some time between enlistment in their home areas and their arrival at the barracks. Their ages ranged from 15 to 41 years. Typical were the cases of two privates called Shoots. 'They came from the same farm . . . [probably] father and son. Their enlistment record was identical. They developed measles one day apart and each lived only ten days' (Steiner, 1977: 85).

Mortality at Benton barracks was unusually high, around 22 per cent of cases. A first-hand description is given by a surgeon of the Third Iowa Cavalry,

D. L. McGugin. '[Measles] seemed ambitious for entire conquest, by seizing every portion of the cuticle . . . the cough was incessant and attended with an expiratory ring . . . the desquamation . . . was not the fine epithelial branny scabs, but rather resembling that following scarlatina' (McGugin, 1865, cited in Steiner, 1977: 85). Illness lasted from four days to six weeks; measles was followed by a succession of complications and sequelae: chronic bronchitis, pneumonia, pleurisy, chronic diarrhoea, and a general debility. Measly boys were long recognizable. Despite this sombre picture, measles cases were not segregated in the camp hospitals, although it was notorious as the 'visitor's disease'. While the experience of the Sixty-Fifth Regiment was severe, it was not unique. Steiner (1977: 85–6) has summarized the impact of measles on four others.

In the Thirty-first Illinois regiment of Colonel John A. Logan composed of rural recruits from the southern part of the state, 500 were ill at one time [from measles] in the Fall of 1861. The surgeon of the new Thirty-eighth Indiana informed the colonel that over 400 of the men had not had the measles and would soon all have it. This proved true. Surgeon Richardson tried to stop an epidemic in the First Maine by ordering out of camp all men who had not had it. Sixty or seventy marched out but the epidemic did not stop because many susceptibles failed to leave. When the disease became bad in the Forty-sixth Illinois, all men who had survived measles were ordered at roll call to step forward three paces. When they proudly did so, they were detailed to nursing duty at the regimental hospital in a nearby house.

CAUSES AND PREVENTION

Causes of High Measles Mortality

The causes identified by Steiner (1977: 109) of the frequent measles outbreaks and associated high mortality in camp include (i) enlistment of active communicable disease carriers, (ii) enlistment and travel during the incubation period of infectious diseases, (iii) contraction of communicable diseases by hospitalized patients and by nurses and doctors, (iv) the use of fever convalescents as cooks, food handlers, nurses, and orderlies, (v) high virulence of the infectious agents (probably the result of repeated rapid passage), and (vi) the low resistance to disease of many recruits.

Seasonality and camp conditions also played their role (Pl. 4.3). Certainly those recruited in winter and confined to unhealthy barracks like Benton and Port Hudson fared less well than those raised in summer and living under canvas. Thus the assistant surgeon of the Eleventh Iowa Regiment, Ingersoll, noted in 1867: 'Benton Barracks appear to me to have been designed and planned, in the most successful way, as a sort of "way-side house" for small-pox, measles, mumps, and home-sickness' (L. D. Ingersoll, cited in Steiner, 1977: 115).

The Twelfth Iowa, chiefly rural men, arrived at Benton Barracks on 30 November 1861 and was assigned to barracks, two companies in space originally designed for one. Within a month, half of the regiment was unfit for duty and 75 had died. Many others remained in the hospital for a time and then had

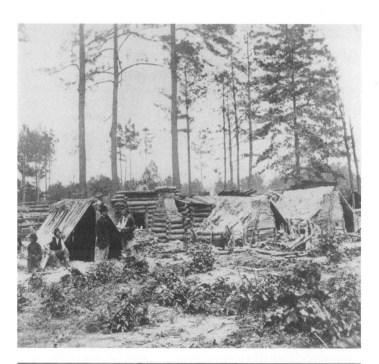

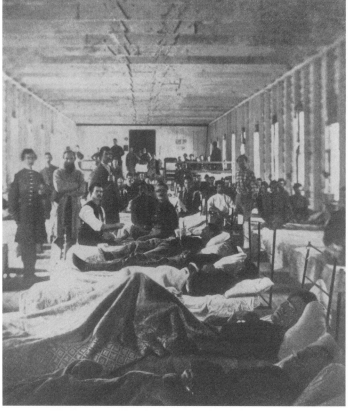

to be discharged from the army on grounds of disability. The regiment's historian, Reed, wrote in 1903 that 'The muster roll shows that no station or battlefield, occupied during the war, was more fatal to the Twelfth than these barracks. The principal diseases were pneumonia, measles, and mumps' (D. W. Reed, cited in ibid. 115).

In offering a prognosis for camp measles, the contemporary observer J. J. Woodward stated: 'This affection is always serious, often fatal either directly or through its sequelae. The prognosis should therefore be guarded' (Woodward, 1964: 273). According to Woodward, it was the characteristically severer nature of camp measles that distinguished it from measles in civilian populations. He wrote:

As it occurs among troops, measles pursues the same general course, and presents, in the main, the same train of symptoms [as witnessed in civilian populations]. Simply it is a much severer affection, and this severity is exhibited chiefly by its assuming a more adynamic character than is usual in private life. (Woodward, 1964, p. 270)

By the term 'adynamic', Woodward was referring to the extremely debilitating nature of the disease. The characteristic manifestations of adynamic camp measles attacks are described by Woodward (1964: 272) as 'frequent and feeble pulse, the great prostration which accompanies the progress of the disease, the subsequent debility, and not unfrequently the occurrence of a brown, dry tongue, as in the case of typhous diseases generally'.

Woodward used the term when describing the worst cases of measles, the so-called 'black measles' characteristic of outbreaks in the deep south. Again, he writes:

The disease [measles] . . . was most formidable, and produced the greatest mortality in the valley of the Mississippi and its tributaries. In this region, and especially in Missouri, and in the army of the Ohio, measles very frequently assumed a typhoid character, and petechial spots made their appearance, constituting what was generally designated as black measles, a condition that was comparatively rare on the Atlantic coast. (ibid. 268–9)

In black measles (*rubeola nigra*), the dusky reddish eruption characteristic of a mild measles attack was replaced by a livid, reddish, or blackish purple, eruption.

The role of measles sequelae. As a rule, few men died from measles alone, but the sequelae of the disease produced fearful results. Measles was perhaps the worst infection from a standpoint of prevalence and complications such as

---

Pl. 4.3. Hospital conditions during the American Civil War

Notes: (Upper) Union front-line hospital at Petersberg *c*.1864 and (lower) Confederate hospital ward, Alexandria Convalescent Camp.
Source: Cliff *et al.* (1993, pl. 5.3, p. 105), from Thompson (1911: 229, 279).

pneumonia and mastoiditis. 'Some surgeons went so far as to say that the bulk of all serious illness was traceable to this particular eruptive fever' (Brooks, 1966: 120).

A special committee appointed by the Provisional Congress to examine the operation of the Quartermaster, Commissary, and Medical Departments reported on 29 January 1862.

It is the peculiar characteristic of measles that the system is left liable to the invasion of the most formidable diseases, upon exposure a short time after undergoing an attack. Fever, pneumonia and diarrhoea . . . follow in the wake of measles where the convalescents are exposed to cold and wet; and when to this we add unsuitable diet, badly-ventilated tents and hospitals, there can be no surprise at the number of sick in the Army, as well as the great suffering and distress. (Cited in Cunningham, 1958: 189)

Other diseases that were observed by medical officers to follow in the wake of measles were ophthalmia, bronchitis, persistent otorrhoea, dysentery, typhoid fever, and phthisis.

If there be any latent tendency to phthisis, it is very apt to be developed. In some dysenteric symptoms are consequent, or a protracted and wasting diarrhoea; some remain in a debilitated condition for months or years, not sick enough to remain in hospital, but not well enough to go on duty; subject to pulmonic symptoms from slight exposure, or to frequent attacks of diarrhoea. (Whittaker, cited in Steiner, 1977: 86)

According to Cunningham (1958: 190), it was asserted early in the war that 'nine out of ten cases of serious illness stemmed from an attack of measles'. Surgeon Bedford Brown was so concerned over the weakening effect of the disease that he proposed furloughs of from two to three weeks' duration for all measles convalescents.

The disease consequent to and traceable to measles cost the Confederate Army the lives of more men and a greater amount of invalidism than all other causes combined; and if this method of general furloughs could have been adopted after an attack of this disease, it would have resulted in preventing a vast loss of life and time, and would have proven a decided means of economy. (B. Brown, cited in ibid. 190)

But, as the war progressed, so the epidemics of measles subsided and its incidence decreased. Nevertheless, the problem was one that continued to plague both armies for the duration of the conflict.

Prevention

There were no effective ways of combating measles. Thus, Woodward (1964: 279) writes:

Measles is to be regarded as a self-limited disease, which terminates in consequence of its own internal laws, and cannot be cut short by any therapeutic measures at present in our possession. The treatment therefore consists essentially in combating the various complications, and in supporting the sinking powers of life, until the violence of the disease is spent.

Surgeons found that the treatment of measles 'involved measures of sanitary supervision rather than clinical instructions or pharmaceutical formulae' (cited in Cunningham, 1958: 188–9). Poor hygiene no doubt contributed heavily to the early outbreaks, and one of the lessons taught by the war was that careful sanitary control was more effective than medication in the treatment of measles. Drugs were of little value in limiting the duration of the disease, and most of them recommended abundant ventilation for those affected. There was, however, some reluctance to give measles patients an abundance of fresh air, due to the fear that the eruption would be 'driven in', as it was termed.

Nevertheless, some experiments in medication proved helpful. One hospital surgeon found that a solution of ammonium acetate 'given in doses of 40 or 50 drops, 3 times a day, in a cup of warm tea, seems to possess a particular eliminating action', while another recommended a tea made from the roots and leaves of sassafras (cited in ibid. 188–9).

One of the most important proposals was that recruits should be kept in camps, almost as quarantine centres, until the epidemic camp diseases had run their course. Thus 'An Alabama Volunteer', as early as December 1861, argued that 'recruits, especially from the country, be kept at least two months in camps of instructions'. By then, the troops would also have acquired some knowledge of drill and camp life, and be prepared for effective service. General Lee made practically the same suggestion nearly a year later (ibid.).

Measles Aetiology

Military camps became laboratories for the development of imaginative hypotheses, and lively debate, regarding the aetiology of measles. One of the most interesting of these hypotheses, propounded by J. H. Salisbury, was the role of 'a peculiar fungus, which developed under straw, under the influence of warmth and moisture' (Woodward, 1964: 274). In support of a fungus–measles relationship, Salisbury recorded the outbreak of measles at Camp Sherman, Newark, Ohio. Measles appeared at Camp Sherman on 4 December 1861, and enquiries apparently failed to trace anyone who could have introduced the disease. It was on this same day that a certain Mr Dille had thrashed some decayed wheat straw. Apparently coincidentally, Mr Dille also developed measles. Of Camp Sherman, Salisbury wrote:

During this time . . . many of the tents were furnished with ticks [mattresses], which were filled with straw for men to sleep on . . . On December 1st, the weather became colder, and snow fell to a depth of about one inch. On the 2d, which was quite warm, this melted and wet the soil and dampened the ticks. December the 4th the measles made its first appearance in Camp Sherman. On the first day there were eight cases, and within a week after there were forty. (Salisbury, 1862, cited in ibid. 277)

However, the hypothesis that measles resulted from infection with a fungus which multiplied in straw met with some opposition. Writing in 1863, Woodward recorded the results of his own experiments.

Since reading Dr. Salisbury's paper, the author . . . has innoculated with the fungus a number of persons, among others himself, Acting Assistent Surgeon Curtis, U.S.A., and Hospital Steward Whitney, U.S.A., without, however, producing any perceptible effect . . . There is a source of error in Dr. Salisbury's observations; they were made during the prevalence of an epidemic of measles. How far were the effects he imagines due to the fungus the result of the epidemic? (ibid. 278–9).

4.4 World War I, 1914–1918

As we saw in Section 4.2, by 1914, the impact of infectious diseases upon armies was greatly diminished as compared with the last half of the nineteenth century. The germ theory of disease, linked to prophylactic measures, had radically altered the picture. In particular, germ theory had given a sound epidemiological basis for improved hygiene, isolation of the sick, and acclimatization of troops entering theatres of war in geographical areas with different spectra of diseases than they had experienced in their homelands. In this section, we illustrate the effect of these different policies, especially hygiene, isolation (quarantine), and acclimatization, by looking at the continuing impact of measles.

4.4.1 Measles in World War I

World War I involved over 30 countries. Its main area of hostilities extended through Europe and Asia Minor from the North Sea to the Persian Gulf. More than 5 million Allied servicemen and 3.3 million of the Central Powers died from wounds, disease, and other causes. Although the historian's focus has largely been upon the great battles such as Verdun and the Somme, there was still a significant loss of life from non-battle causes; and infectious diseases (including measles) played a role. In this section, we look at the quantitative impact of measles upon the forces of two countries on the Allied side, Australia and the United States, before going on to examine the role of measles in the war at sea.

THE AUSTRALIAN EXPERIENCE

Australia's participation in World War I was immediate and wholehearted. As early as 3 August 1914, the Australian cabinet offered to send an 'an expeditionary force of 20,000 men of any suggested composition to any destination desired by the Home Government'. By the end of the war, 416,000 troops had been raised and 330,000 deployed overseas. As a proportion of their population, Australia and New Zealand made a bigger contribution than any other allied country, and their casualty rates (casualties/numbers engaged) of 68 and 58 per cent were also higher (cf. UK 53%, Canada 51%). Australia's official history of the war includes several medical volumes, some of which make direct references to communicable diseases, including measles.

Here, we look first at the impact of measles in three distinct phases of warfare: first, in recruitment camps in Australia; secondly, in transport by sea *en route* to the battlefront; thirdly, in the assembly camps in Egypt and France, and in the theatres of war themselves.

Recruitment Camps in Australia

At the outbreak of war, men rushed to enlist, some selling farms and businesses, or leaving wives and parents to run them. Three-quarters were young men, between 20 and 40 years, and more than a fifth were from farms and outback areas. Tented training camps were set up on racecourses and other open sports grounds on the edge of the cities (Pl. 4.4).

In many ways, the events witnessed in these camps were a rerun of the impact of camp measles in the American Civil War. Official reports raised the question of why measles was so 'remarkably prevalent' among new Australian recruits. Butler (1943) has identified three possible factors: (i) the disease had been controlled in childhood with relative success in Australia. This ensured the presence of a large number of susceptibles in any young adult Australian 'crowd'; (ii) the tendency of the virus, 'given the opportunity of constant intimacy of contact in a susceptible population, to embark on a local career of epidemicity' (Butler, 1943: 681); (iii) the crowding together in the training camps of large numbers of susceptibles. All these factors were cited at one time or another as reasons for profligate measles in the Civil War.

As experience was gained, so the checks against measles and the other contagious diseases were tightened up. In Australia, a threefold camp inspection was eventually held. Men were paraded for medical and dental inspection for the first time within 24 hours of marching into a depot. When news of embarkation

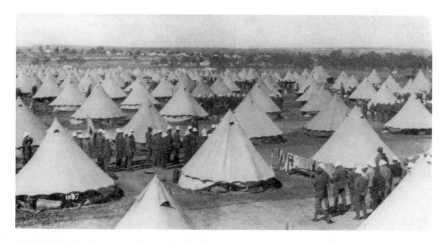

Pl. 4.4. Assembly camps for new recruits in Australia at the start of the Great War

Notes: Broadmeadows Camp, Victoria, in 1914.

Source: Cliff *et al.* (1993, pl. 7.1, p. 146), from Butler (1938, pl. 5, opposite p. 30).

was confirmed, a second inspection parade was held, using the same pro forma nominal roll. A third and final inspection took place within 24 hours of proceeding overseas. This last check was chiefly for the detection of contagious disease (venereal, and scabies) but also covered the detection of contacts of infectious diseases (in particular mumps, measles, and cerebrospinal fever). The medical officer carrying out this final inspection had to sign a certificate stating that the men were (i) medically fit, (ii) fully inoculated and vaccinated, (iii) that the necessary entries had been made in their pay books, and (iv) that they were not contacts of infectious disease (Butler, 1940: 478–9).

Measles on Troopships

Australian troops were hastily gathered together in the months following August 1914 and, by late October, were ready to embark. A convoy of 28 transport ships carrying 20,000 troops (plus a New Zealand contingent in ten transports) sailed from Albany in Western Australia on 1 November. The original destination was Salisbury Plain in southern England. But the preparations for the camps there were so far behind schedule that the convoy was diverted to Egypt, and the ANZAC troops disembarked at Alexandria after a five-week voyage.

The movement of troops from Australia to Europe and the Middle East posed severe epidemiological as well as logistic problems (Pl. 4.5). It involved a

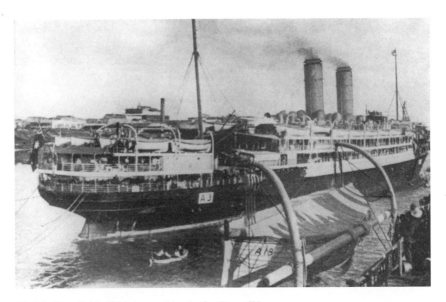

Pl. 4.5. Port Said, 1914: troopships in the Great War

Notes: The transport ship *Orvieto* at Port Said on 2 December, 1914. The *Orvieto* was flagship of the First Australian Convoy that sailed from Albany in Western Australia on 1 November 1914.
Source: Cliff *et al.* (1993, pl. 7.2, p. 147), from Butler (1938, pl. 9, opposite p. 46).

voyage of some 7,000 to 11,000 miles, depending upon the route. At the outbreak of the war, the only guidelines for preserving health on troopships were provided by the old British Admiralty transport regulations. But these were based on a voyage of from three to four weeks. In contrast, the Australian medical service was faced with the difficulty of eight weeks on board under crowded and climatically adverse conditions. The twin problems that had to be faced were (i) how to provide treatment on a voyage for those who fell sick, and (ii) how best to preserve the health of the troops. The latter involved drawing up stringent rules for sleeping accommodation, ventilation, deck spacing, exercise, sleeping, washing, latrines, cooking, and messing.

Experience from the past was an important guide. The Australian medical service, and in particular the Director-General, studied carefully the lessons learnt in the South African (Boer) War, 1899–1902. Then, on the returning troopship, *Drayton Grange*, there had occurred 17 deaths and many cases of serious illness (Table 4.3). Measles itself had led to six deaths and 154 men being treated in hospital. The findings of the subsequent court of inquiry were that 'overcrowding and defective sleeping and hospital arrangements were the chief factors in the calamity, although technically the Board of Trade regulations had been complied with' (Butler, 1938: 35). Butler (1943: 680) noted a direct link between measles on land and sea. From the first convoy in October 1914 until the last sailings at the end of 1918, 'fluctuations in measles on board the Australian transports seem to have reflected generally the epidemic tension in the camps of training'.

Study of Australian records suggests that the amount of contact (taking account of both the duration of contact and its intimacy) was the chief determining factor in the spread of ship epidemics through comparable ship communities; and that a space–time buffer zone, at both ends, between the transport and the camps, was well worthwhile in restricting the spread of

Table 4.3. *Drayton Grange*, 1902: causes of death and sickness

Sickness	Treated in hospital	Deaths
Measles	154	6
Influenza	39	0
'Chest affections'	23	7
Tonsillitis	4	0
Cerebrospinal meningitis	0	1
Dysentery	4	2
Enteric	1	0
Blood poisoning	0	1
Total	225	17

Source: Butler (1938: 35 n. 1).

infectious diseases. Thus the most important modifying influences appear to have been: (i) the early discovery and prompt isolation of the first case; (ii) the facilities for isolating contacts and subsequent cases, and the vigour with which this was carried out. 'In the history of the A.I.F. [Australian Imperial Force] measles, either alone or more often complicated by pneumonia, was responsible for a large proportion of deaths at sea from "disease". In camps and transports over the whole period of the war it was little if any less deadly than cerebro-spinal fever' (ibid. 681). The course of the epidemic on the transports varied considerably from ship to ship: 'It occurred in most outward transport voyages. The peak of the epidemic was usually reached in about the 4th or 5th weeks of the voyage, though energetic action by the S.M.O. sometimes deferred it to the end of the voyage' (ibid.).

Assembly Camps in the Middle East and France

After disembarking at Alexandria, most of the Australian Imperial Force (AIF) went into camp in the desert around Cairo, especially at Mena camp in the shadow of the pyramids. Many of the troops stayed in the Middle East and were involved in fighting with the Ottoman Empire (notably at Gallipoli); others were trans-shipped to Marseilles prior to movement north to take part in the Western Front.

A major outbreak of pleuro-pneumonia, mainly associated with measles, occurred among the troops of the Mena Camp in 1914–15. The most characteristic feature was a fibrinous pleurisy, so dense that it gained a local name 'the Mena shawl'. In these cases, besides the pneumonococcus, the bacillus of Friedlander was prominent. At first, influenza was not regarded as a factor of any significance (but see below), and streptococcal infection was infrequent (ibid. 209).

At the staging camps in Egypt, most of the ordinary infections of temperate zones were fairly common, as well as the various special diseases. The Australian physicians accompanying the troops learned, on the authority of the Dean of the Cairo Medical School, that 'pneumonia was not prevalent in Egypt, and that influenza, though it occurred, was uncommon' (Butler, 1938: 73). Despite this reassurance, influenza ran through the camps unimpeded. In contrast, measles 'elevated by reason of its exanthem to the dignity of isolation' spread less easily. Where it did occur, it often proved fatal when associated with respiratory complications (ibid. 74).

In his official report on the outbreaks in Egypt, Butler (ibid.) cites A. Wright on his reflection on why certain diseases behaved so differently in camps of young troops: 'In the matter of respiratory infections the conditions of war are peculiar. "In peace and civilized conditions the spread of infection from man to man is restricted by the fact that the population is partitioned up into separate rooms and houses. . . . In war all this structural arrangement is swept away."'

Given the medical problems that were occurring in the recruiting camps, considerable thought was given as to how the incidence of infectious diseases might be reduced. Butler (1940: 542–3) comments: 'Cases of many serious infectious diseases—including measles—were brought from the Middle East ... with the Australian and British troops, but failed to gain a hold. The reason why they did not do so reflects the campaign against the major diseases in the war'.

Isolation, at several levels, appears to have been the most promising of the counter-measures to arouse the interest of the military strategists. The transfer of the AIF at the beginning of 1916 from Egypt to the Western Front provides an example, in miniature, of the problem of preventing epidemics of infectious diseases under wartime conditions and, in the 'Marseilles Sieve', of the filtering and isolation policies in action.

The Marseilles Sieve. An account of the holding of the breach is provided by Major H. O. Lethbridge, Australian Army Medical Corps, who was in charge of the Isolation Compound in No. 2 at Moussot, Marseilles. This was a major switching station where Australian and British troops coming from Egypt by ship were disembarked and sent on by rail to the battlefields of northern France.

Almost every transport would send us its quota of infectious diseases so that the importance of this hospital as a filter was great. Where the gravity of the infection warranted, the whole unit or formation was segregated and held up until deemed safe for it to travel north. The fact that most transports took a week (between Egypt and Marseilles) meant that most infections brought from Egypt would have shown up. At one time we had as many as 13 different diseases in the compound, including smallpox, typhus, measles and roseola, mumps, diphtheria, relapsing fever, scarlet fever, scabies, pemphigus contagiosus, cerebro-spinal meningitis, dhobie itch, and chickenpox. (Lethbridge, cited in Butler, 1940: 543)

Measles, along with mumps, posed a particular problem. These diseases provided a constant stream of new infections and because they were so widespread, it was impossible to exclude incubating cases from the drafts for France.

Buffer zones. One solution to the problem was found in the creation of two buffer zones (see Cliff and Haggett, 1989). The first of these was spatial. The spatial separation located new arrivals away from the general depot system until they were clear of infection. The second barrier was time, the interval that separated the medical inspection of the drafts from the date of their departure for the front.

The before and after situations were described by Colonel McWhae (cited in Butler, 1940: 564):

The problems connected with infectious diseases did not arise from dangerous diseases such as cerebro-spinal meningitis but from 'ordinary diseases' such as mumps and measles. Except for a brief period practically all reinforcements from Australia were thoroughly infected with these diseases. Thus during January to March, 1917, 445 cases of mumps, 42 of measles, and 14 of C.S.F. arrived from the transports and cases in

Command Hospitals increased from 300 on January 11th to 802 on March 5th. In this period the control of disease in the depots was in process of evolution. In the early winter months a great proportion of all men in camps were contacts. Effective isolation was impossible, the camps being crowded.

But, within a few months, the situation was being brought under control:

By the end of March, 1917, the depots were reorganised. A thorough attempt was made to keep contacts from drafts. Contacts to the number of 8,600 were isolated, and in May it was possible to accommodate them in tented isolation camps in each training camp, which were placed out of bounds. Contacts of different dates were kept separate and did not mix with their units except in open air training. Nominal rolls showed the date of termination of isolation; cases among contacts were dealt with promptly and their contacts back-dated. The number in each tent was restricted and disinfection of blankets, etc. arranged. (McWhae, cited in Butler, 1940: 564)

The effectiveness of the isolation policy is demonstrated by the fact that almost all cases of mumps and measles occurred among troops already isolated, and very few indeed outside the isolated areas. Instead of large numbers of soldiers being struck off drafts prior to embarkation, it became exceedingly rare for infectious disease to occur in troops who had finished their training. The great success is confirmed by the fact that, from June 1917 to December 1918, not a single case of mumps and only five cases of measles got to France among nearly 100,000 reinforcements (Butler, 1940: 565).

    Part of the success in treating measles was attributed to the simple remedy of providing sufficient space—isolation at the microscale—and adequate ventilation.

By the simple expedient of allowing a space of 2½ feet between each bed and by improving the ventilation of the quarters, the carrier rate, [in C.S.F.] in one instance, fell from 28 to 2 per cent. in 9 weeks, from 28 to 7 per cent. in 6 weeks in another, from 35.8 per cent. to 4.5 per cent. in 6 weeks in a third, and from 28 per cent. to 4.5 per cent. in 5 weeks in a fourth (ibid. 932).

These hospital arrangements are illustrated in Plate 4.6.

Measles in the War Zones

The battle honours of the AIF show that it was heavily involved in a series of major battles including the Dardanelles, First Battle of the Somme, Messines, Passchendaele, Hazebrouck, Gaza, and Damascus. Not surprisingly, the medical accounts of those engagements are dominated by the death and traumatic casualties of battle. The few references to measles are incidental. We learn that, for example, when Australian troops were moved from Egypt to take part in the ill-fated assault on Gallipoli, no special precautions were taken to ensure that incubating cases of measles were excluded among the embarking troops (Butler, 1938: 38). On several vessels outbreaks of measles were found to have commenced: so a case of measles in full exanthem was recorded on the *Orvieto* just after leaving Alexandria for the Dardanelles.

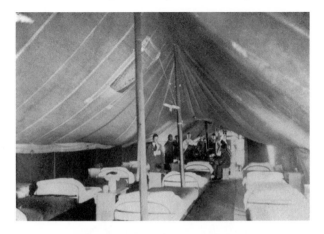

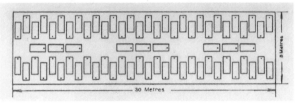

Pl. 4.6. Hospital arrangements in the Great War

Notes: (Upper) A tented ward at No. 3 A.G.H., Abbeville. The marquees are 'brigaded' to form an extended ward. (Lower) Beds arranged in an 'Adrian hut' to accommodate 69 men head to foot to avoid mucous interchange.
Source: Cliff *et al.* (1993, pl. 7.3, p. 150), from Butler (1938, pl. 46 and p. 557).

McWhae (cited in Butler, 1940: 477–8) has described the havoc that infectious diseases played with military planning in the war zones and, in particular, with the deployment of fresh reserves. While it might have seemed a simple matter to send troops a day or two's journey forward from their gathering camps to the front line, in practice it was complicated by epidemic outbreaks. Large numbers of men were struck off the drafts at the last minute. Mumps and measles broke out in the drafts and raged through the Australian Divisions in France. Figure 4.6 illustrates just such a mumps outbreak in the Second ANZAC Corps at the end of 1916.

A more general picture of the role of disease in relation to the pattern of battle casualties is illustrated in Figures 4.7 and 4.8. These graphs plot variations in the evacuations and casualties from the strength of the AIF on the Western Front from April 1916 to December 1918. The non-battle evacuations (white bars) decrease relatively compared with battle casualties (black bars) from late 1916 for the remainder of the war. However, it was only at the times of the big pushes that battle casualties outweighed disease as a cause of evacuation.

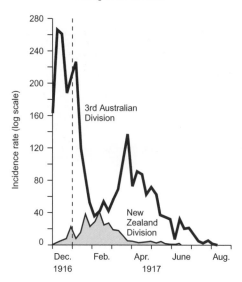

Fig. 4.6. Western Front, December 1916–August 1917: course of a mumps epidemic in the II ANZAC Corps

Source: Cliff *et al.* (1993, fig. 7.1, p. 150), redrawn from Butler (1940, graph 10, p. 556).

Summary

Measles was enormously disruptive of the AIF at all stages—from initial assembly in Australia, on the troopships, in the assembly camps in Africa and in the theatres of war. However, despite its disruptive presence, measles was primarily a non-lethal disease for Australian troops—certainly less so than during the American Civil War. Figures of men made fit for return to duty after measles are difficult to establish, but were probably as high as 94.5 per cent (Butler, 1943: 878). In contrast, the return rate for tuberculosis was only 38.4 per cent. Return-to-duty figures for both British and German armies were lower but, since these were calculated on a different basis, valid comparisons are not possible.

Measles was a cause of mortality when accompanied by secondary respiratory infections. Here, the Australian experience was strikingly similar to the history of severe respiratory infections in American training camps where many fatalities also occurred in similar circumstances. There pleuropneumonia and emphysema were associated with measles. It is the US experience to which we now move.

US EVIDENCE

Unlike Australia, the United States was a late entry as a combatant in World War I. In 1914, President Woodrow Wilson had declared that the United States

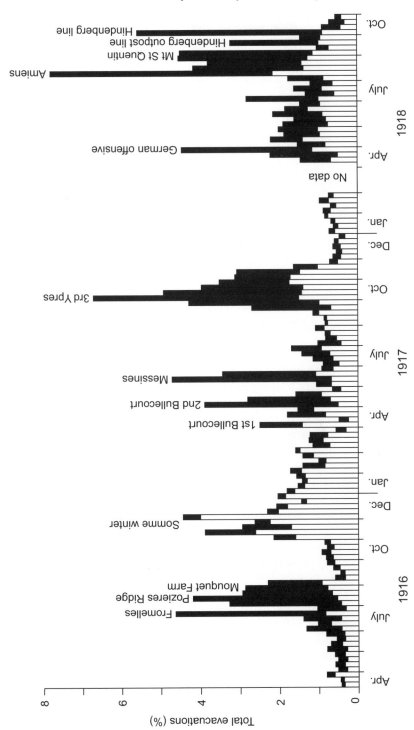

Fig. 4.7. Western Front, 1916–1918, I: percentage of total evacuations (battle in black, non-battle in white) from the army area on the weekly average strength of the Australian Imperial Force (AIF)

Source: Cliff *et al.* (1993, fig. 7.2, p. 150), redrawn from Butler (1940, graph 8, p. 493).

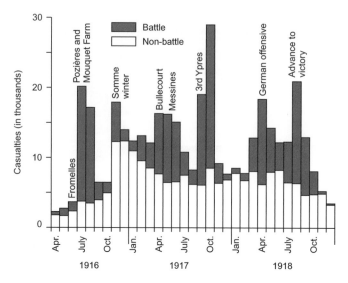

Fig. 4.8. Western Front, 1916–1918, II: total casualties by month (battle in black, non-battle in white) in the Australian Imperial Force (AIF)

Source: Cliff *et al.* (1993, fig. 7.3, p. 151), redrawn from Butler (1940, graph 7, p. 492).

would be 'neutral in fact as well as in name' but, with the German sinking of the *Lusitania* in 1915, military training camps began to be set up. The army was considerably enlarged during 1916 and, in April 1917, the United States declared war on Germany. At its peak, the US armed forces totalled 4.8 million, of whom 1.4 million served with the American Expeditionary Force in France. The US medical history of World War I has been recounted at length, notably in the *Official History Series for World War I: The Medical Department of the United States Army in the World War*. Volume ix is concerned with the impact of communicable diseases, including measles (United States Army, 1928). Shorter but useful accounts appear in Heaton (1963) and Hoff (1958).

Mobilization and Measles

As described more fully in Section 7.4, few diseases were more closely allied to mobilization than was measles. Just as during the Civil War, during the fall and early winter of 1917, when mobilization camps were being organized, barracks and tents were overcrowded and inadequately heated, and it was impossible to supply the men with sufficient warm clothing. These adverse conditions were augmented by an unusually early and severe winter. The draft brought large numbers of individuals together from all walks of life and from every environment: 'The inducted men were principally young adults and included not only the generally immune city boy, but also vast numbers of rural lads who had never before been exposed to the infection' (United States Army, 1928: 411).

Figure 4.9 graphs the monthly trends, from April 1917 until December 1919, in both total admissions to the army and of the subset of these admissions found to be suffering from measles. From this diagram, it can be seen that the peak of measles admissions occurred in November 1917, in the period immediately following US entry into the war. This was followed by a well-marked decline in the admitted-with-measles : mobilization ratio, and parallels our discussion of the Civil War (Sect. 4.3), where the peak for measles admissions was also reached during the first year, in December 1861. As far as measles mortality was concerned in World War I, this also climaxed in November 1917, alongside measles admissions.

Variations by class and race. Both measles admission and measles death rates varied between the officers and other ranks. For admission rates, the officers' rate of 4.7 per 1,000 per annum may be compared with 23.8 for the army as a whole. The officer death rate for measles was also lower: 0.01 compared with 0.57. There are two possible explanations for this pattern: first, officers lived in individual billets or with one or two other officers, and their relationship with the enlisted men did not bring them into close contact with them. Secondly, officers represented an older age group, and as such had had greater opportunity of contracting the disease at some prior date.

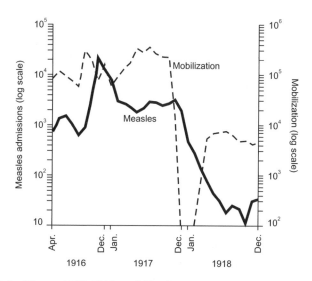

Fig. 4.9. United States, 1917–1919: mobilization and measles

Notes: Number of servicemen succumbing with measles on admission (left vertical axis) compared with numbers mobilized for the United States Army (right vertical axis), April 1917 to December 1919. Note that both vertical axes are plotted on a logarithmic scale.
Source: Cliff *et al.* (1993, fig. 7.4, p. 151), redrawn from United States Army (1928, chart XLVI, p. 415).

Measles was more common among white than among coloured troops but whether this was due to age, diagnosis, or recording differences is not explained. But Puerto Rican troops suffered more than any others in the American Army; measles occurrence was more than three times that among the whites. The Hawaiian troops serving in their own country were the second worse sufferers. It is notable that these two badly affected groups were islanders; their high attack rates probably reflect the population susceptibility that may accumulate as a consequence of the barrier to frequent virus invasions that results from island isolation.

Occurrence by region. Analysis by military camps in the United States reveals substantial geographical differences in the extent to which measles was found (Fig. 4.10). Among white enlisted men, it varied from 1.19 per 1,000 strength at Camp Syracuse, New York, and 7.27 at Camp Dix, New Jersey, to 164.67 at Camp Pike, Arkansas. The highest rates occurred in troops from the southeastern United States.

The northeastern section is thickly settled while the southeastern is sparsely settled. In other words, the bulk of the population in the former have lived in cities and in close proximity, and as such they may be classified as urban. In the southeastern portion there are some large cities, but the bulk of the population may be called rural. A large proportion of the inhabitants in urban States have contracted measles in childhood, while in rural States a large percentage have not been exposed to the disease. (United States Army, 1928: 416)

As Heaton (1963: 33) puts it: 'Measles was essentially a disease of country boys coming for the first time into a densely crowded environment.'

Camp Pike (Arkansas) illustrates Heaton's assertion. Camp Pike stood at the head of the list of rates by camp among admissions. It recruited its quota of troops from southeastern states: Alabama, Arkansas, Louisiana, Mississippi, and Tennessee. Camp Bowie (Texas), which was second, drew its quota from Arkansas, Louisiana, and Texas. Camp Sevier (South Carolina), third, recruited from Alabama, Kentucky, North Carolina, and South Carolina. Camp Wheeler (Georgia), fourth on the list, drew its quota from Alabama, Florida, Georgia, Louisiana, and Mississippi. On the other hand, Camp Grant (Illinois) which drew its admissions principally from Illinois, and Camp Dix (New Jersey) which drew mainly from New York and New Jersey, had two of the lowest rates of measles-infected soldiers among its new recruits. These state-by-state variations in measles admissions and deaths among enlisted white men are mapped in Figure 4.11 and emphasize the higher measles incidence in those from the rural southeast.

The description of the occurrence of measles in Camp Wheeler, Georgia, by Duncan (1918) is typical of many detailed accounts. The construction of the camp was not concluded until November 1917. But the first troops arrived in early September and, by the end of the month, all of the National Guard troops had arrived: among these 11,000 men, the sick report from all causes

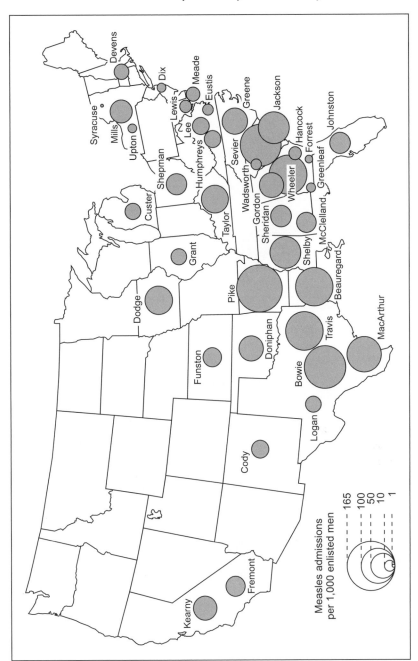

Fig. 4.10. United States, 1917–1919: measles by army camps

Note: Circles are proportional to measles admission rates per 1,000 for white enlisted men, averaged over the period, April 1917 to December 1919.
Source: Cliff *et al.* (1993, fig. 7.5, p. 152), drawn from data in United States Army (1928, chart XLVII, p. 416).

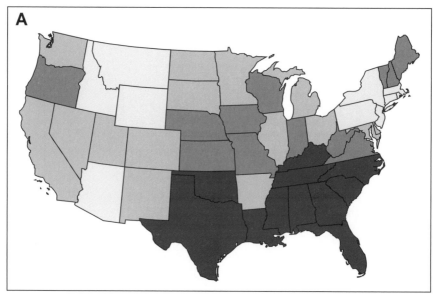

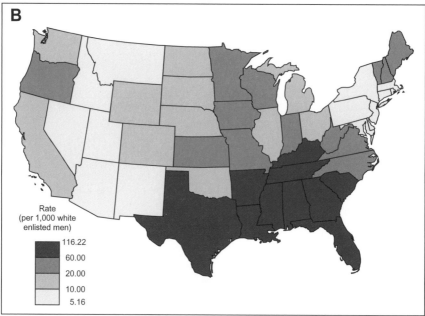

Fig. 4.11. United States, 1917–1919: measles among armed forces by state

Notes: (A) Measles admissions. (B) Measles deaths. Shading is proportional to the rate per 1,000 for white enlisted men, averaged over the period April 1917 to December 1919.

Source: Cliff *et al.* (1993, fig. 7.6, p. 153), redrawn from United States Army (1928, chart XLVIII, p. 418).

was only 3 per cent. On 14 October 1917, the first draft men arrived and, by the end of the month, over 10,000 had arrived. With their arrival, the epidemiological picture changed sharply:

These inducted men brought measles on every train; cases were taken from trains where they had been shut up for from a few hours to 24 hours or more in closed cars filled with men. It can scarcely be wondered that measles got out of control among these men and among the recruits of the various regiments. (Duncan, 1918: 13)

The daily measles admissions which had been seven in mid-October rose to a peak of 174 by late November but, by mid-December, 'the conflagration had burned entirely out'.

Among the American troops serving in France with the American Expeditionary Forces (AEF), there were over 9,000 primary admissions for measles and 358 deaths. When converted to rates, these are well below those in the United States: for admissions, 5.5 per 1,000 per annum as compared with 23.8 and, for deaths, 0.21 as compared with 1.25. The official report suggests that the source of the measles was within the AEF itself and that 'there is no reason to believe that measles was to any noticeable extent due to infections acquired by the soldiers from association with the French civil population' (United States Army, 1928: 427). One factor that might explain the lower incidence in France was the high negative correlation observed between measles incidence and length of army service: soldiers serving in France would probably have met the measles virus in home recruiting camps before sailing for France.

Comparison of Civilian and Military Populations

Comparison of measles incidence in military and civilian populations reveals a general sympathy in the rise and fall of cases in both populations. During 1918, the disease was less common in the United States than it was in 1917, both among civilians and soldiers. However, assessment of the relative incidence in the two populations in 1917–18 must proceed with caution. All ages are encompassed in the civilian occurrence figures (including the childhood ages where measles is most prevalent); in contrast, the Army population is truncated in the younger age groups since recruitment covered those aged 17 and over. Despite this, available data imply that measles was still 18 times more common in the Army than among the civilian population. But it should be noted that the civilian data include only reported cases in the registration area and, undoubtedly, many cases occurred in the civilian population that were never registered.

Problems of Secondary Infection

The official accounts of the war stress that uncomplicated measles was almost never fatal. The gravity of measles lay in the complications caused by certain micro-organisms. Bacterial infections due to pneumococcus, *Corynebacterium diphtheriae*, *Haemophilus influenzae*, *Mycobacterium tuberculosis* and, most particularly, haemolytic streptococcus, are described. According to Heaton (1963: 32–3):

In the First World War, there were 93,629 admissions due to measles among enlisted men in the continental United States and Europe of which bronchopneumonia and lobar pneumonia were complications of measles in 6,283 cases, with 2,186 deaths. Similar data for the entire Army are not available. Suppurative pleurisy, undoubtedly secondary to pneumonia, occurred in 645 cases with 286 deaths. There were 3,926 instances of otitis media, but only 122 of these patients died. Careful studies of the bacteriology of these complications indicated that the hemolytic streptococcus was the causative agent in nearly every case.

Cole and MacCallum (1918) provide a classic study of pneumonia following measles at a base hospital. They give a clear description of interstitial (viral) pneumonia but attributed it to *Streptococcus haemolyticus*, which Bloomfield (1958: 438) considers 'as surely a secondary invader'. Sellars and Sturm (1919) describe the occurrence of the Pfeiffer bacillus in measles cases as common in American cantonments in World War I.

The experience of World War I also throws light on how such secondary infections can occur. At one hospital, the carrier rate for haemolytic streptococcus rose steadily on measles wards from 11 per cent on admission to 57 per cent in patients who had been on the ward from eight to 16 days. If non-carriers of streptococcus with measles were carefully segregated from carriers at the time of admission, the difference in complications was striking; a rate of 6.4 per cent was recorded in non-carriers as opposed to 36.8 per cent among carriers (Heaton, 1963: 32–3). It seems, therefore, that streptococcus was either caught along with the measles virus, or else contracted as a secondary infection following hospitalization after contracting measles; then living in a highly contaminated hospital environment resulted in infection.

Prevention and Control

Munson (1917) appreciated the value of immunity conferred by previous measles attacks and he pioneered a measles control strategy at Fort Wilson Camp, Texas. The statements of soldiers as to whether or not they had previously had measles was used as a basis for quarantining contacts with measles cases. Munson linked these quarantine arrangements with the avoidance of overcrowding in tents, the sunning of bedding and personal effects, and the proper ventilation of sleeping quarters. In this way, outbreaks of measles at Fort Wilson were brought under control.

In some camps, a rapid examination of incoming men was made at the railroad station and suspicious cases were segregated. In others, whole companies were quarantined for 14 days. As in the Australian camps, alternate head and foot sleeping was ordered and enforced during the latter part of the war. Even dust from roads and walks was regarded as a predisposing cause, not only in measles, but also in other infectious diseases; hence roads were sprayed with oil in some camps, with apparently good results in the southwestern camps (United States Army, 1928: 443).

Once troops had caught the disease, treatment was directed at keeping patients comfortable and trying to avoid secondary infections. As the official report reluctantly concluded (ibid. 448):

There were no striking developments in the treatment of measles during the war. Various methods were employed in attempts to minimize complications, but none of them was conspicuously successful, and until the causative agent is identified and a potent protective serum developed, there is little hope there will be any brilliant progress in treatment.

THE WAR AT SEA

A further area of military operation affected by the measles virus was the war at sea. It is useful to draw a distinction between measles outbreaks on board troopships and those which occurred on regular naval vessels. There are epidemiological contrasts between the two situations.

Measles on naval vessels. If the epidemiological experience of troopships was of limited duration, on board serving ships epidemic risks were multiplied through disease seeding by visits to ports and the chance of action. In northern waters, the main troubles were the infections brought from the shore—especially measles, rubella, and mumps. As Butler (1943: 391) comments: 'The difficulties of the medical officer in dealing with the epidemics in the North Sea were not lightened by the fact that the ship frequently spent days at sea under war conditions, with the prospect of action at any time.'

A note in the diary of *Australia*'s senior medical officer gives some indication of the responsibility he carried: 'Returned to port last night. To-day sent 16 cases of measles to Linlithgow Fever Hospital. Sixteen ratings out of a ship which must be ready to go into action at any time, when every man is of value!' (cited in ibid. 391).

The Australian cruiser, *Australia*, arrived to take up its defensive station in the North Sea at midwinter 1914–15. It brought an immediate crop of medical problems in the shape of respiratory tract infections which, however, were successfully overcome as the men became acclimatized and the needs for ventilation were met. Thus, the *Australia*'s sick for the four quarters of 1915 numbered 303, 210, 166, 93. Measles, together with influenza and catarrh, made up most of the large total in the first quarter.

A serious measles epidemic broke out on board the *Australia* on 18 February and lasted until 29 March. The cases were not numerous but made up for this in gravity: 21 occurred; 20 of the patients were native-born Australians, of whom two died from pulmonary complications. Butler (ibid. 391–2) reports that since the disease was of a more severe type than usual, a senior medical officer was sent from the Admiralty to report and advise. The measures already taken were extended, more especially in the daily examination of the whole ship's company, the disinfection of all mess utensils and glasses in the canteen, and greater attention to the ventilation and warming of the ship.

Ships off the Australian coast were also not free from measles but outbreaks appeared less virulent and did not spread so easily.

In the *Encounter* cruising in the Pacific in 1915 a case of measles occurred four days after leaving Sydney. Between July 25th and August 11th five more appeared. The patients were isolated on the cable deck, their mess and the sick bay fumigated, and possible contacts examined daily. The disease was very mild. (ibid. 392)

As the war progressed, concern with hygiene on board reached considerable lengths. The Australian ship, *Brisbane*, refitted at Malta in 1917 and measles (which was rife amongst the children on shore) spread to the boat. In this case the outbreak was dealt with by sending the whole ship's company into camp from 28 March to 11 April while all living spaces in the ship were thoroughly fumigated with formalin. Each cabin and space was closed for 24 hours after spraying and, in the following week, the whole mess deck was painted out. The men returned to a spotless ship.

Lessons from epidemics at sea. A number of writers have commented on the potential epidemiological value of the Australian experience in sea transport and naval vessels in World War I. Thus Butler (1943: 680–1) suggested that, 'In the case of this disease [measles] it is especially regrettable that the absence of exact records of the morbidity on Australian troopship voyages makes an exact study of the 1914–18 experience impossible.'

Cumpston (1919) argued that a troopship is a self-contained highly insulated and concentrated herd. In Australian transports, this herd remained together on the voyage to or from England for a period of eight weeks, far longer than other transports (for example, US and Canadian troops crossing the Atlantic). The herd was reasonably homogeneous in its susceptible history, and used to suffering a wide range of protective and prophylactic expedients and experiments (e.g. shore quarantine, prompt diagnosis and isolation, immunization, and treatment). As Butler (1943: 671) has commented: 'Every new case was reported on pain of severe disciplinary action, a skilled staff, professional and clerical, was often available; and provision could easily have been made for the collecting, assembling, and manipulation of a large number of reasonably comparable experiences.'

OTHER SOURCES OF EVIDENCE

The principal sources of information for this period are of two main types. First, the official histories of World War I (ironically, some of which were not published until after the completion of World War II) usually contain medical volumes. Although the greater part of these are concerned with surgery and the traumas of battle, there is some reference to infectious diseases and thus to measles. In this section, we have for the most part confined ourselves to the

English-language histories and specifically to measles outbreaks among Commonwealth and US troops. Such work as we have undertaken on French and German records suggests that the measles virus was no respecter of nationalities (see e.g. the study of Debré and Joannon, 1926, illustrated in Fig. 4.12).

One instance of measles among the troops from other parts of the Commonwealth is instructive (Macpherson *et al.*, 1922–3, ii). In August 1916, two battalions of the British West India Regiment arrived in France from Egypt. They were employed as ammunition supply companies for the heavy siege artillery. During 1917, other battalions arrived in France as reinforcements direct from the West Indies, together with a contingent of the Bermuda Garrison Artillery. There was an outbreak of measles in the 9th Battalion when it disembarked at Boulogne on 13 August 1917, and it was immediately segregated. Macpherson *et al.* (1922–3, ii. 145) explain:

The men mostly came from Jamaica, where measles was prevalent in one of the camps at Port Royal, so much so that the contingent from the camp which should have been

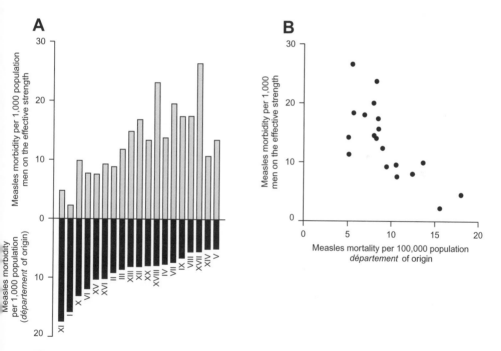

Fig. 4.12. French research on measles rates in relation to army recruitment

Notes: (A) Debré and Joannon's (1926) study of measles morbidity and mortality in French regiments. (B) Measles morbidity tended to be highest among those troops drawn from *départements* of France where measles mortality in the *département* of origin was lowest.
Source: Cliff *et al.* (1993, fig. 7.6, p. 156), drawn from data in Debré and Joannon (1926, p. 116 and fig. 27, p. 117).

embarked was left behind, and a contingent obtained from another camp took its place. On the voyage from Halifax [in Canada] twenty-one cases of measles occurred and were sent to hospital. The battalion landed at Liverpool and entrained direct for Folkestone. No notification was received at Boulogne that measles was prevalent in the battalion, and it was put into camp with large numbers of other troops.

The lack of reporting was strongly resented in France where preparations for the Ypres offensive were under way. The facts were reported to the War Office by the Adjutant-General on 5 September 1917, but the War Office in reply blandly stated that 'as all cases had been isolated from the beginning, the others were not considered to be contacts' (Macpherson *et al.*, 1922–3, ii. 145).

The second type of source is the thousands of regimental and minor histories. We have not used these, but they probably contain useful fragments of information.

TRENDS IN TIME

We have argued that, historically, in times of military mobilization, infectious diseases were a serious problem among new recruits. The case studies we have presented in this and the previous section are consistent with the long-term trends established from Curtin's data in Section 4.2, and they can be translated to other geographical locations. For example, in barracks in France in the mid-nineteenth century, measles was a serious cause of death; 116 out of 1,000 deaths among the soldiers were due to this disease (Christie, 1987: 554). In all conflicts, as in World War I, recruiting camps and depots were recognized as key locations where the incidence of measles could rise rapidly and produce high morbidity rates.

By the time of World War I, measles, like many infectious diseases, had enormous nuisance value logistically in terms of the morbidity it generated, but its role as a camp killer was greatly reduced. Yet, despite the generally reduced mortality, diseases still remained major causes of death in armies where and whenever preventive measures were inadequate or conditions were especially unfavourable. Examples which appear elsewhere in this book include the Cuban Insurrection of 1895–8 (yellow fever; see Sect. 12.3) and the Spanish–American War of 1898 (typhoid fever; see Sect. 7.3). Butler (1940: 542) has drawn attention to a number of severe outbreaks between 1914 and 1918: smallpox in Russia and Turkey, typhus in Serbia and Russia, malaria in the Palestine campaign, dysentery and enteric fever at Gallipoli and in Mesopotamia, epidemic jaundice at the Dardanelles, and measles, mumps, and roseola in all concentration camps. Wound infections occurred universally. Tables 4.4 and 4.5 summarize the relative impact of disease and battle as causes of mortality in US and Russian troops during World War I and show the large proportion of deaths still caused by disease even in 1918.

But it is important to put individual diseases in perspective and to note their comparative decline even though their cumulative burden was often great.

Table 4.4. Losses in World War I: United States

Mode of death	No.
Killed in battle	35,560
Died of wounds	14,720
Died of illness	57,460
Died of other causes	7,920
Total	115,600

Source: Lancaster (1990, table 33.16.3, p. 329).

Table 4.5. Losses in World War I: Russian Empire, 1914–1917

Mode of death	No.
Killed	664,890
Died of wounds with their units	18,378
Died of wounds in the hospitals	300,000
Died of diseases in the hospitals	130,000[1]
Died in captivity	285,000
Sudden deaths	7,196
Reported missing	200,000
Died of gas	6,340
Additional losses from the Caucasian front	50,000
Total dead and missing	1,661,840

Notes: [1] Registered cases: smallpox 2,708; cholera 30,810; relapsing fever 75,429; typhus 21,093. Effects were worse in the Red Army, 1917–20, yielding: smallpox 5,749; cholera 22,465; relapsing fever 780,870; typhus 522,458.
Source: Lancaster (1990, tables 33.16.5 and 33.16.6, p. 330). Modified after Kohn and Meyendorff (1932, table 76), in which there is a discussion of the validity of the statistics.

Until the influenza pandemic of 1918–19 (Sects. 7.4.1, 11.3, 12.5.3), only one sickness achieved general epidemic proportions during World War I, namely trench fever. The limited nature of infections is itself remarkable, given that some 15 million men were serving on both sides on the Franco-Belgian front under conditions which simply 'invited outbreaks of the pestilences characteristic of warfare' (Butler, 1940: 542). As Butler (ibid.) has argued, 'the negative history (as we may term it) of disease in the Great War is more significant than the positive, and the absence of certain diseases more impressive than the prevalence of others'. By the time of World War II, this was even more the case.

4.5 Patterns since 1918

4.5.1 Trends in Time

The long-term decline in the significance of infectious diseases in armies continued. Just as the germ theory of disease revolutionized disease-containment procedures from the 1880s, three major advances in prevention and treatment continued the process after 1918.

The first was the discovery of new antibiotics which prevented secondary infections. Until the introduction of the sulphonamides in 1935, there was no antiseptic capable of attacking bacteria in tissues of the body; in World War II, the sulphonamides were used throughout and, in 1944, penicillin became available. Case-fatality rates were therefore greatly reduced by preventing a range of secondary infections associated with the common respiratory infections—pneumonia, otitis media, mastoiditis, and meningitis, usually of streptococcal origin. Dangerous hospital epidemics of gangrene were avoided altogether. The range of available antibiotics mushroomed after 1945.

The second major advance was the rapid development of vaccines against many of the common infections, so eliminating the susceptible population. Smallpox was eradicated globally by 1979, and a wide range of other infections that beset armies in the past are now controlled by vaccination. These include cholera, hepatitis, measles, mumps, plague, poliomyelitis, rubella, typhus fever, and yellow fever, as well as killers like anthrax and rabies. Much of the global progress has been articulated through the World Health Organization Expanded Programme of Immunization (see Sect. 3.6).

The third advance was the discovery in 1937 that blood could be stored for up to a week in a condition suitable for use in transfusions. This permitted the use of transfusions on a massive scale in World War II. In general, the treatment of shock was greatly improved in World War II.

The real impact of each of these advances was not felt until World War II and after. This is illustrated in Figure 4.13 and Table 4.6. Figure 4.13 shows the recorded number of cases per annum per 1,000 average strength in the US Army in the continental United States. Although there are clearly cycles of dis-

Table 4.6. Measles rates in the US armed forces since 1861

Conflict	Cases per 1,000 man-years	Deaths
Civil War, 1861–5	32.2	2.0
Spanish–American War, 1898	26.1	0.32
World War I, 1914–18	23.8	0.57
World War II, 1939–45	4.7	0.004
Vietnam War, 1966	0.9	0.0

Source: Cliff *et al.* (1993, table 7.5, p. 159), from Black (1984, table 3, p. 407).

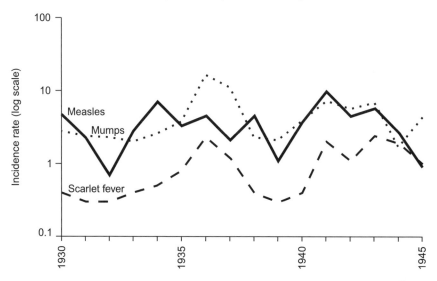

Fig. 4.13. Incidence rates for measles, mumps, and scarlet fever in the US Army based in the Continental United States

Notes: Incidence is measured as the number of cases per annum per 1,000 average strength. The data for 1930–41 are for enlisted men only.
Source: Data from Hoff (1958, table 24, p. 134).

Table 4.7. Royal Naval Hospital, Gosport, 1914–1918 and 1939–1945: measles admissions

World War I	1914[1]	1915	1916	1917	1918			Total	Case rate[3]
Measles admissions	1	194	409	118	158			880	16.0
World War II	1939[2]	1940	1941	1942	1943	1944	1945		
Measles admissions	7	31	90	32	53	10	42	265	2.9

Notes: [1] August–December 1914. [2] September–December 1939. [3] Per 1,000 patients admitted.
Source: Cliff *et al.* (1993, table 7.6, p. 159), from Mellor (1972, table 38, p. 85).

ease activity which coincide with measles cycles in the civil population (Stokes, 1958), the general trend is almost horizontal. But Table 4.6 shows the long-term collapse of measles rates in the US Army from 1861 to 1966. The last date is post-mass vaccination from measles in the US; this had commenced in 1965.

A similar story is told with data for the UK. Table 4.7 shows the vastly reduced case rates per 1,000 patients admitted to the Royal Naval Hospital, Gosport, in World War II when compared with World War I.

Yet within these trends, infectious diseases could still present the same problems as they had done historically when armies assembled or were in confined spaces. The history of infectious diseases among Australian troops in World War II illustrates the point.

4.5.2 Australia, 1939–1945

As in World War I, the official Australian histories of the 1939–45 period are exceptionally full. Australian troops served widely, starting in the Western Desert and, following Japan's entry into the war, increasingly in Southeast Asia and the Pacific.

WAR ON LAND

From March 1942, when the Japanese invaded New Guinea, Australian troops were heavily involved. Walker (1957), in *The Island Campaigns*, has described the impact of measles upon Australian forces fighting the Japanese in the New Guinea campaign.

The 3rd Field Ambulance was assigned the task of supporting the 14th Brigade in the Bootless area. These arrangements were not made easier by an epidemic of measles, which broke out among late arrivals of the 14th Brigade. 'A' Company of the 14th Ambulance set up a measles hospital in Murray Barracks to deal with the outbreak, which soon affected over 200 men. This unit, in addition to setting up action stations in sites occupied in the Moresby area, also had the task of acting as an evacuation centre for patients being transferred to the mainland. (Walker, 1957: 9)

WAR AT SEA

An analysis by Walker (1961: 133) of infectious diseases in the Royal Australian Navy to the middle of 1945 showed that mumps were widespread in some ships in 1939–40, though not serious in degree. In the same year, rubella affected training depots in large numbers but not the seagoing ships.

According to the account of Walker (ibid.), when large numbers of men were carried in a transport, the effect of propinquity was clearly apparent if an epidemic disease was introduced. In *Manoora*, which was conveying 1,100 army officers and men to Western Australia, there was an outbreak of measles accompanied by an epidemic of an influenzal type of cold. This combination imposed a serious strain on the accommodation in the sick bay.

Closed communities, such as ships and Arctic and Antarctic expeditions, often found that they were immune from many of the respiratory epidemics unless some carrier from without intruded into their bounded world. So, in many ships and in large, land-based establishments, which were closed and semi-closed communities, large epidemics of upper respiratory tract infection could and did occur following the introduction of infection. As described in

Walker (ibid. 133–4), the Australian destroyers in the Mediterranean suffered outbreaks of respiratory infections during the winters of 1939–40 and 1940–1 due, in a large measure, to the unsatisfactory ventilation of the ships and to prolonged bouts of bad weather. 'In ships at sea even small outbreaks might be significant because of the limited space available for isolation and the difficulty of replacing personnel, and it was fortunate that opportunities for infection by the most prevalent agents were more limited in the navy than in the other Services' (ibid. 133).

As we have seen, infections did occur, however. At the end of 1941, Surgeon Commander L. Lockwood listed a number which were treated in the fleet while *Hobart* was serving in the Mediterranean:

... amoebic dysentery, bacillary dysentery, catarrhal (infective) jaundice, cerebro-spinal meningitis, malaria, pulmonary tuberculosis, typhoid and paratyphoid fevers, undulant fever, diphtheria, pneumonia, erysipelas, rubella, scarlet fever, smallpox, poliomyelitis, mumps and measles. Of course, ships on the Mediterranean Station had to call at ports in the Middle East where there were health hazards quite apart from those normally expected to produce problems of recognition, prevention and treatment. (ibid.)

4.6 HIV in the US Army, 1985–1989

Relatively high incidence of sexually transmitted diseases (STDs) has been part and parcel of armies and war from time immemorial. As we have already seen in Figure 4.4, nineteenth-century armies in Europe and in the colonies of the European powers were no exception. With the coming of penicillin, treatment was relatively straightforward from World War II. In 1979, however, problems with STDs took on a new dimension when the first case of AIDS (acquired immunodeficiency syndrome) was reported. An international picture of the first decade of the global AIDS/HIV pandemic is provided in Smallman-Raynor, Cliff, and Haggett (1992). There is still no cure for the causative agent of AIDS, the human immunodeficiency virus (HIV). While treatment regimes in times of peace in the advanced economies enable infected individuals to resume a comparatively normal lifestyle, in the developing nations, especially in Africa and in Asian countries like Thailand and Burma, HIV rates in both civil and military populations can reach catastrophic levels.

There is compelling evidence that both national and liberation (rebel) armies in many African countries have played a major role in fuelling the epidemic in that continent. This is studied in Section 10.4. As a preliminary to that work, in this section, we look at the nature of the problem among recruits into the US Army between 1985 and 1989 and see to what extent the patterns of HIV infection in the national population (Sect. 4.6.1) are reflected among army recruits (Sect. 4.6.2).

4.6.1 AIDS in the United States, 1979–1989

In order to interpret patterns of HIV infection among military recruits, it is important to understand the geographical and ethnic distribution of AIDS in the general population of the United States during the 1980s. A detailed account appears in Smallman-Raynor *et al.* (1992: 185–231).

ETHNIC DISTRIBUTION

During the first decade of the global AIDS pandemic, the US epidemic was sharply concentrated among homosexuals, intravenous drug users (IVDUs), and ethnic minorities. Table 4.8 gives the relative risk for AIDS by ethnic group and transmission category in US adults (aged 13 years and over) for the period ending on 31 December 1989. Relative risk (*RR*) is defined as

$$RR = (A_i/P_i)/(A_j/P_j), \tag{4.3}$$

the ratio of the cumulative incidence of AIDS in a group *i* to that in a reference group *j* where *A* and *P* refer to AIDS case totals and population size respectively. Because the absolute majority of US AIDS cases during the 1980s was among Whites, the cumulative AIDS incidence rate for Whites has been chosen as the reference epidemic in Table 4.8 so that, by definition, their relative risk is 1.0.

The top row of Table 4.8 (All cases) shows that, regardless of gender or transmission category, Blacks and Hispanics display an inflated risk for AIDS relative to Whites. For Blacks, the risk is 3.63 times higher than for Whites. For

Table 4.8. Relative risks for AIDS among US adults by ethnicity to 31 December 1989

Transmission route	Relative risk by ethnic classification[1]			
	White	Hispanic	Black	Other
All cases	1.00	3.89	3.63	0.54
By gender				
Males	1.00	3.49	3.27	0.44
Females	1.00	10.80	13.97	1.42
By transmission category				
Homosexual/non-IVDU	1.00	2.10	1.74	0.46
Homosexual IVDU	1.00	3.48	3.38	0.28
Heterosexual IVDU	1.00	20.78	18.86	0.75
Heterosexual contact	1.00	11.89	23.50	1.33
Other/unknown	1.00	3.97	3.50	0.92

Notes: [1] The ethnic classification is specified by US Centers for Disease Control and Prevention and forms the basis for the collection of US data on AIDS and HIV. Whites form the reference epidemic.
Source: Smallman-Raynor *et al.* (1992, table 5.2.1, p. 195).

Hispanics, the factor is 3.89. In contrast, for Others (including Alaskan natives, American Indians, and Asian/Pacific islanders) the risk is approximately half that seen for Whites.

The most dramatic variations occur when individual transmission categories are examined. For heterosexual intravenous drug users (IVDUs), the risk of AIDS is respectively 18.86 and 20.78 times as great in Blacks and Hispanics as in Whites. Although variable, this pattern of raised risk among ethnic minorities is repeated in all other transmission categories and also by gender.

GEOGRAPHICAL DISTRIBUTION

In 1990, approximately 138 million people, representing 57.5 per cent of the total US population, resided in the country's 93 largest (over 500,000 population) Standard Metropolitan Statistical Areas (SMSAs). The locations of these urban agglomerations are indicated by circles on Figure 4.14. The majority are located in the eastern half of the country, especially along the Atlantic seaboard. To the west, a second cluster occurs on the Pacific coast of California. Elsewhere, large SMSAs are only infrequently found.

Together, these SMSAs formed the core locations for the US AIDS epidemic throughout the 1980s. By October 1989, over 85 per cent of the 112,241 AIDS cases reported to the Centers for Disease Control and Prevention resided in these settlements. However, incidence varied dramatically between the SMSAs. To illustrate this, the proportional circles in Figure 4.14 plot the cumulative AIDS incidence rate per 100,000 population for each SMSA by 31 October 1989. In addition, each circle has been shaded according to the probability of that rate occurring by chance. These probabilities have been computed by reducing the rates to standard Normal scores and comparing them to a Normal distribution; the three darkest shading categories denote significantly high incidence at the 1, 5, and 10 per cent levels in a one-tailed test (see Cliff and Haggett, 1988: 25–9). The two lighter shading categories flag whether non-significant incidence rates are above or below the mean.

The average rate for the 93 large SMSAs was 69.1 AIDS cases per 100,000 population. However, it is evident from Figure 4.14 that the distribution is highly skewed. Most metropolitan areas displayed rates well below the national average; significantly high rates were restricted to seven SMSAs in just four states (California, Florida, New York, and New Jersey) and Puerto Rico. The urban AIDS epidemic in the 1980s reached its zenith in San Francisco SMSA, California, where the cumulative rate of 427.3 per 100,000 was almost twice that of the second-ranked SMSA, New York. New York State was the nucleus of a cluster of high incidence SMSAs (New York, Jersey City, and Newark; rates 160 per 100,000) in the extreme northeast of the country. A further cluster of high rates (125 per 100,000) was focused on the two neighbouring Floridan SMSAs of Fort Lauderdale and Miami. Finally, in the Caribbean

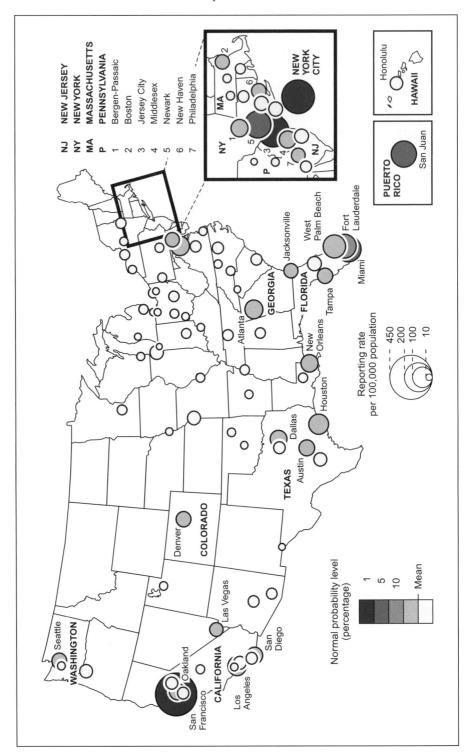

Basin, San Juan SMSA (Puerto Rico) displayed the country's sixth most intense metropolitan epidemic (154.8 per 100,000).

4.6.2 HIV in Military Recruits

Since October 1985, all persons applying for active duty or reserve military service in the United States, the service academies, and the Reserve Officer Training Corps have been screened for HIV infection as part of their entrance medical evaluation. The data are published by Centers for Disease Control and Prevention (CDC, 1990). Applicants are interviewed by recruiting officials about drug use and homosexual activity (both of which are grounds for exclusion from entry into military service). Potential applicants are informed that they will be screened for HIV antibody and therefore we might expect these risk groups to be under-represented.

At the geographical levels of states and SMSAs over 500,000, the military data set gives the number of recruits tested, and the number HIV positive by age, gender, and ethnic groups. To mirror the geographical scales used in the previous subsection, these data are analysed here first at the state level and then for the SMSAs.

STATES

Some 2.49 million applicants were tested over the period, of whom 3,114 (0.12%) were found to be HIV positive. Table 4.9 summarizes the rates by ethnic groups and gender. Although the military data are for HIV whereas the national data examined in the previous section are for AIDS, comparison of Tables 4.8 and 4.9 implies some significant differences as between military recruits and national relative risk. Among applicants for military service, the bias is towards ethnic minorities just as it is in the US population at large. But it is Black males with the greatest rates among the military applicants. Nationally, in terms of relative risk, Hispanics had a somewhat greater relative risk than Blacks, and there was a strong female bias.

The data relating to all applicants and giving the percentage HIV positive by ethnic groups were then subjected to a principal components analysis. Table 4.10 summarizes the results. Two components were extracted with eigenvalues greater than unity, and the loadings are given in Table 4.10. The components

◀

Fig. 4.14. Cumulative AIDS incidence rates in US cities by 31 October 1989

Notes: Proportional circles plot the cumulative AIDS incidence rate per 100,000 population in the 93 largest (population over 500,000) Standard Metropolitan Statistical Areas (SMSAs) at the end of the first decade of the epidemic in the United States. States with significantly high rates have been determined by comparison with a Normal distribution. See text for details.

Source: Redrawn from Smallman-Raynor *et al.* (1992, fig. 5.4C, p. 206).

Table 4.9. United States, 1985–1989: prevalence of HIV antibody in civilian applicants for military service by gender and ethnic group

Gender	Percentage of those tested HIV positive					
	All	White	Hispanic	Black	American Indian, Alaskan	Asian Pacific Islands
Males	0.14	0.06	0.21	0.40	0.11	0.05
Females	0.06	0.02	0.08	0.15	0.04	0.02

Source: Data from CDC (1990, table 2A).

Table 4.10. HIV among US army recruits, 1985–1989: state level. Principal components loadings for percentage of recruits from different ethnic groups diagnosed as HIV positive

Ethnic group (% HIV positive)	Loadings	
	Component 1	Component 2
Whites	0.683	−0.484
Blacks	−0.730	−0.442
Hispanics	0.000	0.753
Indians	0.000	0.000
Asians	0.000	0.000
Cumulative percentage of variance explained	83.5	96.5

split Hispanics (component 2) from Whites and Blacks (component 1). Whites and Blacks are at opposite ends of component 1. These results emphasize the significance of Blacks and Hispanics as vectors of HIV among military applicants.

To illustrate the geographical pattern of HIV infection among potential recruits from different states, Figure 4.15 uses Poisson probability mapping, described in Cliff and Haggett (1988: 25–9), to identify states with significantly high levels of infection. Under the Poisson model, each state is assumed

Fig. 4.15. United States 1985–1989: prevalence of HIV-1 antibody in civilian applicants for military service, I

Notes: Poisson probability mapping has been used to identify states with especially high rates in different ethnic groups. (A) All applicants. (B) Whites. (C) Blacks. (D) Hispanics. Proportional circles give the HIV rate per 100,000 population in the ethnic group concerned. White circles: $p > 0.10$; light grey circles: $p \leq 0.10$; dark grey circles: $p \leq 0.05$; black circles: $p \leq 0.01$.
Source: Data from CDC (1990, table 2A).

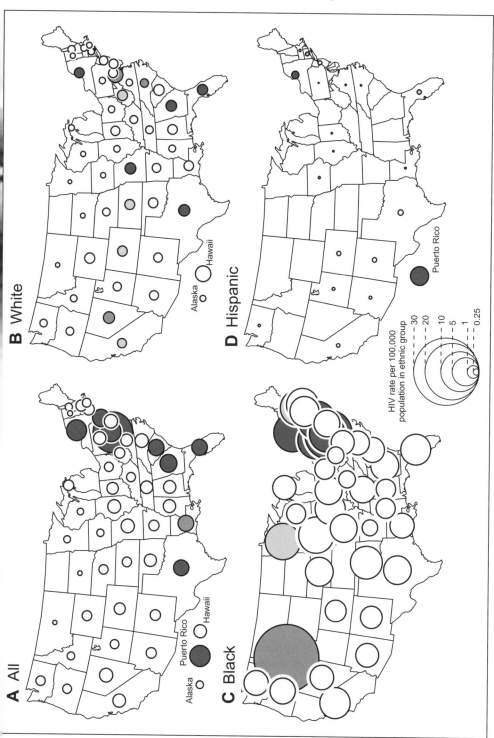

to have an equal and independent chance of having an event (here, an HIV infection) occur in it. Figure 4.15 uses the 10, 5, and 1 per cent probability levels to map states with significantly high levels of infection in different ethnic groups. Proportional circles have been utilized to show rates per 100,000 population for the ethnic group concerned (that is, for Blacks, the rate has been calculated per 100,000 Black population in each state, and so on).

For all recruits, Figure 4.15A shows that infection rates reflect several features of the AIDS pattern mapped in Figure 4.14. The concentration of high rates among the eastern seaboard states is especially marked. The signal difference is the lack of significant values for the Pacific seaboard states. Figures 4.15B–D map states with significantly high rates for the principal ethnic groups. Among Whites (Fig. 4.15B), the emphasis on the eastern seaboard states is reduced, to be replaced by new states with high rates in the central farming (Kansas) and Rocky Mountain states (Nevada, Colorado). The map follows fairly closely the national pattern for AIDS shown in Figure 4.14. The high rates states for Blacks (Fig. 4.15C) are concentrated almost exclusively in the north and northeast. Among Hispanics, the focus of high-rate states in the north and northeast seen for Blacks is repeated.

Figure 4.16 illustrates HIV infection rates among all prospective recruits at the level of SMSAs. The mapping conventions of Figure 4.15 have been followed. The patterns closely echo those for AIDS mapped in Figure 4.14. They confirm the concentration of the epidemic in the major cities of the United States, especially on the east and west coasts.

4.7 Conclusion

The fall in the incidence of infectious diseases among soldiers from 1850 to the present day parallels that in civil populations. As we saw in Sections 4.4 and 4.5, it was the result of better preventive medicine, beginning with the scientific breakthrough of the germ theory of disease in the 1880s. Immunization was central in causing the long-term declining trend of infections. This had successfully commenced with vaccination against smallpox in

Fig. 4.16. United States 1985–1989: prevalence of HIV-1 antibody in civilian applicants for military service, II

Notes: Poisson probability mapping has been used to identify SMSAs with especially high rates among all applicants for military service. Proportional circles give the HIV rate per 100,000 population. White circles: $p > 0.10$; light grey circles: $p \leq 0.10$; dark grey circles: $p \leq 0.05$; black circles: $p \leq 0.01$.
Source: Data from CDC (1990, table 4A).

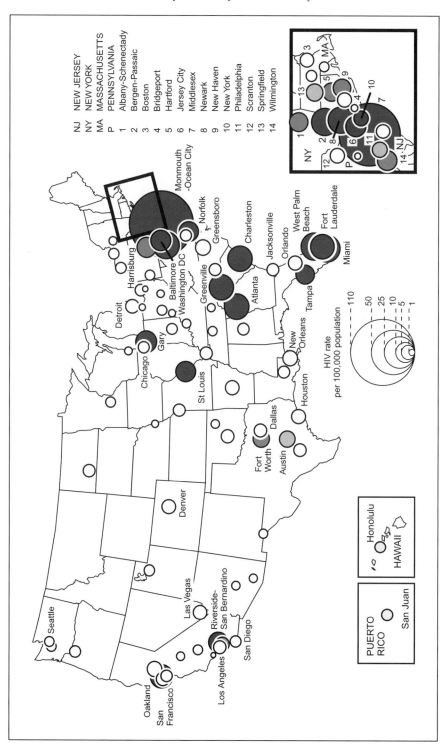

Table 4.11. Chronology of the development of vaccines, 1796–1960

Disease	Date (approx.)	Developer/discoverer
Smallpox	1796	Jenner
Anthrax	1881	Pasteur
Rabies	1885	Pasteur
Diphtheria (antitoxin)	1891	Behring and Kitasato
Tetanus (antitoxin)	1891	Behring and Kitasato
Cholera	1892	Haffkine
Plague	1897	Haffkine
Typhoid	1898	Wright
Tuberculosis (BCG)	1921	Calmette and Guérin
Typhus fever	1933–8	Weigl/Cox
Pertussis	1933–6	Sauer/Kendrick
Yellow fever (17D)	1938	—
Poliomyelitis	1954–6	Salk/Sabin
Measles	1960	Enders

Source: Based on information in Parish (1968, pp. 218–23).

1796;[1] it continued during the late nineteenth and twentieth centuries with an ever-widening range of vaccines against infections (Table 4.11). Vaccination was reinforced with effective direct therapeutic intervention, illustrated in the second half of the nineteenth century by the use of quinine against malaria, drugs against amoebic dysentery, and techniques to prevent the dehydration of cholera victims. The effectiveness of these measures was a beginning enhanced in the twentieth century with a growing armoury of antibiotics like sulphano-mides (1930s), penicillin (1940s), and, thereafter, streptomycin, neomycin, and tetracycline, among many others.

Despite all this progress against infectious disease, sexually transmitted infections remained a persistent problem among the military, highlighted in the present age by HIV. We study this theme in detail in Chapter 10. One other arena in which infectious diseases frequently reign supreme even today is among displaced (refugee) people. Then, the frequent breakdown of hygiene and nutritional standards provides a window for infectious diseases to re-emerge as large-scale killers. It is to this topic that we turn in the next chapter.

[1] Year of Edward Jenner's first experiment with human-to-human vaccination.

5

Mortality and Morbidity in Modern Wars, III: Displaced Populations

We do not understand why saffron flowers before the shrine
Lie dead,
As our sons lie dead along the way.
Along the road to the city.
We do not understand,
Why only death has pity.
Death is all that remains,
The only harvest for what we sowed.
We do not understand,
Why death should be our harvest.

Tara Ali Baig, 'Bengal Famine', 1943[1]

[1] Reproduced in Currey and Gibson (1946: 48–51).

5.1 Introduction

As a threat to life and liberty, wars and political upheavals have served to precipitate the flight of populations since biblical times (Marrus, 1985; Zolberg *et al.*, 1989; UNHCR, 2000). Historically, the basic mechanism of flight, sometimes across national boundaries, and with no surety of safety or asylum in the new land, has operated as a device for the carriage of infectious diseases from one geographical location to another. In Chapter 2, for example, we encountered numerous instances of wartime fugitives who spread bubonic plague, typhus fever, and other war pestilences to their local 'host' populations. At the same time, however, fleeing populations may be forced to enter epidemiological environments to which they are unacclimatized, with the attendant risk of exposure to diseases for which they have little or no acquired immunity. The intensive mixing of the populations in refugee camps or other makeshift forms of shelter, often with poor levels of hygiene, with little or no medical provision, and under conditions of stress and malnutrition, further add to the disease risks of displacement (Prothero, 1994; Kalipeni and Oppong, 1998; UNHCR, 2000).

The epidemiological dimensions of wartime population displacement—variously manifesting in the movements of refugees, evacuees, and other persons who abandon their homes as a consequence of conflict—form the theme of the present chapter. We begin, in Section 5.2, with a brief overview of international developments in the recognition and management of war-displaced populations, the legal meaning which attaches to such classifications as *refugee* and *internally displaced person* (IDP), and theoretical frameworks that have been developed for the study of such groups. International refugees, along with certain other categories of displaced person, have fallen within the mandate of the Office of the United Nations High Commissioner for Refugees (UNHCR) since its inception in January 1951. Drawing on this source, Section 5.3 examines global trends in refugees and other UNHCR-recognized populations of concern during the latter half of the twentieth century, while Section 5.4 reviews epidemiological aspects of the associated population movements.

The remainder of the chapter follows a regional-thematic structure. Section 5.5 explores the intersection of population displacement and infectious disease in the context of civil defence, taking as an example the evacuation of schoolchildren and other 'priority classes' from the militarily vulnerable towns and cities of Britain during World War II. Turning from Europe to the Middle East, Section 5.6 examines long-term patterns of infectious disease activity in the semi-permanent population of Palestinian refugees in the Contested Territories of the West Bank and the Gaza Strip, Jordan, Lebanon, and Syria. Finally, Section 5.7 addresses the explosive outbreaks of louse-borne typhus and cholera that followed on the population disclocation of Burundi and Rwanda, Central Africa, during the civil wars and genocide of the mid-1990s. The chapter is concluded in Section 5.8.

5.2 Background

In Section 2.2, we described one of the earliest historical references to epidemic transmission in a war-displaced population. In 430 BC, with the Peloponnesian Army bearing down on Athens, an estimated 200,000 inhabitants of the surrounding countryside uprooted to the city. When the Plague of Athens appeared in that same year, notes Thucydides, it was the inadequately sheltered refugees from the countryside that 'suffered most' and perished in 'wild disorder' (Thucydides, 2. 52, transl. Jowett, 1900: 138–9). And so, down the ages, those displaced as a consequence of war have ranked amongst the most vulnerable and needy of people. Yet, prior to the nineteenth century, it appears that such populations rarely impinged upon public conciousness. According to Marrus (1985: 7–8), physical limits to the sustainability of large-scale population movements in early societies, coupled with the lack of obligation of host populations to extend any form of protection or support, generally dictated against the survival of refugees *en masse*. Into the nineteenth century, European attention, at least, began to turn to the burgeoning numbers of *émigrés* and other exiles from the revolutionary wars and political upheavals of the time (Marrus, 1985). But it was the early twentieth century, and the massive population dislocation wrought by conflict in the crumbling empires of Tsarist Russia and Ottoman Turkey that finally brought the refugee problem to the forefront of international attention (Marrus, 1985; Zolberg *et al.*, 1989).

5.2.1 International Developments

International efforts to manage and assist refugees can be traced to the aftermath of World War I. In 1921, the International Committee of the Red Cross petitioned the recently established League of Nations to provide assistance to an estimated 1.5 million Russians who had been displaced by ongoing civil war, disease, and famine. The same year, the League of Nations appointed the first High Commissioner for Refugees—Fridtjof Nansen (Pl. 5.1). With provisionally limited tenure, and with duties initially directed to the resettlement or repatriation of the Russian refugees, Nansen's appeals to the League allowed the work of his office to extend to the several million Armenians, Bulgars, Greeks, and Turks who had been displaced in the years after 1912 (UNHCR, 2000).

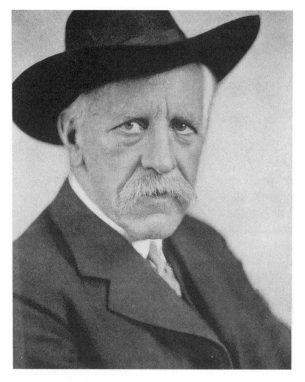

Pl. 5.1. Fridtjof Nansen (1861–1930)

Notes: Norwegian zoologist, Arctic explorer, oceanographer, and humanitarian. On the initiative of the International Committee of the Red Cross, Nansen was appointed by the League of Nations as the first High Commissioner for Refugees in 1921—a post which he held until the year of his death. He was awarded the Nobel Peace Prize in 1922.
Source: © AP Wide World Photos.

OFFICE OF THE UNITED NATIONS HIGH COMMISIONER FOR
REFUGEES (UNHCR)

While the League of Nations responded to inter-war refugee movements through the ad hoc appointment of special High Commissioners and envoys, World War II was to provide the impetus for new international developments. The United Nations Relief and Rehabilitation Administration (UNRRA), established in 1943, took initial responsibility for the post-war repatriation of the many millions of refugees that had resulted from the recent conflict in Europe. But the repatriation programme proved controversial and, from July 1947, the International Refugee Organization (IRO) assumed temporary responsibility for refugees. In January 1951, the remit of the IRO was transferred to the newly created Office of the United Nations High Commissioner for Refugees (UNHCR). Underpinned by the 1951 UN Convention Relating to the Status of Refugees, and with its primary functions formed to include the protection, repatriation, or assimilation of refugees and other populations of concern, UNHCR has retained its international mandate into the twenty-first century (UNHCR, 2000).

5.2.2 Categories of Displaced Person

In common parlance, a refugee (from the French *réfugier*, to take refuge) is a person who, for reasons of war, persecution, famine, or some other disaster, has been compelled to abandon his or her home in search of sanctuary. In international law, however, a complex legal framework has developed around the meaning of the term 'refugee' and the particular status which it affords. Here, we first consider the definition of a refugee in international law, before turning to the related, but legally distinct, concept of 'internally displaced person'. Standard surveys of the issues addressed in this subsection include Grahl-Madsen (1966, 1972) and Chimni (2000), while UNHCR (2000) provides an historical perspective on institutional developments.

REFUGEES

In international law, the term 'refugee' is reserved for a displaced person who has been forced across an international border. As defined in Article 1 A(2) of the 1951 UN Convention Relating to the Status of Refugees—which came into force on 22 April 1954—a refugee is any person who

[as a result of events occurring before 1 January 1951 and] owing to well-founded fear of being persecuted for reasons of race, religion, nationality, membership of a particular social group or political opinion, is outside the country of his nationality and is unable or, owing to such fear, is unwilling to avail himself of the protection of that country; or who, not having a nationality and being outside the country of his former habitual residence as a result of such events, is unable or, owing to such fear, is unwilling to return to it. (Cited in UNHCR, 2000: 23)

While the 1967 Protocol to the Convention made some technical adjustments to this original statement, including the removal of the temporal limitation 'before 1 January 1951', subsequent conventions and declarations have expanded the 1951 definition to meet specific regional circumstances.

1. *Africa.* In 1969, the Organization of African Unity's (OAU) Refugee Convention extended the basic 1951 UN definition to include

every person who, owing to external aggression, occupation, foreign domination or events seriously disturbing public order in either part or the whole of his country of origin or nationality, is compelled to leave his place of habitual residence in order to seek refuge in another place outside his country of origin or nationality. (Cited in UNHCR, 2000: 55)

The OAU Refugee Convention came into force in 1974 and, since that time, the 1951 UN Convention, the 1967 UN Protocol and the 1969 OAU Convention have provided the legal framework for UNHCR activities in Africa (ibid.).

2. *Latin America.* In response to the particular circumstances that pertained in Central America during the 1970s and 1980s, the 1984 Cartagena Declaration on Refugees expanded the 1951 UN definition to include those who flee their country 'because their lives, safety or freedom have been threatened by generalized violence, foreign aggression, internal conflicts, massive violation of human rights or other circumstances which have seriously disturbed public order' (cited in ibid. 123). As UNHCR (ibid.) notes, although the Cartagena Declaration—and the definition of a refugee which it contains—is not legally binding on its signatories, most countries of Central and South America apply the definition as a matter of routine.

Stateless Persons

It is important to note that the legal instruments of the United Nations draw a distinction between 'refugees' and 'stateless persons'. Although the two categories are classically related, the rights of stateless persons were first addressed in the 1954 UN Convention Relating to the Status of Stateless Persons. According to Article 1 of the Convention, a stateless person is simply defined as one 'who is not considered as a national by any State under the operation of its law' (cited in Batchelor, 1995: 232).

INTERNALLY DISPLACED PERSONS (IDPS)

The international tools to protect refugees do not cover internally displaced persons (IDPs)—those who, according to the UN Secretary-General on Internally Displaced Persons, 'have been forced to flee their homes suddenly and unexpectedly' but 'who are within the territory of their own country' (cited in Chimni, 2000: 406). Although the International Committee of the Red Cross has traditionally assisted such persons, and the UNHCR's involvement with IDPs dates back to the 1960s, the internally displaced have usually been viewed as falling under the jurisdiction of the state concerned. Moreover, while the number of internally displaced has apparently escalated in recent years, reaching an estimated 20–5 million worldwide in 1999 (UNHCR, 2000: 214), the protection of IDPs is frequently complicated by the difficulties of distinguishing them from the civil popuations with which they mix. As a consequence, there is some debate as to whether IDPs should be seen as a special category of person or whether they should be included in the general classification of 'vulnerable people' (UNHCR, 2000).

5.2.3 Theoretical Frameworks

A number of researchers have attempted to classify the movements of refugees and internally displaced persons, and to describe, theorize, and model the

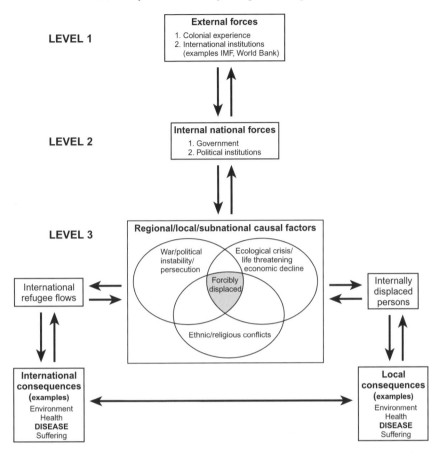

Fig. 5.1. Conceptual framework for the analysis of population displacement in Africa
Source: Redrawn from Kalipeni and Oppong (1998, fig. 1, p. 1640), originally based on Wood (1994, fig. 2, p. 614).

social, political, and cultural settings in which such forced population displacements occur (see e.g. Kunz, 1973, 1981; Peterson, 1975; Zolberg *et al.*, 1989; Wood, 1994). As Wood (1994: 608) notes, however, such efforts have not been wholly successful, not least because 'involuntary migrations are based on complex decision-making processes and diverse causal factors'. Accepting these difficulties, Figure 5.1 is based on the work of Wood (1994) and Kalipeni and Oppong (1998) and provides a conceptual framework for the refugee situation in one world region (Africa). The diagram shows schematically how subnational (Level 3) factors of war/political instability, ethnic/religious conflict, and ecological crisis/economic decline may, in concert with national (Level 2) and international (Level 1) forces, interact to generate internal population displacement and international refugee movements. As the lower level of the model indicates, these movements may have severe ramifications for health, disease, and the environment both at local and international levels. We return to a consideration of the intersection of war-associated population displacement, health, and disease in Section 5.4.

5.3 Global Patterns of Displacement, 1950–1999

To examine global patterns of population displacement in the era of the UNHCR, 1950–99, we draw on geo-coded counts of refugees and other displaced populations as published in Annexes 2 and 3 of the agency's *The State of the World's Refugees 2000* (UNHCR, 2000). Our consideration begins with an examination of global and world regional trends in refugees, before turning to the distribution of other categories of displaced person.

5.3.1 Refugees

GLOBAL AND WORLD REGIONAL TRENDS

Figure 5.2A is based on information included in UNHCR (2000) and plots end-of-year estimates of the global number of refugees, 1950–99. Principal geographical foci of UNHCR activities in each decennial period are indicated on the chart while, for reference, Table 5.1 lists a sample of war-associated refugee movements during the 50-year observation interval. Taken together, two features of Figure 5.2A and Table 5.1 are noteworthy. First, from an initial focus in Europe during the 1950s, the geographical compass of refugees has rapidly expanded to include large—in some instances, massive—international displacements in the continents of Africa (1960s onwards), Asia (1970s onwards), and the Americas (1980s). Secondly, in association with this geographical expansion, the 1970s marked the beginning of a steep upwards trend in the estimated number of refugees, from some 2.5 million in 1970, to in excess of 18.3 million in the early 1990s. Thereafter, the number declined to about 11.7 million in 1999.

The post-1960s increase in the estimated number of refugees is examined for each of six world regions (Africa, Asia, Europe, Latin America/Caribbean, North America, and Oceania) in Figure 5.2B. As the graph shows, the overall pattern is dominated by Asia and Africa, with the annual totals peaking in the early 1990s (Asia) and the mid-1990s (Africa) at around 8.5 million and 6.8 million respectively. In addition, the graph shows a sharp increase in the number of refugees in Europe (largely associated with political upheavals and conflicts in the Soviet Union and the former Yugoslavia) during the 1990s. Elsewhere, in Latin America/Caribbean, North America, and Oceania, the regional counts of refugees remained at comparatively low (≤1.2 million) annual levels throughout the observation period.

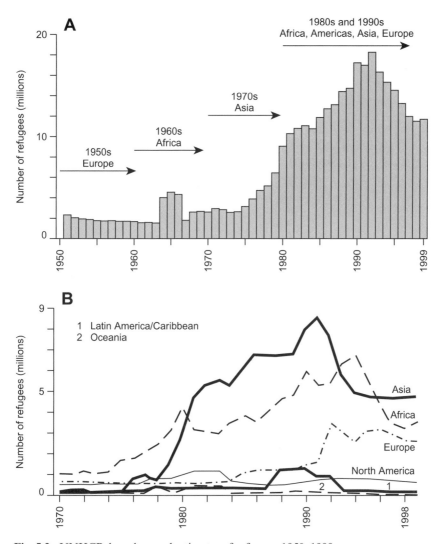

Fig. 5.2. UNHCR-based annual estimates of refugees, 1950–1999

Notes: (A) Global estimates of the number of refugees, 1950–99, with the principal geographical focus of UNHCR activities in each decennial period indicated. (B) World regional estimates of the number of refugees, 1970–99. All data relate to 31 December of the given year. Palestinian refugees, under the mandate of the United Nations Relief and Works Agency for Palestinian Refugees (UNRWA), have been excluded from all estimates.

Source: Data from UNHCR (2000, annex 3, p. 310).

Table 5.1. Sample war-associated refugee flows, 1950–1999

Country or region

Origin	Asylum	Year of arrival	Conflict	No. of refugees
Hungary	Austria	1956–7	Hungarian Revolt	173,000
Ruanda (Rwanda)	Central Africa	1960–1	Ruandan Civil War	120,000
Nigeria	West Africa	1967–70	Biafran War	50,000
East Pakistan (Bangladesh)	India	1971	Pakistani Civil War	9,900,000
Indochina	Thailand	1975–9	Civil Wars	280,000
Ethiopia (Eritrea)	Sudan	1976–84	Ethiopian–Eritrean War	500,000
Afghanistan	Pakistan	1978–80	Afghan Civil War	2,500,000
Afghanistan	Iran	1979–80	Afghan Civil War	2,000,000
Kampuchea	Thailand	1979–81	Kampuchean Civil War	300,000
Ethiopia	Somalia	1979–80	Ethiopian–Eritrean War	700,000
El Salvador and Nicaragua	Honduras	1983–6	Civil Wars	37,000
Ethiopia	Sudan	1984–5	Ethiopian–Eritrean War	340,000
Sudan	Ethiopia	1987–8	Sudanese Civil War	320,000
Somalia	Ethiopia	1987–8	Somalian Civil War	305,000
Mozambique	Malawi	1987–8	Mozambican Civil War	555,000
Burundi	Rwanda	1988	Civil War	50,000
Liberia	Guinea	1990	Liberian Civil War	300,000
Liberia	Côte d'Ivoire	1990	Liberian Civil War	200,000
Somalia	Ethiopia	1990–1	Somalian Civil War	200,000
Sudan	Ethiopia	1990	Sudanese Civil War	40,000
Kuwait and Iraq	Jordan	1990	Gulf War	750,000
Mozambique	Malawi	1990–2	Civil War	250,000
Azerbaijan	Armenia	1990–2	Armenian–Azerbaijani War	290,000
Armenia	Azerbaijan	1990–2	Armenian–Azerbaijani War	200,000

Iraq	Iran	Kurdish revolt	1991	1,100,000
Iraq	Turkey	Kurdish revolt	1991	450,000
Sierra Leone	Guinea	Sierra Leonean Civil War	1991	185,000
Ethiopia	Sudan	Ethiopian–Eritrean War	1991	51,000
Somalia	Kenya	Somalian Civil War	1991–2	320,000
Croatia and Bosnia–Herzegovina	Other former Yugoslav republics	Croatian War of Independence and Bosnian Civil War	1991–3	750,000
Croatia and Bosnia–Herzegovina	Western Europe	Croatian War of Independence and Bosnian Civil War	1991–3	512,000
Georgia	Russia	Georgian Civil Wars	1991–3	140,000
Somalia	Yemen	Somalian Civil War	1992	50,000
Sudan	Kenya	Sudanese Civil War	1992	20,000
Myanmar	Bangladesh	Burmese Guerrilla War	1992	250,000
Mozambique	Zimbabwe	Mozambican Civil War	1992	60,000
Tajikistan	Afghanistan	Tajikistan Civil War	1993	60,000
Togo	Ghana	Civil War	1993	120,000
Togo	Benin	Civil War	1993	120,000
Burundi	Tanzania	Burundian Civil War	1993	350,000
Burundi	Rwanda	Burundian Civil War	1993	370,000
Rwanda	Tanzania	Rwandan Civil War	1994	400,000
Rwanda	Burundi	Rwandan Civil War	1994	100,000
Rwanda	Zaire	Rwandan Civil War	1994	1,000,000
Serbia (Kosovo)	Albania	Kosovo Uprising	1999	426,000
Serbia (Kosovo)	Macedonia	Kosovo Uprising	1999	228,000

Source: Data from Toole and Waldman (1990, table 1, p. 3297), Toole (1997, table 14-1, p. 198), and UNHCR (2000).

Relative Changes: Biproportionate Scores

To further examine the space–time concentration of refugees plotted in Figure 5.2B, the 30 (year) × 6 (world region) matrix of estimated refugee counts was analysed using the method of biproportionate scores (Cliff and Haggett, 1988: 212–14). The method is described in Appendix 5A but, in essence, biproportionate scores permit an assessment of *relative* changes in levels of refugee activity by region and time period. Following the computational procedure outlined in the appendix, the histograms in Figure 5.3 plot, for each world region, biproportionate scores from 1970 (top) to 1999 (bottom). Here, the scores have been scaled to a base of 100; scores in excess of 100 mark a relative excess of refugees in space and time while scores below 100 mark a relative deficit.

Periodic sharp increases in the values of the biproportionate scores—of greater or lesser duration—are a prominent feature of Figure 5.3 and highlight the essential fluidity of the refugee situation in the various world regions. For regions of the Old World, the upper histograms identify repeated phases of relatively intense refugee activity in Africa (mid-1970s, early to mid-1980s, and mid-1990s), the explosive rise in Asia from the early 1980s and a bipolar temporal distribution in Europe (early to mid-1970s and mid- to late 1990s). For regions of the New World, the lower histograms depict periods of relatively intense refugee activity in Latin America/Caribbean (1970s, mid-1980s to early 1990s), North America (early to mid-1970s), and, finally, Oceania (late 1970s to early 1980s).

Interpretation

Taken together, the refugee patterns in Figures 5.2 and 5.3 and Table 5.1 track the changing global environment of war and political unrest in the latter half of the twentieth century. Although complex, the major regional developments may be summarized as follows:

(i)   1960s, decolonization and the colonial and civil wars of Africa;
(ii) 1970s, unrest in South Asia and military and political upheavals in Indochina;
(iii) 1980s, the growth of Superpower proxy wars in Africa, Asia, and Latin America;
(iv) 1990s, the end of the Cold War and an upsurge in ethnic and civil wars in Eastern Europe and Central Africa.

5.3.2 Other Populations of Concern

As noted in Section 5.2.2, refugees comprise only one form of displaced population. In addition to refugees, international attention also focuses on asylum seekers, internally displaced persons (IDPs), as well as refugee and IDP returnees and other populations whose legal position (including such categories as 'humanitarian status' and 'temporary protection') varies from one

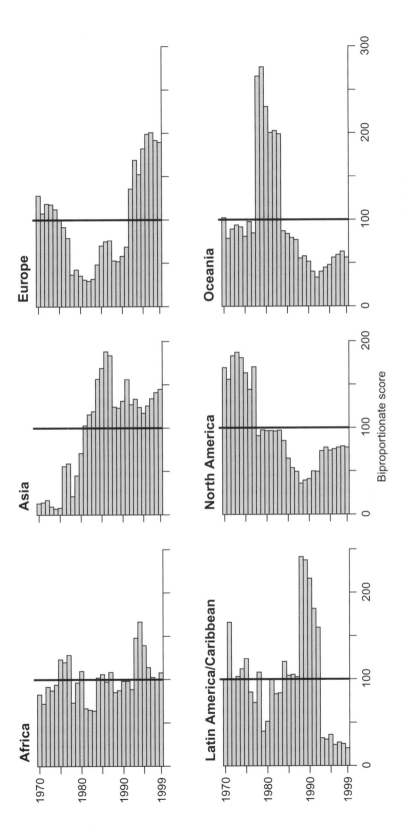

Fig. 5.3. World regional distribution of refugees and biproportionate scores, based on UNHCR annual estimates, 1970–1999

Notes: For each year, the histograms plot the world regional concentration of refugees. Scores in excess of 100 (indicated by the heavy vertical lines) mark a relative excess of refugees in time and space, while scores below 100 mark a relative deficit.

country to another. These various groups, along with refugees, are gathered together by the UNHCR under the umbrella term *populations of concern* (UNHCR, 2000).

GEOGRAPHICAL PATTERNS, 1999

Figure 5.4 is based on information collated by UNHCR (2000) and plots, as proportional circles, the global distribution of UNHCR-recognized populations of concern to the end of 1999. Here, the percentage proportion of the population classified as refugees is indicated by the shaded sectors while, for reference, Table 5.2 gives a regional breakdown of the other constitutent population categories. As the table indicates, there were in excess of 22.3 million people of concern to UNHCR at the end of 1999, of whom some 50 per cent fell into categories other than 'refugee'. Of the non-refugee groupings, major regional foci are identified in Figure 5.4 as Eastern, Middle, and Western Africa, South-Central and Western Asia, most of Europe, and North America.

While Table 5.2 identifies IDPs as numerically the most important category of displaced person other than refugees, UNHCR recognizes that the listed total of about 4.1 million IDPs represents a gross understatement of the true extent of internal displacement. By way of illustration, Table 5.3 is again based on information included in UNHCR (2000) and lists, in rank order, those countries of the world with estimated IDP populations of 0.5 million or more in 1999. Headed by the war-torn African states of Sudan (4.0 million IDPs) and Angola (1.5–2.0 millions IDPs), the estimated total level of internal displacement in the 18 sample states of Table 5.3 ranges up to 18.6 million. As noted in Section 5.2.2 above, the global population of IDPs at this time may have approached 25 million (UNHCR, 2000).

Table 5.2. World regional distribution of refugees and other populations of concern[1] to the UNHCR, 31 December 1999

| Region | Refugees | Asylum seekers | Returned refugees | Others of concern | | | Total |
				IDPs[2]	Returned IDPs[2]	Other	
Africa	3,523,050	60,990	932,780	762,900	941,100	37,000	6,257,820
Americas	710,680	607,130	5,970	0	0	21,200	1,344,980
Asia	4,781,750	24,650	627,740	1,724,800	10,600	149,350	7,318,890
Europe	2,617,650	532,700	950,200	1,593,100	376,700	1,278,900	7,349,250
Oceania	64,500	0	0	0	0	0	64,500
Total	11,697,630	1,225,470	2,516,690	4,080,800	1,328,400	1,486,450	22,335,440

Notes: [1] 'Populations of concern' is an umbrella term for various categories of person (including refugees, internally displaced persons, asylum seekers, and others) to whom the operations of the UNHCR are directed. [2] Internally displaced persons.
Source: Data from UNHCR (2000, annex 2, pp. 306–9).

return to their homelands or to be resettled elsewhere' (UNHCR, 2000: 108). Within this broad specification of function, camps vary greatly in size, character, and degree of permanancy. For the most part, however, camps are intended to be of a temporary nature and are constructed to these ends (ibid.).

As noted by Van Damme (1995), camp conditions may have deleterious effects on the physical, mental, and social well-being of the inhabitants. Refugees in camps are often dependent on food aid and this may be deficient in quality and/or quantity, thereby resulting in the occurrence of malnutrition and avitaminoses such as beriberi and scurvy. By analogy with military camps (see Ch. 8), high-level population mixing, overcrowding, and insanitary conditions may serve to promote the rapid spread of infectious diseases such as measles, acute respiratory tract infections, cholera, dysentery, and diarrhoeal diseases, especially in the initial 'emergency phase' of a refugee situation. In longer-term settings, the effective delivery of humanitarian assistance may be further compromised by the 'militarization' of camps and the establishment of militia control (Van Damme, 1995; UNHCR, 2000). Notwithstanding these observations, however, UNHCR (2000) maintain that refugee camps offer the safest and materially most secure option for the delivery of assistance to displaced populations.

5.4.1 Mortality Patterns

Comprehensive overviews of mortality during late-twentieth-century refugee/IDP crises are provided by Michael J. Toole and Ronald J. Waldman (Toole and Waldman, 1990; Toole, 1997). We draw on their evidence in the present section.

EMERGENCY PHASE MORTALITY

There are many problems associated with the estimation of mortality among displaced populations in emergency situations, not least the lack of accurate and reliable surveillance data (Toole, 1997). Where information is available, however, studies frequently reveal elevated levels of mortality in the weeks and months that immediately follow the onset of an emergency (Shears *et al.*, 1987; Toole and Waldman, 1990; CDC, 2001*e*). By way of illustration, Table 5.4 relates to sample refugee and IDP movements in the years 1978–95 and gives the crude mortality rate (CMR) (per 1,000 per month) in the displaced population (1). In addition, the table gives a baseline estimate of the CMR (2), variously formed for local host or non-displaced populations, along with the ratio of rates (1):(2). Here, a ratio in excess of parity marks a relatively high CMR in the displaced population, while a ratio less than parity marks a relatively low CMR.

With few exceptions, Table 5.4 records substantially inflated CMRs for both refugees and IDPs. In extreme instances, such as Cambodian refugees in

Table 5.4. Estimated crude mortality rates (CMRs) for sample refugee and internally displaced populations, 1978–1995

Year (month)	Country		Crude mortality rate (per 1,000 per month)		
	Host	Origin	Displaced (1)[1]	Baseline (2)[2]	Ratio (1):(2)
Refugees					
1978 (June–Dec.)	Bangladesh	Burma	6.3	1.7	3.7:1
1979 (Oct.)	Thailand	Cambodia	31.9	0.7	45.6:1
1980 (Aug.)	Somalia	Ethiopia	30.4	1.8	16.9:1
1985 (Jan.–Mar.)	Sudan (East)	Ethiopia	16.2	1.7	9.5:1
1987 (Jan.–June)	Malawi	Mozambique	1.0	1.7	0.6:1
1989 (Feb.–Apr.)	Ethiopia	Somalia	6.6	1.9	3.5:1
1990 (July)	Ethiopia	Sudan	6.9	1.7	4.1:1
1991 (June)	Ethiopia	Somalia	14.0	1.8	7.8:1
1991 (Mar.–May)	Turkey/Iraq	Iraq	12.6	0.7	18.0:1
1992 (Mar.)	Kenya	Somalia	22.2	1.8	12.3:1
1992 (Mar.)	Nepal	Bhutan	9.0	1.3	6.9:1
1992 (June)	Bangladesh	Myanmar	4.8	0.8	6.0:1
1992 (June)	Malawi	Mozambique	3.5	1.5	2.3:1
1992 (Aug.)	Zimbabwe	Mozambique	10.5	1.5	7.0:1
1993 (Dec.)	Rwanda	Burundi	9.0	1.8	5.0:1
1994 (May)	Tanzania	Rwanda	1.8	1.8	1.0:1
1994 (June)	Burundi	Rwanda	15.0	1.8	8.3:1
1994 (July)	Zaire	Rwanda	102.0	1.8	56.7:1
Internally displaced persons					
1988 (July)	Sudan (El Meiram)		90.0	1.7	52.9:1
1990 (Jan.–Dec.)	Liberia		7.1	1.2	5.9:1
1991 (Mar.–May)	Iraq		12.6	0.7	18.0:1
1991 (Apr.)–92 (Mar.)	Somalia (Merca)		13.8	2.0	6.9:1
1992 (Apr.–Nov.)	Somalia (Baidoa)		50.7	2.0	25.4:1
1992 (Apr.–Dec.)	Somalia (Afgoi)		16.5	2.0	8.3:1
1992 (Apr.)–93 (Mar.)	Sudan (Ayod)		23.0	1.6	14.4:1
1992 (Apr.)–93 (Mar.)	Sudan (Akon)		13.7	1.6	8.6:1
1992 (Apr.)–93 (Mar.)	Bosnia (Zepa)		3.0	0.8	3.8:1
1993 (Apr.)	Bosnia (Sarajevo)		2.9	0.8	3.6:1

Notes: [1] Recorded mortality rate in displaced populations. [2] Baseline rate (non-displaced) populations.

Source: Data from Toole and Waldman (1990), table 2, p. 3298) and Toole (1997, table 14-3, p. 203 and Table 14-4, p. 207).

Thailand (Oct. 1979), Rwandese refugees in Zaire (July 1994), and IDPs in Sudan (July 1988), CMRs exceed the baseline rate by a factor of 45 or more. A factor of between three and ten, however, is more typical of the sample. Inasmuch as a difference exists between the two categories of displaced population in Table 5.4, the marginally higher average CMR ratio for IDPs (14.8) than refugees (12.0) may reflect the more severe difficulties—including access to, and adequacy of, humanitarian assistance—often encountered by the former population (Toole, 1997).

Post-emergency Trends

The highest levels of mortality among refugees and IDPs typically occur in the emergency phase of the displacement, with a decline in the weeks and months following the implementation of relief operations. To illustrate this, Figure 5.5 is redrawn from Toole and Waldman (1990) and plots the monthly CMR (per 1,000 per month) during the year after the establishment of sample war-associated refugee camps in Africa (northwestern Somalia, 1980–1 and Sudan, 1985) and Asia (Thailand, 1979–80). For all three locations, mortality dropped progressively over the observation period, albeit at different rates, to reach relatively low levels (<2.0 per 1,000 per month) between two (Thailand) and 12 (Sudan) months after the establishment of the camps. For refugees at an additional African location (eastern Ethiopia, 1988–9), however, Figure 5.5

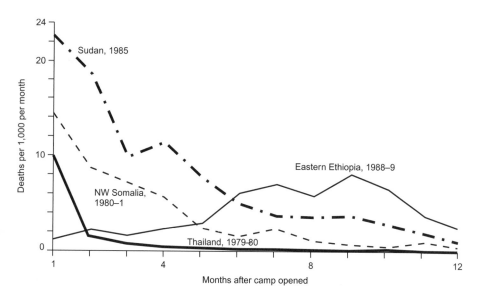

Fig. 5.5. Monthly crude mortality rates (per 1,000 per month) in sample refugee camps of Africa and Asia

Source: Redrawn from Toole and Waldman (1990, unnumbered fig., p. 3298).

Table 5.5. Communicable disease risk factors in refugee and other relief camps

Water and sanitation	Crowding		Poor shelter
	Non-vector	Vector	
Gastroenteritis[1]	Measles[1]	Typhus fever	Pneumonia[1]
Dysentery[1]	Meningitis	Relapsing fever	
Cholera	Tuberculosis	Malaria	
Poliomyelitis	Diphtheria		
Typhoid fever	Whooping cough		
Hepatitis	Scabies		
Bilharzia	Trachoma		

Note: [1] Main causes of morbidity and mortality associated with malnutrition in most camps.
Source: Shears *et al.* (1987, table V, p. 317).

illustrates an aberrant pattern of rising mortality over the first nine months of the observation period.

CAUSES OF DEATH

Leading causes of death in the emergency phase of late-twentieth-century refugee/IDP crises caused by war have included diarrhoeal diseases and measles, while a range of other infectious diseases (notably, acute respiratory infections, hepatitis, malaria, and meningitis) have also contributed to overall patterns of mortality; see Table 5.5. Additionally, protein-energy malnutrition has operated as both a direct cause of death and, more frequently, as an exacerbating factor in the severity of such conditions as dysentery, gastroenteritis, measles, and pneumonia. Demographically, these factors have usually manifested as disproportionately high rates of mortality among young children (aged <5 years) and, to a lesser extent, older children and adult females (Toole and Waldman, 1990; Toole, 1997).

Table 5.6 lists sample countries in which diarrhoeal diseases (cholera and dysentery due to *Shigella dysenteriae* type 1), measles, and certain other infectious diseases (malaria, hepatitis E, and meningococcal meningitis) were recorded as major causes of mortality among displaced populations during the 1970s, 1980s, and 1990s. We briefly consider each category of disease in turn, before examining the issue of nutritional deficiency.

Diarrhoeal Diseases

Of the diarrhoeal diseases, cholera (ICD-10 A00) and dysentery (ICD-10 A03) have ranked among the most pervasive killers of refugees and IDPs in Africa and Asia (Table 5.6). In these regions, major epidemics of cholera have been associated with case-fatality rates of up to 30 per cent. Likewise, epidemics of dysentery associated with *Shigella dysenteriae* type 1 have yielded case-fatality

Table 5.6. Sample countries in which diarrhoeal diseases, measles, and certain other infectious diseases were recorded as leading causes of death among displaced populations, 1970s–1990s

Diarrhoeal diseases			Other leading infectious causes of mortality		
Cholera	Dysentery[1]	Measles	Malaria	Hepatitis E	Meningococcal meningitis
Africa					
Burundi	Burundi	Ethiopia	Ethiopia	Ethiopia	Burundi
Malawi	Kenya	Malawi	Kenya	Kenya	Ethiopia
Swaziland	Malawi	Somalia	Malawi	Somalia	Sudan
Zaire	Rwanda	Sudan	Mozambique		Zaire
Zimbabwe	Tanzania	Zimbabwe	Somalia		
	Zaire		Sudan		
Asia					
Afghanistan	Bangladesh	Bangladesh	Thailand		Thailand
Bangladesh	Nepal	Nepal			
Nepal					
Turkey					
Central America					
		Honduras			

Note: [1] Due to *Shigella dysenteriae* type 1.
Source: Based on information in Toole and Waldman (1990) and Toole (1997).

rates of up to 10 per cent in vulnerable age groups (Toole, 1997). The combined spread of cholera and dysentery in one war-displaced population (Rwandese refugees in eastern Zaire, 1994) is examined further in Section 5.7.

Measles

Epidemic outbreaks of severe measles (ICD-10 B05) have been documented as a leading cause of infant and childhood mortality in the refugee/IDP populations of Africa, Asia, and Central America (Table 5.6). Desenclos *et al.* (1990), for example, note that measles accounted for up to 8.6 per cent of total mortality in some cohorts of El Salvadorian and Nicaraguan children (aged <5 years) resident in Honduran refugee camps, 1984–7. For the same age group, Porter *et al.* (1990) document case-fatality rates of 15–22 per cent during a measles epidemic among Mozambican refugees in Malawi, 1988–9. High measles attack rates in refugee populations have been attributed to: (i) low levels of immunization; (ii) inappropriate immunization; (iii) low levels of circulating measles antibody in mothers; and (iv) rapid loss of maternally derived antibodies among young infants in tropical areas (see Desenclos *et al.*, 1990; Porter *et al.*, 1990). While such factors have contributed to further measles outbreaks among African (Malawi and Zimbabwe) and Asian (Nepal) refugees during the 1990s, mass vaccination coverage under the WHO's Expanded Programme on Immunization (EPI) has effectively limited the dissemination of the disease among refugees and IDPs in some settings (Toole, 1997).

Other Infectious Diseases

Of the other infectious diseases listed in Table 5.6, the movement of displaced populations to, and through, areas of endemic malaria (ICD-10 B50–54) has occasionally resulted in high malaria mortality rates in refugee camps of both Africa and Asia. Both regions have also witnessed the epidemic spread of meningococcal meningitis (ICD-10 A39.0) among refugee populations while, in Africa at least, significant outbreaks of hepatitis E (ICD-10 B17.2) were recorded among refugees in Ethiopia, Kenya, and Somalia during the early 1990s (Toole and Waldman, 1990; Toole, 1997).

To the causes of death in Table 5.6 can be added other infectious diseases which, under localized circumstances, have had a severe impact on the health and mortality of war-displaced populations. Examples are examined further in Sections 5.7 and 13.5.4 and include: epidemic louse-borne typhus (ICD-10 A75.0) in Burundi (Raoult *et al.*, 1998); visceral leishmaniasis (ICD-10 B55.0) in southern Sudan (Zijlstra *et al.*, 1991); and diphtheria (ICD-10 A36) in the states of the former Soviet Central Asia (Usmanov *et al.*, 2000).

Nutritional Deficiencies

As noted above, the severity of infectious diseases in displaced populations may be exacerbated by protein-energy malnutrition arising from prolonged food shortages. Within relief camps, malnutrition may be further exacerbated by lack of food and/or the occurrence of infectious diseases such as measles, while scurvy and other avitaminoses may result from vitamin-deficient food rations. The recorded prevalence of nutritional deficiencies has occasionally reached very high levels in young children. Among those aged less than 5 years, for example, Toole (1997) notes levels of acute malnutrition approaching 50 per cent for Sudanese refugees in Ethiopia (1990) and Mozambican refugees in Zimbabwe (1992). Even higher levels have been recorded among the internally displaced children of such countries as Somalia (1992).

LONG-TERM REFUGEE CAMPS

Although the risk of infectious diseases tends to be greatest in the emergency phase of a refugee/IDP crisis, infectious conditions remain a potent threat in longer-term camps. Referring to the period June 1987 to May 1988, for example, Elias *et al.* (1990) describe how disease monitoring and surveillance helped avert a potentially severe epidemic of dengue haemorrhagic fever in a decade-old Cambodian refugee camp on the Thai–Cambodian border. Monitoring of hospital discharge data also allowed the early identification of outbreaks of common childhood infections, including acute respiratory illnesses such as pneumonia and bronchitis, while pathological examination revealed the high prevalence of canine rabies in the camp. Such findings underscore the continued disease risk in long-term refugee camps, and the need for ongoing disease surveillance and monitoring in such settings (Elias *et al.*, 1990).

5.4.2 Responses

Many of the common causes of mortality in displaced populations are preventable. As Shears *et al.* (1987: 317) observe: 'epidemics and high mortality are not inevitable consequences in refugee camps but result from predictable diseases for which attack rates and fatality rates may be reduced by planned prevention and treatment'. In addition to providing for the basic needs of the displaced (including protection, potable water, adequate nutrition, sanitation, and shelter), Toole (1997: 209–10) recommends that relief programmes should include the prompt implementation of six key health components:

(*a*) a health information system for nutrition monitoring and disease surveillance;
(*b*) measures of diarrhoeal disease control, treatment, and education;
(*c*) immunization against measles and other diseases in the Expanded Programme on Immunization (EPI);
(*d*) basic curative care, with special reference to maternal and child health;
(*e*) selective feeding programmes for vulnerable and malnourished groups;
(*f*) measures of endemic disease control and epidemic preparedness.

In turn, the successful implementation of these components demands that host countries—and international relief agencies—have adequate technical and manpower resources to mount a timely and appropriate response to humanitarian crises.

5.5 Wartime Evacuation in the United Kingdom, 1939–1945

In this and the following two sections, we explore specific instances of the spread of infectious diseases with wartime population displacement. Formal UNHCR-based definitions of the various categories of displacement (including 'refugees' and 'internally displaced persons') are provided in Section 5.2.2. Our examination begins here with a special instance of internal population displacement that predates the establishment of the UNHCR, namely: population evacuation in World War II.

CIVIL DEFENCE AND EVACUATION IN THE UNITED KINGDOM, 1939–1945

As a strategy of civil defence, the wartime evacuation of civil populations from militarily vulnerable areas represents a formal, state-sanctioned and directed,

mechanism for mass internal population displacement. Such was the circumstance in the United Kingdom during World War II. On 1 September 1939—
just two days before the Anglo-French declaration of war on Nazi Germany,
and in anticipation of an extended aerial bombardment of its great cities—the
British Government activated plans for the voluntary evacuation of schoolchildren and other designated 'priority' classes from urban areas of the country. The evacuation was, in the words of the Rt Hon. Walter Elliot, Minister of
Health, 'a great national undertaking',[2] involving the initial dispersal of inner-
city residents to many hundreds of rural locations across England, Scotland,
and Wales (Titmuss, 1950: 562). For the British public, at least, this was an
urban exodus of almost unprecedented proportions (Glover, 1940). But it was
merely the first phase of an ongoing operation which, during the six years of
World War II (1939–45), provided for the dispersal of some 4 million evacuees
and re-evacuees (Titmuss, 1950: 355–6). To these can be added countless others
who, either unwilling or unable to avail themselves of the official evacuation
scheme, found private sanctuary in the British countryside.[3]

While the evacuation of 1939–45 brought issues of inner-city deprivation to
the wide attention of a wartime public, the particular significance of the dispersal as a stimulus for social and welfare reform continues to provide fertile
ground for debate among historians of British social policy (see e.g. Welshman,
1999). In the present section, we examine a more immediate but, at the time, no
less contentious or uncertain aspect of the dispersal: the extent to which the
associated population flux gave rise to epidemics of infectious diseases among
evacuees and, more particularly, their hosts (Glover 1939–40; Stocks, 1941,
1942). Drawing on the study of Smallman-Raynor *et al.* (2003), the account to
follow will demonstrate a basic epidemiological principle: the geographical *dispersal* of highly concentrated (urban) populations—like the geographical *concentration* of widely dispersed (rural) populations (see Sect. 12.2)—serves as an
efficient mechanism for the historical propagation of war epidemics in civil
populations.

5.5.1 Background to the Dispersal

THE EVACUATION SCHEME

Details relating to the origin and development of the 1939–45 evacuation
scheme are provided elsewhere (Titmuss, 1950: 23–44; Smallman-Raynor *et al.*
2003) but, as implemented in September 1939, the plan was based on a three-
category division of the local authority areas of England, Scotland, and Wales.
A total of 81 areas which were considered vulnerable to air attack, and from

---

[2] Rt. Hon. Walter Elliot, 31 Aug. 1939, cited in *The Times* (London, 1 Sept. 1939), p. 7.
[3] Although information relating to the number of 'unofficial' evacuees is generally lacking, Titmuss
(1950, app. 2, pp. 543–9) estimates that some 2 million people were privately evacuated between June and
September 1939.

which movements were organized, were termed *evacuation areas*, while a total of 1,100 'safe' areas, to which the evacuees were moved, were termed *reception areas*; all other areas were classified as *neutral areas*. Movements from the evacuation areas were undertaken on a voluntary basis, with eligibility for evacuation limited to four priority classes: unaccompanied schoolchildren (aged 5–15 years); younger children accompanied by mothers or other guardians; pregnant women; and certain categories of disabled person. As for billeting in the reception areas, the majority of evacuees were lodged in the private residences of local populations; alternative arrangements, with accommodation in hospitals, camps, and other facilities, were made for those with illness and disability (see Glover, 1939–40; Padley and Cole, 1940).

Beginning with the evacuation of unaccompanied schoolchildren on 1 September 1939, followed by accompanied children and other priority classes on subsequent days, the entire evacuation process was all but complete by 4 September. Some impression of the magnitude of the operation can be gained from Table 5.7. Of the estimated 3.64 million people who were eligible for evacuation (Glover, 1939–40), upwards of 1.47 million, including almost 827,000 unaccompanied schoolchildren, availed themselves of the scheme.[4] The level of uptake, however, varied by evacuation area. By way of illustration, Figure 5.6 plots the percentage proportion of schoolchildren who were transferred from the principal urban evacuation zones of Great Britain in September 1939. As the map shows, levels of evacuation varied from in excess of 60 per cent in some towns and cities of Northern England to substantially less than 30 per cent in the Midlands. All told, some 42 per cent of schoolchildren were evacuated from the London area.

In the absence of the anticipated aerial bombardment of British cities, the latter months of 1939 witnessed a gradual 'drift-back' of evacuees from the reception areas; by January 1940, the number of evacuees still remaining in the reception areas had fallen to an estimated 520,000 (Ministry of Health, 1946: 108). Subsequent waves of evacuation, albeit on a much smaller scale than that of September 1939, accompanied the German invasion of France (May 1940) and the onset of the London Blitz (Sept. 1940–May 1941) (Titmuss, 1950: 355–69). Thereafter, evacuation movements continued at a very low level, with the geographical pattern reflecting the particular areas of the country which had been targeted for attack by the *Luftwaffe*. The relative calm, however, was shattered in the summer of 1944 when the terror instilled by the V1 'flying bomb' gave rise to a sudden eruption in evacuation activity. Between June and September of that year, some 1.25 million people were removed to the safety of the reception areas (Ministry of Health, 1946: 108–9; Titmuss, 1950: 424–30).

---

[4] The exact numbers involved in the evacuation of September 1939 are not known with any certainty. Thus, on 7 September 1939, the Prime Minister, Neville Chamberlain, informed Parliament that 1,475,000 children and mothers had been evacuated. A week later, on 14 September, the Minister of Health, Walter Elliot, placed the figure at 1,400,000. For a consideration of the numbers involved in the evacuation, see Padley and Cole (1940: 42–3); Ministry of Health (1946: 107); Titmuss (1950: 103–9).

Table 5.7. Dispersal of September 1939: total number of evacuees by priority class

Priority class	Number of evacuees			
	England		Scotland	Total
	London[1]	Provinces		
Unaccompanied schoolchildren	393,700	371,200	62,059	826,959
Children accompanied by mothers	257,000	169,500	97,170	523,670
Expectant mothers	5,600	6,700	405	12,705
Others[2]			15,432[4]	110,057
Total	94,625[3]			1,473,391

Notes: [1] Includes metropolitan area. [2] Includes teachers, helpers, and disabled persons. [3] Disaggregated counts for London and the provinces not available. Total includes 5,270 disabled persons. [4] Includes 1,787 disabled persons.
Source: Data from Titmuss (1950: 103 and app. 9, p. 562), reproduced from Smallman-Raynor *et al.* (2003, table 1, p. 399).

But, as the allied armies advanced northwards through Europe, the bombing decreased and, by early September 1944, aerial attacks on the United Kingdom had all but ceased.

EVACUATION AND INFECTIOUS DISEASES

The epidemiological risks posed by the evacuation scheme were to prompt considerable concern among members of the medical community. As early as 6 May 1939–some four months before the first wave of evacuation—an editorial commentary in *The Medical Officer* warned of the 'definite danger of serious disturbance of the epidemiological balance of the [reception] districts', adding that the danger arose from the 'difference between the immunity values of town and country populations' (Anonymous, 1939a: 174). As the editorial explained,

the removal of numbers of children from large centres of population and their billeting in the midst of populations without adequate experience of the effects of circulating infections entails a definite risk of an increase in the incidence of epidemic diseases in the billeting areas, because these communities are not protected by the immunising effects of repeated subinfective dosage derived from the reservoir of the circulating infections (Anonymous, 1939a: 174).

Local health officials concurred. 'It would seem probable', the Medical Officer of Health for Lambeth, Ashley G. G. Thompson, informed readers of *The Medical Officer* 'that epidemics of diphtheria, scarlet fever, cerebro-spinal meningitis and infantile paralysis [poliomyelitis] will be started among the country population' (Thompson, 1939: 192). James A. Forrest, Medical Officer

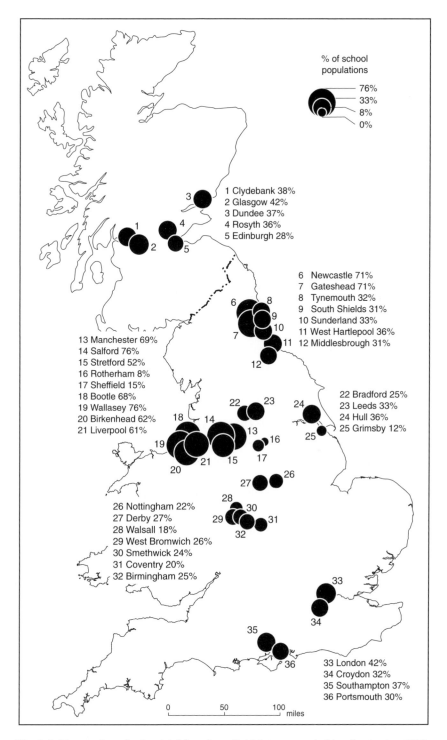

% of school
populations

76%
33%
8%
0%

1 Clydebank 38%
2 Glasgow 42%
3 Dundee 37%
4 Rosyth 36%
5 Edinburgh 28%

6 Newcastle 71%
7 Gateshead 71%
8 Tynemouth 32%
9 South Shields 31%
10 Sunderland 33%
11 West Hartlepool 36%
12 Middlesbrough 31%

13 Manchester 69%
14 Salford 76%
15 Stretford 52%
16 Rotherham 8%
17 Sheffield 15%
18 Bootle 68%
19 Wallasey 76%
20 Birkenhead 62%
21 Liverpool 61%

22 Bradford 25%
23 Leeds 33%
24 Hull 36%
25 Grimsby 12%

26 Nottingham 22%
27 Derby 27%
28 Walsall 18%
29 West Bromwich 26%
30 Smethwick 24%
31 Coventry 20%
32 Birmingham 25%

33 London 42%
34 Croydon 32%
35 Southampton 37%
36 Portsmouth 30%

0   50   100
miles

Fig. 5.6. Evacuation of schoolchildren from British towns and cities, September 1939

Notes: Proportional circles plot the number of evacuees as a percentage proportion of all school-children in the sample evacuation areas.

Source: Smallman-Raynor *et al.* (2003, fig. 1, p. 400), originally based on information in Titmuss (1950, app. 5, pp. 550–1).

of Health for Hebburn, Co. Durham, was equally apprehensive: 'As far as the "droplet spread" infectious diseases are concerned,' he wrote, 'it seems to me to be almost inevitable that severe epidemics . . . will be generated in the reception areas' (Forrest, 1939: 201). It was *The Lancet*, however, that provided the most measured consideration of the likely geographical dimensions of the disease risk:

Children from crowded cities, which may be considered as permanent epidemic centres of the common infectious diseases, are carrying specific organisms into rural districts which may be, but often are not, permanent epidemic areas for those same organisms. The result will depend not so much on whence the emigrants came as on where they have gone . . . [T]hus, though all reception areas must expect some increase in the number of cases of infectious disease . . . it is only in the most rural areas that real trouble is likely to arise . . . (Anonymous, 1939*b*: 605)

Despite the warnings, however, no general measures were introduced to prevent the outbreak of epidemic diseases in the reception areas (Padley and Cole, 1940: 87–95; Titmuss, 1950: 14–15). Rather, the official response was restricted to the provision of extra hospital facilities for infectious conditions (Glover, 1939–40: 401) while, as a precautionary measure, two diseases (measles and whooping cough) were added to the list of notifiable conditions (Anonymous, 1939*c*; MacNalty, 1940); efforts to immunize against a further disease (diphtheria) were stymied by the difficulties of acquiring the parental consent of unaccompanied children (Anonymous, 1939*d*: 792; Glover, 1939–40: 407).

Preliminary Surveys of Infectious Disease Activity
Several weeks into the first phase of evacuation, and with concerns over the threat of infectious diseases still rife (see e.g. Anonymous, 1939*e*), it was with some satisfaction that the Minister of Health could inform the House of Commons of the reportedly low incidence of infectious diseases in the reception areas:

We have returns of the incidence of infectious diseases in the reception areas for the first two months since the outbreak of war. The salient fact stands out that there has been no outbreak of epidemics within those two months. Not only that, but the figures for the epidemic diseases are lower than those of the corresponding period of 1938. This is a very fine result. (House of Commons, 2 Nov. 1939)[5]

The same broad conclusions were reached by Dr J. Alison Glover of the Royal Society of Medicine. In his Presidential Address to the Section of Epidemiology and State Medicine on 5 April 1940, Glover observed that the first four months of evacuation (Sept.–Dec. 1939) had been accompanied by 'remarkably low' levels of infectious disease activity (Glover, 1939–40: 405).

---

[5] Parliamentary Debates, 5th ser., *House of Commons Official Report. Fourth Session of the Thirty-Seventh Parliament of the United Kingdom of Great Britain and Northern Ireland, 3 George VI. Twelfth Volume of Session 1938–9* (London, 1939) 352 HC Deb., 5th ser., col. 2183.

This, he concluded, could be attributed to a series of factors which—somewhat ironically—had seemed 'so darkly to cloud the success of evacuation' and which included: (i) the sub-maximal levels of evacuation uptake; (ii) the rapid drift-back of some evacuees; (iii) the degree of epidemiological protection provided by the 'double-shift' schooling system that had been adopted in many reception areas; and (iv) the much-maligned closure of schools in evacuation and neutral areas (Glover, 1939–40: 411).

Notwithstanding these observations, the latter months of 1939 were to witness mild epidemics of chickenpox and rubella (Glover, 1939–40: 409; Anonymous, 1940: 660–1) while, during the early months of 1940, influenza and cerebrospinal meningitis began to spread across Britain (Glover, 1940: 631; Councell, 1941: 570). However, as E. G. Baxter concluded in his report to the Fabian Society:

There is . . . no evidence as to the extent to which these epidemics have been connected with evacuation . . . Nor can we say how these epidemic diseases have struck among the population of the reception areas, though reports, again drawn from general observation, suggest quite definitely that the country children have suffered far more than the evacuees, and this may suggest that the gloomy prophecies as to the medical effects of mingling populations possessing different kinds of resistance to disease are, to a very small extent, coming true. (Padley and Cole, 1940: 95)

The Work of Percy Stocks

Spurred by the preliminary nature of the early reports, the most detailed analytical study of the association between evacuation and infectious disease activity was conducted by Dr Percy Stocks (Pl. 5.2). Biographical details are given elsewhere (Reid *et al.*, 1975) but, in his wartime capacity as Chief Medical Statistician in the General Register Office, London, Stocks undertook a comparative analysis of the incidence of a series of infectious diseases (diphtheria, measles, scarlet fever, and whooping cough) in the evacuation, reception, and neutral areas of England and Wales during the period up to mid-1941. The full results of his investigations were published in consecutive volumes of the *Journal of the Royal Statistical Society* in 1941–2 (Stocks, 1941, 1942).

Drawing on more complete information than had been available to previous analysts,[6] Stocks was able to demonstrate that the initial evacuation of September 1939 was temporally associated with inflated levels of reported disease activity in some reception areas. The evidence, however, varied by disease, time period, and geographical location. Moreover, as Stocks noted, any

---

[6] In a generous response to the investigations of Stocks, for example, J. Alison Glover was to emphasize the preliminary nature of his own enquiries: 'Dr. Percy Stocks's admirable paper . . . must have special appeal to anyone, like myself, who was rash enough to try to give an outline of the epidemiology of the first four months' evacuation, while still without detailed information with regard to diphtheria and scarlet fever to which Dr. Stocks has had access, and which he has now marshalled with his unrivalled skill' (J. A. Glover, in discussion of Stocks, 1941: 337).

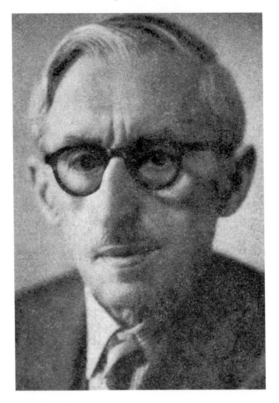

Pl. 5.2. Percy Stocks (1889–1974)

Notes: British physician and medical statistician who was appointed to the position of Chief Medical Statistician, General Register Office, in 1933. While working in the GRO during the early years of World War II, Stocks undertook a seminal study of the impact of evacuation on the spread of such infectious diseases as diphtheria, measles, scarlet fever, and whooping cough. The results of his investigation were published in the *Journal of the Royal Statistical Society* in 1941–2. *Source*: Reid *et al.* (1975: 65).

interpretation of the results was complicated by a failure to separate (i) the disease signal associated with evacuation from (ii) the disease signal associated with the regular, background, cycle of epidemiological activity (Stocks, 1941: 312). A further complication arose from the fact that, during the first wave of evacuation at least, many schools in evacuation areas were closed. This had the effect of reducing levels of mixing among susceptible and infected children, possibly leading to damped case rates in evacuation areas (see: Glover, 1939–40: 411; Stocks, 1940). Given that no data were collected on this at the time, there is no obvious way of quantifying the impact of the damping effect.

Prompted by the inconclusive nature of the original analysis, the following sections re-examine the evidence for an evacuation-related upsurge in two of

Stocks's diseases (diphtheria and scarlet fever) in the reception areas of a single city (London) during the entire period of the war, 1939–45. In so doing, the general epidemic curve (disease signal (ii), above) is filtered from the data, thereby permitting an assessment of the specific role of evacuation as a factor in disease activity (disease signal (i)). The study is supplemented by a parallel analysis of a third disease (poliomyelitis) whose postulated epidemiological link to the evacuation (Thompson, 1939) went unexplored at the time.

5.5.2 Study Site and Data

THE STUDY SITE: LONDON AND RECEPTION COUNTIES

Although, as shown in Figure 5.6, the evacuation of 1939–45 involved the dispersal of schoolchildren and others from many industrial towns and cities of Britain, two principal considerations have informed the selection of London as the basis for the present analysis. First, in numerical terms, London formed the epicentre of the national evacuation scheme. Table 5.7 indicates that almost 50 per cent of all British schoolchildren evacuated at the start of World War II were of London origin; subsequent waves of evacuation—including those associated with the Blitz (1940–1) and the V1 attacks (1944)—merely served to consolidate the primacy of London as a source of evacuees and re-evacuees (Titmuss, 1950: 355–6). Secondly, from an epidemiological perspective, London contained some of the most densely populated areas of the country and, *ceteris paribus*, these areas were likely to have had a relatively high incidence of communicable diseases capable of geographical transfer to the reception areas.

Against this background, Figure 5.7 identifies the principal counties (shaded) to which London evacuees were dispersed during the course of the war. As the map shows, the evacuees were strewn over much of southern and eastern Britain. The majority, however, were transferred to proximal locations in the southeast of England (dark shading in Figure 5.7) (T. L. Crosby, 1986: 28–9). For the purposes of the present analysis, therefore, the study is limited to a conterminous area of southeastern England defined by the following 14 counties: Bedfordshire, Berkshire, Buckinghamshire, Cambridgeshire, Essex, Hertfordshire, Kent, Middlesex, Norfolk, East Suffolk, West Suffolk, Surrey, East Sussex, and West Sussex. These 14 reception counties, together with the London evacuation area, form the geographical framework for our analysis.

THE DATA: THE REGISTRAR GENERAL'S *RETURNS*

To examine the epidemiological impact of evacuation on the reception counties for London, the analysis draws on the disease counts collated by the General Register Office (GRO), London, and published in the Registrar General's *Weekly Return of Births and Deaths*[7] and *Quarterly Return of Births,*

---

[7] Registrar General, *Weekly Return of Births and Deaths in London and in . . . Other Large Towns . . .* (and similar titles). London: HMSO.

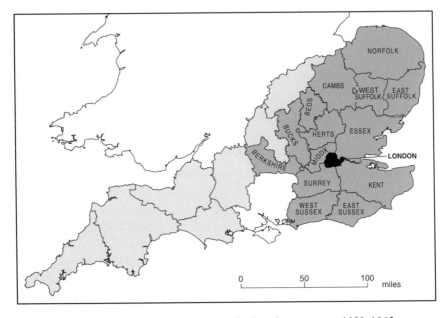

Fig. 5.7. Counties serving as reception areas for London evacuees, 1939–1945

Notes: The principal counties to which London evacuees were transferred have been shaded in light and dark tones; counties included in the present analysis are identified by the dark shading. *Source*: Smallman-Raynor *et al.* (2003, fig. 2, p. 403).

Deaths and Marriages[8] for England and Wales. Full details are given in Smallman-Raynor *et al.* (2003) but, in brief, the *Returns* were used to form quarterly time series of morbidity for each sample disease (scarlet fever, diphtheria, and poliomyelitis) and geographical area (London and 14 reception counties) over a 68-quarter observation period, 1933–49. To permit a comparative analysis of disease activity in war and peace, each of the resulting quarterly series was then sectioned into various time slices. The principal time slices which form the basis of the summary information on disease incidence in Table 5.8 were as follows:

(1) 1933 (qr. 1)–1939 (qr. 2), a 26-quarter period of peace immediately preceding the onset of the Anglo-French declaration of war on Germany (3 Sept. 1939);

(2) 1939 (qr. 3)–1945 (qr. 3), a 25-quarter period of war, ending with the capitulation of Japan and the termination of the war in the Pacific (14 Aug. 1945); and

(3) 1945 (qr. 4)–1949 (qr. 4), a 17-quarter period of demobilization and post-war reconstruction.

[8] Registrar General, *Quarterly Return of Births, Deaths and Marriages Registered in the Divisions, Counties, and Districts of England and Wales . . .* (and similar titles). London: HMSO.

Table 5.8. Cases of diphtheria, poliomyelitis, and scarlet fever recorded in the Registrar General's Returns, 1933–1949

County/area	Diphtheria cases[1]			Poliomyelitis cases[1]			Scarlet fever cases[1]		
	1933–9[2]	1939–45[3]	1945–9[4]	1933–9[2]	1939–45[3]	1945–9[4]	1933–9[2]	1939–45[3]	1945–9[4]
Bedfordshire	3,044 (47.27)	736 (9.97)	94 (1.89)	18 (0.28)	32 (0.43)	3 (0.06)	3,110 (48.30)	4,588 (62.16)	1,982 (39.82)
Berkshire	1,783 (21.13)	1,252 (12.54)	125 (1.91)	83 (0.98)	103 (1.03)	13 (0.20)	3,786 (44.87)	5,108 (51.15)	1,449 (22.18)
Buckinghamshire	1,238 (16.15)	1,095 (11.64)	118 (1.93)	19 (0.25)	102 (1.08)	14 (0.23)	3,536 (46.12)	4,628 (49.21)	1,708 (27.88)
Cambridgeshire	142 (3.70)	277 (7.07)	27 (0.98)	12 (0.31)	21 (0.54)	2 (0.07)	1,881 (48.95)	1,302 (33.24)	882 (32.02)
Essex	15,996 (32.73)	3,897 (10.03)	755 (2.32)	463 (0.95)	136 (0.35)	21 (0.06)	39,904 (81.65)	20,315 (52.29)	12,557 (38.57)
Hertfordshire	71,654 (13.82)	1,179 (8.29)	159 (1.62)	62 (0.52)	65 (0.46)	25 (0.26)	5,749 (48.05)	6,260 (44.03)	2,223 (22.71)
Kent	7,588 (21.43)	2,872 (9.64)	475 (1.91)	179 (0.51)	188 (0.63)	13 (0.05)	19,793 (55.91)	14,258 (47.88)	7,539 (30.27)
London	56,274 (52.27)	9,786 (16.28)	2,145 (3.89)	559 (0.52)	244 (0.41)	36 (0.07)	83,022 (77.11)	26,682 (44.38)	20,119 (36.47)
Middlesex	12,645 (25.06)	4,482 (9.29)	718 (1.90)	281 (0.56)	213 (0.44)	45 (0.12)	36,151 (71.66)	23,406 (48.51)	13,496 (35.70)
Norfolk	2,921 (22.39)	1,279 (11.07)	167 (1.94)	70 (0.54)	54 (0.47)	1 (0.01)	6,697 (51.34)	6,271 (54.26)	2,606 (30.30)
Suffolk, East	1,072 (13.76)	684 (10.60)	293 (5.67)	43 (0.55)	31 (0.48)	5 (0.10)	4,605 (59.12)	3,149 (48.79)	1,112 (21.53)
Suffolk, West	122 (4.53)	334 (12.16)	38 (2.06)	25 (0.93)	12 (0.44)	1 (0.05)	996 (36.97)	1,390 (50.59)	424 (22.94)
Surrey	6,591 (18.52)	2,988 (8.63)	499 (1.91)	169 (0.47)	150 (0.43)	17 (0.06)	20,850 (58.59)	16,627 (48.02)	8,573 (32.77)
Sussex, East	1,771 (12.11)	1,010 (8.53)	288 (2.86)	83 (0.57)	59 (0.50)	10 (0.10)	5,654 (38.67)	4,805 (40.57)	2,194 (21.79)
Sussex, West	1,052 (16.15)	381 (5.75)	66 (1.29)	55 (0.84)	56 (0.84)	3 (0.06)	3,407 (52.31)	3,068 (46.27)	1,399 (27.32)
England and Wales	390,118 (36.74)	231,709 (24.24)	31,144 (4.38)	4,802 (0.45)	4,216 (0.44)	536 (0.08)	744,728 (70.14)	503,796 (52.69)	283,597 (39.92)

Notes: [1] Average quarterly case rate (per 100,000 population) in parentheses. [2] 1933 (q. 1)–1939 (q. 2). [3] 1939 (q. 3)–1945 (q. 3). [4] 1945 (q. 4)–1949 (q. 4). Case totals are given for London and a sample of 14 counties that received London evacuees during World War II.
Source: Smallman-Raynor *et al.* (2003, table 2, p. 406).

As described in subsequent sections, additional subdivisions of the war period (2) were undertaken to permit an analysis of disease activity associated with the major phases of evacuation. For all subdivisions, disease rates were formed on the basis of demographic information drawn from the Registrar General's *Returns*.

5.5.3 Evidence over Time

Our analysis of the epidemiological impact of evacuation begins with a longitudinal examination of the time series for scarlet fever, diphtheria, and poliomyelitis. Two basic issues are addressed.

(1) *Levels of disease activity.* To what extent did the evacuation result in raised levels of disease activity in the reception counties of London?
(2) *Levels of epidemiological integration.* Underpinning question (1), to what extent did the population flux engendered by the evacuation result in a strengthening, or otherwise, of the epidemiological integration of London and the reception counties?

We examine each question in turn. Our consideration begins with a brief note on the time series under analysis.

TIME SERIES COMPONENTS

As described in Section 5.5.1, analyses of the impact of evacuation on patterns of disease activity are complicated by the need to separate the disease signal associated with the dispersal from the regular, background, pattern of disease activity. As regards the latter, the three diseases considered in the present study are characterized by both annual (seasonal) and supra-annual (cyclical epidemic) peaks in incidence.

Seasonality. In the United Kingdom, diphtheria and scarlet fever have historically tended to peak in the early winter months while, for poliomyelitis, the epidemiological record reveals a seasonal peak in summer/early autumn (Cliff *et al.*, 1998: 202–4).
Epidemic cycles. Superimposed upon the seasonal peaks of disease activity, major epidemics occur periodically. The periodic wavelength is disease- and population size-specific but, in major cities of the United Kingdom, biennial cycles were common in the first half of the twentieth century for all three diseases (Cliff *et al.*, 1998: 180–5).

While these seasonal and cyclical effects may be identified and filtered from the data using classical methods of time series analysis, and this is done later in the present section, the different approach of using ratios of time series was initially employed.

LEVELS OF DISEASE ACTIVITY: SERIES RATIOS

One epidemiological expectation of the evacuation is that the dispersal should have resulted in an increase in disease activity in the reception zones relative to the evacuation zones. To examine this expectation in the context of London and the reception counties, the 68-quarter time series of case rates for a given disease and reception county was used in the numerator of a simple ratio calculation, in which the corresponding time series of case rates for London formed the denominator. In this manner, the computational process yielded 14 (reception counties) × 68 (quarters) time series of ratios for each of the three sample diseases. Here, ratios greater than unity imply greater disease intensity in the reception county than in London, and vice versa. The specification of relative disease intensity in this manner allows for any seasonal/cyclical effects provided that it can be assumed that these time series components are approximately similar in London and the reception counties. As the geographical units are proximal and the climatic regime does not differ greatly, the assumption of a common epidemic curve is probably not unreasonable.

Results

Figure 5.8 plots the response envelope for the 14 reception counties by showing the median, maximum, and minimum ratios obtained across the set of series in each quarter for (A) scarlet fever, (B) diphtheria, and (C) poliomyelitis. To assist in the interpretation, the intervals associated with the two main phases of evacuation (1939–40 and 1944–5) have been highlighted while, for reference, the pecked horizontal lines on each graph mark ratios of unity.

An outstanding feature of Figure 5.8 is the sharp increase in the ratio values for scarlet fever (Fig. 5.8A) and diphtheria (Fig. 5.8B) during the evacuation period of 1939–40. Starting from generally low (<1.0) values in the pre-war period, consistent with higher disease rates in London, the ratios rise steeply with the onset of evacuation and are indicative of a relative upsurge in disease activity in the reception counties. Thereafter, the ratio values fall away in the inter-evacuation period, rising to a secondary peak with the evacuation of 1944–5. Poliomyelitis (Fig. 5.8C) shares the same broad features as scarlet fever and diphtheria, but with the signal associated with the evacuation of 1939–40 slightly lagged in time.

Discussion: Surface Analyses

Interpretations of the evacuation-induced changes in relative disease activity graphed in Figure 5.8 are subject to one well-documented epidemiological effect of the dispersal: the marked reduction in levels of disease incidence in London during the evacuation of 1939–40 (see: Anonymous, 1939*d*; Glover, 1940; Stocks, 1940). Some impression of the phenomenon, which was attributed by contemporary observers to the impact of population contraction and school closure on levels of population mixing (Glover, 1940; Stocks, 1940), can

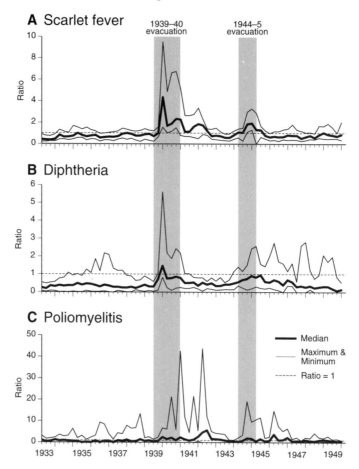

Fig. 5.8. Quarterly time series of infectious disease activity, London and reception counties, 1933–1949

Notes: Line traces plot the maximum, median, and minimum disease time series, with reception county rates expressed as a ratio of the London rate to remove the effect of the epidemic curve. (A) Scarlet fever. (B) Diphtheria. (C) Poliomyelitis. The intervals associated with the two main phases of evacuation (1939–40 and 1944–5) have been highlighted. For reference, the pecked horizontal lines on each graph mark ratios of unity.

Source: Smallman-Raynor *et al.* (2003, fig. 3, p. 408).

be gained from the surfaces in Figure 5.9. To form the surfaces, the time series for each disease and geographical area were divided into two periods: 1933 (q. 1)–1939 (q. 2) and 1939 (q. 3)–1940 (q. 4). In each time period, the average quarterly incidence rate (per 1,000 population) was calculated for the 14 reception counties to define the z axis in a three-dimensional plot in which the x and y axes were the ranks of the cartesian coordinates of the geographical centroids

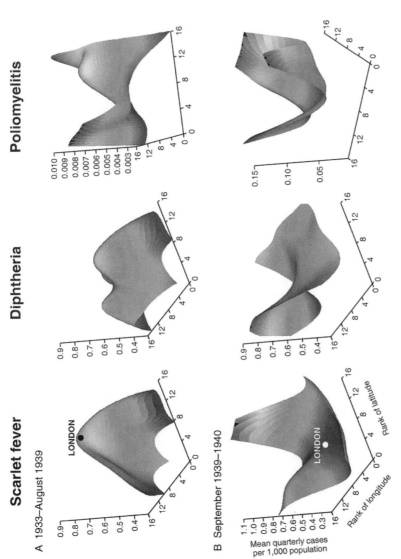

Fig. 5.9. Surfaces showing the average quarterly incidence (per 1,000 population) of scarlet fever, diphtheria, and poliomyelitis in London (centre of surface) and the reception counties

Note: Surfaces are shown for the periods prior to (A) and during (B) the evacuation of 1939–40.

Source: Smallman-Raynor *et al.* (2003, fig. 4, p. 409).

of the counties. Using ranks, London (the evacuation zone) is in the centre of each surface, with the evacuation counties forming a surrounding necklace.

The dramatic change in the shape of the surfaces between the two time periods emphasizes the impact of the 1939–40 evacuation on disease rates. The change from the 'dome' shape of the pre-war period, when London had the highest disease rates, to the 'bowl' of the evacuation era in which London lies in the base of the bowl highlights the transfer of the main pockets of disease from the evacuation area to the reception counties. The change is especially marked for scarlet fever (Fig. 5.9A) and diphtheria (Fig. 5.9B); for poliomyelitis (Fig. 5.9C), the change is still present but less prominent. It is apparent, however, that the temporal reconfiguration of the surfaces is not solely the product of increased levels of disease activity in the reception counties. For scarlet fever, for example, the repositioning of London was associated with a fall in average quarterly disease levels from in excess of 0.7 per 1,000 (1933–9) to somewhat less than 0.4 per 1,000 (1939–40).

LEVELS OF EPIDEMIOLOGICAL INTEGRATION:
TIME SERIES DECOMPOSITION

An alternative way of allowing for the epidemic curve in the disease time series is to filter out trend and seasonal components using classical time-series methods (Chatfield, 1980; Box *et al.*, 1994). Accordingly, Figure 5.10 shows the quarterly time series for each of the reception counties and London, based on case rates per 1,000 population, after removal of trend and seasonal components; a model which assumed a linear trend and additive seasonal components was fitted to filter these components (Box *et al.*, 1994). The filtered time series for London are plotted as the heavy line traces in Figure 5.10, while the 14 reception counties are represented by the fine line traces. As with the ratios approach, the raised rates for scarlet fever (Fig. 5.10A) and diphtheria (Fig. 5.10B) in the reception counties, compared with London, are strongly marked for the 1939–40 evacuation. This is also apparent for the 1944–5 evacuation period, but the contrast is less pronounced. Finally, the filtered time series in Figure 5.10C reveal no marked evidence of an evacuation-related increase in poliomyelitis activity.

Phase Relationships: Method

While Figure 5.10 provides information on the temporal course of the three diseases, other techniques are required to determine whether evacuation was associated with a fundamental change in the *epidemiological integration* of London and the reception counties. To examine this latter issue, we employ one powerful technique for measuring spatial associations in geo-coded time series, namely cross-correlation analysis. Details of the technique are given later in Section 6.7.3. For the purposes of the present analysis, each of the filtered time series of disease-incidence rates for London was treated as the reference series,

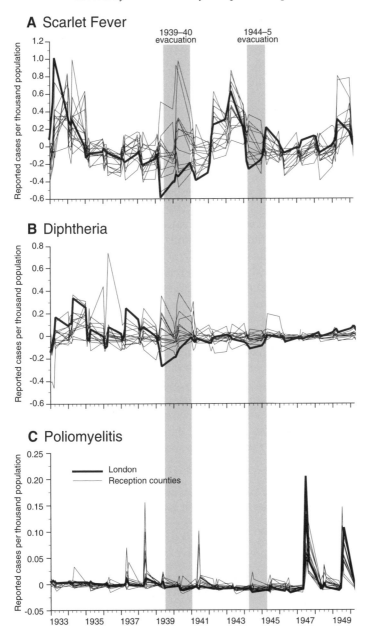

Fig. 5.10. Disease time series, 1933–1949, for London (heavy line trace) and reception counties after the removal of trend and seasonal components

Notes: (A) Scarlet fever. (B) Diphtheria. (C) Poliomyelitis.

Source: Smallman-Raynor *et al.* (2003, fig. 5, p. 411).

against which the corresponding time series for the 14 reception counties were systematically compared. To compare levels of epidemiological integration in war and peace, the cross-correlation analysis was conducted for three time periods (the pre-war period, 1933–9; the war period, 1939–45; and the entire observation period, 1933–49), thereby yielding a total of (14 reception counties × 3 diseases × 3 time periods =) 126 cross-correlation functions (CCFs). By analogy with Section 6.7.3, we define the short-term lead or lag of a reception county with respect to London as the value of k at which the correlation r_k is a maximum.

Phase Relationships: Results

For each time period, Figure 5.11 maps the leads and lags, in quarters, between the various reception counties and London for (A) scarlet fever, (B) diphtheria, and (C) poliomyelitis. Given the anticipated direction of the evacuation-induced transfer of disease (i.e. from London to the reception counties), reception counties that were in-phase with ($k=0$) or lagged ($k>0$) London have been shaded; reception counties which led London ($k<0$) have been left unshaded. For reference, Table 5.9 summarizes the average correlations, $\bar{r}_k$, and average lags, $\bar{k}$, between London and the reception counties for the periods of peace (1933–9) and war (1939–45).

According to Table 5.9 and Figure 5.11, the transition from peace to war was associated with a complex pattern of continuity and change in the epidemiological bonding of London and the reception counties. For both the pre-war and war periods, Table 5.9 shows that the average correlations for scarlet fever were higher than for diphtheria and poliomyelitis, indicative of a more tightly bonded epidemiological system for scarlet fever than the other diseases. Importantly, however, Table 5.9 also reveals that the war had a differential impact on the three diseases. So, while the epidemic bonding for scarlet fever changed but

Table 5.9. Lead–lag relationships between London and reception counties by time period and disease

Disease	Time period	
	1933–9[1]	1939–45[1]
Scarlet fever	0.69 (0.86)	0.67 (0.69)
Diphtheria	0.56 (0.31)	0.38 (−0.09)
Poliomyelitis	0.47 (−0.14)	0.57 (0.50)

Notes: [1] Table values are the average correlations, $\bar{r}_k$, and average lag (in parentheses), $\bar{k}$, computed from the individual maximum correlation coefficients, r_k, in the cross-correlation functions (CCFs) between London and the reception counties. The averages have been calculated over the 14 $\{r_k\}$ and $\{k\}$ for each disease and time period.
Source: Smallman-Raynor *et al.* (2003, table 3, p. 414).

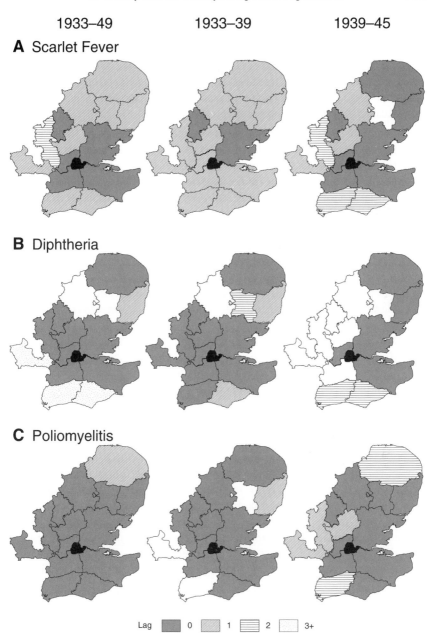

Fig. 5.11. Leads and lags of reception counties with respect to London, by disease and time period

Notes: Lag 0 = London and reception county in-phase. Shaded reception counties lagged London by the number of quarters shown; reception counties which led London are unshaded. (A) Scarlet fever. (B) Diphtheria. (C) Poliomyelitis.

Source: Smallman-Raynor *et al.* (2003, fig. 6, p. 413).

little in the peace–war transition, it weakened for diphtheria but strengthened for poliomyelitis.

The differential impact of the war on epidemiological integration is further highlighted by the lead–lag structures in Figure 5.11. For the pre-war period (1933–9), the maps for all three diseases show that the reception counties were primarily in-phase with, or lagging, London. During the war (1939–45), however, the lead–lag relationships changed significantly.

1. Scarlet fever (Fig. 5.11A). There was a general tendency for the reception counties to move from a lagging (pre-war) to an in-phase (war) pattern; the change is reflected in the inter-period reduction of the average lag, $\bar{k}$, in Table 5.9 and implies that evacuation served to increase the speed of spatial disease transmission from London to the reception counties.
2. Diphtheria (Fig. 5.11B). Reception counties to the east of London remained in-phase in the transition from peace to war, while reception counties to the north and west of London switched from in-phase to leading. This switch, which is marked by the change of sign of the average lag, $\bar{k}$, in Table 5.9, is counter-intuitive for the northern and western counties since it implies a diffusion process from the reception counties to London—reversing the initial direction of population movement caused by evacuation.
3. Poliomyelitis (Fig. 5.11C). For both the pre-war and war periods, the dominant tendency was for reception counties to be in-phase with, or lagging, London and this is consistent with disease propagation from the capital to the reception counties.

Summary

While the evacuation had a marked impact upon the epidemiological integration of London and the reception counties, it is evident that the nature of the impact varied by disease. For scarlet fever, the findings imply that evacuation was associated with an increase in the speed of disease transmission from London while, for poliomyelitis, the evacuation served to enhance the epidemiological interdependence of London and the reception counties. The evidence for diphtheria is ambiguous but, for the northern and western reception counties, the results of the cross-correlation analysis are consistent with a simple transmission model in which the return of evacuees served to carry the infection back into London.

5.5.4 Evidence over Space

To this point, the analysis of disease activity in the London reception zones has been restricted to the insights provided by geographically aggregated (county-level) morbidity statistics. By adopting the census-based classification of 'urban districts' and 'rural districts' included in the Registrar General's

Returns,[9] the present section uses geographically disaggregated data to examine the epidemiological impact of evacuation in the urban and rural sectors of the 14 reception counties.[10] In so doing, a classic technique in the spatial analysis of epidemiological data is employed: Poisson probability mapping (see Sect. 4.6.2).

POISSON PROBABILITY MAPPING

One way of determining which reception counties display significantly high, or significantly low, incidence of a disease in a given time period is to compare the observed case levels with those expected under a simple Poisson process (see e.g. Cliff and Haggett, 1988: 28–9). Here, the ideas of 'significantly high' and 'significantly low' are articulated by determining the chance of obtaining cases levels at least as big or at least as small as those recorded if the disease-generating process is spatially random. The important assumptions underlying the Poisson are that:

(*a*) there are no interactions between counties;
(*b*) there is no possibility of clusters of disease incidence within counties;
(*c*) there is no tendency for neighbouring counties to display similar traits.

The assumptions imply that the counties are acting independently of each other and each county has an equal and independent chance of having an event (i.e. a case of a disease) occurring in it. The main role of the Poisson is to act as a 'no dependence' or spatially random benchmark against which data may be tested.

Method

Under the assumptions of the Poisson process, the probability, $P(X = x)$, of observing a certain number, x, of deaths from a given disease in a sub-area (urban or rural) of a particular reception county is given by

$$P(X = x) = [\exp(-\lambda)\lambda^x]/x!, \quad x = 0, 1, 2, \ldots \tag{5.1}$$

where the parameter, λ, is the expected, or mean, number of deaths in that sub-area. The probability of observing at least as many cases as x is obtained by solving and summing equation (5.1) from x to ∞; see Cliff and Haggett (1988: 28–9) for further details.

For the purposes of the present analysis, the Poisson parameter, λ, was estimated from the London data so that the metropolis formed the comparison location against which disease levels in the urban and rural districts of the

---

[9] For further details of the classification of urban and rural administrative districts, see Registrar General (1931), *Census of England and Wales, 1931: Preliminary Report, Including Tables of Population Enumerated in England and Wales (Administrative and Parliamentary Areas) and in Scotland, the Isle of Man and the Channel Islands on 26/27 April, 1931*. London: HMSO.

[10] To form the geographically disaggregated series, each of the original series was sectioned in space to yield further series for (i) urban administrative districts and (ii) rural administrative districts.

reception counties were assessed. The time window of data, 1933–49, was divided into five sections: (*peace*) 1933–9 (end of q. 2); (*evacuation*) 1939 (start of q. 3)–1940; (*war*) 1941–3; (*evacuation*) 1944–5; (*peace*) 1946–9. Sectioned in this manner, Poisson probabilities were generated from equation (5.1) for each disease, time period, and urban/rural sub-area of the 14 reception counties. The resulting probabilities give the chance of obtaining, under the null hypothesis, observed case levels as high or higher than those recorded for counties exceeding expectation, and as small or smaller for counties below expectation.

Results

The graphs in Figure 5.12 plot, for rural (left) and urban (right) areas of the reception counties, the Poisson probabilities for (A) scarlet fever, (B) diphtheria, and (C) poliomyelitis. For illustrative purposes, the line traces for all 14 reception counties have been plotted for scarlet fever in rural areas (Fig. 5.12A, left). In the remaining graphs, the maximum, median, and minimum line traces have been drawn in the manner of Figure 5.8. The horizontal pecked lines denote significantly high and low disease counts at the $p = 0.10$ level.

Figure 5.12A reveals a distinctive pattern for scarlet fever. For both urban and rural areas, the sharp rise in probabilities during the two main periods of evacuation (1939–40 and 1944–5) is consistent with a high incidence of the disease in the reception areas as compared with London. Between the two probability peaks, the probability trough is coincident with the mid-war period of quiescence in evacuation from the capital. While the same broad pattern—albeit far less exaggerated—can be deciphered for diphtheria (Fig. 5.12B), the pattern is absent for poliomyelitis (Fig. 5.12C).[11]

When the graphs for urban and rural areas are contrasted, a further feature of Figure 5.12 emerges. Notwithstanding the expectations of wartime epidemiologists and others, there is little evidence to suggest that the epidemiological effect of the evacuation was more pronounced in rural districts of the reception counties. So, for all three diseases, the probabilities for urban areas generally run at similar, or higher, levels than the corresponding probabilities for rural areas. Such a finding is consistent with the observations of Stocks (1941: 321–3) and suggests that, in practice, the rural 'immunity deficit' highlighted by *The Lancet* in 1939 (Anonymous, 1939*b*) had little discernible impact on urban–rural differentials in disease activity.

---

[11] In interpreting the evidence for poliomyelitis in Fig. 5.12C, we note that a fundamental property of the poliomyelitis virus is its extreme sensitivity to climatic conditions. As indicated in Sect. 5.5.3, the disease is strongly seasonal with virtually all cases occurring during the late summer and early autumn. Cases outside of this period are exceedingly rare. It is possible that, in forming Fig. 5.12C, the aggregation of disease counts from quarters into time blocks and into 'urban' and 'rural' smoothes the data so much that it masked a rapid response to the virus by children in the reception areas. To investigate this possibility, Poisson probabilities were recalculated on a county basis for each quarterly period, 1933–49. Although not shown, the probabilities display a clear, dramatic rise at the beginning of the evacuation period (Sept. 1939), persisting through 1940. A similar rise in the probabilities occurred in 1944, coincident with the wave of evacuation catalysed by the V1 bombing campaign.

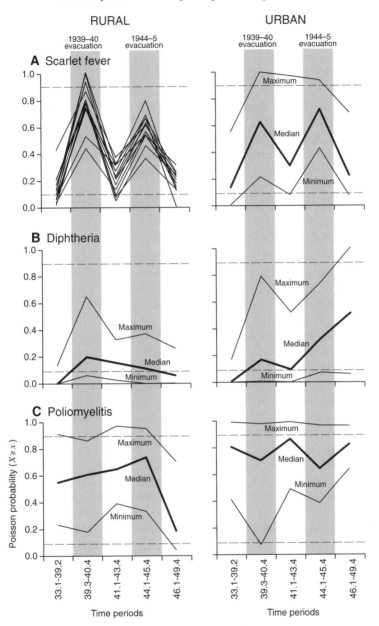

Fig. 5.12. Poisson probabilities for rural and urban areas of reception counties, 1933–1949

Notes: (A) Scarlet fever. (B) Diphtheria. (C) Poliomyelitis. The line traces for all 14 reception counties are plotted for scarlet fever in rural areas (A, left). In the remaining graphs, maximum, median, and minimum probabilities across the 14 reception counties are plotted. Pecked lines mark significantly high and low case levels at the $p = 0.10$ level.

Source: Smallman-Raynor *et al.* (2003, fig. 7, p. 416).

5.5.5 Summary

Writing in the *Report of the Chief Medical Officer, 1939–45*, the words of CMO Sir Wilson Jameson were to kindle the common post-war perception that evacuation had little (if any) discernible impact on epidemic activity. 'Many', Sir Wilson recalled, 'had prophesied that evacuation in 1939 would cause an increased spread of infectious disease'. 'Yet,' he concluded, 'there was less than usual' (Ministry of Health, 1946: 2). Such a perspective was informed by a general downward trend in morbidity and mortality from a number of common childhood infections, of which diphtheria—the subject of a concerted immunization campaign from 1941—displayed the most pronounced reduction (ibid. 3).

Framed by this post-war perception, and with the advantage of modern computing capacity to hand, three principal findings emerge from the investigation of scarlet fever, diphtheria, and poliomyelitis:

1. *Levels of disease activity.* Although the exact details vary by disease, the general thrust of both the temporal and spatial evidence is to confirm that evacuation often led to inflated levels of disease activity in the reception counties as compared with London. Some impression of the inflation can be gained by recognizing that, during the evacuation of 1939–40, the maximum quarterly disease incidence rate in the reception counties exceeded the rate for the metropolis by a factor of five or more (see Fig. 5.8). The incidence of scarlet fever was especially affected by the evacuation; diphtheria displayed similar behaviour patterns to scarlet fever, but in reduced form. Patterns for poliomyelitis proved to be more variable, although evidence of raised incidence in the reception areas was found when temporally and spatially disaggregated data were analysed.

2. *Levels of epidemiological integration.* Consistent with the above finding, the population flux engendered by the evacuation served to increase epidemiological integration by (i) accelerating the speed of disease propagation from London (scarlet fever) and (ii) enhancing the epidemiological interdependence of London and the reception counties (poliomyelitis). The evidence for the third disease (diphtheria) is counter-intuitive but, for the northern and western reception counties, it is consistent with a simple transmission model in which the return of evacuees served to carry the infection back to London.

3. *Urban–rural differentials in disease activity.* Contrary to the expectations of wartime medical officers, evacuation-related increases in disease activity were no more pronounced in rural, as compared with urban, districts of the reception counties. This finding suggests that factors other than rural immunity deficits—factors including absolute and relative differentials in the billeting (and, hence, mixing) of evacuees in urban and rural areas—may have played a critical role in the determination of disease levels in the reception zones (see Stocks, 1941: 321–3).

While the evacuation from London operated as a principal mechanism in the wartime mixing of schoolchildren in southern England, it is acknowledged that other factors may have contributed to the observed patterns of disease activity. As Figure 5.6 shows, for example, some of the larger south coastal settlements (Portsmouth and Southampton) also represented a source of evacuees and, while the scale of the associated movements from these locations was comparatively small, they too may have had some impact on the disease patterns identified above. Wartime trends in population realignment and mixing, other than those associated with evacuation, may also have influenced the results, while more sensitive analyses of disease activity (according to age, evacuation status, and case fatality) are precluded by the lack of relevant data in the Registrar General's *Returns*.

Subject to these uncertainties, the findings outlined above serve to emphasize the complexity of the evacuation–disease relationship during World War II. As we have already noted in our introduction to the analysis, however, a general principle also emerges: *notwithstanding the inconclusive nature of the wartime literature, the geographical dispersal of highly concentrated (urban) populations—like the geographical concentration of widely dispersed (rural) populations—has served as an efficient mechanism in the historical propagation of war epidemics in civil populations.* The role of wartime population concentration as a mechanism for epidemic transmission is examined in Section 12.2.

While this section has focused upon the role of urban–rural dispersals in spreading infectious agents, other studies have now begun to investigate how this process might also have led to raised incidence of cancers caused by infectious agents. For example, in their historical study of the rural incidence of childhood leukaemia, 1945–9, Kinlen and John (1994) document a significantly raised level of leukaemia in those rural areas which, in previous years, had recorded a high ratio of evacuees to local children. While the current status of knowledge precludes the establishment of a cause–effect relationship, Kinlen and John (1994) postulate that the evacuation-related mixing of children from rural and urban locations may have promoted the transmission of an infectious agent involved in the aetiology of childhood leukaemia.

5.6 Palestinian Refugees

On 29 November 1947, the UN General Assembly adopted—by a majority of 33 votes to 13 (10 abstentions)—recommendations that the British mandate in Palestine should be terminated, and that the newly independent land should be partitioned into separate Jewish and Arab states. With the immediate rejection of the UN resolution by Palestinian Arab leaders, the ensuing two years of civil unrest and international conflict were to result in the dislocation of a UNestimated 726,000 Palestinians[12] in a pre-war population of 1.2–1.3 million (Morris, 1987). While many refugees settled in the Gaza Strip and the West Bank, almost 300,000 moved to other territories in neighbouring Jordan, Lebanon, and Syria; see Figure 5.13 for locations. Half a century on, and with further wars and natural growth having served to swell the displaced population by several millions, the same five locations (Gaza Strip, West Bank, Jordan, Lebanon, and Syria) remain home to the majority of Palestinian refugees.

5.6.1   UNRWA and Palestinian Refugees

Official organizations for the assistance of Palestinian refugees can be traced to the early days of the refugee crisis. In 1948, at the height of the Arab–Israeli War (1948–9), the United Nations established the delivery of relief through UNRPR (United Nations Relief for Palestinian Refugees). The remit of UNRPR was transferred to UNRWA (United Nations Relief and Works Agency for Palestinian Refugees in the Near East) in 1949 and, since that time, UNRWA has provided for the health, education, and welfare of registered refugees (Lilienfield *et al.*, 1986; UNRWA, 2002). Palestinian refugees who receive assistance from UNRWA are excluded from the mandate of the UNHCR and, as such, are not bound by the definition of refugees given in Section 5.2.2 (UNHCR, 2000: 20).

REGISTERED REFUGEES AND REFUGEE CAMPS

Table 5.10 is based on information collected by UNRWA and gives, by field of asylum, the distribution of the 3.74 million registered refugees in June 2000. The table indicates that the majority of refugees were resident in Jordan (42%) and the Gaza Strip (22%), with the West Bank (16%), Lebanon (10%), and Syria (10%) accounting for the remainder. Approximately one-third of the refugees (1.21 million) were housed in the 59 official Palestinian refugee camps (Table 5.10), and these are mapped by population size in Figure 5.13. As the map shows, the largest camps (>40,000 refugees) were located in the densely populated Gaza Strip, northwestern Jordan, and southern Lebanon. Elsewhere, in the West Bank and Syria, individual camps did not exceed about 20,000 refugees. Regarding the nature of the camps, marked variations existed in terms of age, urban/rural location, and level of consolidation. Longer-established settlements, at least, had some degree of infrastructural regularization while, within the camps, UNRWA maintained health centres, supplementary feeding centres and schools, along with sanitary, construction, and maintenance services (Lilienfield *et al.*, 1986; UNRWA, 2002).

---

[12] In fact, the exact number of Palestinian Arabs displaced by the unrest of 1947–9 is not known with certainity. As Morris (1987: 298–9) notes, other estimates vary from about 520,000 (Israeli sources) to upwards of 1 million (Arab sources).

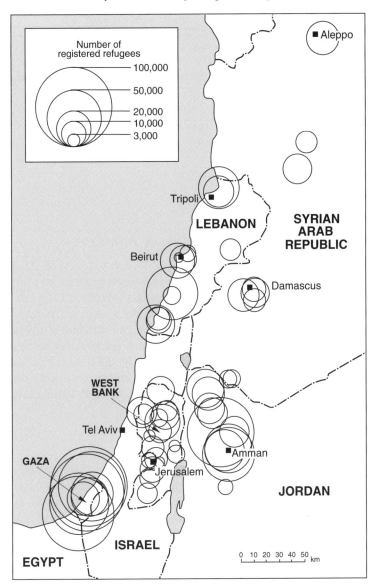

Fig. 5.13. Location of Palestinian refugee camps, June 2000

Notes: Circles mark the locations of the 59 official Palestinian refugee camps in the Gaza Strip, West Bank, Jordan, Lebanon, and Syria. The area of each circle has been drawn proportional to the registered camp population in June 2000.
Source: Redrawn from UNRWA (2001*b*).

Table 5.10. Distribution of registered Palestinian refugees, June 2000

	Field of UNRWA operation					
	Jordan	West Bank	Gaza Strip	Lebanon	Syria	Agency-wide
Registered refugees	1,570,192	583,009	824,622	376,472	383,199	3,737,494
No. of camps	10	19	8	12	10	59
Camp population	280,191	157,676	451,186	210,715	111,712	1,211,480

Source: UNRWA (2001*a*).

5.6.2 Infectious Disease Patterns

During the decades since its inception, UNRWA has been responsible for the development and implementation of a comprehensive programme of primary health care and preventive medicine for Palestinian refugees. Elements of the programme are described by UNRWA (2002) and encompass: (i) intensive disease surveillance and control strategies, including mass immunization against WHO Expanded Programme on Immunization (EPI) target diseases; (ii) maternal and child care; (iii) environmental health; and (iv) health education. Framed by these operations, the present section examines historical patterns of infectious disease activity in the population of registered Palestinian refugees, 1960–87.

DISEASE DATA

To examine disease patterns in registered refugees, we draw on the annual counts of morbidity collated by UNWRA for 12 sample diseases (chickenpox, diphtheria, dysentery, enteric fever, hepatitis, measles, meningitis, mumps, poliomyelitis, scarlet fever, trachoma, and respiratory tuberculosis) in the five fields of asylum (Gaza Strip, West Bank, Jordan, Lebanon, and Syria), 1960–87.[13] Here, our selection of diseases and time interval has been conditioned by the requirement of a complete (12 disease × 5 field × 28 year =) 1,680-unit matrix of morbidity,[14] with the end-point of the observation period fixed to the onset of unrest associated with the first Palestinian Intifada (1987–93). For reference, the total number of reported cases of each disease is given by geographical area in Table 5.11.

---

[13] The authors are grateful to Dr Fathi Mousa of UNRWA for providing the data analysed in this section.

[14] Even then, disease-surveillance data for refugees in the West Bank are not available in a systematic fashion until 1968.

Table 5.11. Reported cases of 12 sample diseases, registered Palestinian refugees (1960–1987)

Disease	Field of asylum[1]					
	Jordan	West Bank[2]	Gaza	Lebanon	Syria	All fields
Chickenpox	47,258	19,719	33,702	39,378	27,962	168,019
Diphtheria	42	3	1	6	25	77
Dysentery	67,383	8,866	103,192	88,517	66,335	334,293
Enteric fever	838	4	605	259	4,403	6,109
Hepatitis	3,591	2,226	8,474	2,537	3,813	20,641
Measles	43,933	4,616	35,006	23,963	14,032	121,550
Meningitis	94	8	82	48	57	289
Mumps	46,532	19,256	26,448	29,091	26,559	147,886
Poliomyelitis	234	18	367	174	114	907
Scarlet fever	148	1	0	3	216	368
Trachoma	135,872	488	76,355	9,833	5,861	228,409
Tuberculosis (respiratory)	1,875	169	2,772	1,756	542	7,114
Total	347,800	55,374	287,004	195,565	149,919	1,035,662

Notes: [1] Case totals for some annual units of the observation period (1960–87) are based on back-calculations from disease rates (per 100,000 registered refugees). [2] Disease counts not available for years prior to 1968.
Source: Data from UNRWA.

AGGREGATE ANALYSIS

The original disease matrix was first summed across the set of 12 sample dis-eases to yield an aggregate annual series of disease activity for each of the five fields of asylum, 1960–87. The resulting five series, formed to a rate per 100,000 registered refugees, are plotted as the line traces in Figure 5.14A; a sixth (heavy) line trace gives the total disease rate for the set of geographical units. Consis-tent with the documented success of UNRWA's programme of preventive medicine (Lilienfield *et al.*, 1986), the graph shows a long-term downward trend in infectious disease activity for each field of asylum. The reduction, however, is most prominent in the years prior to the Arab–Israeli conflict of 1973, with a general tendency towards stabilization thereafter.

To identify periods when infectious disease activity was relatively important in each field of asylum, the aggregate annual disease rates in Figure 5.14A were standardized across the set of geographical units using biproportionate scores. The resulting annual scores are plotted by field in Figure 5.14B. As in Section 5.3, the graphs have been formed so that scores in excess of 100 identify periods of relatively raised disease activity.

Figure 5.14B identifies marked variations in the periods when disease activ-ity was relatively important in the five fields of asylum. For two fields (Jordan and Lebanon), high scores (>150) correlate with the onset of civil wars in the

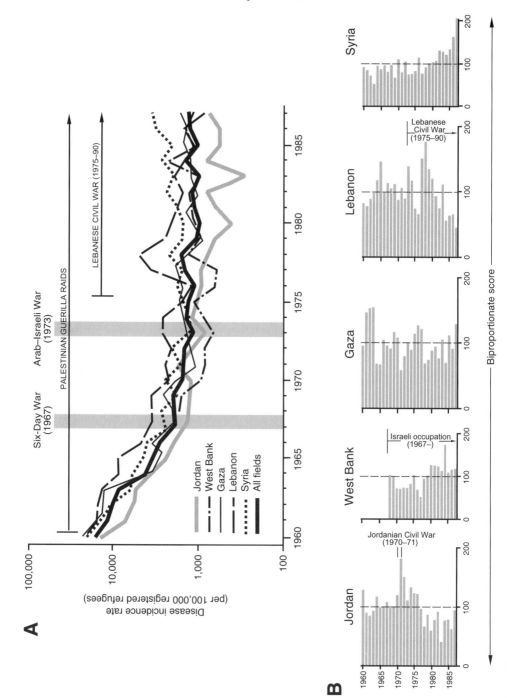

early 1970s (Jordanian Civil War, 1970–1) and the mid-1970s (Lebanese Civil War, 1975–90) and are suggestive of the deleterious epidemiological conse-quences of these episodes on refugee health. Thereafter, while the scores for both Jordan and Lebanon drop to generally low levels (<100) during the 1980s, a corresponding increase in disease activity for two other fields (Syria and the West Bank) is reflected in Figure 5.14B by the rise in scores to consistently high values (>100). Finally, for the Gaza Strip, Figure 5.14B illustrates a see-saw pattern, with the early and late 1960s, the mid-1970s, and the mid-1980s being marked out as phases of relatively increased disease activity.

DISEASE-SPECIFIC ANALYSIS

For each of the 12 sample diseases, the line traces in Figure 5.15 plot the annual incidence rate (per 100,000 registered refugees) across the five fields of asylum. To assist interpretation, the bar chart on each graph is again based on biproportionate scores and gives the number of fields of asylum in which the disease was relatively important in a given year. Large counts (to a maximum value of 5) identify years in which the disease was of geographically wide-spread importance. Conversely, small counts identify years in which the disease was of geographically limited importance.

Incidence rates (Fig. 5.15, line traces). Consistent with the aggregate results in Figure 5.14A, the most striking feature of Figure 5.15 is the long-term downward trend in levels of recorded activity for most diseases. The pattern is especially evident for diphtheria, dysentery, enteric fever, measles, meningitis, poliomyelitis, trachoma, and tuberculosis. Achievements in the control of chickenpox, hepatitis, and mumps, on the other hand, were far less signal, while recorded levels of scarlet fever increased sharply during the 1980s.

Relative geographical importance (Fig. 5.15, bar charts). As judged by the bar charts in Figure 5.15, observed changes in the levels of disease activity were associated with shifts in the relative geographical importance of the sample diseases. In particular, diseases of periodically widespread geographical importance in the period up to the mid-1970s, such as measles, meningitis,

---

Fig. 5.14. Infectious disease activity in the population of registered Palestinian refugees, 1960–1987

Notes: All graphs are based on a sample of 12 infectious diseases (chickenpox, diphtheria, dysen-tery, enteric fever, hepatitis, measles, meningitis, mumps, poliomyelitis, scarlet fever, trachoma, and respiratory tuberculosis) for which records were available over the 28-year observation period. (A) Aggregate annual disease incidence rate (per 100,000 registered refugees) by geographical field of asylum. (B) Biproportionate scores of infectious disease activity for each field of asylum; scores in excess of 100 (indicated by the vertical pecked lines) mark years in which the corresponding fields recorded relatively high levels of disease activity.

Source: Data from UNRWA.

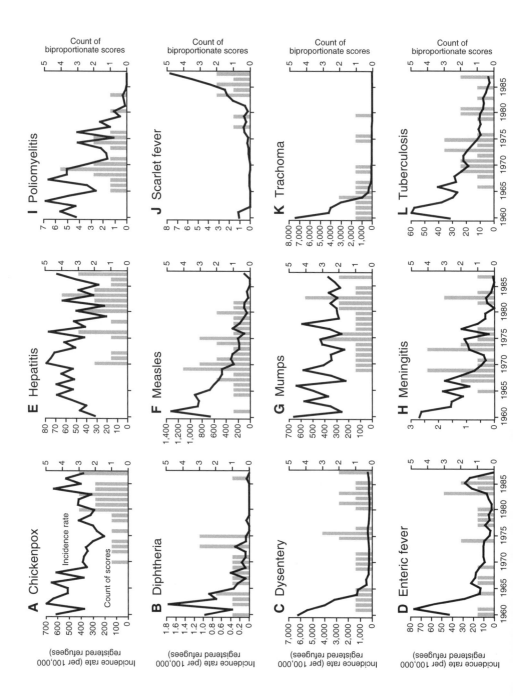

poliomyelitis, and tuberculosis were joined and, from the 1980s, supplanted by conditions such as chickenpox, hepatitis, mumps, and scarlet fever.

Geographical Variation

To examine further geographical variability in disease incidence rates across the five fields of asylum, the coefficient of variation, *CV*, was computed. *CV* was defined as

$$CV = 100(s/\bar{x}), \tag{3.1 bis}$$

where, for a given disease, $\bar{x}$ and s are the arithmetic mean and standard deviation respectively of the incidence rates (per 100,000 registered refugees) in the five fields in each year. The coefficient is large where there is relatively high variation in relation to the mean, and small when the variation is relatively low.

Figure 5.16 plots these coefficients of variation in a standardized format by setting the *CV* for each disease in the first year (1960) equal to 100, and indexing later values with respect to first values. The *CV* for the aggregate rate of 12 diseases is plotted on each graph for reference. In contrast to the epidemic curves plotted in Figure 5.15, which showed a general decrease in levels of disease activity over time, the graphs in Figure 5.16 indicate an overall tendency for geographical variability in disease rates to have increased over time. With four notable exceptions (diphtheria, dysentery, mumps, and scarlet fever), the rising trends imply that some fields of asylum had made much more rapid progress in disease control than others.

5.6.3 Palestinian Refugees and the Lebanese Civil War

In the foregoing discussion, we noted how levels of disease activity among Palestinian refugees had been adversely affected by local conflicts in their fields of asylum. So, Figure 5.14B identified a marked increase in disease activity among Palestinian refugees in Jordan during the Jordanian Civil War (1970–1) while a similar, and more protracted, feature was identified for Palestinian refugees in the Lebanon during the Lebanese Civil War (1975–90). In this

◄————————————————————————————————————

Fig. 5.15. Sample epidemic curves, registered Palestinian refugees (1960–1987)

Notes: Line traces plot the annual rate (per 100,000 registered refugees) for 12 infectious diseases in the aggregate population of Palestinian refugees. To identify periods of particular epidemiological significance associated with a given disease, biproportionate scores were computed across the matrix of 12 (diseases) × 28 (years) for each field of asylum (Jordan, West Bank, Gaza, Lebanon, and Syria). For years in which infectious disease activity was relatively important in a given field (defined as scores > 100 in Fig. 5.14B), individual diseases with biproportionate scores in excess of unity were identified. In this manner, the bar chart on each graph plots the count of disease-specific scores in excess of unity for a given year, to an annual maximum of 5 (= number of fields of residence).
Source: Data from UNRWA.

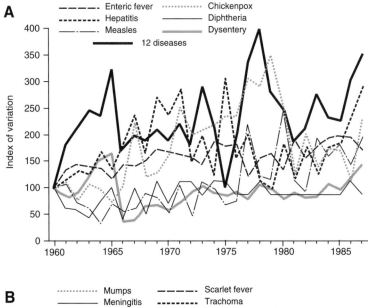

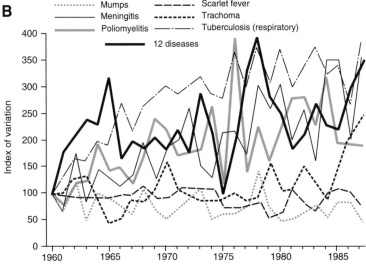

Fig. 5.16. Geographical variation in the annual incidence of sample infectious diseases, registered Palestinian refugees (1960–1987)

Notes: The coefficient of variation, *CV*, has been used as a measure of the relative dispersion in annual disease incidence rates (per 100,000 registered refugees) across the five geographical fields of residence (see explanation in text). Each disease has been standardized on an initial value of 100 in the first year (1960), and subsequent values have been indexed with respect to this initial value.

section, we examine further the correspondence between the Lebanese Civil War and infectious disease patterns in the resident population of Palestinian refugees.

BACKGROUND: THE LEBANESE CIVIL WAR (1975–1990)

Civil war began in the Lebanon in 1975 and lasted throughout our observation period, eventually to end with the withdrawal of rival militias in 1990. The war left the country and its health system shattered. In excess of 144,000 people (mostly civilians) are believed to have died as a consequence of the fighting, while an additional 200,000 persons were wounded. Countless others 'disappeared' during the course of the hostilities. At the same time, poverty, a lack of drugs and vaccines all contributed to an upsurge in infectious diseases. Outbreaks of typhoid and paratyphoid fevers were recorded in the early 1980s (World Health Organization, 1984). Diarrhoeas, respiratory and childhood infections also assumed a position of public health importance among the war-affected populations (Armenian, 1989; Armenian *et al.*, 1989), while the 1980s and 1990s witnessed an epidemic upsurge in tuberculosis (Bahr *et al.*, 1991).

DISEASE TRENDS IN PALESTINIAN REFUGEES

One way to examine the epidemiological impact of the Lebanese Civil War on resident Palestinian refugees is to compute the local annual disease rate per 100,000 registered refugees as a ratio of the corresponding disease rate for Palestinian refugees in all fields of asylum. Formed in this manner, ratios in excess of unity mark years in which the disease rate for refugees in the Lebanon was higher than the rate for the entire refugee population. The resulting disease ratios, computed for each of the 12 sample diseases, are plotted as the heavy line traces in Figure 5.17. In addition, owing to the military involvement of neighbouring Syria, the broken line traces plot the equivalent disease ratios for Palestinian refugees resident in that country. Ratios of unity are marked on each graph by the broken horizontal line while, for reference, the period corresponding to the war has been highlighted.

When examined for Palestinian refugees in the Lebanon, a striking feature of Figure 5.17 is the relative upsurge in a broad range of diseases (chickenpox, dysentery, enteric fever, hepatitis, measles, mumps, poliomyelitis, and respiratory tuberculosis) with the onset of the war in the mid-1970s. For some diseases, this upsurge is set against a previously stable (enteric fever and measles) or downward (hepatitis) trend in relative disease activity. For other conditions, such as diphtheria, meningitis, scarlet fever, and trachoma, the war appears to have had a small, or negligible effect, on disease activity.

For Palestinian refugees in Syria, Figure 5.17 indicates that the onset of the war was also associated with a relative upsurge in some diseases (notably chickenpox, dysentery, and hepatitis), although the overall effect was much less dramatic and less sustained than that witnessed for the refugees in the

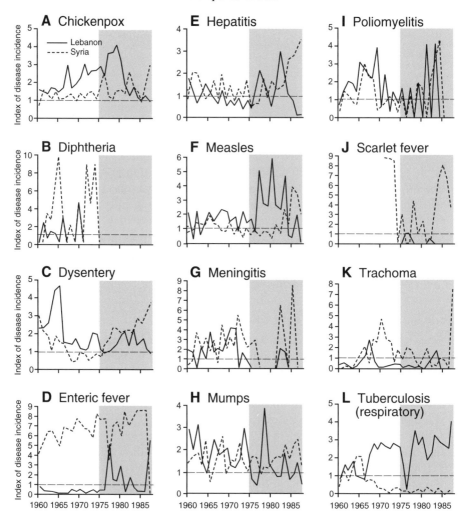

Fig. 5.17. Impact of the Lebanese Civil War (1975–1990) on infectious disease activity among registered Palestinian refugees in the Lebanon and Syria, 1960–1987

Notes: The graphs plot an index of annual incidence for 12 sample diseases in the Lebanon (full line traces) and Syria (broken line traces). The index has been formed as the ratio of the field-specific disease incidence rate to the aggregate rate for all registered Palestinian refugees in the Middle East. Horizontal broken lines mark ratios of unity. The period corresponding to the Lebanese Civil War has been highlighted on each graph.

Source: Data from UNRWA.

Lebanon. Rather, the line traces for refugees in Syria highlight the relative rise in disease activity towards the end of the observation period—a period that coincided with a general deterioration in the economic and political stability of the country (Hilan, 1993).

5.6.4 Summary

Our examination of sample infectious diseases in the population of registered Palestinian refugees, 1960–87, has shown:

(*a*) a long-term downward trend in infectious disease activity in each of the five fields of asylum. This finding corresponds with the development of a comprehensive programme of preventive medicine by UNRWA (Lilienfield *et al.*, 1986; UNRWA, 2002);

(*b*) between-field variations in the periods of relative importance of infectious disease activity. Although details vary by time interval and location, periods of raised disease are positively correlated with episodes of civil war, economic and political instability in the fields of asylum. The onset of the Lebanese Civil War of 1975–90 had a particularly deleterious epidemiological impact on Palestinian refugees in that country;

(*c*) notwithstanding stark successes in the control of many of the sample diseases, certain infectious conditions (notably chickenpox, hepatitis, and mumps) persisted in the refugee population. To these latter diseases can be added scarlet fever, which displayed a marked rise in reported activity during the 1980s;

(*d*) for the majority of diseases studied, there was a long-term increase in the geographical variability of reported activity. Given findings (*a*)–(*c*), the observed increase in geographical variability almost certainly reflects between-field variations in the success of control strategies for individual diseases.

5.7 Ethnic Conflict, Displacement, and Disease in Central Africa

In Section 5.3, we observed how population displacement in Africa had reached unprecedented levels during the 1990s. As an annual average for the decade, UNHCR-based estimates indicate there to have been some 5 million refugees in Africa (UNHCR, 2000, annex 3, p. 310),[15] representing almost 1 per cent of the entire population of the continent. To these can be added many millions more who were forcibly displaced within their countries of nationality or habitual residence. As Table 5.1 indicates, a long series of wars in such places as Ethiopia, Liberia, Mozambique, Sierra Leone, Somalia, Sudan, and Togo contributed to the overall pattern of displacement. Among the largest of the movements, however, were those resulting from the ethnic conflicts that erupted in the neighbouring states of Burundi and Rwanda, Central Africa, during 1993 and 1994. All told, the two conflicts yielded well over 2 million international refugees (Table 5.1) while the number of internally displaced persons (IDPs)

[15] Based on end of year estimates.

still stood at 1.4 million in late 1999 (Table 5.3). The movements spawned outbreaks of dysentery, malaria, acute respiratory infections, and meningitis. Most prominent among the epidemiological events, however, were explosive camp-based epidemics of louse-borne typhus (IDPs in Burundi) and cholera (Rwandese refugees in eastern Zaire). Again, UN-based definitions of IDPs and refugees are outlined in Section 5.2.2.

LOUSE-BORNE TYPHUS: BURUNDIAN IDPS

The assassination of President Melchior Ndadaye of Burundi on 21 October 1993 precipitated a fierce civil war between the country's Hutu and Tutsi tribal groups; see Figure 5.18 for the location of Burundi. By the end of the year, hostilities had resulted in the internal displacement of an estimated 130,000 persons, with the number growing to 800,000—representing some 13 per cent of the entire population of Burundi—during the events of the next several years (Table 5.3). Many hundreds of thousands of others, either unwilling or unable to find sanctuary in Burundi, fled across international borders into neighbouring Rwanda, Tanzania, and Zaire (Table 5.1).

The population movements were, from the outset, accompanied by the spread of infectious diseases. As early as December 1993, the sentinel surveillance system of Burundi had detected a substantial increase in the occurrence of dysentery and malaria while, over the border in Rwanda, non-bloody diarrhoea and respiratory tract infections added to the health problems of the Burundian refugees (CDC, 1994a). The most marked epidemic event, however, occurred in 1996–7 with the spread of louse-borne typhus fever in the camps of the displaced in Burundi.

Preliminary Evidence (1995–1996)

Clinical and epidemiological details of classic louse-borne typhus are given in Appendix 1A. The disease occurs sporadically in the highlands of Sub-Saharan Africa, with countries of Central (Burundi and Rwanda), East (Ethiopia), and West (Nigeria) Africa serving as the main endemic foci. As regards the occurrence of the disease in Burundi, an outbreak, associated with some 9,000 reported cases, occurred in 1974–5. Thereafter, the annual incidence of the disease fell to low levels, with no documented cases between 1990 and 1994 (World Health Organization, 1997). From November 1995, however, a fever of unknown origin, in association with a proliferation of body lice, began to spread in an overcrowded prison camp in the northern province of N'Gozi (see Fig. 5.18). The prison outbreak escalated to a peak in January 1996 and, from thereon, an epidemic of typhus fever (known locally as *sutama*) began to take hold in the country's internally displaced population (Bise and Coninx, 1997; Raoult *et al.*, 1998). While several thousand cases were reported in 1996, the major period of epidemic transmission occurred in 1997 (World Health Organization, 1997).

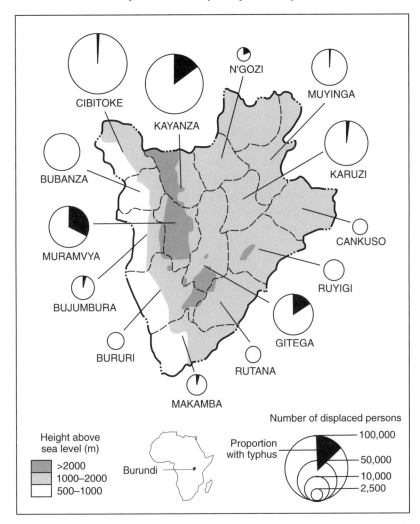

Fig. 5.18. Epidemic louse-borne typhus among residents of camps for the internally displaced in Burundi, Central Africa, January–September 1997

Notes: Proportional circles plot the number of internally displaced persons (IDPs) by province, while the black segments mark the percentage proportion of IDPs diagnosed with typhus. Shaded areas of the map mark land above 1,000 metres and 2,000 metres.
Source: Drawn from data in Raoult *et al.* (1998, fig. 1, p. 354 and table 3, p. 356).

Dimensions of the Epidemic (1997)

The proportional circles in Figure 5.18 are based on information included in Raoult *et al.* (1998) and plot, by province, the distribution of some 700,000 internally displaced persons in Burundi during 1997. At this time, most of the displaced were resident in 28 large camps; the majority of camps were located away from towns and cities; many lacked any form of health care. Based on information for these constituent camps, the shaded sectors in Figure 5.18 indicate the percentage proportion of the displaced population in which typhus fever was diagnosed between January and September 1997. All told, 43,971 cases were recorded in the camps, with the highest levels of disease activity in (i) the central highland provinces of Gitega, Kayanza, and Muramvya and (ii) the small refugee population of N'Gozi. While the disease remained largely restricted to the central and northern highland provinces, cases of typhus fever in the lower-lying capital province, Bujumbura, are believed to have resulted from the migration of people from the highlands. Whether the epidemic ultimately developed from a single source, or resulted from a series of localized independent outbreaks, however, remains unknown (Raoult *et al.*, 1998).

While the highland provinces of Burundi are recognized as a focus of the causative agent of typhus fever, *Rickettsia prowazekii*, certain predisposing factors appear to have resulted in particularly high levels of disease activity among the displaced in those provinces. Such factors included poor sanitation, a cold climate and the consequent need for several layers of clothing, thereby promoting conditions favourable to body louse infestation.

Epidemic Control

Although disease activity in the principal foci of the epidemic (Gitega, Kayanza, and Muramvya provinces) began to decline in April–May 1997 (Fig. 5.19), substantial difficulties were encountered in the control of the epidemic. Owing to the ongoing hostilities, supplies of insecticides did not become widely available until July. Even then, delousing operations were complicated by the transient nature of the camp populations. Under such circumstances, Raoult *et al.* (1998) warn against over-reliance on insecticides for the control of typhus fever. Rather, a combination of delousing and antibiotic treatment is recommended as the optimum control strategy.

CHOLERA: RWANDESE REFUGEES IN EASTERN ZAIRE

In early April 1994, long-standing ethnic tensions in Rwanda erupted into genocide. Within three months, an estimated 800,000 people—mainly ethnic Tutsis—had perished at the hands of Hutu extremists and other *génocidaires*. By mid-July, however, resurgent Tutsi forces had begun to reassert control in Rwanda, precipitating the flight of 2 million or more ethnic Hutus. While some fled to western Tanzania (580,000 refugees), northern Burundi (270,000), and Uganda (10,000), the majority (1.2 million) moved to Goma and proximal locations in eastern Zaire (UNHCR, 2000) (see Fig. 5.20). For the latter contingent, the mortality rates that accompanied the displacement were, in the words of the Goma Epidemiology Group (1995: 343), 'almost unprecedented in refugee populations'. 'The world', the same source adds, 'was simply not prepared for an emergency of this magnitude.'

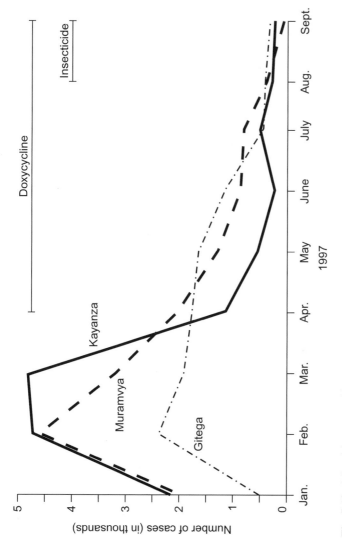

Fig. 5.19. Monthly count of louse-borne typhus fever in the camps of internally displaced persons in three central highland provinces of Burundi, January–September 1997

Notes: The period associated with the administration of antibiotic (doxycycline) treatment and insecticides is indicated. The locations of the three provinces (Gitega, Kayanza, and Muramvya) are indicated in Fig. 5.18.

Source: Redrawn from Raoult *et al.* (1998, fig. 2, p. 355).

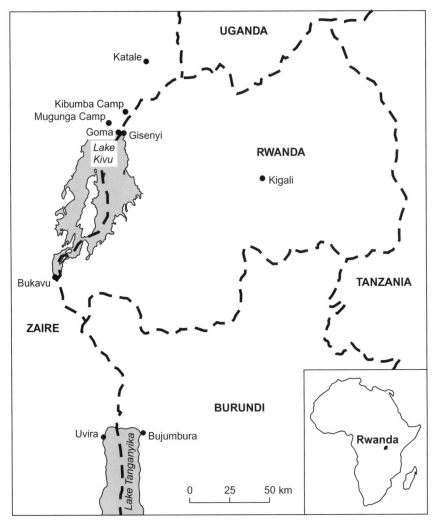

Fig. 5.20. Map showing the location of Rwandese refugee camps in eastern Zaire, 1994
Source: Redrawn from Goma Epidemiology Group (1995, fig. 1, p. 339).

Death Rates among Refugees in Zaire

Some impression of the level of mortality sustained by Rwandan refugees in eastern Zaire can be gained from Table 5.12. For a month-long period from the beginning of the displacement (14 July), the lower row of the table is based on a body count of refugees and gives the crude mortality rate (per 10,000 per day) associated with an estimated refugee population of between 0.5 and 0.8 mil-

Table 5.12. Estimated crude mortality rate for Rwandan refugees in Zaire, 1994

	Survey period	Estimated population	Estimated crude mortality rate[1]	Estimated percentage mortality
Katale survey	14 July–4 Aug.	80,000	41.3	8.3
Kibumba survey	14 July–9 Aug.	180,000	28.1	7.3
Mugunga survey	14 July–13 Aug.	150,000	29.4	9.1
Body count (all areas)	14 July–14 Aug.	500,000–800,000	31.2–19.5	9.7–6.0

Note: [1] Expressed per 10,000 per day.
Source: Goma Epidemiology Group (1995, table 1, p. 340).

lion.[16] The total body count of 48,347 yields a mortality rate of 19.5–31.2 per 10,000 per day, consistent with the death of up to 10 per cent of refugees during the first month of the crisis. The results of population surveys in the camps at Katale, Kibumba, and Mugunga, in which many of the refugees were eventually settled (Fig. 5.20), provide similar high estimates of crude mortality (Table 5.12) (Goma Epidemiology Group, 1995).

Epidemic Cholera, July–August 1994

Surveys indicate that an overwhelming proportion of all deaths (85–90%) were associated with cholera and other diarrhoeal diseases. The first case of cholera was diagnosed in the refugee population on 20 July, to be followed by an explosive outbreak of the disease associated with *Vibrio cholerae* O1 (biotype El Tor) in the days that followed. Details are sketchy but, between 14 July and 12 August, some 62,000 cases of diarrhoeal disease were reported from the refugee health facilities in eastern Zaire, of which an estimated 35,000 were attributable to cholera. Allowing for those cholera cases that did not present to health facilities, the Goma Epidemiology Group (1995) place the actual cholera case-load at 58,000–80,000—equivalent to an attack rate of up to 16 per cent (Goma Epidemiology Group, 1995; Van Damme, 1995).

Unfortunately, detailed information on the geographical distribution of cholera is unavailable (Goma Epidemiology Group, 1995). However, some 57 per cent of all reports of diarrhoeal disease in the seven days to Wednesday 27 July (marking the epidemic peak) originated from health facilities in and around the town of Goma. Untreated water from Lake Kivu, near which the Goma refugees were originally located, is suspected to have operated as a principal source of infection. With the transmission of the disease further fuelled by overcrowding, poor personal hygiene, and lack of adequate sanitation, it

---

[16] As described by the Goma Epidemiology Group (1995: p. 340), the estimate of 0.5–0.8 million is based on water and food ration distribution figures and on agency-based mapping exercises.

seems that cholera spread so rapidly that vaccination would have had no tangible effect on the course of the epidemic (Goma Epidemiology Group, 1995).

Epidemics of other diseases followed on the heels of cholera. Some 15,500 clinical cases of dysentery (caused by *Shigella dysenterae* type 1) were diagnosed between 8 and 14 August while, during the first 16 days of the month, morbidity surveillance also detected 83 laboratory-confirmed cases of meningitis due to *Neisseria meningitidis*. By this time, however, the international relief response had begun to take effect and disease-control measures were successfully implemented.

Subsequent Cholera Outbreaks

The cholera outbreak of July–August 1994 was followed in subsequent years by further outbreaks of the disease among the Rwandan refugees.

Returnees (November 1996). Between 16 and 24 November 1996, some 350,000 refugees from five camps in eastern Zaire re-entered Rwanda through Gisenyi (Fig. 5.20). Health personnel of Médecins Sans Frontières (MSF) undertook 15,675 consultations along the route of the returnees, of which 8,916 were for watery diarrhoea. Sample tests indicated that an unknown, but probably substantial, proportion of diarrhoeal disease was attributable to infection with *Vibrio cholerae* O1 (Brown *et al.*, 1997).

Refugees in Zaire (April 1997). In April 1997, a cholera outbreak was reported among 90,000 Rwandan refugees located between Kisangani and Ubundu, some 450 km northeast of Goma. During a 16-day period, 4 to 19 April, a total of 545 cholera patients were admitted to the treatment centre (attack rate 0.9%), of which 67 (12.3%) died. Several factors contributed to the inflated mortality during the outbreak, including (i) lack of adequate food, shelter, or access to health care in the months prior to the appearance of cholera and (ii) logistic difficulties associated with accessing isolated camps by relief personnel. Although intervention strategies (surveillance, health education, provision of potable water, aggressive oral rehydration therapy, and the construction of latrines) may have been effective in preventing the further spread of the disease, such activities ceased on 21 April 1997 when the refugees were dispersed by unidentified militias (CDC, 1998).

5.8 Conclusion

This chapter has examined the epidemiological dimensions of wartime population displacement. Whatever the specific cause or category of displacement, be it the voluntary movement of childhood evacuees in Britain during World War II, or the forced movement of legally defined 'refugees' and 'internally displaced persons' in the post-1950 era, all have been intimately associated with the geographical transmission of infectious diseases.

In the context of British evacuees during World War II, the particular epidemiological threat rested with the mixing of populations from two very different epidemiological environments. The majority of evacuees were schoolchildren from London and other large cities; locations where some of the more common infectious diseases of childhood were endemic, where levels of acquired immunity to such infections were correspondingly high, and from which the dangers of disease exportation to other locations were rife. In marked contrast, the rural areas to which the evacuees were dispersed were too sparsely populated to maintain many infectious diseases in endemic form; exposure to childhood infections occurred on a relatively infrequent basis, and levels of acquired immunity among the local children were correspondingly low. Under these circumstances, the urban–rural transfer of evacuees served as an efficient mechanism in the propagation of infectious diseases such as diphtheria, scarlet fever, and, to a lesser extent, poliomyelitis.

The global dynamics of population displacement have changed significantly during the last 50 years, as have international responses to them. Over time, the priority concerns of international agencies such as UNHCR have expanded to encompass Europe (1950s), Africa (1960s), Asia (1970s), and the multi-continent challenges of the superpower proxy wars (1980s). The proxy wars ended in the early 1990s, but maintained internal momentum without superpower support. Whatever the war and whatever the geographical setting, however, refugees and IDPs in the modern era have often fallen victim to a common set of ailments: diarrhoeal diseases, measles, acute respiratory tract infections, and malnourishment. Malaria, hepatitis, and meningitis have occasionally appeared and, on rare occasions, diseases such as typhus fever have been recorded. For the most part, however, the disease pattern is predictable and, given adequate resources for the timely implementation of humanitarian relief, the resulting mortality is preventable (Shears *et al.*, 1987; Toole, 1997). As Toole and Waldman (1990: 3299) note, 'it is not the *type* of illness but rather the *incidence* and *high mortality rates* that make these [displaced] populations remarkable' (emphasis in original).

Appendix 5A

Biproportionate Scores (Section 5.3.1)

Suppose a matrix of observations $\{x_{ij}\}$ is available in which m years form the rows (denoted by i) and n regions the columns (denoted by j). Each cell of the matrix gives the value of the variable of interest (e.g. the estimated number of refugees) for a particular year in a given region. If we wish to assess the relative importance of years across the set of regions, the matrix must be standardized in some way. A variety of methods exist to achieve this. One of the most common is to use row and column totals to generate expected values in each region and then to examine departures of the actual values from

Table 5.A1. Biproportionate scores: hypothetical data for the count of refugees in two years and five regions

Year	Regions					Total
	1	2	3	4	5	
Part (A) Original data						
1	800	400	200	100	50	1550
2	80	40	20	10	5	155
Total	880	440	220	110	55	
Part (B) First iteration scores						
1	258	129	65	32	16	500
2	258	129	65	32	16	500
Total	516	258	130	64	32	
Part (C) Second iteration scores						
1	100	100	100	100	100	500
2	100	100	100	100	100	500
Total	200	200	200	200	200	

these expectations. A particularly powerful alternative is to use biproportionate scores, and we illustrate the computational procedures using the data in part (A) of Table 5.A1.

In step one of the standardization procedure, the values are scaled so that each row sum is equal to the number of columns in the matrix, here five. This is achieved by calculating the row sums in the original data (e.g. 1550 in the case of year 1) and then dividing these totals by five to give a scaling factor for each row of the data matrix. For the first row, this procedure yields $1550/5 = 310$ and, for the second row, $155/5 = 31$. The adjusted scores are then obtained by taking the values in each row of the original data matrix and dividing them by their corresponding scaling factor. This step produces the matrix given in Table 5.A1(B) where, to eliminate decimal points, all values have been multiplied by 100.

The standardization process then continues by scaling the columns of the matrix given in part (B) so that each column sum is equal to the number of rows in the matrix, here two. This yields the matrix given in Table 5.A1(C) where again all values have been multiplied by 100. The process of adjustment is continued, operating alternately on rows and columns until the adjusted matrix converges; that is, the values in the matrix cease, within some margin of error set by the researcher, to change. We can express this process formally as

$$\begin{bmatrix} x_{11} & x_{12} & x_{13} & \cdots & x_{1n} \\ x_{21} & x_{22} & x_{23} & \cdots & x_{2n} \\ \vdots & \vdots & \vdots & \vdots & \vdots \\ \vdots & \vdots & \vdots & \vdots & \vdots \\ x_{m1} & x_{m2} & x_{m3} & \cdots & x_{mn} \end{bmatrix} \begin{bmatrix} n+e \\ n+e \\ \vdots \\ \vdots \\ n+e \end{bmatrix} =$$

$$= \begin{bmatrix} m+e & m+e & \cdots & m+e \end{bmatrix} \quad (5.A1)$$

where *e* is an allowable tolerance term. In the simple example given in Table 5.A1, convergence has already occurred by the end of the second cycle but, in large matrices with irregular relationships between the regions, a substantial number of iterations may be required.

In the matrix recorded in part (C) of Table 5.A1, the columns give the *relative* importance of each year in a given region; the rows show the *relative* importance of a given year across the regions. A value of unity (100) in the biproportionate matrix is the expected value under an exponential model. Cell values greater than unity are relatively more important; cells with values less than unity are relatively less important. Thus, the large scores (>100) for Africa, Asia, and Europe during the latter years of the 1990s (Fig. 5.3), when compared with the low scores (<100) for elsewhere, highlight the Old World concentration of refugee activity at this time.

PART III

A Regional Pattern of War Epidemics

Introduction to Part III

In Part III of this book, our treatment switches from the longitudinal time-based analysis of Part II to a series of regional case studies in which a number of repeating themes linking war and epidemic diseases are examined.

Theme 1: Military mobilization at the outset of wars has long served as a fertile breeding ground for epidemics. The enlistment and concentration of large numbers of raw recruits, often from disparate geographical locations, usually under conditions of great urgency, and occasionally with inadequate attention to the health and well-being of the new muster, provides conditions ripe for the rapid—sometimes, explosive—spread of infectious diseases. For example, as we have seen in Section 4.4.1, the rush of young Australian men—many from isolated farms and outback areas—to enlist during World War I (1914–18) resulted in epidemics of measles in local recruitment camps and later on board troopships and in the assembly camps for the Western Front (Butler, 1943). At about the same time, in the English counties of Berkshire, Hampshire, and Wiltshire, Reece (1916: 75) noted how the overcrowding of young men 'joining the colours' resulted in the local transmission of meningococcal (cerebrospinal) meningitis among both the recruits and the civilians with which they were billeted. During World War II (1939–45), primary atypical pneumonia reached epidemic proportions among fresh musters of the US Army (Anonymous, 1945*a*) while, in more recent times, respiratory diseases have continued to blight newly mobilized units of US troops (Gray *et al.*, 1999).

Theme 2: Military camps of all kinds provide opportunities for the spread of epidemic diseases. The historical circumstances are summarized by Joseph Janvier Woodward (Pl. 4.2) who, in his classic treatise *Outlines of the Chief Camp Diseases of the United States Armies* (1863), observed how

Crowding is a condition present in all great encampments. Thousands of men are frequently, from military necessity, aggregated together in a comparatively limited space . . . [U]nder such circumstances the immense population, resembling that of a great city, congregated upon an area even less than that which a city of equal population would occupy, is deprived of all those advantages of drainage and sewerage which great cities usually enjoy in civilized countries. But not only is the actual population per acre too great for health, the men are crowded together in their tents in a most unhealthy fashion. (Woodward, 1863: 45)

In the privations of war, such unhealthy conditions may affect troops in field and siege camps, as well as military detainees in prisoner of war (POW), labour, and internment camps. In turn, military camps may seed epidemics in contiguous civil populations.

Theme 3: Emerging and re-emerging diseases have long been a feature of war. As we have already observed in Chapter 2, wars of the late Middle Ages were afflicted by such apparently 'new' conditions as English sweating sickness, venereal syphilis, and louse-borne typhus fever. Somewhat later, Asiatic cholera emerged as a disease of nineteenth-century wars while, in the twentieth century, deployed forces in World War II (1939–45) and the Korean War (1950–3) were beset by such seemingly novel diseases as 'Balkan grippe', Korean haemorrhagic fever, and Japanese encephalitis. The localized civil wars of more recent years, too, have played an important role in the disease emergence–re-emergence complex. An illustration is provided by the epidemic resurgence of visceral leishmaniasis in Sudan (Seaman *et al.*, 1996), diphtheria in Tajikistan (Usmanov *et al.*, 2000), and louse-borne typhus in Burundi (Raoult *et al.*, 1998).

Theme 4: Sexually transmitted diseases (STDs) have been a scourge of both military personnel and the wars in which they have been deployed since time immemorial. The venereal nature of gonorrhoea was known to Hippocrates in the fourth century BC (Rothenberg, 1993), and we may reasonably infer that this disease contributed to the documented problem of prostitution in the army camps of classical Greece and Rome (Hinrichsen, 1944). In more recent times, the pan-European spread of venereal syphilis in the aftermath of the Italian War of Charles VIII (1494–5) provides one of the most dramatic—if controversial—instances of the intersection of armies, STDs, and war (see Sect. 2.3.3). As a scourge of modern wars, STDs accounted for some 1.23 million admissions in the US Army during World War II (Reister, 1976) while, in more recent times, the advent of HIV/AIDS has introduced a new dimension to the problem of STDs and war.

Theme 5: Island epidemics hold a prominent place in war history. From the War of the Grand Alliance (1688–97) to the Cuban Insurrection (1895–8), yellow fever was a formidable foe of the European armies that ventured to the tropical islands of the Caribbean Basin (Sect. 2.6.2). Elsewhere, the mysterious fever that broke out on the Dutch island of Walcheren during the British Expedition of 1809–10 ranks as one of the greatest medical disasters to have befallen the British Army (Sect. 2.4.5) while, as Burnet and White have commented, the outbreak of poliomyelitis which accompanied the raising of the siege of Malta in 1942–3 'may be said to pose the central problem for the understanding and eventual control of poliomyelitis' (cited in Cliff *et al.*, 2000: 424). On a much grander geographical scale, a series of diseases endemic to South Pacific islands—malaria, filariasis, dengue, and scrub typhus—served as a major drain on the fighting strength of US forces in the Pacific War (1942–5), thereby threatening the success of General MacArthur's island campaigns.

Each of the themes can be played out in a number of geographical theatres. In this book, we take the great world regions of Pan America (Ch. 7), Europe (Ch. 8), Asia and the Far East (Ch. 9), Africa (Ch. 10) and Oceania (Ch. 11). The intersection of regions and themes we have chosen from the 25 combinatorial

Table III.A. Matrix of regional–thematic examples

Region	Theme					
	1. Military mobilization	2. Camps	3. Emerging and re-emerging diseases	4. Sexually transmitted diseases	5. Island epidemics	Additional themes
Pan America	Chapter 7 American Civil War (1861–5) Spanish–American War (1898) World War I (1914–18) World War II (1939–45)	American Civil War (1861–5) Spanish–American War (1898) World War I (1914–18) World War II (1939–45)	World War I (1914–18) World War II (1939–45)		Cuban Insurrection (1895–8)	Chapter 12 Cuban Insurrection (1895–8) *Theme: epidemiological integration and war*
Europe		Chapter 8 Crimean War (1853–6) Franco-Prussian War (1870–1) World War II (1939–45)	World War II (1939–45)		World War II (1939–45)	World War I (1914–18) World War II (1939–45) *Theme: civilian epidemics*
Asia/Far East		World War II (1939–45) Korean War (1950–3)	Chapter 9 World War II (1939–45) Korean War (1950–3) Vietnam War (1960–75)			Chapter 12 World War II (1939–45) *Theme: POWs and forced labour*
Africa		South African War (1899–1902)	Ugandan Civil War (1978–9)	Chapter 10 French Colonial Wars in N. Africa World War II (1939–45) Ugandan Civil War (1978–9)	World War II (1939–45)	Chapter 12 South African War (1899–1902) *Theme: population reconcentration*
Oceania		World War II (1939–45)	World War I (1914–18) World War II (1939–45)		Chapter 11 Samoan Wars (1848–99) Taranaki Wars (1860–72) World War I (1914–18) World War II (1939–45)	

Notes: The matrix highlights those wars that are examined in Part III of the book. For a specific region, the shaded cells identify the sample wars examined by theme in Chapters 7 to 12. Most of the examples have direct or indirect relevance to more than one theme and, where appropriate, these are indicated in the unshaded cells of the matrix.

possibilities is summarized as the highlighted cells in Table III.A. Although examples could be found of each theme in each region, on grounds of length alone we have not tried to be exhaustive. Instead our strategy has been to select three or four wars—including where possible one from the nineteenth century and one from the twentieth century—which are both intrinsically interesting and which clearly illustrate the particular theme under examination. Inevitably, other selections could have been made, and we hope that readers will be able to add to the matrix of examples treated here. Finally, a set of additional themes at the epidemiological intersection of war and infectious disease is examined in Chapter 12 (Table III.A).

To study the regional examples which we report, several geographical techniques are used to follow the time–space tracks of epidemics linked to different wars. As a prelude to Part III, therefore, Chapter 6 illustrates the full range of techniques employed in the regional chapters by applying them to a single war-related epidemic: the great epidemic of cholera which spread in the latter stages and immediate aftermath of the Philippine–American War (1899–1902). It is to this chapter that we now turn.

6

Tracking Epidemics

'You will not apply my precept,' he said, shaking his head. 'How often have I said to you that when you have eliminated the impossible, whatever remains, *however improbable*, must be the truth?'

Sherlock Holmes to Watson in *The Sign of Four*, chapter 6,
'Sherlock Holmes gives a demonstration'

6.1 Introduction

In studies of past, present, and likely future disease distributions, the 'added value' provided by the geographer lies in three main areas: detecting spatial concentrations of disease; isolating the processes (environmental, social, demographic, and pathogenic) which cause these disease hotspots; and in enhancing our understanding of the space–time dynamics of disease spread. This is as true of war-related epidemics as of any others.

Within geography, there is a long-standing tradition of mapping disease. In this early history, the incidence maps of yellow fever produced in 1798 are often given pride of place (Robinson, 1982). These were, however, pre-dated by maps of topics as diverse as hospital capacities and the distribution of dressing-stations on a battlefield, through to maps of pestilential swamps and other hostile medical environments. But, so far as most epidemiological reports were concerned, such maps were usually incidental.

The breakthrough in disease mapping occurred in the middle of the nine-teenth century with the cholera map produced by Dr John Snow to accompany the second edition of his prize-winning essay *On the Mode of Communication of Cholera* (1855*a*). What set Snow's work apart was not the cartography (dot maps, which were a well-established cartographic device, to show the geographical distribution of individual cholera deaths), but his inductive rea-soning from the map. By showing what he termed the 'topography of the out-break', Snow was able to draw inferences about the central source of infection.

The use of mapping as an important device for suggesting hypotheses of medical interest may be traced through to the present day. For war and disease, the classic example is the *Seuchen Atlas*. This atlas of epidemic disease (Zeiss, 1942–5; Anderson, 1947) was conceived by the German army as an adjunct to war, enhancing its ability to mount military campaigns. The atlas was produced as separate sheets over the years 1942–5. Its distribution was confined to mili-tary institutes and to those German university institutes involved in training medical students. The scope of the atlas was not global but confined largely to those areas where the Army High Command expected to be fighting. As a consequence the atlas was divided into eight sections: (1) general maps, (2) Near East, (3) Trans-Caspian region, (4) Eastern Europe, (5) Baltic region, (6) Central Europe, (7) Mediterranean region, and (8) North and West Africa. Each map showed the way in which epidemic diseases 'nest' in a region with the goal of the cartographic methods being to 'record on the geomedical map those disease-promoting geofactors which are crucial in determining the distribution or restriction of the relevant disease' (Barrett, 2000: 514). By geo-factors, the atlas included animal reservoirs, vegetation zones, soil formations, and climatic areas.

As the thrust of the *Seuchen Atlas* shows, many quintessentially geographical questions may be posed about war-related epidemics: how may we detect 'hot spots' of spatially raised incidence of disease in war zones? What causes such spatial concentrations? For transmissible diseases, what are the geographical corridors that will be followed as diseases spread from one area to another in times of war? How rapidly will the disease move? Will there be directional biases? How do we handle the issue of geographical scale so that models of disease at the micro-scale of individuals may be meshed with those for families, communities, cities, regions, and countries? To what extent may results worked out for one war-related disease be applied to another? How may ideas on the geographical incidence and spread of war-related epidemics be incorporated into mathematical models which can be used as forecasting tools to break the war–disease manifold in future conflicts? And can these approaches be used to devise spatial containment strategies in the event of biological warfare?

In this chapter, we present a number of methods employed by geographers to study time–space patterns of disease incidence and spread. The techniques are explored in the context of the great cholera epidemic which struck the Philippine Islands in two waves between 1902 and 1904 at the end of the Philippines Insurrection (1899–1902) against American rule. The material presented is based upon Smallman-Raynor and Cliff (1998*a*, 1998*b*, 2000, 2001*a*) where full details of historical sources are given. The methods described are used in subsequent chapters to study in different regional settings the several aspects of the war–disease interface outlined in the introduction to Part III of this book.

6.2 Cholera and the Philippine–American War, 1902–1904

6.2.1 Background

The socio-demographic context of the 1902–4 cholera epidemic in the Philippine Islands, including the particular relationship of the epidemic to population upheavals engendered by the fated insurrection against US annexation (Philippine–American War, 1899–1902), has been outlined in an earlier study (Smallman-Raynor and Cliff, 1998*a*). As described in Appendix 1A, classic Asiatic cholera which caused the epidemic of 1902–4 is a severe, often rapidly fatal, diarrhoeal disease produced by the bacterium *Vibrio cholerae*. Transmission of the bacterium usually occurs via the ingestion of faecally contaminated water and, less commonly, food. At least until the beginning of the twentieth century, the Philippine Islands lacked the conditions necessary to maintain the cholera bacterium in endemic form. Thus, the 1902–4 cholera epidemic in the Philippines—like the five cholera epidemics that had preceded it—resulted from the importation of the *vibrio* to the archipelago.

The Study Site

The Philippines archipelago consists of some 7,100 islands strewn over half a million square miles of ocean; see Figure 6.1. At about the time of the

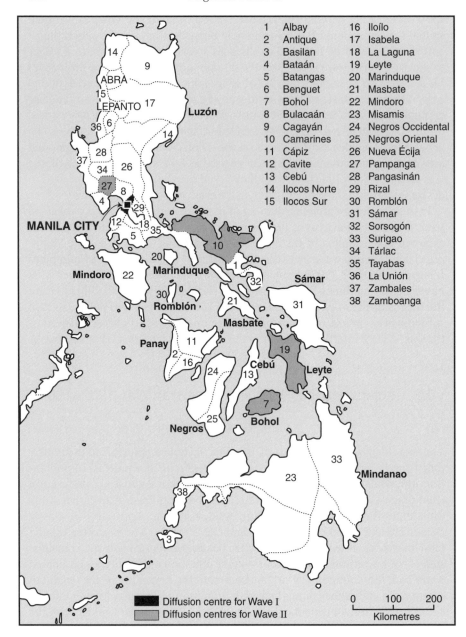

1	Albay	16	Iloílo
2	Antique	17	Isabela
3	Basilan	18	La Laguna
4	Bataán	19	Leyte
5	Batangas	20	Marinduque
6	Benguet	21	Masbate
7	Bohol	22	Mindoro
8	Bulacaán	23	Misamis
9	Cagayán	24	Negros Occidental
10	Camarines	25	Negros Oriental
11	Cápiz	26	Nueva Écija
12	Cavite	27	Pampanga
13	Cebú	28	Pangasinán
14	Ilocos Norte	29	Rizal
15	Ilocos Sur	30	Romblón
		31	Sámar
		32	Sorsogón
		33	Surigao
		34	Tárlac
		35	Tayabas
		36	La Unión
		37	Zambales
		38	Zamboanga

Diffusion centre for Wave I
Diffusion centres for Wave II

0   100   200
Kilometres

Fig. 6.1. The Philippine Islands

Notes: The map indicates the location of islands and provinces referred to in the text. The diffusion centres for the two cholera waves are also marked.

Source: Smallman-Raynor and Cliff (2001*a*, fig. 2, p. 290).

epidemic, in 1903, some 5 per cent of the islands were inhabited by a population totalling 7.6 millions. Almost half resided on the northern island of Luzón; only seven other islands (Bohol, Cebú, Leyte, Mindanao, Negros, Panay, and Sámar) recorded populations in excess of 100,000. Manila City, situated on the west coast of Luzón, was the largest settlement (1903 population 220,000), chief port, and trading centre. Elsewhere, the settlement pattern was characterized by scattered villages and towns of less than 40,000 inhabitants.

As a country of oceanic islands, settlements in the Philippines were doubly isolated; externally from the rest of the world, and internally from each other. Internal isolation was not only by way of the sea, from one island to another, but also, because of the rugged and mountainous nature of much of the terrain, from settlement to settlement on a single island.

THE WAR CONTEXT

The Insurrection gravely impaired the epidemiological protection afforded by natural isolation. The Insurrection began on 4 February 1899 and officially ended some 38 months later in April 1902. During this period, over 100,000 US troops were deployed to combat the rural guerrilla forces. Many of the troops were stationed in an interconnected network of some 500 garrison towns, and these towns became the focus for migrants seeking protection from the war in the countryside. Large-scale population movements and congregation were further fuelled by agricultural dislocation, the disruption of food supply lines, and the US strategy of forced population concentration to combat the guerrilla fighting. Thus, when cholera appeared in the archipelago in the penultimate month of the war, March 1902, the isolation of many settlements had been eroded by three years of military occupation, conflict, population displacement, and congregation. The situation was compounded by population dispersal in the immediate aftermath of the Insurrection. This cocktail of factors led to the beginning of a two-year cholera epidemic across the islands which attacked the population in two spatially congruent but temporally distinct waves (Figs. 6.1 and 6.2).

6.2.2 Data Sources

During the course of the 1902–4 cholera epidemic, officers of the United States Public Health Service (USPHS), stationed in the Philippines, were directed to submit reports of the progress of the disease to the USPHS Surgeon-General in Washington, DC. These reports were published in the weekly *Public Health Reports* (Washington: Government Printing Office) (see Pl. 1.2H), and Figure 6.2 is drawn from these data. The horizontal axis has been formed by coding the first week of the epidemic (week ending 22 Mar. 1902) as week 1, with subsequent weeks numbered sequentially thereafter, up to and including week 99. The two infection waves (denoted Wave I and Wave II) are defined by the

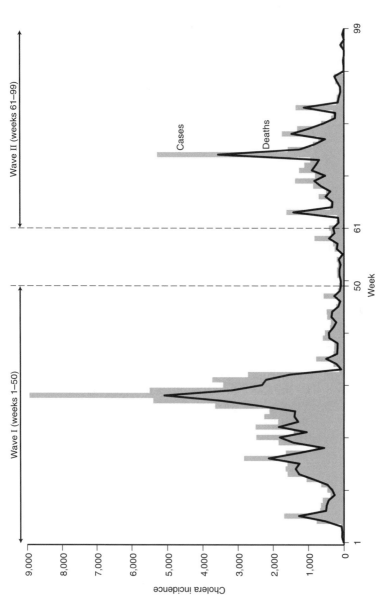

Fig. 6.2. National series of cholera cases (histograms) and deaths (line traces) by week, Philippine Islands, March 1902–February 1904

Notes: The series are based on the weekly counts of morbidity and mortality recorded in the *Public Health Reports* for 570 infected municipalities. The horizontal axis has been formed by coding the first week of the epidemic (ending 22 Mar. 1902) as week 1, with subsequent weeks numbered sequentially thereafter up to, and including, week 99 (ending 6 Feb. 1904). The graph defines two waves of infection; summary details of each wave are given in Table 6.1.

Source: Smallman-Raynor and Cliff (2001*a*, fig. 1, p. 289).

Table 6.1. Reported cholera cases and deaths by island in Waves I and II of the 1902–1904 epidemic in the Philippines

	Cases[1]		Wave II		Deaths[1]		Wave II	
	Wave I		Wave II		Wave I		Wave II	
Philippines	71,221	(93.2)	26,267	(34.4)	47,548	(62.2)	19,896	(26.0)
Islands								
Bohol	1,911	(70.9)	438	(16.2)	1,274	(47.3)	291	(10.8)
Cebú	2,288	(35.0)	10,815	(165.4)	1,323	(20.2)	8,096	(123.8)
Leyte	569	(14.6)	564	(14.5)	396	(10.1)	465	(11.9)
Luzón	30,271	(84.1)	8,498	(23.6)	22,517	(62.5)	6,287	(17.4)
Masbate	188	(43.0)	272	(62.2)	116	(26.5)	143	(32.7)
Mindanao	2,271	(88.9)	1,839	(71.9)	1,137	(44.5)	1,483	(58.0)
Mindoro	283	(87.5)	0	(0.0)	262	(81.0)	0	(0.0)
Negros	5,011	(102.6)	911	(18.6)	3,328	(68.1)	689	(14.1)
Panay	27,713	(350.6)	1,840	(23.2)	16,691	(211.2)	1,352	(17.1)
Other islands[2]	716	(19.2)	1,090	(29.3)	504	(13.5)	1,090	(29.3)

Notes: [1] Rates per 10,000 population (1903 census) are shown in parentheses. [2] Basilan, Marinduque, Romblón, and Sámar.
Source: Smallman-Raynor and Cliff (1998*b*, table 1, p. 191).

vertical pecked lines. Wave I (weeks 1–50) spread in the closing stages and immediate aftermath of the Philippine–American War. It persisted for 50 weeks, expiring in the last week of February 1903 (week 50, ending 28 Feb.). It reached a peak in early October (week 29) and was associated with a reported total of 71,221 cases and 47,548 deaths. Wave II (weeks 61–99) spread in the period of reconstruction that followed the Philippine–American War. It began in mid-May 1903 (week 61, ending 16 May), lasted 39 weeks to early February 1904 (week 99, ending 6 Feb.), and was associated with a reported total of 26,267 cases and 19,896 deaths. Summary details of each wave are given in Table 6.1.

6.3 Map Sequences

6.3.1 Textual Accounts: Reconstruction of National Diffusion Routes

The simplest way of tracing the spread of an epidemic is through sequential mapping. In the case of the Philippines cholera epidemic, the US *Public Health Reports* contain, in addition to numerical data, textual descriptions of the spread of the epidemic which are here abstracted and organized to form a time-sequenced account of the diffusion of Wave I. With such qualitative evidence, it is often possible using the cartographic devices of dated circles and vectors to visualize the sequence and corridors of spread of a disease. Figure 6.3 shows these mapping techniques for Wave I at the local scale of Batangas and La Laguna (Fig. 6.3A) and the island wide scale (Fig. 6.3B) of the Philippines.

In a period of less than 12 months, Wave I of the cholera epidemic (Mar. 1902–Feb. 1903) had been introduced to the Philippines, spread hundreds of kilometres from its point of introduction to reach the most remote islands of the archipelago, and faded away. Figure 6.1 serves as a location map for islands and provinces referred to in the following account. A telegram dated 24 March 1902 provided the first evidence of cholera in the islands. The informant was the Chief Quarantine Officer for the Philippines, J. C. Perry, and the message was unequivocal: 'Cholera is now present at Manila; 18 cases'.[1] In fact, the first cases had appeared a few days earlier, on the 20 March, in the Farola district of the city. It is unlikely at this point in time that the ultimate source of cholera in Manila will ever be known, although contemporary accounts speculated on its importation with fresh vegetables from Canton, China, where cholera had been present for some time.

Whatever the source of the disease, emergency measures were immediately invoked in the city. Public health surveillance was intensified, all suspicious cases were admitted to hospital, contacts were sent to the city's detention camp, infected houses were cleansed and placed under guard, all green vegetables were destroyed, wells and cisterns were closed, and distilled water stations established. To prevent onwards spread from Manila to the provinces, a cordon was thrown around the city, ferry boat and rail traffic was halted, and a permit system was introduced to control the movements of individuals.

By mid-April it had become evident that these efforts to quarantine Manila from the rest of the archipelago had failed. The dispatches from the Chief Quarantine Officer recount how the disease was first carried to two towns on Manila Bay, Orión and Hagonoy, by escapees aboard local *bancas* (a type of native sailing vessel). Further localized spread from Manila occurred down the Pasig River and into Lake Laguna de Bay, with the lakeside towns of Calamba, Biñan, and Santa Cruz infected by early May. From La Laguna province, the bacterium spread overland to Batangas with onwards carriage to Calapán on

--→

Fig. 6.3. Diffusion of Wave I of the cholera epidemic, Philippine Islands, March 1902–February 1903

Notes: (A) The local scale in the provinces of Batangas and La Laguna. Circles are shaded by week of first registration of cholera, with the week indicated in numerical form for each locality. (B) The macro-scale of the islands in which vectors trace the reconstructed routes of spread and the solid circles denote the municipalities infected in the three weeks (25 Apr.–9 May, 1903) prior to the onset of the second wave.

Sources: (A) Smallman-Raynor and Cliff (2000, fig. 5, p. 50); (B) Smallman-Raynor and Cliff (1998b, fig. 2, p. 193).

[1] United States Public Health Service, *Public Health Reports*, xvii (Washington, 1902), p. 716.

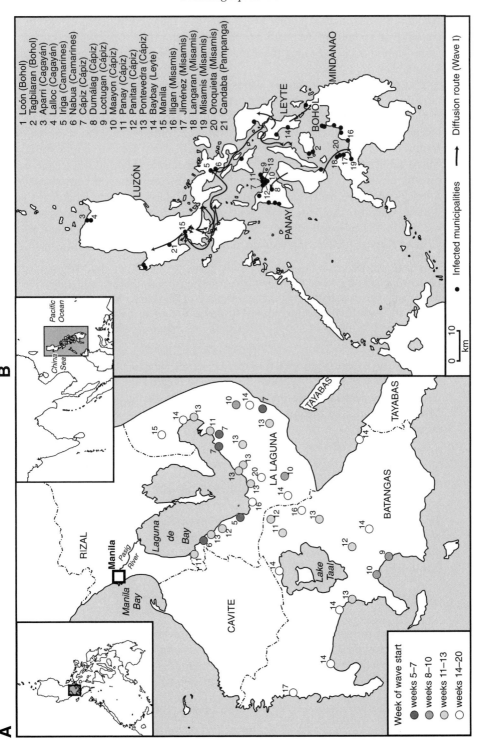

the adjacent island of Mindoro. From Mindoro, the bacterium was carried by *banca* to the island of Marinduque in July. Meanwhile, northwards spread from Manila occurred along the Pangasinán railway, eventually reaching La Unión province by June.

To set against this contagious 'wave-like' expansion outwards from Manila, as early as April 1902 we obtain the first impression of long-distance carriage of the bacterium by the United States Army. A dispatch from the Chief Quarantine Officer recounts how a troopship, headed from Manila, carried the bacterium to the port city of Nueva Cáceres, southeastern Luzón, in mid-April. This establishment of Nueva Cáceres as an epidemic bridgehead was to play a pivotal role in the subsequent appearance of the disease in the southern islands. By early May, the bacterium had appeared in Tacloban, Leyte Island, with Nueva Cáceres the suspected source. From here, the disease spread rapidly to the adjacent islands, the arrival of the disease in the island of Cebú in August 1902 having been documented in particular detail:

> . . . a banca arrived at Tobogan [*sic*], on this island [Cebú], with a dead Filipino on board from Carigara, Leyte, and requested permission to enter that port and to inter the dead man. This was refused by the presidente . . . [T]he banca had gone, after this refusal, to Catmón, where it was allowed to land and the body buried. Following this, within a few days (the exact time not known), several cases of death occurred preceded by vomiting and diarrhea.[2]

Although no source is reported for Negros Island, some link to the outbreak in adjacent Cebú must be suspected. But, once in Negros, the disease spread by native sailing vessel to the populous island of Panay by late August 1902 and Misamis province on the far southern island of Mindanao by January of the following year.

6.4 Epidemics in Space

Textual evidence will take us only so far in unravelling the tracks followed by war-related epidemics. In the remainder of this chapter we show how, when quantitative data are available, statistical methods may be used to add substantially greater insights into the patterns and processes of epidemic spread.

6.4.1 Types of Diffusion Processes

Accounts of the space–time tracks followed by infectious diseases usually recognize three main types of diffusion process. A *contagious process* describes the situation in which the disease moves from its centre of introduction to its physically nearest neighbouring centres. These, in their turn, transmit the disease to

---

[2] United States Public Health Service, *Public Health Reports*, xvii (Washington, 1902), pp. 2074–5.

their geographically nearest neighbours, and so on. In this manner, the disease spreads in a wave-like manner outwards from its point of introduction. Alternatively, a *hierarchical process* describes the situation in which the disease moves progressively through the urban hierarchy. Typically, the initial point of introduction of a disease is the largest urban centre. Then, urban centres next in size follow, and so on, through to the smallest settlements. Finally, a *mixed process* describes the situation in which the spread pattern contains components of both contagious and hierarchical diffusion.

6.4.2 Autocorrelation on Graphs

One way of determining which of the above models best characterizes the spread of a war-related epidemic is to use the technique of autocorrelation on graphs. In this technique, the area over which spread is being studied is treated as a *topological graph* consisting of a set of nodes (the geographical units which comprise the study area) and the links between them. These links are constructed to create a network or *graph* which corresponds to the diffusion process being examined.

The spatial degree goodness-of-fit between any diffusion graph and the case rate of a disease observed in a set of geographical units can be assessed by computing the spatial autocorrelation coefficient, I. Technical details are given in the chapter appendix (Sect. 6A.1). Here we note that the I coefficient increases as the degree of correspondence between a given graph and cholera case rates in the nodes of the graph increases. Appendix 6A.1 also shows that I may be tested for statistical significance against the Normal distribution.

To illustrate the methodology, I was calculated for each of the 99 weeks of the national epidemic from March 1902 to February 1904. Figure 6.4 plots, as bar charts, the weekly time series of reported cholera cases per 10,000 population for the Philippine Islands as a backcloth for line traces of the weekly series of I for the contagion[3] (Fig. 6.4A) and hierarchy (Fig. 6.4B) diffusion graphs. For both charts, the horizontal line set at 1.65 marks statistically significant I coefficients at the $p = 0.05$ level (one-tailed test for positive spatial autocorrelation); values above this level represent periods when the actual diffusion process corresponded significantly with the diffusion graph. Finally, the time intervals associated with Waves I and II are indicated by the vertical broken lines.

Figure 6.4A shows that the MST graph (contagious spread) was important throughout the first half of Wave I; in the interval of relative epidemiological calm prior to Wave II; and, finally, during the first half of Wave II. At other times, the MST graph was of low or no statistical significance. Figure 6.4B shows that the hierarchy graph (hierarchical transmission) was of only fleeting importance in the later stages of both waves.

---

[3] The contagion graph was configured as a minimum spanning tree (MST). An MST is the simplest graph such that all nodes are linked.

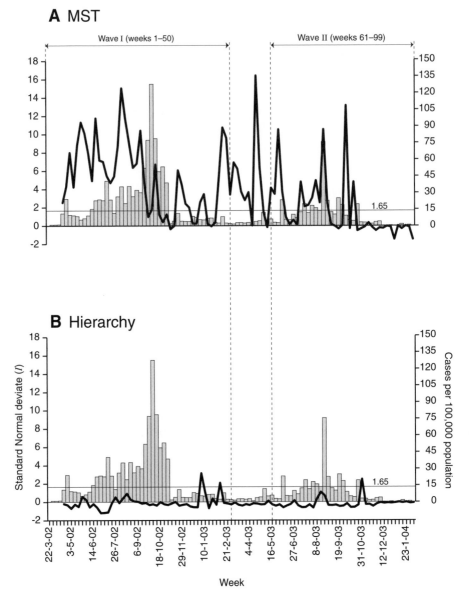

Fig. 6.4. Cholera diffusion at the national level, Philippine Islands, March 1902–February 1904

Notes: Bar charts plot the weekly cholera case rate per 10,000 population. Corresponding values of the spatial autocorrelation coefficient, *I*, as a standard Normal deviate for different diffusion graphs are superimposed as line traces. (A) MST graph. (B) Population hierarchy graph. Horizontal lines at 1.65 mark the *p* = 0.05 significance level in a one-tailed test for positive spatial autocorrelation.

Source: Smallman-Raynor and Cliff (1998*b*, fig. 4, p. 198).

BETWEEN-WAVE COMPARISONS

One implication of Figure 6.4 is that, while contagious spread was very much more important than hierarchical diffusion, the processes varied in importance by stage of the wave cycle. To examine this further, Figure 6.5 replots the series of *I* for Waves I and II for the contagion (Fig. 6.5A) and hierarchy (Fig. 6.5B) graphs. To define the horizontal axes, the week of peak cholera morbidity for each wave was called week zero; weeks before and after the peak were coded with reference to this origin. Again, the horizontal lines at 1.65 mark statistical significance of the *I* coefficient at the $p = 0.05$ level (one-tailed test for positive spatial autocorrelation).

QUALITATIVE COMPARISONS

Figure 6.5A shows that contagious spread was statistically significant in the build-up (pre-peak), peak, and late fade-out (post-peak) stages of both waves. Two further features of the build-up/peak stages are also evident from Figure 6.5A:

(*a*) Contagious spread was most important in the very early stages of the build-up of Wave I. Thereafter, the trace declined (indicative of a weakening in contagious spread) as the infection wave developed to a peak. In contrast, the trace for Wave II ascended to a peak (a strengthening of contagious spread) with increasing disease incidence.

(*b*) Relative to the apexes of the line traces, autocorrelation generally ran at a much higher level in Wave I than in Wave II. This implies a more strongly structured contagious process for Wave I.

Figure 6.5B, which relates to the hierarchy graph, displays the same broad differences in timing described for the MST graph. However, with the exception of the final week of fade-out for Wave II, the *I* coefficients lie well below the $p = 0.05$ level of statistical significance.

INTERPRETATION

These findings are consistent with the hypothesis that, although war may not materially alter disease-diffusion processes, it may change the timings of those processes. Large-scale population movements in the immediate aftermath of the Philippine–American War would account for the strongly structured, early, and widespread spatial transmission of Wave I; almost 60 per cent of municipalities had been seeded with the cholera *vibrio* at eight weeks (the phase difference between the time series of *I* for the MST graph and the time series of case rates) prior to the wave peak. Wave II, which began over a year after the end of the war, was not subject to the same large-scale population movements, and spatial transmission was less strongly structured and much slower; less than 25 per cent of municipalities had been affected at eight weeks prior to the wave peak.

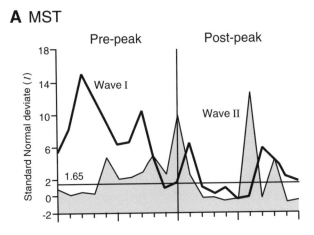

A MST

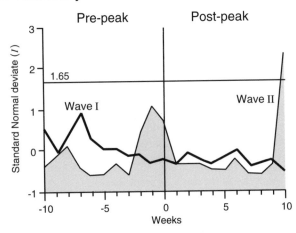

B Hierarchy

Fig. 6.5. Comparison of cholera diffusion for Waves I and II at the national level, Philippine Islands

Notes: For each wave, values of the spatial autocorrelation coefficient, *I*, as a standard Normal deviate are plotted as line traces for different diffusion graphs. (A) MST graph. (B) Population size hierarchy graph. The time scale on the horizontal axes is in weeks either side of the week of peak disease intensity for each wave. Vertical lines indicate wave peaks, coded as week zero. Horizontal lines at 1.65 mark the $p = 0.05$ significance level in a one-tailed test for positive spatial autocorrelation.

Source: Smallman-Raynor and Cliff (1998*b*, fig. 5, p. 199).

As described in Smallman-Raynor and Cliff (1998*a*, 1998*b*), futher analysis of the data using autocorrelation on graphs at the spatial scales of islands and provinces showed that, at all spatial scales, contagious spread was more important than hierarchical diffusion in the development of both waves, and that the contagion was stronger in Wave I than in Wave II.

6.5 Epidemics in Time and Space

A fundamental question that can be asked about the spread of Waves I and II relates to the velocity at which the two waves developed in the population of the Philippines. Did the waves differ in their velocity in the same geographical areas? If so, were these differences related to variations in the nature and strength of the underlying spread processes?

6.5.1 Lag Maps

One measure of wave velocity is the average or expected length of time to infection, denoted $\bar{t}$, for an area in an epidemic wave. The computation of $\bar{t}$ and other measures of wave velocity are given in the chapter appendix (Sect. 6A.2). As defined there, for rapidly moving waves $\bar{t}$ will tend to be small, whereas for slowly moving waves $\bar{t}$ will be relatively large.

To compare the velocities of the two infection waves in each province and island, Figure 6.6 plots the average times to infection, $\bar{t}$, for Wave I (horizontal axis) against Wave II (vertical axis). The result for the nation is also shown. If there was no difference in the velocities of the two waves, points would lie on the pecked line drawn at 45°. Points above the 45° line identify geographical areas in which Wave II developed more slowly than Wave I, while points below the 45° line mark areas where Wave II developed more rapidly.

In Figure 6.6, the many points above the 45° line indicate the general tendency for Wave II to have developed at a slower rate than Wave I. This pattern is evident for the nation, four of the seven islands, and two-thirds of the provinces. In contrast, areas in which Wave II developed more rapidly than Wave I are few in number and, notably, include the highly populated island of Luzón.

6.5.2 Disease Centroids

A second way of examining the spatial progress of epidemic waves is to map the trajectory followed by the geographical centre of disease activity as the wave unfolds. Technical details of the way in which the geographical centre is constructed are given in the chapter appendix (Sect. 6A.3). Here, to illustrate the method, Figure 6.7A plots the location of the centre of cholera activity in Wave

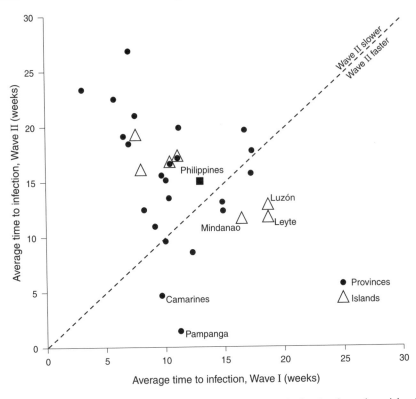

Fig. 6.6. Comparison of the velocity of Waves I and II at the levels of province, island, and nation, Philippine Islands

Notes: For each area, the graph plots the average time to infection, $\bar{t}$, for Wave I (horizontal axis) against that for Wave II (vertical axis). Points above the 45° line represent areas for which the velocity of Wave II was less than that for Wave I. Points below the line represent areas for which the velocity of Wave II was greater than for Wave I.
Source: Smallman-Raynor and Cliff (1998*b*, fig. 8, p. 206).

I on a weekly basis from April to October 1902 in the neighbouring provinces of Batangas and La Laguna. The position of the cholera centre in a given week is indicated by a circle, with the week identified numerically; as before, all weeks have been indexed to the first week of the epidemic (week 1, ending 22 Mar.), with week 5 (ending 19 Apr.) denoting the start in the observation area. To capture the general direction of movement of the disease, vectors link the position of the cholera centres in successive weeks.

The trajectory of Wave I can be divided into two broad periods: (1) weeks 5–23, shown by the solid lines; and (2) weeks 24–30 (pecked lines).

1. *Weeks 5–23* (solid vectors) This period was associated with an initial focus of cholera occurrence in La Laguna, followed by a north–south drift to

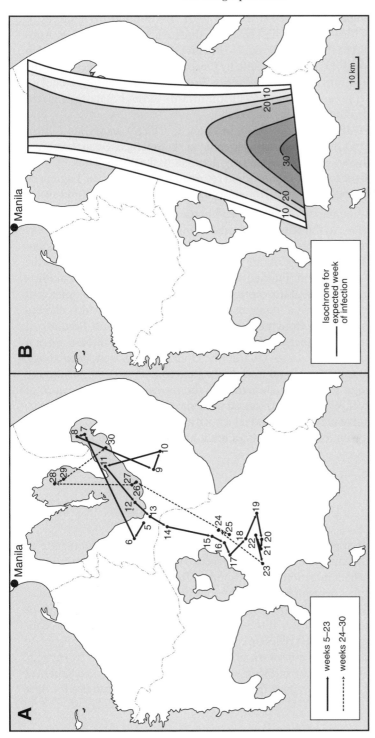

Fig. 6.7. The spread of cholera in Batangas and La Laguna, Wave I, 1902

Notes: (A) Location of the geographical centre of cholera activity by weekly period, April to October 1902. The locations of the disease centre are indicated by circles, with the corresponding week identified in numerical form; weeks have been indexed to the first week of the epidemic (week 1, ending 22 Mar.), with week 5 (ending 19 Apr.) denoting the start of the epidemic in the observation area. Vectors link the position of the cholera centre in successive weeks. (B) Average trend in Figure 6.7A, showing the expected week of infection from the start of the epidemic.

Source: Smallman-Raynor and Cliff (2000, fig. 6, p. 52).

southern Batangas. As plotted in Figure 6.3A, the southwestern shores of Laguna de Bay formed the earliest centre of disease activity (weeks 5–6, Apr.) with a rapid shift to the east in weeks 7–11 (May). Cholera incidence peaked in La Laguna in week 13 (mid-June) and, by the following week, the centre of the wave had shifted into northern Batangas. From here, the centre of cholera activity began a progressive movement southwards through Batangas, reaching its southerly limits in weeks 20–3 (July).

2. *Weeks 24–30* (broken vectors) In August, Chief Quarantine Officer Perry could report the abatement of the epidemic in Batangas. Soon thereafter, the centre of cholera activity began a rapid retreat to the north. Thus, by week 26 (mid-Sept.), the focus of the wave had returned to the vicinity of Laguna de Bay and was to remain there until the end of the observation period (mid-Oct.).

Figure 6.7B summarizes the main trend in the progression of Wave I by fitting a *trend surface* to the centroids plotted in Figure 6.7A. Details of the way in which the trend surfaces can be constructed are given in the chapter appendix (Sect. 6A.3). In Figure 6.7B, for five-weekly intervals, the lines depict the expected time of infection (indexed to week 1 of the epidemic) in Batangas and La Laguna. The diagram captures two key features of the spread of Wave I. First, it identifies a 'compression-like' movement in which cholera pushed into central areas from the east and the west of the region. Secondly, it underscores the importance of the north–south drift of the disease. Such a feature is consistent with Chief Quarantine Officer Perry's view, cited above, that the disease spread overland from La Laguna to Batangas. Application of this methodology to Wave II showed that the movements of the centre of cholera activity in Waves I and II shared the same average patterns, namely: (i) a compression-like movement in which cholera pushed inwards to the central sector of the region, coupled with (ii) a predominant north–south drift of the disease.

6.6 Complex Epidemic Spaces

A conventional approach to disease mapping is to plot the phenomenon of interest in Euclidean space (Cliff and Haggett, 1988). But, in times of war, the spaces within which infectious diseases spread from person to person can display great complexities which reflect individual contact networks at local levels, inter-city movements at meso-levels, through to inter-country movements of troops, civilians, and refugees at the coarsest geographical scales. In this context, a mapping system that relies on conventional 'box space' is unrealistic. By 'box space' we refer to the network of points and areas bounded by eastings and northings (on a planar surface) or latitude and longitude (on a spherical surface); these provide an inert framework or spatial infrastructure for data recording.

An alternative approach is to construct the disease-diffusion space with multidimensional scaling (MDS). This allows the data to force the spatial framework into position. In its simplest form, the idea of 'forced space' is exemplified by isodemographic maps, where areas with large populations are distended to occupy large spatial extents on the map and vice versa (Dorling, 1995). The same broad notion—that the properties of an entity can be used to define the structure of a spatial representation—has been posited as one starting-point for contemporary geographical reconceptualizations of space and time (Massey, 1999). Such conceptualizations may yield insights into epidemic processes which may not be apparent from disease mapping in conventional Euclidean space.

6.6.1 The MDS Mapping Concept

The concepts which underpin MDS mapping are straightforward. On a conventional geographical map, the relative locations of points correspond to their (scaled) geographical locations. In MDS mapping, the relative locations correspond instead to their degree of similarity on some variable measured for them. For example, we might map points into a time space; locations separated by short travel times will appear close together in such a space, while centres linked by long travel times will be widely separated. In general terms, the greater the degree of similarity between places on the variable measured, the closer together the places will be in the MDS space. Conversely points which are dissimilar on the variable will be widely separated in the MDS space, irrespective of their geographical location on the globe. The MDS problem is to find a configuration of n points in m-dimensional space such that the interpoint distances in the configuration match the experimental (dis)similarities of the n objects as accurately as possible. This may be viewed as an issue of statistical fitting, and technical details of the procedure are given in the chapter appendix (Sect. 6A.4). For geographical problems, lower order spaces ($1 \leq m \leq 3$), which enable combinations of time, space, and time–space mapping to be undertaken, are particularly useful. By their nature, higher dimensional ($m \geq 4$) 'maps' can be enormously complex and commonly have no straightforward geographical interpretation.

This basic idea can be extended to the mapping of points from geographical space into a wide range of different spaces which are significant for our understanding of the geographical incidence and spread of disease in wartime. For example, if we are studying disease attack rates per unit of population, MDS will map those areas with similar rates in close proximity even if they are widely separated geographically. Thus MDS might be used to define an 'invasion space' which could form a backcloth for mapping the incidence of disease to determine whether areas invaded early in a conflict have similar epidemiological behaviour.

6.6.2 Cholera Spaces

In this section, we use MDS to construct the cholera diffusion spaces associated with the epidemic of 1902–4 at the spatial scales of provinces and islands. Within these spaces, units that are similar in terms of their weekly case rates per 10,000 population will appear close together in the space, irrespective of their geographical locations in the Philippine Islands. Conversely, units that are dissimilar in terms of their cholera activity will appear widely separated, even though they may be geographically proximal. The Pearson product moment correlation coefficient, r, was used to measure similarity; the greater the degree of similarity between any pair of geographical units in their time series of reported case rates, the larger the value of r. We focus upon two-dimensional MDS cholera 'maps' which may be compared with the conventional spread maps of Figures 6.3 and 6.7 to assess the extent to which geographical (dis)similarities in disease activity reflected the spatially contagious process that dominated the transmission of the epidemic. To seed the MDS computational procedure, longitude/latitude (x, y) coordinates of the province and island centroids were supplied.

COMPARING ARBITRARY SPACES

Once a disease space has been constructed by MDS, we will wish to compare this new space with other spaces. For example, as outlined above, we might wish to determine how map-like the diffusion space is by comparing the result with a conventional geographical map. Close correspondence might be expected if contagious diffusion driven by distance is the dominant process. Other comparator spaces might be population size of units (hierarchical diffusion) or mobilization spaces.

Generalized Procrustes analysis, GPA (Gower, 1975; Rohlf and Slice, 1990; Goodall, 1991), provides a vehicle for comparing arbitrary multidimensional configurations. GPA registers forms by removing translational and rotational differences between them, and then scales them such that they best fit. Modern software to carry out Procrustes analysis is *Morphologica* (O'Higgins and Jones, 1999). A less elaborate approach for two-dimensional spatial comparisons, used in this chapter, is to employ the affine correlation defined in Tobler (1965) and Ahuja and Coons (1968). Technical details are given in the chapter appendix (Sect. 6A.5).

For each MDS configuration, the affine correlation coefficient was computed between (i) province/island coordinates (u_i, v_i) in MDS space and (ii) the longitude and latitude coordinates (x_i, y_i) of province/island centroids. The closer the MDS coordinates are to the true longitudes and latitudes (i.e. the more map-like the configuration and, hence, the stronger the spatial effects in disease occurrence), the higher will be the affine correlation.

RESULTS

Figures 6.8 and 6.9, which relate to the geographical levels of province and island respectively, plot the two-dimensional minimum-stress MDS configurations for the entire epidemic (A), Wave I (B), and Wave II (C). Each province/island is represented by a circle whose area has been scaled to the reciprocal of its geographical distance from the origin of the epidemic; the circles relating to Luzón Island and its constituent provinces have been shaded, while Manila province is represented by a square symbol. Finally, the goodness-of-fit (stress) criterion for each configuration is given in Table 6.2, along with the average affine correlation, $\bar{R}$, between (i) province/island coordinates (u_i, v_i) in MDS space and (ii) the corresponding longitude and latitude coordinates (x_i, y_i) of province/island centroids.

The configurations in Figures 6.8 and 6.9 have two common features:

(*a*) They display a wide spread of data points around the origins of the spaces, indicative of underlying differences in the cholera time series at the levels of provinces and islands.

(*b*) At both spatial levels, a fundamental reconfiguration of the cholera spaces occurred between Wave I and Wave II. The reconfiguration was associated with a reduction in the importance of spatial effects in cholera transmission. At the province level, the configuration for Wave I (Fig. 6.8B) mirrors the configuration for the entire epidemic (Fig. 6.8A). For both solutions, the index province (Manila) is positioned to the right of the space, and is surrounded by a group of geographically proximal provinces (represented by the relatively large circles) on Luzón Island. Away from this main grouping, geographically more remote provinces (represented by the relatively small circles) stretch across the space as a constellation of data points. In contrast, for Wave II (Fig. 6.8C), the main cluster of Manila and its geographically proximal provinces has disintegrated, to be replaced by a roughly circular orbit of provinces around the origins of the space.

A between-wave reduction in the map-like nature of the configurations is confirmed in Table 6.2. The average affine correlation falls from $\bar{R} = 0.26$ (Wave I) to $\bar{R} = 0.08$ (Wave II); a similar between-wave reduction is also observed in Table 6.2 for the island configurations (Figs. 6.9B and 6.9C), with a fall in the average affine correlation from $\bar{R} = 0.49$ (Wave I) to $\bar{R} = 0.27$ (Wave II). Table 6.2 also shows that, when examined for corresponding time periods, the affine correlations run at a consistently higher level for islands than provinces. While this may reflect scale effects arising from the modifiable areal unit problem (Openshaw, 1984), the results imply that spatial effects in cholera transmission were more important for islands than provinces.

The declining importance of wave-like spread over the duration of the epidemic at both province and island scales is reinforced in Figure 6.10 which

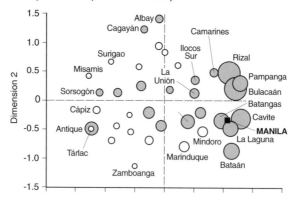

A Epidemic (weeks 1–99)

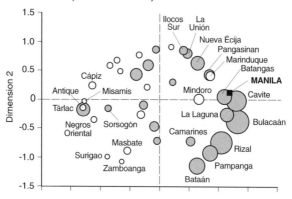

B Wave I (weeks 1–50)

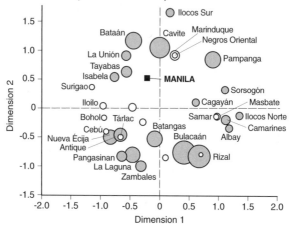

C Wave II (weeks 61–99)

Fig. 6.8. Two-dimensional minimum-stress MDS configurations for cholera in the provinces of the Philippine Islands, 1902–1904

Notes: (A) Entire epidemic, March 1902 to February 1904 (weeks 1–99). (B) Wave I, March 1902 to February 1903 (weeks 1–50). (C) Wave II, May 1903 to February 1904 (weeks 61–99). See text for mapping conventions.

Source: Smallman-Raynor and Cliff (2001*a*, fig. 5, p. 300).

plots the average affine correlations $\{\bar{R}\}$. A histogram of the national series of weekly cholera case rates (per 10,000) forms the backcloth. The curves in Figure 6.10 follow a common pattern. They attain their highest values (i.e. spatial effects were most important) in the build-up and peak phases of Wave I. Thereafter, the traces display a long-term decline (a general weakening of spatial effects), but with secondary peaks at the onset and termination of Wave II. Finally, the tendency for the $\{\bar{R}\}$ to run at higher levels for islands than provinces again implies that spatial effects were more strongly structured for islands than provinces.

6.7 Time Series and Epidemic Models

So far, this chapter has focused upon methods for examining cross-sectional or spatial patterns formed by epidemics. Often, however, the primary focus will be changes over time (as in Part I of this book), commonly with the aim of building qualitative or quantitative models of these changes. Sometimes the models may be for forecasting so that past experiences can be used to throw light on likely futures for war-related epidemics—as, for example, simulating the likely disease results of biological warfare. In this section, we explore some of the ways in which time-based analysis may be developed.

6.7.1 Susceptible–Infective–Removed (SIR) Models

The basic mechanism whereby epidemic waves of infectious diseases are generated is shown in Figures 6.11 and 6.12. In Figure 6.11, at any time t, we assume that the total population in a region can be divided into three classes: the population at risk or susceptible population of size S_t, the infected population of size I_t, and the removed population of size R_t. The removed population is taken to be composed of people who have had the disease, but who can no longer pass it on to others because of recovery, isolation on the appearance of overt symptoms of the disease, or death. The infected element in a population is augmented by the homogeneous mixing of susceptibles with infectives ($S \times I$) at a rate determined by a diffusion coefficient (β) appropriate to the disease. The infected element is depleted by recovery of individuals after a time period at a rate controlled by the recovery coefficient (μ). As Figure 6.11 shows, the addition of further parameters to the model, such as the birth rate, γ, allows more complex models to be generated.

The formal articulation of Figure 6.11 into a mathematical model handles three types of transition (Table 6.3):

(a) A susceptible being infected by contact with an infective.

(b) An infective being removed. We assumed that infection confers life-long immunity to further attack after recovery, which is reasonable for many infectious diseases.

A Epidemic (weeks 1–99)

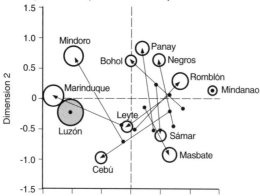

B Wave I (weeks 1–50)

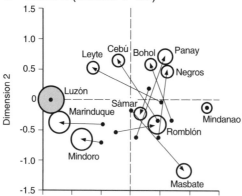

C Wave II (weeks 61–99)

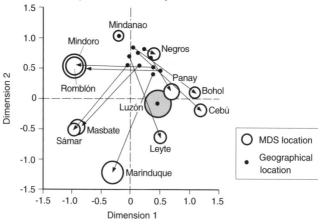

Table 6.2. Cholera in the provinces and islands of the Philippine Islands, 1902–1904: average affine correlations, $\bar{R}$, associated with the two-dimensional minimum-stress MDS solutions

Time interval	n	MDS (two-dimensions)	
		Stress	$\bar{R}$
Provinces			
Epidemic (weeks 1–99)	38	0.27	0.31
Wave I (weeks 1–50)	38	0.19	0.26
Wave II (weeks 61–99)	38	0.23	0.08
Islands			
Epidemic (weeks 1–99)	12	0.18	0.46
Wave I (weeks 1–50)	12	0.15	0.49
Wave II (weeks 61–99)	12	0.20	0.27

Source: Data from Smallman-Raynor and Cliff (2001*a*, table II, p. 296).

(*c*) A susceptible 'birth'. This can come about either through a child growing up into the critical age range (that is, reaching about six months of age).

As formulated, this model is aspatial. However, as we have already seen for cholera in the Philippines, the entrainment of disease with war implies geographical spread of infection between areas; and it can also be shown (Bartlett, 1957) that infectious diseases persist only in regions above a certain population size (the *critical community size*). These endemic disease reservoirs act as sources of infection for small areas below the critical community size.

◄─────────────────────────────────────

Fig. 6.9. Two-dimensional minimum-stress MDS configurations for cholera in 12 islands of the Philippine Islands, 1902–1904

Notes: (A) Entire epidemic, March 1902 to February 1904 (weeks 1–99). (B) Wave I, March 1902 to February 1903 (weeks 1–50). (C) Wave II, May 1903 to February 1904 (weeks 61–99). See text for mapping conventions. The diagram shows the difference between the conventional geographical locations of the islands in latitude–longitude space and their locations in MDS space. To achieve this, the most northerly (Luzón) and southerly (Mindanao) islands have been used as 'anchors' to pin the two map coordinate systems together, with the locations in geographical space shown by solid circles. The vectors give the mismatch between the two coordinate systems by pointing to the corresponding position of each island in MDS space. This is analogous to Tobler's (1976) concept of forcing functions down the gradient of which the diffusion process flows. The greater length of the vectors in Wave II reflects the more chaotic cross-currents of the spread process. *Source*: Smallman-Raynor and Cliff (2001*a*, fig. 6, p. 301).

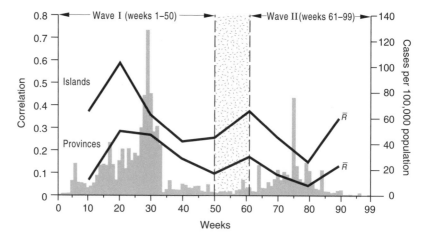

Fig. 6.10. Two-dimensional minimum-stress MDS configurations for cholera in the Philippine Islands, March 1902–February 1904

Notes: For 20-week overlapping periods, the lower line trace plots the average affine correlations ($\bar{R}$) between (i) the MDS coordinates of provinces and (ii) the geographical position (longitude and latitude) of province centroids. The upper line trace plots the equivalent information for islands. The national series of weekly cholera cases rates (per 10,000 population) is plotted as a histogram.

Source: Smallman-Raynor and Cliff (2001*a*, fig. 8, p. 303).

Table 6.3. Mass action models: transition types and rates

Transition	Rate
1. $S \to S-1; I \to I+1; R \to R$	βIS
2. $S \to S; I \to I-1; R \to R+1$	μI
3. $S \to S+1; I \to I; R \to R$	γ

These ideas lead to the qualitative model for the generalized persistence of disease in a set of regions as shown in Figure 6.12. In large areas such as cities above the critical community size threshold, like community A, a continuous trickle of cases is reported. These provide the reservoir of infection which sparks a major epidemic when the susceptible population, S, builds up to a critical level. This build-up occurs only as children are born, lose their mother-conferred immunity, and escape vaccination or contact with the disease. Eventually the S population will increase sufficiently for an epidemic to occur. When this happens, the S population is diminished and the stock of infectives, I, increases as individuals are transferred by infection from the S to the I population. This generates the D-shaped relationship over time between sizes of the S and I populations shown on the end plane of the block diagram.

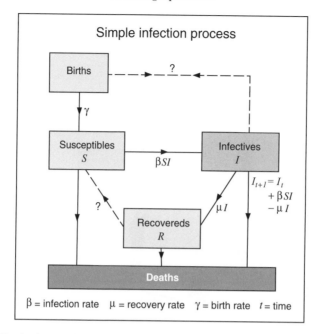

Fig. 6.11. Basic elements in the *SIR* model

Notes: *S*: susceptibles; *I*: infectives; *R*: recovereds; γ: births; β: infection (diffusion) rate; μ: recovery rate.

In smaller communities with populations below the critical community size (settlements B and C in Figure 6.12), epidemics can only arise when the disease agent is reintroduced by the influx of infected individuals (so-called index cases) from reservoir areas. These movements are shown by the broad arrows in Figure 6.12. In such smaller communities, the *S* population is insufficient to maintain a continuous record of infection. The disease dies out and the *S* population grows in the absence of infection. Eventually the *S* population will become big enough to sustain an epidemic when an index case arrives. Given that the total population of the community is insufficient to renew the *S* population by births as rapidly as it is diminished by infection, the epidemic will eventually die out.

It is the repetition of this basic process which generates the successive epidemic waves witnessed in most communities. Of special significance is the way in which the continuous infection and characteristically regular Type I epidemic waves of endemic communities break down as population size diminishes into first, discrete, but regular Type II waves in community B and then, secondly, into discrete and irregularly spaced Type III waves in very small communities like C. Thus disease-free windows will automatically appear in both time and space whenever population totals are small and geographical densities are low.

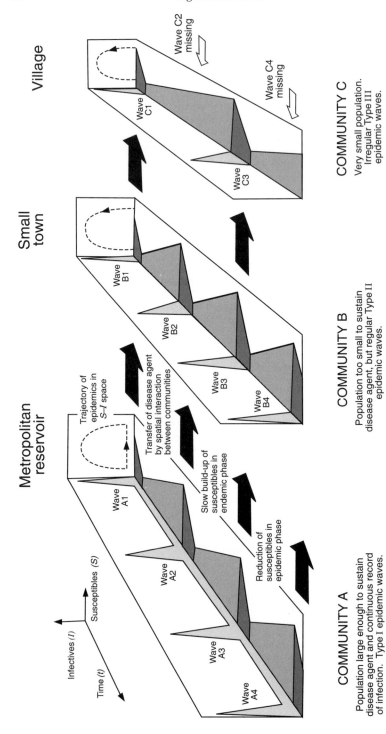

Fig. 6.12. Conceptual view of the spread of a communicable disease in communities of different population sizes

Source: Haggett (2000, fig. 1.9, p. 25).

6.7.2 Cholera in the Philippines: Wave I Incidence and Wave II Spread Processes

An implication of Figure 6.12 is that, in geographical settings, later epidemic waves will reflect in part the downstream effects of earlier waves. We investigate this effect for the two cholera waves at the province scale in the Philippines using regression analysis and the MST and population hierarchy graphs defined in Section 6.4.

The dependence of Wave II of the cholera epidemic upon the prior spread of Wave I was emphasized by contemporary observers. Thus, writing of the attenuated spread of cholera in Iloilo during 1903, Chief Quarantine Officer Heiser commented that 'After the terrible epidemic . . . suffered last year [1902, Wave I] it would seem that most of the susceptible material had been used up.'[4] In that province, the reporting rate for Wave I exceeded 590 cases per 10,000 population with a death rate of some 350 per 10,000. Under such circumstances, the spatial transmission of Wave II was conditional on the geographical distribution of much reduced susceptible populations.

To examine statistically the influence of disease incidence in Wave I on the spread processes of Wave II, the regression model

$$\bar{I}_i = \beta_0 + \beta_1 x_i + e_i \tag{6.1}$$

was postulated. Here, x_i is a measure of disease intensity in province i for Wave I, $\bar{I}_i$ is the average spatial autocorrelation coefficient, I, defined in Section 6.4 for a given wave phase and diffusion graph for Wave II, e_i is an error term, and β_0 and β_1 are parameters to be estimated.

One complication of the regression model in equation (6.1) is the selection of a suitable measure of disease intensity, x_i, for Wave I. Although cholera rates per 10,000 population form one possible measure, case rates are not independent of the processes that underlay the spread of Wave I. Under these circumstances, the statistical parameters of the regression model would partly reflect the association between the spread processes of Waves I and II. To remove this confounding effect, for each diffusion graph and phase of wave development, Wave I case rates (per 10,000 population) were first regressed on the $\{\bar{I}_i\}$ for Wave I. The residuals from these regressions formed the independent variable, x_i, in the corresponding solutions of equation (6.1).

Ordinary least squares solutions of equation (6.1) are summarized for the province level in Table 6.4. For each phase of wave development (col. 2) and diffusion graph (col. 3), the table gives the estimated intercept ($\hat{\beta}_0$) and slope ($\hat{\beta}_1$) coefficients with their associated Student's t-statistics in parentheses, the coefficient of determination, R^2, and the associated F-ratio. Statistically significant values at the $p = 0.05$ level (two-tailed test) are indicated by an asterisk.

---

[4] United States Public Health Service, *Public Health Reports*, xviii (Washington, 1903), p. 1742.

Table 6.4. Results of regressions of $\bar{I}_i$ (Wave II) on residual cholera case rates per 10,000 (Wave I) at the level of province

Model	Phase	Process	$\hat{\beta}_0 (t)$	$\hat{\beta}_1 (t)$	$R^2(F)$
1	Epidemic[1]	MST	0.35 (2.60*)	−0.08 (−0.39)	0.01 (0.15)
2	Epidemic[2]	Hierarchy	0.07 (0.95)	0.53 (3.67*)	0.43 (13.36*)
3	Build-up[1]	MST	0.52 (3.27*)	0.29 (1.21)	0.07 (1.47)
4	Build-up[3]	Hierarchy	0.10 (1.56)	0.57 (4.37*)	0.52 (19.12*)
5	Fade-out[1]	MST	−0.04 (−0.30)	−0.30 (−1.55)	0.13 (2.39)
6	Fade-out[1]	Hierarchy	−0.02 (−0.09)	0.13 (0.27)	0.01 (0.08)

Notes: * Significant at the $p = 0.05$ level (two-tailed test). [1] Two extreme outliers omitted. [2] Four extreme outliers omitted. [3] Three extreme outliers omitted.
Source: Smallman-Raynor and Cliff (1998b, table 2, p. 205).

Table 6.4 shows that, for each phase of wave development, the statistical parameters of all models associated with the MST graph (models 1, 3, and 5) are low and non-significant. In contrast, for the epidemic and build-up stages, models 2 and 4 record a strong and positive association between the $\{\bar{I}_i\}$ for the hierarchy graph and $\{x_i\}$. No similar association is identified for the fade-out phase in model 6.

These results imply that levels of hierarchical spread in the build-up to Wave II were, in part, a product of the level of disease intensity in Wave I. As hypothesized in the introduction to this subsection, one possible explanation for the relationship rests with the decline of the susceptible population (through death and immunity) arising from Wave I. Large reductions in the susceptible population may have served to pin Wave II to the upper tiers of the urban hierarchy, where absolute levels of susceptibility were generally higher and the likelihood of hierarchical contacts was increased.

6.7.3 Cholera in the Philippines: Cross-Correlation Analysis

The second feature of Figure 6.12 is propagation of infection between areas (shown by the solid black arrows). This raises the question of whether we can identify how regions interact with each other when an epidemic diffuses through them. Cross-correlation analysis provides a method for characterizing such interactions, and we apply this to examine the spatial interactions between provinces in the second cholera wave. Statistical details of cross-correlation analysis are given in the chapter appendix (Sect. 6A.6).

For the 39-week duration of Wave II, the cholera case rate (per 10,000 population) for each of the 39 provinces was treated as a time series. Let r_k denote the correlation between any pair of series at lag k. The value of k at which the maximum correlation occurs is conventionally taken as the lead or lag of one time series with respect to another. If $k = 0$, the series being compared are said to be in phase; $+k$ ($k > 0$) signifies that the second series (the comparison series) lags the first series (the reference series), and $-k$ ($k > 0$) that the comparison series leads the reference series. Finally, a plot of the correlation coefficient, r_k, against the lag k yields the cross-correlation function (CCF).

An assumption of the present analysis is that one or more of the eight seed provinces for Wave II plotted in Figures 6.3B and 6.13 served, directly or indirectly, as the source of cholera in the remainder of the archipelago. The spatial associations implied by this assumption were examined by computing the ($8 \times 31 =$) 248 CCFs, where each of the eight seed provinces formed the reference series against which the 31 other (non-seed) provinces were compared (comparison series).

RESULTS

The results of the analysis are summarized in Figure 6.13. Each of the 39 provinces is identified on the left-hand map by a numerical code placed at its geographical centroid. On the right-hand map, seed provinces are denoted by shaded circles. Vectors link each non-seed province to the seed with which it shared the largest CCF value at lags $0 \leq k \leq 6$. The restriction of the analysis to lags $0 \leq k \leq 6$ is a logical extension of the assumption that the seed provinces served as the cholera sources for the rest of the archipelago. Reciprocal links mark in-phase ($k = 0$) associations, while out-of-phase ($1 \leq k \leq 6$) associations are represented by unidirectional links. Solid vectors identify provinces for which the highest CCF value was shared with one of its three geographically nearest seeds; broken vectors relate to seeds which were ranked fourth to sixth nearest. Vector weights define the strength of the associations. Provinces for which no vectors are shown fall outside the mapping conventions of seed proximity (i.e. seeds ranked seventh or eighth nearest) and/or strength of association (maximum $k < 0.40$).

Figure 6.13 identifies three regionally discrete cells: (i) a northern cell, centred on the seed provinces of Manila and Pampanga; (ii) a central cell, centred on the Camarines seed; and (iii) a southern cell, centred on the island seeds of Bohol and Leyte. All three cells are characterized by tight bonding between geographically proximal units, with the Camarines cell distinguished by a preponderance of reciprocal links. The three remaining seeds (Cápiz, and the geographically remote provinces of Cagayán and Misamis) are detached from the overall pattern.

INTERPRETATION

It is important to note that the vectors in Figure 6.13 do not represent the diffusion corridors of Wave II. Rather, they identify pairs of seed/non-seed provinces that are very similar in terms of their time-series behaviour. However, assuming that Wave II spread from one or more of the seed provinces, the

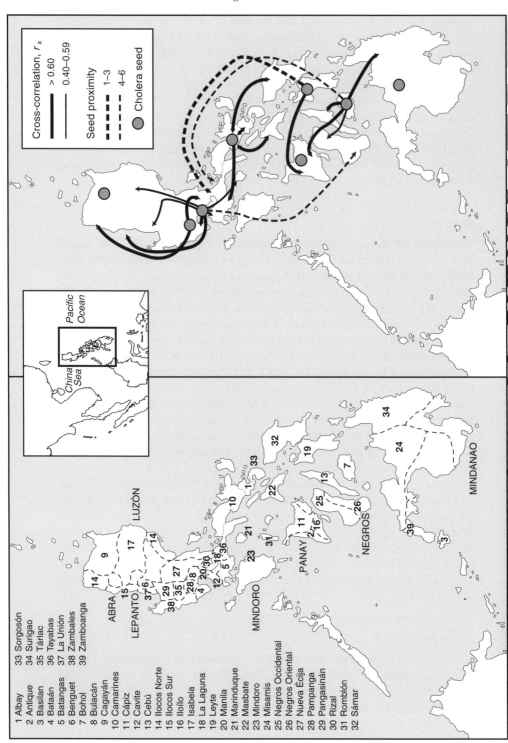

tight regional bonding of geographically proximal series over short lags is consistent with the following simple model: Wave II evolved from three independent centres of infection (Manila/Pampanga, Camarines, and Bohol/Leyte), with each centre serving as the initial point of infection for a regional cell. The regional component to this model contrasts sharply with the diffusion pattern reconstructed previously for Wave I (see Sect. 6.3). That diffusion pattern, which is traced by the vectors in Figure 6.3B, was characterized by an interregional drift of the disease from a single origin at Manila.

6.8 Conclusion

This chapter has presented a number of geographically valuable techniques for unravelling the space–time tracks of war-related epidemics. These range from simple time-sequence maps, through statistical methods for assessing the location and velocity of epidemic waves, to alternative conceptualizations of epidemic spaces and models which can be used to forecast the spread of epidemics. These methods are all used in subsequent regional chapters to examine different facets of the war–disease interface.

So far as the cholera epidemic associated with the Philippines Insurrection at the turn of the twentieth century is concerned, the methods we have described enable us to reach five conclusions:

(a) *The nation-wide development of Wave I was characterized by an inter-regional drift of the disease from a single starting-point at Manila. In contrast, Wave II erupted from three independent centres of infection, with each centre serving as the initial point of infection for a discrete regional cell.* While military movements had played a vital role in the interregional spread of Wave I, the tight bonding of the regional cells for Wave II may represent a reassertion of the regional isolation of the island communities characteristic of the era prior to the Philippine–American War (1899–1902).

Fig. 6.13. Associations between provinces in terms of similarity of cholera activity in Wave II, based upon cross-correlations (CCFs) between the weekly series of morbidity rates per 10,000 population

Notes: The left-hand map identifies provinces. On the right-hand map, seed provinces are identified by shaded circles. Vectors link each non-seed province to the seed with which it shared the largest correlation at lags $0 \leq k \leq 6$. Reciprocal links mark in-phase ($k = 0$) associations, while out-of-phase associations are represented by unidirectional links. Solid vectors identify provinces for which the largest CCF value was shared with one of its three geographically nearest seeds. Broken vectors relate to seeds ranked fourth to sixth nearest. Vector weights define the strengths of the associations.

Source: Smallman-Raynor and Cliff (1998*b*, fig. 3, p. 195).

(*b*) *Contagious spread dominated the nation-wide development of both waves,*
but there were marked differences in the strength and velocity of spread;
hierarchical diffusion played only a minor role in the later stages of each
wave. It may be hypothesized that the strongly structured, early, and
widespread contagious transmission of Wave I resulted from large-
scale population interaction in the immediate aftermath of the
Philippine–American War. Removed in time from the war, Wave II was
not subject to the same levels of population interaction; spatial transmission was less strongly structured and geographical seeding was slower. For both waves, hierarchical transmission was limited by the lack of a
well-developed urban hierarchy.

(*c*) *The spread processes for islands and provinces weakened between Wave I*
and Wave II. This finding is consistent with the national level result in (*b*).

(*d*) *At the province level, the geographical structure of spread processes*
altered between Wave I and Wave II. However, levels of disease incidence
in Wave I, directly influenced by the war, have a statistical link to the
operation of hierarchical spread in the build-up to Wave II.

(*e*) *Wave II developed at a slower rate than Wave I in many areas at all*
geographical scales. For provinces, the reduction in wave velocity was
associated with a weakening of the structure of the underlying spread
processes. The evidence of (*b*) and (*c*), above, points to a similar explanation for the levels of island and nation.

These five points emphasize the complexity of epidemiological spread
processes in the two years that followed the Philippine–American War. However, a general principle also emerges: the disruption brought about by war,
through increased population flux, will probably strengthen existing geographical corridors of disease spread and amplify speed of propagation as compared
with levels prevailing in peace.

Appendix 6A

This appendix outlines the mathematical and computational details of the various techniques described in this chapter.

6A.1 Autocorrelation on Graphs (Section 6.4.2)

The autocorrelation on graphs approach requires us to construct graphs consisting of
nodes to represent the geographical units (e.g. medical districts), and lines or edges con-
necting the nodes. The connections are made so that the pattern of edges mimics the
corridors of disease spread which correspond with the diffusion model we wish to test.
For example, to check for the existence of contagious and hierarchical effects in the
spread of a disease, appropriate graphs are:

(1) A nearest neighbour graph defined by setting each element, w_{ij}, in a matrix **W** equal to 1 if medical districts i and j are nearest neighbours as judged by, say, the straight-line distance in miles between them, and $w_{ij} = 0$ otherwise (cf. the MST graph A in Figs. 6.4 and 6.5).

(2) A hierarchical graph in which $w_{ij} = 1$ if, irrespective of its geographical position, medical district j is the next larger or next smaller district in population size to i, and $w_{ij} = 0$ otherwise (the hierarchy graph of Figs. 6.4 and 6.5).

To determine the goodness-of-fit between a graph and the attack rate of a given disease, two spatial autocorrelation statistics are available (Cliff and Ord, 1981: 1–65). The simplest, the so-called BW statistic, tests a binary coding of the nodes (e.g. presence/absence of the disease, above/below the median attack rate). Moran's I statistic enables interval-scaled variate values (e.g. rate per 100,000 population) to be studied. We outline each in turn.

BW Join Counts

The BW statistic is defined as

$$BW = \frac{1}{2} \sum_{i=1}^{n} \sum_{\substack{j=1 \\ i \neq j}}^{n} w_{ij}(x_i - x_j)^2. \tag{6.A1}$$

The $\{w_{ij}\}$ are drawn from graphs (1) and (2) above; $x_i = 1$ if vertex i is colour-coded B (presence) and $x_i = 0$ if the vertex is coded W (absence).

The sampling distribution of BW under the null hypothesis of no spatial auto-correlation in the variate may be tested for significant departure from its null value as a standardized Normal (z) score for roughly 20 or more nodes (see Cliff and Ord, 1981: 36–41). This standardized score marks the degree of correspondence between any graph and the transmission path followed by a diffusion wave: the larger (negative) the score, the greater the correspondence between the hypothetical and the actual diffusion paths.

Moran's I

Following Cliff and Ord (1981: 17–21), we define I as

$$I = \left(\frac{n}{S_0}\right) \sum_{i=1}^{n} \sum_{\substack{j=1 \\ i \neq j}}^{n} w_{ij} z_i z_j \bigg/ \sum_{i=1}^{n} z_i^2 \tag{6.A2}$$

where n is the number of nodes, x_i is the disease rate per 100,000 population at node i, and $z_i = x_i - \bar{x}$. The $\{w_{ij}\}$ are drawn from graphs (1) and (2) above. In addition, $S_0 = \sum_{i=1}^{n} \sum_{j=1}^{n} w_{ij}, \bar{x} = 1/n \sum_{i=1}^{n} x_i$, and we adopt the convention that $w_{ij} = 0$. I may be tested for significance as a standard Normal deviate, and the expectation and variance under the null hypothesis of no spatial autocorrelation are given in Cliff and Ord (1981: 21). As the correspondence between a given graph and the spatial pattern of rates increases, I becomes larger. The line traces plotted in Figure 6.4 are the standard Normal deviates for I for each week of the epidemic.

6A.2 Epidemic Velocity (Section 6.5)

The concept of epidemic velocity has attracted theoretical attention because of its importance for possible preventive measures; the spread of slow-moving waves may be simpler to check than that of rapidly moving waves. Basic references are Mollison (1991) and van den Bosch *et al.* (1990). If we are dealing with a simple spatial process where the epidemic spreads with a well-defined wavefront (as in the case of the studies by Mollison, 1977), then the physical concept of distance travelled over time may be appropriate. However, where the wavefront is not a well-defined line, and where the susceptible population through which the epidemic moves is both discontinuous in space and has sharp variations in density, then alternative definitions of velocity must be sought.

Lag Maps (Section 6.5.1)

One approach is to calculate *lag maps* or *charts* from the average time to infection for each geographical area, i, in a study region. Denote the first week in which cholera associated with Wave I or Wave II appeared in the Philippines as $t = 1$. The subsequent weeks of the wave may then be coded serially as $t = 2, 3, \ldots ,$. Then the average time to infection, $\bar{t}$, is defined as

$$\bar{t} = \frac{1}{n} \sum_{t=1}^{T} t x_t \tag{6.A3}$$

where x_t is the number of reported cases at time t and $n = \Sigma x_t$ for all t. We can interpret $\bar{t}$ as the average or expected length of time to infection for an area in a wave. For rapidly moving waves, $\bar{t}$ will be small, whereas for slowly moving waves, $\bar{t}$ will be relatively large. It is the values of $\bar{t}$ for the various provinces and islands of the Philippines in Waves I and II which are plotted in Figure 6.6.

Further insights into epidemic velocity may be obtained from the moments of the frequency distribution of reported cases in time. The rth central moment about $\bar{t}$ may be written as

$$m_r = \sum_{i=1}^{T} \left[(t - \bar{t})^r x_t \right] \big/ n, \tag{6.A4}$$

so that m_2 is the variance in time of case occurrence. The standard measures of skewness and kurtosis, $\sqrt{b_1}$ and b_2, are then defined as $\sqrt{b_1} = m_3 / m_2^{3/2}$ and $b_2 = m_4 / m_2^2$.

The characteristic epidemic curve for infectious diseases of the sort considered in this book follows a Normal distribution. Compared with this benchmark, fast-moving waves will peak early, implying small values for both $\bar{t}$ and the standard deviation, $s = \sqrt{m_2}$. An early concentration of cases would also result in a large value for the Pearson kurtosis coefficient, b_2, and a positively skewed frequency distribution. A slow-moving wave might be expected to peak late in time (large $\bar{t}$) and to have cases more evenly spread over the duration of the wave (large s, small b_2). These characteristics are illustrated in Figure 6.A1.

6A.3 Disease Centroids (Section 6.5.2)

Suppose we define a centroid for a map to show the mean centre of reported disease incidence at time t. Time changes in the position of the centroid may then be monitored to

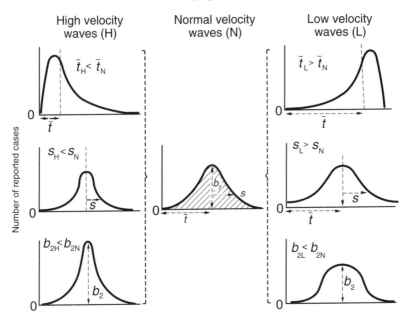

Fig. 6.A1. Characteristic case frequency distribution for normal, high, and low velocity epidemic waves

Source: Cliff *et al.* (2000, fig. 6.18, p. 273).

determine both direction and velocity of spread. Kuhn and Kuenne (1962) give an appropriate centroid statistic. Assume that data are recorded for areas. The location of the jth areal unit whose disease incidence is to be measured may be given a horizontal cartesian coordinate u_j and a vertical map coordinate v_j (say for its geographical centre). Let the reported number of cases for the jth unit be I_j. Choose an initial location for the centroid at a map coordinate position $\hat{U}, \hat{V}$. The centroid of the distribution is now located by an iterative search procedure based upon repeated solution of the equations

$$\hat{U}_{k+1} = \sum_{j=1}^{n} I_j u_j d_{j(k)} / \sum_{j=1}^{n} I_j d_{j(k)}, \text{ and } \hat{V}_{k+1} = \sum_{j=1}^{n} I_j v_j d_{j(k)} / \sum_{j=1}^{n} I_j d_{j(k)}. \tag{6.A5}$$

until $\hat{U}_{(k+1)} - \hat{U}_{(k)} < \varepsilon$ and $\hat{V}_{(k+1)} - \hat{V}_{(k)} < \varepsilon$ where ε is a pre-specified convergence error level. In these equations, d_j is the distance between the latest centroid and the jth area. The new centroid is denoted by the subscript $(k + 1)$. As shown in Figure 6.7A, by plotting centroids for successive time periods and linking them in sequence, the general direction of movement can be captured.

Centroid results may be generalized using polynomial trend surfaces. Let t denote the month ($t = 1, 2, \ldots$) in which the centroid is at location $\hat{U}_t, \hat{V}_t$. Then the trend surface model

$$t = \sum_{i=0}^{m} \sum_{j=0}^{n} \beta_{ij} \hat{U}_t^i \hat{V}_t^j + \varepsilon_t \qquad t = 1, 2, \ldots \tag{6.A6}$$

may be fitted using standard multiple regression techniques. The quadratic surface fitted to the points of Figure 6.7A is plotted in Figure 6.7B. Other, more sophisticated methods of surface fitting include distance-weighted least squares and Kriging (Stein, 1999).

6A.4 Multidimensional Scaling (Section 6.6)

The essential idea behind multidimensional scaling (MDS) is most readily illustrated using a geographical analogy. When a conventional map of a portion of the earth's surface is drawn, some distortion results in transforming a curved segment of the globe onto a flat piece of paper. The particular map projection used will determine the nature and extent of the scale or directional distortion introduced. But, subject to these known errors, all the map projections in common use attempt to ensure that the locations of points on the map systematically reflect their relative positions on the globe.

If, however, we use MDS to represent points on the globe, a space is constructed in which the locations of the points correspond not to their (scaled) geographical locations but to their degree of *(dis)similarity* on some variable measured for them. MDS attempts to find a configuration of n points in an m-dimensional space such that the interpoint distances in the configuration best reflect the observed (dis)similarities of the n objects. This may be viewed as a problem of statistical fitting.

Two subsidiary questions arise from the above discussion:

(*a*) How shall we measure '(dis)similarity'?
(*b*) What value of m should be selected?

We consider each in turn.

The (Dis)Similarity Matrix

The MDS method uses a *dissimilarity matrix* which defines the degree of correspondence between locations in terms of some variables. As an example using binary data, let $X(i \times j)$ be a matrix of presences and absences of infectious diseases for disease i in area j. A number of similarity coefficients for dichotomous data are documented in Gower (1985). They are all metric and produce symmetric positive semi-definite (Gramian) matrices and are suitable for use in MDS. From the alternatives given in Gower, $S6$ (Tanimoto's dichotomy coefficient) is especially useful in disease studies. $S6$ is defined for any pair of variables from the following table.

x_j

		1	0	Totals
x_i	1	a	b	$a+b$
	0	c	d	$c+d$
Totals		$a+c$	$b+d$	

Then

$$S6 = \frac{a+d}{a+2(b+c)+d}. \tag{6.A7}$$

$S6$ gives the proportion of pairs where the values of both variables agree, standardized by all possible patterns of agreement and disagreement.

Using *S*6, we now define a similarity matrix, $\mathbf{S} = \{s_{ij}\}$. The elements s_{ij} are the values for *S*6 calculated for all diseases and areas, and reflect the similarity between locations in terms of their patterns of recorded presence/absence of diseases. From $\mathbf{S}$, a matrix $\mathbf{D}$ $(=\{\delta_{ij}\})$ of dissimilarities ($\delta_{ij} = K - s_{ij}$ for some constant K) can be obtained. This matrix of dissimilarities serves as the basis for MDS. The dissimilarities are fixed given quantities and we wish to find the m-dimensional configuration whose distances 'fit them best'. The locations of the points in the configuration are selected to preserve the rank ordering of the relative distances of the experimental dissimilarities.

The final distance metric may be regarded as a monotone transformation of the rank ordering. By adopting as our central goal the requirement of a monotonic relationship between the observed dissimilarities and the distances in the configuration, the accuracy of a proposed solution can be judged by the degree to which this condition is approached. For a proposed configuration, we perform a monotonic regression of distance upon dissimilarity and use the residual sum of squares, suitably normalized, as a quantitative measure of fit, known as the *stress*, S ($0 \leq S \leq 1$; small values of S denote a good fit or low stress). We seek to minimize stress.

Denote the n points of the configuration by $x_1, \ldots, x_n$, and let $x_i = [x_{i1}, x_{i2}]^T$, where the second subscript denotes the space dimension. Let d_{ij} be the (euclidean) distance between the points x_i and x_j. Then we define the stress, S, of the fixed configuration x_1, $\ldots, x_n$ to be

$$S_{(x_1,\ldots,x_n)} = \underset{d_{ij} \text{ statisfying} M}{\text{minimum}}\left[\sum_{i<j}\left(d_{ij} - \hat{d}_{ij}\right)^2 \middle/ \sum_{i<j} d_{ij}^2 \right] \qquad (6.\text{A}8)$$

where M is the monotonicity condition.

The Monotonicity Condition

In MDS, two forms of the monotonicity condition are commonly used as follows:

1. Weak monotonicity (Kruskal, 1964*a*). Here, the distances fitted in the monotone regression (the $\hat{d}_{ij}$ in equation (6.A8)) meet the condition

whenever $\delta_{ij} < \delta_{rs}$ then $\hat{d}_{ij} \leq \hat{d}_{rs}$. $\qquad (6.\text{A}9)$

That is, weak monotonicity allows unequal data to be fitted by equal disparities.

2. Strong monotonocity (Guttman, 1968). In this case the distances are required to be strongly monotone with the data. That is

whenever $\delta_{ij} < \delta_{rs}$ then $\hat{d}_{ij} < \hat{d}_{rs}$. $\qquad (6.\text{A}10)$

Because this criterion does not allow unequal data to be fitted by equal disparities, it almost always results in a final configuration with higher stress than with approach (1). A full comparison of the criteria appears in Lingoes and Roscam (1973). We have used the weak monotonicity condition in this book.

The exact form of M also depends upon how we deal with ties in the dissimilarity values. For *primary* treatment of ties, M is the condition

whenever $\delta_{ij} < \delta_{rs}$ then $\hat{d}_{ij} \leq \hat{d}_{rs}$. $\qquad (6.\text{A}11)$

In this case, when $\delta_{ij} = \delta_{rs}$ no condition is imposed on $\hat{d}_{ij}$, $\hat{d}_{rs}$. For *secondary* treatment of ties, M is the condition whenever $\delta_{ij} < \delta_{rs}$ then $\hat{d}_{ij} \leq \hat{d}_{rs}$ and whenever $\delta_{ij} = \delta_{rs}$ then $\hat{d}_{ij} = \hat{d}_{rs}$.   (6.A12)

In practice, secondary treatment of ties is computationally much easier and faster than primary treatment of ties. It should be noted, however, that the method employed to deal with ties will affect the shape of the resulting configuration. The stress is invariant under translation and uniform stretching and shrinking of the configuration. We therefore normalize each configuration by first placing its centre of gravity or centroid at the origin and then stretching or shrinking so that the mean squared distance of the points from the origin equals 1.

Computatation

Computationally, therefore, MDS consists of two main problems. The first is to find the configuration with minimum stress; this is done iteratively from an initial configuration of objects in the space. From a given configuration a new one, with lower stress, is obtained by using the method of steepest descent. Let

$$\nabla\Sigma = \left(\frac{\partial\Sigma}{x_{11}}, \ldots, \frac{\partial\Sigma}{x_{nm}} \right) \tag{6.A13}$$

denote the gradient vector (evaluated at the current configuration). Then the new configuration has

$$x_{iv}^{new} = x_{iv} - \phi \frac{\partial\Sigma / x_{iv}}{|\nabla\Sigma|}, \quad i = 1, 2, \ldots, n; v = 1, 2, \ldots, m, \tag{6.A14}$$

where ϕ is a step size. At each step of the iterative process, the secondary computational problem of monotone regression is tackled—that of finding the values of $\hat{d}_{ij}$ from the fixed known values d_{ij} of the distances in the current configuration. Kruskal (1964a, 1964b) provides details of a possible algorithm for the determination of the $\hat{d}_{ij}$ and gives suggestions for the step size, ϕ.

Other Measures of Similarity

Although we have used $S6$ in this book when dealing with dichotomous data, we have employed other correlation coefficients as our measures of similarity: Spearman's rank correlation coefficient, ρ, when dealing with ranked variables, and (as in Sect. 6.6) Pearson's product moment correlation coefficient, r, with interval and ratio scaled data.

Value of M

The stress between the MDS and observed configurations reduces monotonically as m increases. However, multidimensional spaces are frequently difficult to interpret. Moreover, as with the MDS examples in this chapter, we frequently wish to see how similar an MDS configuration is to a conventional geographical map. In these circumstances we set $m = 2$.

A further property of MDS which enhances our ability to see how map-like an MDS configuration is arises from the solution algorithm. As noted above under 'Computation', the procedure starts from an initial configuration which can be specified by the researcher, and iterates from this to the minimum-stress configuration. If we seed the MDS algorithm with the geographical coordinates of a set of areas (e.g. longitude and latitude) then, by comparing the initial and MDS maps, we have a direct measure of the degree to which the MDS and conventional maps coincide. We can quantify the goodness-of-fit between the two using the *affine correlation coefficient* (low correlation = poor fit and vice versa).

6A.5 The Affine Correlation Coefficient (Section 6.6.2)

The two-dimensional correspondence between any initial MDS configuration (such as latitude and longitude), defined by the coordinates (x, y), and the final configuration in an MDS space, specified by the coordinates (u, v), may be determined using the affine correlation coefficient (see Tobler, 1965). This is based upon the affine tranformation familiar from GIS (geographical information systems). The closer the MDS coordinates are to the true latitude/longitudes, the higher will be the spatial correlation (and the more 'map-like' the MDS configuration). In its full form, given two sets of coordinates, the affine transformation handles all aspects of the tranformation (scaling, shear, rotation, translation, projection, and overall scaling); see Ahuja and Coons (1968) for details. Thus it is possible to compare the relationship between the same set of objects mapped in two different coordinate systems.

Let $x_i, y_i; u_i, v_i$ denote the rectangular coordinates of the ith point in the two point patterns we wish to compare (here the longitudes and latitudes of the centroid of the ith state and the corresponding coordinates in the MDS space, respectively). In addition, let $W_i = (u_i, v_i)'$ and $Z_i = (x_i, y_i)'$ represent the ith observation pair, $i = 1, 2, \ldots, n$, where the primes denote the transpose. The objective is to use least squares methods to estimate the coefficients A and B in the transformation

$$\hat{W}_i = A + BZ_i. \tag{6.A15}$$

The regression can be considered as a mapping from the xy plane to the uv plane.

Treating the observations as the components of vectors in this way means the constants become

$$A = (a_1, a_2)' \quad \text{and} \quad B = \begin{pmatrix} b_{11} & b_{12} \\ b_{21} & b_{22} \end{pmatrix}, \tag{6.A16}$$

and the equation to be minimized is

$$\sum_{i=1}^{n} (\hat{W}_i - W_i) \cdot (\hat{W}_i - W)'. \tag{6.A17}$$

The complete affine transformation is therefore of the form

$$\begin{pmatrix} \hat{u}_j \\ \hat{v}_j \end{pmatrix} = \begin{pmatrix} a_1 \\ a_2 \end{pmatrix} + \begin{pmatrix} b_{11} & b_{12} \\ b_{21} & b_{22} \end{pmatrix} \begin{pmatrix} x_i \\ y_i \end{pmatrix}. \tag{6.A18}$$

The *affine correlation*, which is an overall measure of the degree of correlation between the two point patterns, is given by

$$R_{WZ} = \frac{\sigma_u^2 (r_{xu}^2 + r_{yu}^2 - 2r_{xu}r_{yu}r_{xy}) + \sigma_v^2 (r_{xv}^2 + r_{yv}^2 - 2r_{xv}r_{yv}r_{xy})}{(\sigma_u^2 + \sigma_v^2)(1 - r_{xy}^2)}. \tag{6.A19}$$

This is not symmetric and so $R_{WZ} \neq R_{ZW}$. Accordingly, we generally quote in this chapter and elsewhere in this book, $\bar{R}$, the arithmetic average of R_{WZ} and R_{ZW}.

6A.6 Cross-Correlation Analysis (Section 6.7.3)

Cross-correlation analysis proceeds by computing the correlation coefficient, r_k, between any pair of time series to determine the value of k at which the maximum correlation occurs. This value of k is conventionally taken as the lead or lag of the one series with respect to the other. Let x_{it} denote the death rate for disease i in time period t and x_{jt} denote the corresponding value for disease j. Then the cross-correlation at lag k, r_k, is given by

$$r_k = \mathrm{corr}[x_{it}, x_{j,t+k}] = \sum [(x_{it} - \bar{x}_i)(x_{j,t+k} - \bar{x}_j)] \Big/ \Big[\sum (x_i - \bar{x}_i)^2 \sum (x_j - \bar{x}_j)^2\Big]^{1/2}$$

(6.A20)

where $\bar{x}_i$ and $\bar{x}_j$ are the means of the time series.

In the notation of equation (6.A20), the $\{x_{it}\}$ are termed the reference series and the $\{x_{it}\}$ the comparison series. If $k = 0$, the reference and comparison series are said to be in phase; $+k$ ($k > 0$) signifies that the comparison series lags the reference series, and $-k$ ($k > 0$) that the comparison series leads the reference series. Finally, a plot of the correlation coefficient, r_k, against the lag k yields the cross-correlation function (CCF).

7

Pan America: Military Mobilization and Disease in the United States

In the flames stood & view'd the armies drawn out in the sky
Washington Franklin Paine & Warren Allen Gates & Lee:
And heard the voice of Albion's Angel give the thunderous command:
His plagues obedient to his voice flew out of their clouds
Falling upon America, as a storm to cut them off

William Blake, 'America: A Prophecy' (plate 14, 1793)

7.1 Introduction

In the previous chapter, we outlined a number of methods employed by geographers to study time–space patterns of disease incidence and spread. In this and the next four chapters we use these methods to explore five linked themes in the epidemiological history of war since 1850 (Table III.A). We begin here with Theme 1, military mobilization, taking the United States as our geographical reference point.

Military mobilization at the outset of wars has always been a fertile breeding ground for epidemics. The rapid concentration of large—occasionally vast—numbers of unseasoned recruits, usually under conditions of great urgency, sometimes in the absence of adequate logisitic arrangements, and often without sufficient accommodation, supplies, equipage, and medical support, entails a disease risk that has been repeated down the years. The epidemiological dangers are multiplied by the crowding together of recruits from different disease environments (including rural rather than urban settings) while, even in relatively recent conflicts, pressures to meet draft quotas have sometimes demanded the enlistment of weak, physically unfit, and sometimes disease-prone applicants. The testimony of Major Samuel D. Hubbard, surgeon to the Ninth New York Volunteer Infantry, US Army, during the Spanish–American War (1898) is illustrative:

I examined all the recruits for this regiment . . . Practically all the men belonged to one class . . . They were whisky-soaked, homeless wanderers, the majority of whom gave Bowery lodging houses as their places of residence . . . Certainly the regiment was composed of a class of men likely to be susceptible to disease . . . The regiment was hastily recruited, and while the greatest care was used to get the best, the best had to be selected from the worst. (Hubbard, cited in Reed *et al.*, 1904, i. 223)

But the problem of mobilization and disease is not restricted to new recruits. As part of the broader pattern of heightened population mixing, regular service personnel may also be swept into the disease milieu while, occasionally, infections may escape the confines of hastily established assembly and training camps to diffuse widely in civil populations.

Against this background, the case studies of mobilization and disease presented in this chapter draw on the detailed epidemiological records of the United States Army. From the main phases of military mobilization embraced by our time window, 1850–1990, we select two nineteenth-century (Civil War, 1861–5 and Spanish–American War, 1898) and two twentieth-century (World War I, 1914–18 and World War II, 1939–45) wars for scrutiny. Adopting a chronological structure, Section 7.2 uses the statistical information included in *The Medical and Surgical History of the War of the Rebellion (1861–65)* (Surgeon-General's Office, 1870–88) to examine geographical patterns of recruitment and disease in one of the first great military mobilizations of the modern period—the American Civil War. While upwards of 3.7 million men were raised during the Civil War (Kreidberg and Henry, 1975), the US Army was so reduced in the following decades that, when war was declared on Spain in April 1898, there were scarcely 28,000 regulars to fight an estimated 400,000

Spaniards under arms (Bayne-Jones, 1968). The spread of the epidemic of typhoid fever that accompanied the US mobilization against Spain in 1898, and which debilitated the commands of the newly established US Volunteer Army, forms the theme of Section 7.3. Finally, moving into the twentieth century, Section 7.4 examines the occurrence of infectious diseases in the home camps of the US Army during the world wars. The chapter is concluded in Section 7.5.

7.2 Recruiting Fields in the American Civil War (1861–1865)

In this section, we extend our examination of measles in the American Civil War (Sect. 4.3) to a consideration of the broader epidemiological consequences of the mobilization of the Union and Confederate armies. A discussion of the impact of infectious diseases on individual campaigns is provided by Steiner (1968).

7.2.1 Background: Mobilization

The American Civil War (also called the War between the States and the War of the Rebellion) lasted from 1861 to 1865. It involved the federal government of the United States and 11 southern states which asserted their right to secede from the Union. The secession of the Southern states (in date order, South Carolina, Mississippi, Florida, Alabama, Georgia, Louisiana, Texas, Virginia, Arkansas, Tennessee, and North Carolina; see Fig. 7.1 for locations) in 1860–1 and the ensuing outbreak of armed hostilities was the culmination of decades of growing sectional friction over the related issues of slavery, trade and tariffs, and the doctrine of the rights of states. This friction arose out of basic differences between the economies of the Northern and Southern states. The North had a growing manufacturing sector and small farms using free labour, while the South's economy was based on large plantations using slave labour. In the 1840s and 1850s, the Northern states wanted to prohibit slavery in the Western territories that would eventually become new states. The Southern states opposed all efforts to block the expansion of slavery and feared that the stance taken by the North would eventually endanger existing slave-holdings in the South itself.

By the 1850s, some Northerners had begun calling for the complete abolition of slavery, while several Southern states threatened to secede from the Union as a means to protect their right to keep slaves. When Abraham Lincoln, the candidate of the anti-slavery Republican Party, was elected president in late 1860, the Southern states carried out their threat and seceded. Organized as the Confederate States of America, the Southern states, under President Jefferson Davis, counted on patriotism, the strategic advantage of interior lines of communication, and the international importance of their chief cash crop, cotton, to win a short war of independence. The Northern states of the federal Union, under President Abraham Lincoln, commanded more than twice the population of the Confederacy and possessed even greater advantages in manufacturing and transportation.

DISEASE DATA

The disease history of the war is recorded in seven volumes of *The Medical and Surgical History of the War of the Rebellion (1861–65)*, prepared for the US Congress under the direction of Surgeon-General Joseph K. Barnes of the US Army (Surgeon-General's Office, 1870–88); see Plate 1.2C. The detailed investigation was carried out by J. J. Woodward, Assistant Surgeon-General in the US Army (Pl. 4.2).

Volume i, upon which the analyses of this section are based, consists of a series of statistical tables presenting a summary view of the monthly reports made to the Surgeon-General during the Rebellion covering the sickness of the Army, mortality, and discharges from service. The data are divided ethnically into White Troops and Coloured Soldiers. At the start of the conflict, data were collected on printed forms for 143 diseases. The broad disease classes were: fevers; eruptive fevers; diseases of organs of the digestive system; diseases of the brain and nervous system; disease of the urinary and genital organs including venereal infections; disease of the circulatory system; disease of the fibrous and muscular structures; abscesses and ulcers; wounds and injuries; eye diseases; ear diseases; all other diseases. By 1862, the Army Board felt the classification was inadequate and recommended a change to a system based upon that devised for the British Army by William Farr, then Registrar General:

Class I   Zymotic diseases (miasmic, enthetic, dietic diseases)
Class II   Constitutional diseases (diathetic and tubercular diseases)
Class III   Parasitic diseases
Class III   Local diseases (diseases of the nervous system, eye, ear, organs of circulation, respiration, digestion, urinary and genitalia, bones and joints, integumentary system)
Class V   Wounds, accidents, and injuries (wounds including accidents and injuries, homicide, suicide, execution of sentence).

The zymotic diseases included epidemic, endemic, and contagious diseases supposedly induced by some agent.

The data were also collected on a regional basis:

Atlantic   New England, Appalachia, and Atlantic seaboard from Maryland to Florida.
Central   The area between the Appalachians and the Rockies drained by the Mississippi and its tributaries.
Pacific   Rockies and Pacific seaboard.

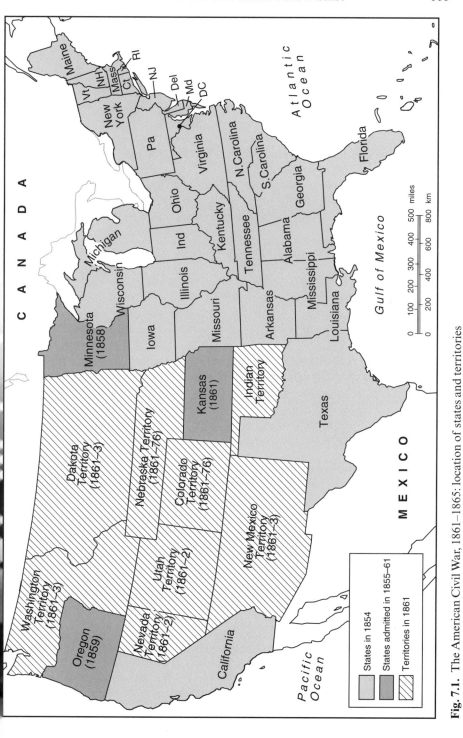

Fig. 7.1. The American Civil War, 1861–1865: location of states and territories

Source: Drawn from data in *Encyclopaedia Britannica*, Britannica CD 99Multimedia Edition.

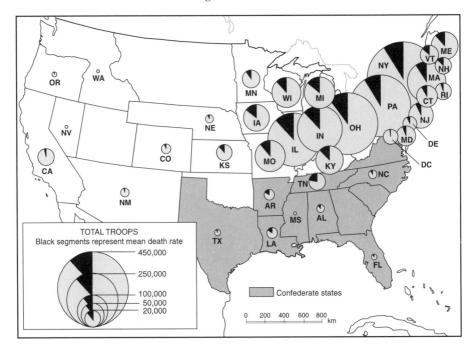

Fig. 7.2. The War of the Rebellion

Note: Proportional circles give total troops raised by states and territories, along with the mean annual death rate.

Source: Drawn from data in Surgeon-General's Office (1870–88, v and vii *passim*).

7.2.2 General Mortality and Morbidity

War began in Charleston, South Carolina, with the firing of Confederate artillery on Fort Sumter on 12 April 1861. Both sides quickly began raising and organizing armies. Figure 7.2 uses proportional circles to show the estimated totals of troops raised by the various states and territories over the course of the conflict, along with the estimated mean annual death rate which each experienced.

MOBILIZATION

The history of the mobilization is reviewed by Kreidberg and Henry (1975: 83–140). In their words, the conflict was

the last of the old wars as well as the first of the modern wars by 20th century standards. Its modernity extended from the comprehensiveness of its mobilization to the grim tragedy of its final casualty lists. The problems of Civil War mobilization in both the United States and the Confederate States were problems of mobilization for modern warfare. (ibid. 83)

Union Army

One striking feature of military mobilization in the northern states was the ultimate size of the army raised. From a regular force of little over 16,000 officers
and men at the outbreak of hostilities, a series of proclamations and calls in the
following weeks and months succeeded in raising the strength of the Army to
800,000. Further calls for volunteers were issued in 1862, 1863, and 1864 such
that, by the end of the war, the total number mustered into the Union Army
probably approached 2.2 million[1] (out of a Northern population of 22
million).

The first few months of mobilization were accompanied by a plethora of
logisitic problems. Lacking in preparedness, and with little planning for the
management of large numbers of new recruits, arrangements for the provision
of food, clothing, and shelter had to be improvised. As for procedures regarding the selection of recruits, the first call of 15 April 1861 merely informed the
mustering officers that they should 'receive no men under the rank of commissioned officer who is in years apparently over forty-five or under eighteen, or
who is not in physical strength and vigor' (cited in Kreidberg and Henry, 1975:
98). While the formal requirement of a physical examination was introduced
from 3 August 1861, it would seem that many medical inspections were inadequately conducted (or even overlooked) in the haste of the recruitment drive
(see ibid. 98 n. 32).

The Confederacy

As Kreidberg and Henry (1975: 129–34) note, there is no complete compilation
of the size of the Confederate Armies, although it is generally accepted that the
aggregate total strength was about 1 million (out of a Southern population of
9 million, including 3.5 million slaves). In general terms, the problems of mobilization which confronted the Confederacy paralleled those of the Union.
With many states having placed themselves on a war footing after secession in
early 1861, authorization for the call-out of the militia, the acceptance of
100,000 volunteers, and the organization of a 10,600-strong regular army was
given by Provisional Congress on 6 March 1861. A call for a further 400,000
volunteers was authorized some five months later, on 8 August, while numbers
were further boosted by the general Conscription Act (authorizing the draft of
all white males aged 18–35 years) of 16 April 1862 (Kreidberg and Henry, 1975:
129–38).

LOSSES

While the exact mortality and morbidity experienced by the Union and Confederate sides will never be known, the data which are available show that the
disease history of the war repeats a theme familiar from Section 4.3: greater
loss of life and morbidity from disease than from the consequences of battle

---

[1] The estimate of 2.7 million sometimes quoted includes re-enlistments.

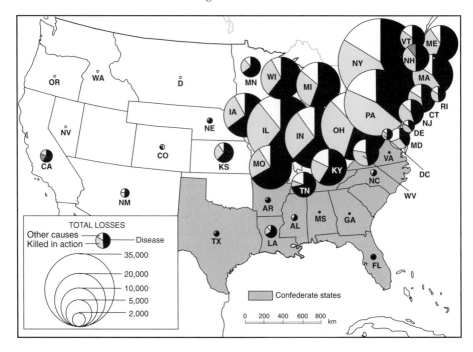

Fig. 7.3. Mortality among Union and Confederate troops in the War of the Rebellion

Note: Proportional circles show battle deaths, and deaths from disease and other causes, 1861–5.
Source: Drawn from data in Surgeon-General's Office (1870–88, v and vii *passim*).

(Steiner, 1968, 1977). Figure 7.3 summarizes this by using proportional circles to show, for each state and territory, the estimated total losses over the course of the war from disease, battle, and other causes. Losses from disease commonly reached 50 per cent and more of state totals. But, if the proportions plotted in Figure 7.3 look stark, Figure 7.4 illustrates the even more catastrophic situation for those unlucky enough to be captured alive and put in prison camps. Among officers (Fig. 7.4B), death rates from disease often approached 50 per cent. Among the regular troops (Fig. 7.4A), it was much worse, with generally a better than 75 per cent chance of dying from disease before liberation (Pl. 7.1).[2]

In the remainder of this subsection we look at the general patterns and causes of mortality and morbidity in more detail, focusing upon Union forces for which more data are available.

[2] Of all the prison camps established during the war, the Confederate military prison camp at Andersonville, Ga. (Camp Sumter) stands as the most notorious. For graphic descriptions of the conditions endured by prisoners at Andersonville, and the diseases from which the prisoners died, see McElroy (1879) and Chipman (1911). On Union prison camps, see Frohman (1965).

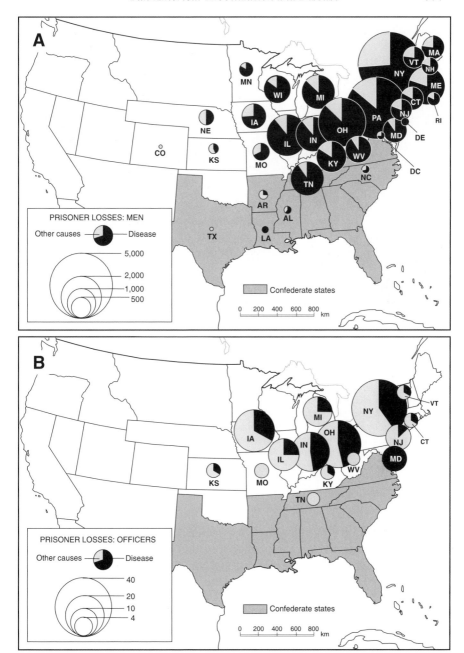

Fig. 7.4. Mortality among Union and Confederate prisoners in the War of the Rebellion

Notes: Proportional circles show deaths from disease and other causes among prisoners. (A) Men. (B) Officers.

Source: Drawn from data in Surgeon-General's Office (1870–88, v and vii *passim*).

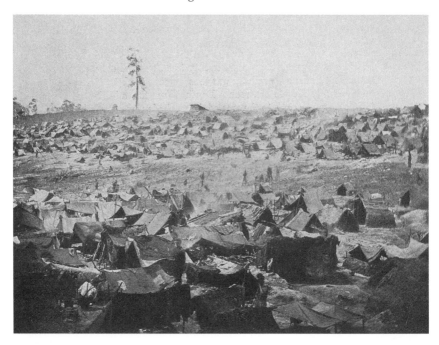

Pl. 7.1. Prisoner of war camp at Andersonville, Georgia, American Civil War (1861–1865)

Notes: Andersonville camp as it appeared in August 1864. The camp, established by the Confederate Army to accommodate Union prisoners, covered an area of 27 acres and was enclosed by a 20-foot stockade. For the eight months from February to September 1864, McElroy (1879: 316) records a mortality rate of 23.3 per cent among the 40,611 incarcerated Union soldiers. The leading causes of death included diarrhoea, dysentery, and scurvy. The Prison Keeper, Captain Henry Wirz, was later tried by a US military court and executed.
Source: Thompson (1911: 75, lower).

Mortality

Table 7.1 shows the agreed figures for Union troops reported at the time, although it is estimated that the tabulated mortality among white troops is deficient by 24.7 per cent (Surgeon-General's Office, 1870–88, v. 3). Over the course of the conflict, the average annual mortality rate per 1,000 mean strength among white troops was 53.48 and 143.4 among coloureds. Remarkable features include the ratio of disease : battle deaths—over 4 : 1—among all troops, reaching 20 : 1 among coloured volunteers. The Surgeon-General's Office estimated over the conflict that, among coloured troops, there was an annual rate of 15 violent deaths and 133 deaths from disease per 1,000 strength. In the regular army, the rates were 27 violent and 32 disease deaths per 1,000 strength. Among white volunteers, the figures were 33 and 55 per 1,000 mean strength (Woodward, in Surgeon-General's Office, 1870–88, i., pp. xl–xli). Thus not only

Table 7.1. Mortality among Union troops in the American Civil War, 1861–1865

Cause	Regulars		White volunteers		Coloured volunteers		Total	
	No.	%	No.	%	No.	%	No.	%
Killed in battle	1,355	23.7	41,369	15.6	1,514	4.5	44,238	14.5
Died of wounds and injuries	1,174	20.5	46,271	17.4	1,760	5.3	49,205	16.2
Suicide, homicide, and execution	27	0.5	442	0.2	57	0.2	526	0.2
Died of disease	3,009	52.6	153,995	58.1	29,212	87.5	186,216	61.2
Unknown causes	159	2.8	23,188	8.7	837	2.5	24,184	7.9
Total	5,724	1.9	265,265	87.2	33,380	11.0	304,369	100.0

Source: Woodward in Surgeon-General's Office (1870–88, i., p. xxxvii).

Table 7.2. Annual sickness and mortality among Union white and coloured troops per 1,000 mean strength

Troops	Year ending 30 June											
	1861		1862		1863		1864		1865		1866	
	Cases	Deaths	Cases	Deaths	Cases	Deaths	Cases	Deaths	Cases	Deaths	Cases	Deaths
White	3,822	10.8	2,983	49	2,696	63	2,210	48	2,273	56	2,362	42
Coloured							4,092	211	3,205	140	2,797	94

Source: Woodward in Surgeon-General's Office (1870–88, v, table I, p. 6).

did all troops die disproportionately often from disease rather than in battle, but coloured troops suffered dramatically more disease-related mortality than whites.

MORBIDITY

Among white troops, 5,417,360 cases of specified disease and 7,187 cases of unspecified disease (total 5,424,547 exclusive of 400,933 cases of wounds, accidents, and injuries in Class V) were recorded. Among coloured troops, 605,017 cases were reported. However, while both figures are underestimates, the belief is that rates quoted are unlikely to be substantially affected. The average annual case rate per 1,000 of mean strength was 2,435 among white troops and 3,299 among coloureds. The annual rates are given in Table 7.2.

Diseases

Table 7.3 summarizes the comparative frequency and mortality from disease among white and coloured troops. For mortality and morbidity, there is a

Table 7.3. Impact of disease upon Union forces: white troops, 1 May 1861–30 June 1866; coloured troops, 1 July 1863–30 June 1866

Disease (White troops)	Cases per 1,000 mean strength	Deaths per 1,000 mean strength	Cases per 1,000 cases of all disease	Deaths per 1,000 of total disease deaths	Disease (Coloured troops)	Cases per 1,000 mean strength	Deaths per 1,000 mean strength	Cases per 1,000 cases of all disease	Deaths per 1,000 of total disease deaths
Diarrhoea, dysentery	3,675.93	80.71	292.23	292.1	Diarrhoea, dysentery	2,518.14	105.81	254.4	245.97
Malarial fever	2,698.78	17.38	214.55	62.91	Malarial fever	2,488.73	39.08	251.47	69.93
Digestion	1,306.1	8.83	103.83	32.04	Digestion	887.77	15.19	89.7	35.31
Bronchitis, catarrh	901.57	2.53	71.67	9.16	Bronchitis, catarrh	531.91	4.07	53.75	9.46
Rheumatism	590.71	1.01	46.96	3.67	Rheumatism	525.5	3.67	53.1	8.55
Boils, abscesses	440.17	0.46	24.99	1.67	Other miasmic diseases	396.9	8.98	40.13	20.88
Syphilis, gonorrhoea, orchitis	423.85	0.29	33.69	1.05	Nervous system	391.53	12.75	39.56	29.04
Other miasmic diseases	404.6	5.33	32.16	19.28	Lung, pleura inflammation	381.27	86.62	38.52	210.35
Nervous system	394.29	9.49	31.34	34.33	Eruptive fevers	276.86	55.08	27.27	128.04
Eye and ear	272.75	0.02	21.68	0.06	Scurvy	265.28	6.07	26.8	14.11
Continued fevers	268.16	59.91	16.55	216.82	Syphilis, gonorrhoea, orchitis	233.22	0.5	23.56	1.16
Eruptive fevers	240.83	23.26	14.85	84.19	Boils, abscesses	192.37	0.42	19.44	0.98
Other respiratory	235.32	2.97	18.71	10.74	Eye and ear	158.33	0.03	16.6	0.07
Lung, pleura inflammation	215.78	32.73	17.15	118.47	Other respiratory	151.03	6.35	15.26	14.75
Typho-malarial fevers	115.65	8.67	9.19	31.37	Typho-malarial fevers	123.16	20.35	12.44	47.31
Itch	74.39	0	5.91	0	Continued fevers	68.98	37.36	6.97	86.84
Scurvy	71.22	0.82	5.66	2.96	Itch	51.63	0	5.22	0
Urino-genital	69.28	0.92	5.51	3.32	Urino-genital	49.34	2.05	4.98	4.76
Circulatory organs	58.22	3.54	4.63	12.81	Circulatory organs	25.5	7.31	2.58	16.98
Consumption	31.3	11.29	2.49	40.85	Consumption	21.77	18.94	2.2	44.04
Bones, joints	18.73	0.1	1.49	0.36	Bones, joints	15.54	0.23	1.57	0.55
Diphtheria	16.87	1.53	1.34	5.53	Diphtheria	12.69	0.95	1.28	2.22

Source: Smart in Surgeon-General's Office (1870–88, v, table II, p. 11).

strong correlation between the indices for white and coloured troops (0.98 for cases/1,000 mean strength; mortality 0.87; 0.98 for disease-specific cases per 1,000 cases of all diseases; 0.87 for disease-specific mortality per 1,000 deaths from all diseases). Diarrhoea and dysentery, malarial fever, digestion, bronchitis and catarrh, and rheumatism occupy the first five positions for both. Diarrhoea, dysentery, and malaria occurred with great frequency (one to four episodes per soldier), yielded high mortality, and were in a league of their own. Thus diarrhoea and dysentery together appeared on more than 25 per cent of all the entries upon the sickness reports, while malaria and typho-malaria accounted for about another quarter of all cases of disease. Among the fevers, the continued fevers (e.g. scarlet fever, typhus, typhoid, pneumonia), eruptive fevers (e.g. smallpox, measles) and sexually transmitted diseases appear mid-table and affected roughly one in four soldiers. Malarial fevers caused nearly one-tenth of the total deaths. Especially high mortality rates among cases were caused by the eruptive fevers. Nearly one-tenth of the total deaths arose from them, from a case rate of only 14.8 of every 1,000 cases of disease. In order of gravity, the continued fevers, mainly typhoid, took second place (216 deaths in every 1,000 from disease from only 16.5 cases in every 1,000 cases of disease). To the miasmic diseases (poisonous vapours thought to infect the air) were attributed more than half of the cases per 1,000 cases of disease and nearly three-quarters of the disease mortality.

Table 7.4 compares case and mortality rates as between white and coloured troops by calculating the ratios of data columns 3:7 and 4:8 of Table 7.3. The results have then been sorted by data column 1 of Table 7.4. Ratios greater than 1 imply greater impact upon coloured troops. For cases, there is relatively little difference between the troops. But coloured troops suffered significantly disproportionate mortality.

7.2.3 Recruitment and Disease

During the War, the link between recruitment and disease became as familiar to soldiers as did the excess of disease over battle as the principal cause of mortality and morbidity. Raw recruits from the countryside comprised classic virgin soil populations exposed to new disease environments. As we saw in Section 4.3, the so-called eruptive fevers—smallpox, measles, scarlet fever, and erysipelas—which were ordinarily infections of childhood were not necessarily so among those coming from remote rural areas away from the viruses and streptococci of the cities. As such, the farm boy proved a fertile field for microbial multiplication (Brooks, 1966: 120). As noted in Section 7.2.2, during the war, the average annual mortality rate per 1,000 mean strength among the Union's white troops was 53.48, compared with 143.4 among coloureds. In contrast, from 1840 to 1858 (peacetime), the average annual death rate from all diseases per 1,000 strength among white troops in the US Army was 18.98. Thus the transition from peace to war saw a tripling among white soldiers of

Table 7.4. Disease ratios, coloured : white Union troops

Disease	Cases[1]	Mortality[2]
Scurvy	4.73	4.77
Lung, pleura inflammation	2.25	1.78
Eruptive fevers	1.84	1.52
Typho-malarial fevers	1.35	1.51
Nervous system	1.26	0.85
Other miasmic diseases	1.25	1.08
Malarial fever	1.17	1.11
Rheumatism	1.13	2.33
Bones, joints	1.05	1.53
Diphtheria	0.96	0.40
Urino-genital	0.90	1.43
Consumption	0.88	1.08
Itch	0.88	1.00
Diarrhoea and dysentery	0.87	0.84
Digestion	0.86	1.10
Other respiratory	0.82	1.37
Boils, abscesses	0.78	0.59
Eye and ear	0.77	1.17
Bronchitis, catarrh	0.75	1.03
Syphilis, gonorrhoea, orchitis	0.70	1.10
Circulatory organs	0.56	1.33
Continued fevers	0.42	0.40

Notes: [1] Cases per 1,000 cases of all diseases. [2] Deaths per 1,000 deaths from all diseases.

the death rate from disease, while Barnes has estimated the excess mortality among white troops because of the War to be 44.15 per 1,000 strength annually (Surgeon-General's Office, 1870–88, v. 9).

7.2.4 Temporal Patterns

The front loading of sickness and mortality to the principal periods of recruitment in the early stages of the war is illustrated in Figure 7.5. This shows the prevalence of disease and mortality among white and coloured troops of the US armies during and immediately following the war per 1,000 of strength present. With the exception of the flat curve for white mortality, the other line traces decline steadily over the duration of the conflict. The sick rate of the coloured troops was highest immediately after their enrolment in 1863 when nearly half of the command was reported as having been taken sick during each of the months July, August, and September. In subsequent years, the general health of the coloured troops improved so markedly that during the last quarter of the year to June 1866, their sick rates were somewhat lower than those of white troops.

Death rates among the coloured troops followed a parallel course to morbidity—high at first, about 25 per 1,000 of strength monthly during the first four months of service but declining thereafter to a minimum of 3.18 per 1,000 in May 1866. However, at no point during their service did the mortality rate for coloured troops fall below that of the white commands.

The same declining trend was found for some of the principal diseases. Figure 7.6, which traces the prevalence of continued fevers (typhoid, typhus, and typho-malarial fever) among white troops, shows the same long-term declining trends plotted for all diseases in Figure 7.5.

7.2.5 Regional Patterns

Table 7.5 gives the regional distribution of sickness and mortality per 1,000 mean strength. This shows that each region suffered disproportionate case rates[3] in the first year it was affected by the conflict, and confirms the excess suffering of coloured troops. Figure 7.7 makes the point for the continued fevers. As Smart commented: 'The commencement of service was in all instances characterized by the highest ratio of sickness' (Surgeon-General's Office, 1870–88, v. 11). Rates fell through 1864 and were more variable thereafter. This variability is attributed by Smart to the arrival of more virgin soil troops among recruits.

The diminished sick rate [from 1861–4] must be attributed to the weeding out by death and discharge for disability of the inferior material necessarily present in all new levies. The term of service of many regiments expired during the third year of the war, when the hardy veterans composing them were in many instances replaced by raw troops who, in becoming inured to active service, swelled the sick rates during the fourth year. (Smart, in Surgeon-General's Office, 1870–88, v. 20)

Just as virgin-soil troops experienced raised disease and mortality rates, so environment also affected incidence. The high death rate of troops in the Central region is a feature of Table 7.5 where the military Departments of Tennessee and the Gulf were especially afflicted. These low ground areas suffered especially from malaria. Unfavourable environmental conditions produced the highest rate in the war, 4,012, during the third year by the continued exposure of troops in the malarious regions of the Department of North Carolina. In contrast, favourable environmental and virgin soil factors combined in 1863 when the lowest rate, 1,293, was furnished by the high grounds of Western Virginia and a low rate of 1,563 was given by the veterans of the Army of the Potomac. Most of the troops involved in the great battles beginning with Gettysburg in 1863 and ending at Petersburg in June 1864 spent 'the greater portion of this period . . . in what was regarded by the troops as a

---

[3] In 1861, only two months of service were embraced by the data collection date, and this is reflected in the low mortality rates.

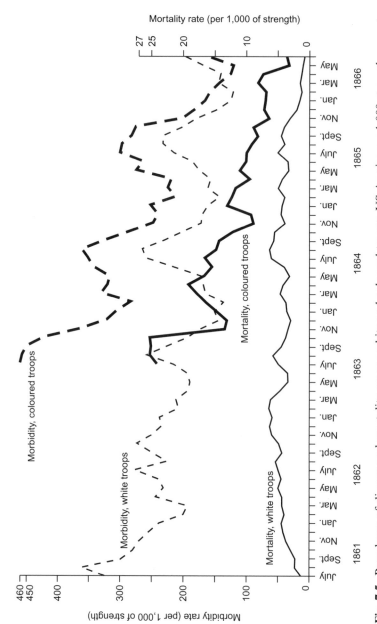

Fig. 7.5. Prevalence of disease and mortality among white and coloured troops, US Armies per 1,000 strength present, monthly 1861–1866

Source: Redrawn from Surgeon-General's Office (1870–88, v, graph facing p. 24).

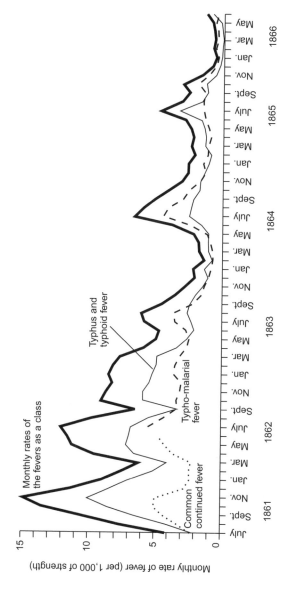

Fig. 7.6. Prevalence of continued fevers among white troops per 1,000 strength present, monthly 1861–1866

Source: Redrawn from Surgeon-General's Office (1870–88, v, graph facing p. 199).

Table 7.5. Regional distribution of sickness and mortality from disease per 1,000 mean strength (year ending 30 June)

Region	1861 Cases	1861 Deaths	1862 Cases	1862 Deaths	1863 Cases	1863 Deaths	1864 Cases	1864 Deaths	1865 Cases	1865 Deaths	1866 Cases	1866 Deaths
White troops												
Atlantic	3,930	11.4	2,719	32	2,553	42	2,137	33	2,221	53	2,292	42
Central	3,432	7.2	3,495	81	2,841	85	2,262	58	2,328	61	2,549	48
Pacific			2,171	10	2,133	9	1,816	11	1,864	12	1,749	14
Total white	3,822	10.8	2,983	49	2,696	63	2,210	48	2,273	56	2,362	42
Coloured troops												
Atlantic							3,461	83	3,122	111	2,574	100
Central							4,373	269	3,248	156	2,842	93
Total coloured							4,092	211	3,205	140	2,797	94

Source: Smart in Surgeon-General's Office (1870–88, v, table V, p. 18).

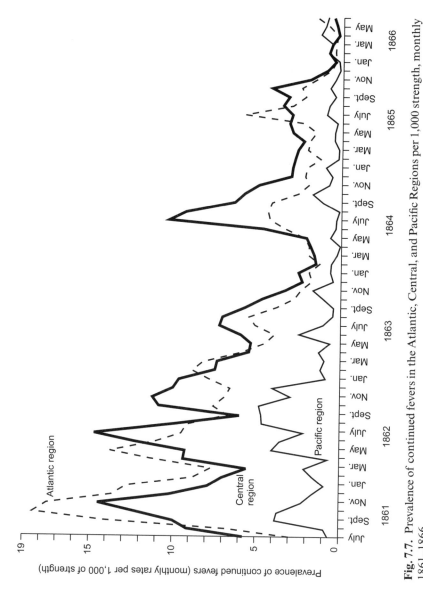

Fig. 7.7. Prevalence of continued fevers in the Atlantic, Central, and Pacific Regions per 1,000 strength, monthly 1861–1866

Source: Redrawn from Surgeon-General's Office (1870–88, v, graph facing p. 202).

picnic in summer quarters on the Rapidan, or hutted during the succeeding winter and spring in a healthy locality' (Smart, in Surgeon-General's Office, 1870–88, v. 20).

Returning to Figure 7.5, the largest monthly rate of cases among white troops occurred in August 1861, shortly after the enlargement of the army to meet military necessities. Exposure, fatigue, altered diet, and a different disease environment coincided with the period of greatest annual prevalence of malaria. The prominence of sickness in April (Central region), July (Atlantic), and October (Atlantic) 1862 was attributed to the prevalence of diarrhoea (Fig. 7.7). Diarrhoea, dysentery, and malaria accounted for over a half of all disease cases reported (507 per 1,000 in white troops). The concurrence of the periods of maximum prevalence of these three sicknesses gives prominence to the autumn months in general. The large autumn and small spring elevations in Figure 7.7 are attributed by Smart (Surgeon-General's Office, 1870–88, v. 24) to:

(*a*) autumn/winter 1861, typhoid;
(*b*) November 1862–March 1863, typhoid, diarrhoea, dysentery, malaria;
(*c*) all autumns, diarrhoea, typhoid, and malaria.

7.2.6 Seasonality

The radar charts in Figure 7.8A–C plot the monthly sickness from disease per 1,000 mean strength among the white troops of the US Army on a regional basis and for each year of the conflict. The charts have been plotted on the same scale and show the substantially greater rates experienced in the first year of the conflict when the 'virgin soil' problem was significant. The Pacific region was the theatre least affected by the conflict and experienced lower rates of sickness throughout the war.

Figure 7.8A–C suggests no obvious seasonality in sickness. However, Figure 7.8D plots the seasonal distribution of each region as a difference from the monthly average for the year. Thus a value of zero denotes equality with the monthly average. Plotted in this way, there is a marked pattern of seasonality each year, with strong peaks of excess sickness in April, August, and December (cf. Sect. 7.2.4).

7.2.7 Summary

Soldiers in the American Civil War experienced substantially higher morbidity and mortality from disease than they had during the preceding two decades of peace, and coloured troops suffered disproportionately more than white troops. For all troops, there was a much greater chance of dying from disease than in the heat of battle. The excess morbidity and mortality which

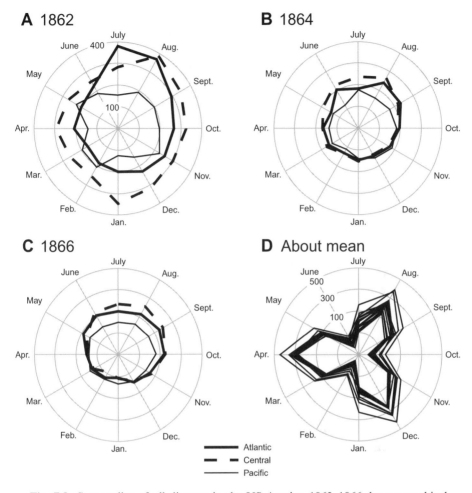

Fig. 7.8. Seasonality of all diseases in the US Armies, 1862–1866, by geographical region

Notes: (A) 1862. (B) 1864. (C) 1866. (D) 1862–6. In D, monthly values are expressed as deviations from the mean rate in a given year. No attempt is made to identify years and regions because of the similarity by time and location when the seasonal distribution is plotted in this way. Charts A–C are on the same scale. The scale of D differs because of the method of calculation.

accompanied the transition from peace to war may be attributed to a mixture of factors including poor camp conditions especially in some regions, inadequate food and hygiene, and limited medical treatment. Equally apparent was the way in which the virgin soil populations of the new recruits suffered in particular, leading to especially high rates in the early months of the war and whenever military necessity led to the raising of new armies.

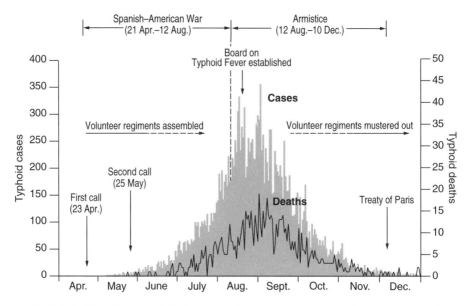

Fig. 7.9. Daily series of typhoid fever cases (bar chart) and deaths (line trace) in sample regiments of the US Volunteer Army during the Spanish–American War, May–December 1898

Source: Smallman-Raynor and Cliff (2001*b*, fig. 1, p. 73).

7.3 Mobilization and Typhoid Fever in the Spanish–American War (1898)

Many of the factors that contribute to the risk of epidemics among newly mobilized forces were to reconverge on the soil of the United States during the Spanish–American War of 1898. Beginning with a first call for volunteers in late April 1898, and swelled by a second call in late May, over 150,000 new recruits were massed in an interconnected system of state assembly camps and national training camps that extended across the eastern United States. Minor outbreaks of camp diseases (cerebrospinal meningitis, measles, mumps, and pneumonia) were to follow. But these outbreaks were dwarfed by an epidemic of typhoid fever that spread through the volunteer encampments (Fig. 7.9). At the height of the epidemic, some 250 to 350 volunteers were struck down by typhoid fever each day; all told, about 24,000 volunteers contracted the disease, and 2,000 died (Reed *et al.*, 1904).

The typhoid epidemic of 1898 was a defining event in the development of hygiene and sanitation in the US Army (Bayne-Jones, 1968: 123–46; Cirillo, 2000). As Cirillo (2000) observes, the epidemic awakened the highest levels of the US military command to basic issues of camp hygiene and disease. Investigations into the cause of the epidemic paved the way for a reorganization of the

Army Medical Department, along with the establishment of the Department of Military Hygiene within the Military Academy at West Point. Military hygiene was effectively promoted to the core curriculum of US military science, with courses in sanitation forming a prerequisite for commission. Fresh insights into the epidemiology of typhoid fever, too, emerged from the inquiries. Not least, healthy carriers, human contacts, and flies were all established as mechanisms in the transmission of the disease (Bayne-Jones, 1968; Cirillo, 2000).

The present section examines the geographical patterns and processes by which typhoid fever spread in the system of state assembly camps and national training camps of the United States during the summer of 1898. Our account draws on the study of Smallman-Raynor and Cliff (2001*b*).

7.3.1 Background to the Epidemic

The aetiology, epidemiology, and clinical course of typhoid fever are reviewed in Appendix 1A. In this subsection, we provide a brief outline of the process of US mobilization during the Spanish–American War, the nature of the camp system in which the volunteer forces were quartered, and the circumstances that promoted the spread of typhoid fever in the assembled contingents.

THE WAR CONTEXT AND US MOBILIZATION

The origins and course of the Spanish–American War (Apr.–Aug. 1898), and its relationship to the Cuban Insurrection against Spain (Feb. 1895–Aug. 1898) (see Sect. 12.3), have been outlined in classic studies by Lodge (1899), Wilson (1900), and Chadwick (1911).[4] Underpinned by a broad range of economic, strategic, humanitarian, and ideological considerations, US military engagement with Spain was precipitated when, on 20 April 1898, the United States issued a demand for the withdrawal of Spanish forces from Cuba. Four days later, on 24 April, Spain responded with a declaration of war and, the following day, the US Congress backdated the official start of the war to 21 April. After a series of successful US military operations on Spanish possessions in the Caribbean (Cuba and Puerto Rico) and Western Pacific (Philippine Islands), an armistice was declared on 12 August 1898. The Treaty of Paris was concluded on 10 December and, with US ratification of the treaty on 6 February 1899, the control of Cuba, Puerto Rico, and the Philippine Islands passed to the United States.

US Mobilization

One prominent feature of the US mobilization against Spain was the rapidity with which a large volunteer army was assembled and mustered into military

---

[4] For other perspectives on the Spanish–American War, see Millis (1931), Foner (1972), Trask (1981), Offner (1992), and Smith (1994).

service. On the eve of the war, the strength of the regular US Army barely exceeded 28,000 officers and men to combat an estimated 400,000 Spaniards under arms. To rectify the imbalance, on 23 April 1898, a first call for volunteers secured the federal draft of the 116,000-strong state militias; a month later, on 25 May, a second call brought the total number of volunteers to in excess of 200,000 (Foner, 1972; Kreidberg and Henry, 1975; Trask, 1981). For the vast majority of these new recruits, an initial period of assembly at local (state) camps and assignment to one of five *c.*30,000-strong Army corps (First, Second, Third, Fourth, and Seventh) was followed by regimental transfer to national training camps in the east and southeast of the United States; most of the remainder, assigned to the Eighth Army Corps and ultimately destined for the Philippine Islands, were dispatched to the west coast (Kreidberg and Henry, 1975).

THE CAMP SYSTEM

As noted earlier in this section, the national training camps to the east and southeast of the United States—and the state assembly camps to which they were linked—formed the focus of the 1898 typhoid fever epidemic in the US Volunteer Army. The locations of the national encampments, proximal to embarkation points for the Caribbean theatre, are mapped in Figure 7.10; the positions of state assembly camps and transit camps referred to in subsequent sections are also indicated.

As Figure 7.10 shows, the system of assembly and training camps spanned much of the east, north central, and southeast of the country. However, many of the campsites were transitory in nature and their number and occupancy waxed and waned with the daily movements of regiments. For detailed information on daily occupancy, we are largely dependent on the regimental data included in Reed *et al.* (1904). According to this source, the state assembly camps rarely exceeded a few thousand men at any given time. The national encampments, however, were of far greater proportions. Camp Thomas, situated at Chickamauga Park (area 24 km²) in northeastern Georgia, was the largest national encampment and, at its daily maximum in late June and early July 1898, is reported to have been occupied by volunteer regiments with a combined mean strength in excess of 46,000. Although somewhat smaller in size, both Camp Alger (Dunn Loring, Virginia) and Camp Meade (Harrisburg, Pennsylvania) had occupancies of at least 21,000 at some stage, while Camp Cuba Libre (Jacksonville, Florida) exceeded 19,000. Yet other national camps,

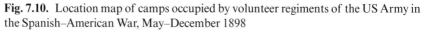

Fig. 7.10. Location map of camps occupied by volunteer regiments of the US Army in the Spanish–American War, May–December 1898

Note: Camp names and spellings are in accordance with the 1904 *Report on the Origin and Spread of Typhoid Fever* (Reed *et al.*, 1904).
Source: Smallman-Raynor and Cliff (2001*b*, fig. 2, p. 75).

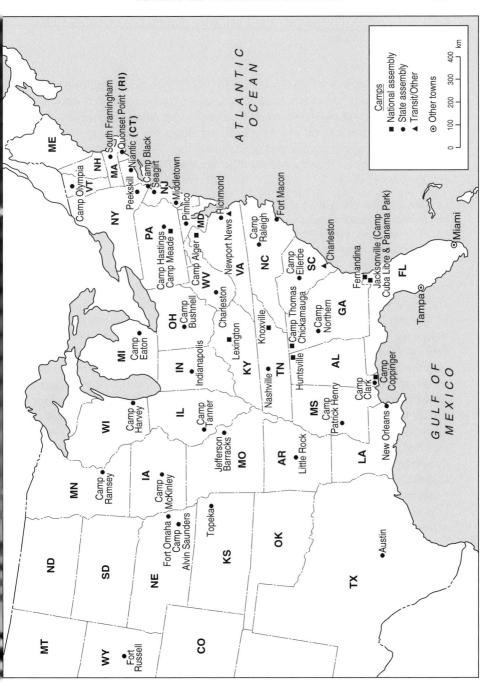

such as Knoxville (Tennessee) and Lexington (Kentucky), exceeded 10,000 men at their maximum.

Sanitary Conditions

Graphic descriptions of the overcrowded and insanitary conditions that greeted many volunteers at the state encampments, and which were to promote the spread of typhoid fever, are provided by regimental physicians. For example, commenting on the sewerage arrangements at Camp Bushnell (Columbus, the state encampment of Ohio; see Fig. 7.10 for location) in April 1898, Lieutenant J. J. Erwin, Assistant Surgeon of the Tenth Ohio Volunteer Infantry, testified:

look any time you would into the fields around that camp and you would see fifty to one hundred to two hundred men defecating . . . The sinks [latrines] were at length provided, and a week or ten days thereafter the rumor passed around that they were infested with 'crabs,' and the men deserted the closets for the fields again.[5]

The campsite of the Tenth Ohio had already been polluted by other regiments, the ground being 'literally covered' with faecal matter; geology, poor drainage, and heavy rains merely conspired to wash the effluent into the low-lying tents of the command (Reed *et al.*, 1904, i. 399). But, if similarly unhealthy conditions were to be found at some other state camps such as Camp Tanner (Springfield, Illinois; see Reed *et al.*, 1904, i. 21), the epidemiological risks were magnified at the national camps. At Camp Thomas—one of the principal foci of the typhoid epidemic—the construction of regimental latrines was hindered by the thin top soil and limestone geology of Chickamauga Park. The shallow privies flooded in heavy rains, with the waste flowing over the campsites of neighbouring commands, and onwards for the main water supply. Overcrowded tents, sometimes with earth floors and pitched on the sites of abandoned latrines, became contaminated as did blankets and other equipage. Insufficient supplies of disinfectants, exposure to contaminated dust, inadequate bathing facilities, an abundance of flies, and the difficulties of distancing kitchens from human waste added further to the health hazard.[6] Similar, if less extreme, conditions prevailed at other national encampments.

7.3.2 Data: The Reed–Vaughan–Shakespeare Report

On 18 August 1898—within days of the declaration of an armistice in the war with Spain and at the very height of the typhoid epidemic in US volunteer regiments (Fig. 7.9)—Special Order 194 of the Adjutant-General's Office, US War Department, provided for

a board of medical officers, to consist of Maj. Walter Reed, surgeon, US Army, Maj. Victor C. Vaughan, division surgeon, US Volunteers, and Maj. Edward O. Shakespeare,

---

[5] Evidence presented to the Board on Typhoid Fever, cited in Reed *et al.* (1904, i. 396).
[6] See e.g. the testimony of regimental surgeons and officials presented to the Board on Typhoid Fever and cited in Reed *et al.* (1904, i. 1–283).

brigade surgeon, US Volunteers . . . for the purpose of making an investigation into the cause of the extensive prevalence of typhoid fever in the various military camps within the limits of the United States.[7] (see Pl. 7.2)

After an initial tour of inspection of the national encampments in the east and southeast of the United States,[8] followed by an exhaustive examination of regimental and hospital sick reports for the volunteer organizations of the Army corps,[9] the preliminary findings of the Board on Typhoid Fever were published in abstract form in 1900 (Reed *et al.*, 1900).[10] An Act of Congress provided for the preparation of a full report, and this was finally published in 1904 as the *Report on the Origin and Spread of Typhoid Fever in US Military Camps during the Spanish War of 1898*, volumes i and ii (Reed *et al.*, 1904) (see Pl. 1.2D).

It is convenient to divide the information contained in the *Report* into two categories: numerical data and textual accounts.

1. *Numerical data.* As described in Section 7.3.3, the epidemic began in the volunteer regiments during the early days of May 1898 and, although typhoid deaths were to persist into 1899, the epidemic was substantially over by the end of 1898. For the 245-day period, 1 May to 31 December, the two volumes of the *Report* provide (i) systematic listings (vol. i) and/or graphical portrayals (vol. ii) of the daily counts of typhoid cases and deaths in the regiments and (ii) information on the mean strengths and daily locations of these commands.

2. *Textual accounts.* In volume i of the *Report*, the numerical data are supplemented by textual accounts of epidemic progress in each regiment. The accounts are drawn from a variety of sources, but include: (i) statements abstracted from regimental sick reports; (ii) the testimony of regimental surgeons; and (iii) personal observations of the members of the Board on Typhoid Fever.

For the purposes of the analysis to follow, we use the numerical counts of typhoid fever contained in the *Report* to examine the processes by which the epidemic spread through the system of military encampments occupied by volunteer regiments of the US Army. Where appropriate, the textual accounts are used to flesh out the numerical evidence.

---

[7] Special Order 194 (sect. 40), issued by H. C. Corbin, Adjutant-General, US War Department; cited in Reed *et al.* (1904, i., p. xiii).

[8] The tour of inspection began in the third week of August 1898 and included: Camp Alger, Va. (20 Aug. 1898); Fernandina, Fla. (26 Aug.); Camp Cuba Libre, Fla. (28 Aug.); Huntsville, Ala. (7 Sept.); Camp Thomas, Ga. (10 Sept.); Knoxville, Tenn. (14 Sept.); and Camp Meade, Pa. (30 Sept.). Victor C. Vaughan's autobiography *A Doctor's Memories*, published in 1926, provides some flavour of the tour. See also Bean (1982: 87–95).

[9] Vaughan and Shakespeare were discharged from the Army in June 1899, but continued their systematic examination of regimental and hospital sick reports at the Army Medical Museum, Washington, until June 1900.

[10] A year earlier, in 1899, the Board had presented a preliminary report of their findings under the title *Preliminary Report on Typhoid in Military Camps of the United States. To: The Surgeon-General of the Army*, Washington, 25 Jan. 1899. The report was reproduced in 1940 in the *Army Medical Bulletin*, 53: 73–103.

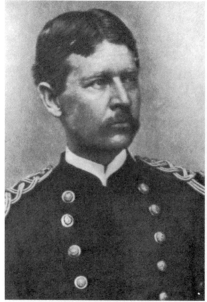

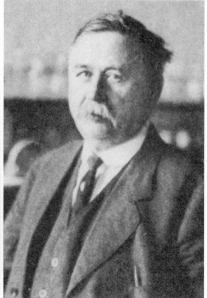

A

B

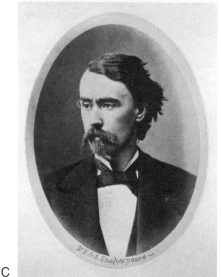

C

Pl. 7.2. Appointed members of the Board on Typhoid Fever, and authors of the *Report on the Origin and Spread of Typhoid Fever in US Military Camps during the Spanish War of 1898* (Washington: Government Printing Office, 1904)

Notes: (A) Walter Reed (1851–1902): US Army medical officer, bacteriologist, and chair of the Board. (B) Victor C. Vaughan (1851–1929): biochemist, bacteriologist, and medical officer with the US Volunteers during the Spanish–American War. (C) Edward O. Shakespeare (1846–1900): bacteriologist, physician, and medical officer with the US Volunteers during the Spanish–American War. *Sources*: (Pls. A and B) Bordley and Harvey (1976, figs. 48 and 23, pp. 199 and 112); (Pl. C) Library of the College of Physicians of Philadelphia.

THE NUMERICAL DATABASE

Full details relating to the construction of the numerical database are given in Smallman-Raynor and Cliff (2001*b*: 76–8), where issues of data quality are also discussed. In brief, for 89 sample regiments (*n*) encamped at a total of 69 different geographical locations (*N*) during the 245-day (*t*) observation period, the counts of typhoid cases[11] were abstracted from the Reed–Vaughan–Shake-speare *Report* to form a three-dimensional 89 (regiment) × 69 (camp) × 245 (days) matrix of disease activity. Further matrices of typhoid activity were then formed by dividing the original matrix into the constituent regiments and encampments of the four corps (First, Second, Third, and Seventh Army Corps) to which the sample commands were attached. Finally, for each of the matrices, the daily counts were combined by seven-day period[12] and summed across the *n* regiments to yield *N* camps × 35 weeks matrices of typhoid cases and typhoid case rates (per 10,000 mean strength) for (i) the entire set of 89 reg-iments and (ii) each of the four Army corps. The total number of regiments and encampments associated with each of the four Army corps is given in Table 7.6. Summary details of the typhoid epidemic in each Army corps are also provid-ed in the table, while Table 7.7 provides an overview of the distribution of typhoid cases by encampment. The *N* × 35 matrices of weekly typhoid cases and typhoid case rates (per 10,000 mean strength) comprise the main plank of the statistical analyses in this section.

7.3.3 Spread Reconstructions

ORIGINS OF THE EPIDEMIC: STATE ASSEMBLY CAMPS

Although cases of typhoid fever had appeared in commands of the regular army soon after the declaration of war (see Reed *et al.*, 1904, i. 500–1), one important feature of the epidemic in volunteer regiments was the role of newly enlisted men in the temporally coincident—but apparently independent—introduction of the disease to a plethora of state assembly camps. The *Condensed Sick Report* for the First Pennsylvania Volunteer Infantry, prepared by Major and Surgeon William G. Harland and dated May 1898, provided the first unequivocal evidence of typhoid fever in the volunteer forces: a prospec-tively diagnosed case at Camp Hastings, the state assembly camp of Pennsyl-vania, on 12 May (Reed *et al.*, 1904, i. 88–94); see Figure 7.10 for location. In

---

[11] As described by Smallman-Raynor and Cliff (2001*b*: 76), the *Report* makes frequent—sometimes scathing—reference to the apparent failure of medical personnel to recognize, diagnose, and record cases of typhoid fever. Under such circumstances, one outstanding action of the Board was to engage in a sys-tematic examination of the many thousands of medical records relating to all suspicious cases of typhoid fever. In this manner, the *Report* draws a distinction between *recognized* cases of typhoid fever (i.e. cases *prospectively* diagnosed and reported by attendant physicians) and *probable* cases of typhoid fever (cases *retrospectively* diagnosed by the Board on Typhoid Fever) (see Reed *et al.*, 1904, i., xviii). Although the potential for error in the retrospective diagnoses cannot be excluded, and this was recognized by the authors of the *Report*, all typhoid data examined in the present study relate to the combined counts of recognized and probable typhoid fever.

[12] The aggregation of daily disease counts by seven-day (weekly calendar) period represented a bal-ance between the need for (i) sufficient numbers of typhoid cases to avoid statistical instabilities in the computation of disease rates and (ii) sufficient time intervals to permit an examination of temporal pat-terns in the epidemic spread process. Weekly calendar periods (Sunday to Saturday) were formed by dividing the 245-day observation period into 35 seven-day units, beginning with the period Sunday 1 to Saturday 7 May (week 1) and ending with the period Sunday 25 to Saturday 31 December (week 35).

Table 7.6. Typhoid fever in volunteer regiments of the United States Army, 1898

Army Corps	No. of regiments (n)	No. of camps (N)[1]	Mean Strength	All deaths[2]	Typhoid fever		Epidemic start[3]	Epidemic end[4]	Epidemic peak[5]
					Cases[2]	Deaths[2]			
First	24	26	29,919	520 (173.8)	5,966 (1,994.1)	404 (135.0)	8 May	14 Dec	1 Sept
Second	32	34	36,183	457 (126.3)	4,649 (1,284.9)	388 (107.2)	14 May	28 Dec	1 Sept
Third	16	22	19,291	438 (227.0)	4,071 (2,110.3)	393 (203.7)	21 May	11 Nov	15 Aug
Seventh	17	21	19,969	434 (217.3)	4,004 (2,005.1)	361 (180.8)	14 May	29 Dec	13 Sept
Total	89	69	105,362	1,849 (175.5)	18,690 (1,773.9)	1,546 (146.7)	8 May	28 Dec	1 Sept

Notes: [1] Number of different camps occupied in the period 1 May–31 December 1898. [2] Rate per 10,000 mean strength in parentheses. [3] Date of presentation of the first identified case of typhoid fever. [4] Date of presentation of the last identified case of typhoid fever. [5] Date of maximum typhoid morbidity.
Data refer to a sample of 89 regiments of the First, Second, Third, and Seventh Army Corps.
Source: Smallman-Raynor and Cliff (2001*b*, table 1, p. 77), based on data abstracted from Reed *et al.* (1904, i and ii).

Table 7.7. Cases of typhoid fever in camps occupied by volunteer regiments of the US Army in the Spanish–American War, 1898

Camp	Typhoid cases	First case	Last case	Epidemic peak[1]
National training camps[2]				
Camp Thomas	5,437	17 May	14 Sept.	16 Aug.
Camp Alger	727	21 May	8 Sept.	25 Aug.
Camp Cuba Libre	3,400	25 May	6 Nov.	13 Sept.
Camp Meade	2,244	10 Aug.	18 Nov.	19 Sept.
Other camps[3]/unknown	6,882	8 May	29 Dec.	30 Aug.

Notes: [1] Date of peak typhoid morbidity. [2] National training camps that served as the initial rendezvous for volunteer regiments of the First, Second, Third, and Seventh Army Corps. [3] Includes state assembly camps, national training camps (other than Camps Thomas, Alger, Meade, and Cuba Libre), transit camps, and camps in Cuba and Puerto Rico.
Source: Smallman-Raynor and Cliff (2001*b*, table 2, p. 77), based on data abstracted from Reed *et al.* (1904, i and ii).

fact, by this date, Camp Hastings had already played host to two probable cases of the disease in the Sixteenth Pennsylvania.[13] Almost simultaneously, sporadic cases of typhoid fever began to appear in newly formed regiments at Camp Harvey (Milwaukee, Wisconsin) on 11 May, Camp Bushnell (Columbus, Ohio) on 14 May, Camp Tanner (Springfield, Illinois) on 15 May, and Camp Black (Hempstead, New York) on 18 May (ibid. 17–21, 32–8, 312–18, 320–1, 573–85).

But, if these state camps yielded the first clinical evidence of typhoid fever, many other camps were actively incubating the disease. By the final week of May, epidemiological evidence suggests that *Salmonella typhi* had entered—if not widely colonized—the state assembly camps of Georgia (Camp Northern), Iowa (Camp McKinley), Mississippi (Camp Patrick Henry), Nebraska (Camp Alvin Saunders), and South Carolina (Camp Ellerbe), among others (further details in Table 7.8).

Figure 7.9, above, charts the development of the typhoid epidemic from these beginnings. For the 245-day period, 1 May to 31 December 1898, the bar graph plots the aggregate daily counts of typhoid cases in the 89 sample regiments analysed. For reference, the line trace is based on supplementary information included in the *Report* and plots, for a subset of 49 regiments, the aggregate daily counts of typhoid deaths.[14] As Figure 7.9 shows, after an initial period of slow growth in May and June, the epidemic grew rapidly in July, to

[13] Two cases of unusually prolonged 'diarrhoea', retrospectively diagnosed as typhoid fever, presented at Camp Hastings, Pennsylvania, on 8 and 10 May. These cases represent the earliest evidence of typhoid fever in volunteer organizations. See Reed *et al.* (1904, i. 28–32).
[14] Daily mortality counts are unavailable for 40 of the 89 sample regiments included in the present study.

reach a peak in the August and early September of the armistice. Thereafter, and with the progressive demobilization of the volunteer regiments, the epidemic subsided in October and November, but with disease activity lingering to the end of the year.

EPIDEMIC FOCI: NATIONAL TRAINING CAMPS

While the ultimate origins of the epidemic can be traced to a disparate set of state assembly camps, the decision of the US War Department to override the original recommendations of the Commanding General of the Army[15] and to concentrate the volunteers in a handful of national training camps[16] served not only to focus the epidemic spatially but also to supercharge its spread. Pivotal to this process were four national training camps, variously designated as the initial reception points for the volunteer commands: (i) Camp Thomas (Chickamauga Park, Georgia), the rendezvous for regiments of the First and Third Corps; (ii) Camp Alger (Dunn Loring, Virginia) for first call regiments of the Second Corps; (iii) Camp Meade (Harrisburg, Pennsylvania) for second call regiments of the Second Corps; and (iv) Camp Cuba Libre (Jacksonville, Florida) for the Seventh Corps. The locations of the four camps are given in Figure 7.10.

Table 7.8 is based on the textual evidence included in the *Report* and lists those regiments posited by the Board on Typhoid Fever to have carried typhoid fever from state assembly camps to the four national training camps. For each of the national camps, the table gives the state (source) camp and the infected (index) regiment, the date of arrival of the regiment at the national camp, and the associated date of the first clinical evidence of typhoid fever. Again, Figure 7.10 serves as a location map.

Table 7.8 implicates no less than 62 volunteer regiments originating from a total of 29 different state assembly camps in the initial spread of typhoid fever to the national training camps. The timing and extent of the seeding process varied from one training camp to another. The largest of the national camps, Camp Thomas, was seeded most heavily, with 27 infected regiments of the First and Third Army Corps reaching the campsite in the 16 days to 31 May 1898. By the same date, infected regiments—albeit far fewer in number—had also entered Camps Alger and Cuba Libre. Finally, and considerably later in the epidemic, the establishment of Camp Meade in August 1898 was accompanied by an influx of infected commands that had assembled in response to the second call for volunteers.

---

[15] On 26 April 1898, the Commanding General of the Army, Maj. Gen. Nelson A. Miles, recommended to the Secretary of War, Russell A. Alger, that the volunteer regiments should be retained in state camps for a period of some two months, where they would be equipped, organized, and prepared for active service (Kreidberg and Henry, 1975: 156).

[16] The factors that influenced the decision to concentrate the volunteer regiments in national training camps are outlined by Alger (1901: 26–8). See also: Kreidberg and Henry (1975: 166) and Trask (1981: 158–9).

Table 7.8. Geographical sources of typhoid fever in US national assembly camps during the Spanish–American War, 1898

Probable source of infection	Regiment	Date of arrival at national camp	Date of first typhoid case[1]
Camp Thomas (Chickamauga, Georgia): First and Third Army Corps			
Camp Harvey, Wis.	3rd Wisconsin Vol. Inf.	15 May	24 May
Camp Bushnell, Oh.	4th & 6th Ohio Vol. Inf.	16 & 18 May	17 & 18 May
Indianapolis, Ind.	158th Indiana Vol. Inf.	16 May	6 June
Camp Hastings, Pa.	16th, 1st, & 5th Pennsylvania Vol. Inf.	17, 18, & 20 May	8, 12 & 19 May
Camp Eaton, Mich.	31st Michigan Vol. Inf.	17 May	1 June
Camp Tanner, Ill.	3rd & 5th Illinois Vol. Inf.	17 May	17 & 16 May
Camp Ramsey, Minn.	14th Minnesota Vol. Inf.	18 May	27 May
Charleston, W. Va.	1st West Virginia Vol. Inf.	20 May	6 June
Topeka, Kan.	21st Kansas Vol. Inf.	20 May	21 May
Peekskill, NY	2nd & 9th New York Vol. Inf.	21 & 26 May	1 & 10 June
Jefferson Barracks, Mo.	1st & 5th Missouri Vol. Inf.	21 & 27 May	31 May & 6 June
Camp Alvin Saunders, Nebr.	2nd Nebraska Vol. Inf.	22 May	26 May
Camp Ramsdell, NH	1st New Hampshire Vol. Inf.	22 May	24 May
Nashville, Tenn.	3rd Tennessee Vol. Inf.	24 May	9 June
Camp Olympia, Vt.	1st Vermont Vol. Inf.	24 May	26 May
Lexington, Ky.	2nd & 3rd Kentucky Vol. Inf.	26 May & 2 June	26 & 9 June
Little Rock, Ark.	1st & 2nd Arkansas Vol. Inf.	27 & 30 May	2 & 4 June
Camp McKinley, Ia.	52nd Iowa Vol. Inf.	31 May	8 June
Camp Patrick Henry, Miss.	1st Mississippi Vol. Inf.	31 May	1 June
Camp Ellerbe, SC	1st South Carolina Vol. Inf.	7 June	May
Camp Northern, Ga.	1st Georgia Vol. Inf.	17 June	6 June
Camp Alger (Dunn Loring, Virginia): Second Army Corps			
Camp Hastings, Pa.	6th & 8th Pennsylvania Vol. Inf.	18 & 19 May	29 & 15 May
Camp Black, NY	65th New York Vol. Inf.	20 May	20 May
Camp Bushnell, Oh.	7th Ohio Vol. Inf.	21 May	16 May
Camp Tanner, Ill.	6th Illinois Vol. Inf.	21 May	15 May
South Framingham, Mass.	6th Massachusetts Vol. Inf.	22 May	2 June
Not stated	New York Vol. Cav. (Troops A & C)	23 May	30 May
Nashville, Tenn.	2nd Tennessee Vol. Inf.	29 May	29 May
Richmond, Va.	3rd Virginia Vol. Inf.	5 June	22 June
Camp Eaton, Mich.	34th Michigan Vol. Inf.	9 June	Not known

Table 7.8. (*cont.*)

Probable source of infection	Regiment	Date of arrival at national camp	Date of first typhoid case[1]
Camp Cuba Libre (Jacksonville, Florida): Seventh Army Corps			
Camp Tanner, Ill.	2nd, 4th, & 9th Illinois Vol. Inf.	23 & 29 May & 8 Aug.	25 May, 11 & 2 July
Camp Harvey, Wis.	1st Wisconsin Vol. Inf.	24 May	21 June
Richmond, Va.	2nd & 4th Virginia Vol. Inf.	3 & 7 June	2 & 11 June
Camp Patrick Henry, Miss.	2nd Mississippi Vol. Inf.	21 June	8 June
Fort Omaha, Nebr.	3rd Nebraska Vol. Inf.	22 July	26 July
Camp Ellerbe, SC	1st & 2nd South Carolina	29 July & 16 Sept.	May & 20 June
Indianapolis, Ind.	161st Indiana Vol. Inf	14 Aug.	16 July
Jefferson Barracks, Mo.	6th Missouri Vol. Inf.	15 Aug.	1 Aug.
Camp Meade (Harrisburg, Pennsylvania): Second Army Corps			
Camp Bushnell, Oh.	10th Ohio Vol. Inf	19 Aug.	16 July
Middletown, Del.	1st Delaware Vol. Inf.	20 Aug.	21 May
Charleston, W. Va.	2nd West Virginia Vol. Inf.	30 Aug.	10 July
Pimlico, Md.	1st Maryland Vol. Inf.	9 Sept.	2 Aug.
Niantic, Conn.	3rd Connecticut Vol. Inf.	10 Sept.	14 Aug.
Camp Black, NY	203rd & 202nd New York Vol. Inf.	12 & 14 Sept.	27 July & 30 Aug.
South Framingham, Mass.	5th Massachusetts Vol. Inf.	12 Sept.	2 Aug.
Camp Eaton, Mich.	35th Michigan Vol. Inf.	16 Sept.	2 Aug.
Camp Ramsey, Minn.	15th Minnesota Vol. Inf.	18 Sept.	3 Aug.
Seagirt, NJ	4th New Jersey Vol. Inf.	9 Oct.	2 Aug.

Notes: [1] Includes cases retrospectively identified by the Board on Typhoid Fever.
All information relates to the regiments of the First, Second, Third, and Seventh Army Corps.
Source: Smallman-Raynor and Cliff (2001*b*, table 3, p. 79), based on data abstracted from Reed *et al.* (1904, i).

Some flavour of the seeding of the national training camps can be gained from the testimony of military physicians. For example, commenting on the role of regiments of the Third Army Corps in the initial introduction of the typhoid bacillus to Camp Thomas, Colonel John Hoff, Chief Surgeon of the Corps, reported that

Typhoid fever was brought in in the very beginning with the troops [*sic*] . . . Three regiments . . . came on the ground with what was practically a disabling sick list. These three regiments were the First Mississippi and the First and Second Arkansas. The record of the First Mississippi begins on the 12th of June and total of sick for that day was 64 . . . The Arkansas regiments came into this camp in practically the same condition as did the Mississippi regiment . . . Typhoid fever gradually spread from the infected regiments and soon there were cases in every regiment of the Corps . . . I believe the water supply became infected about the latter part of July.[17]

As implied by the quote from Hoff, and as described in more detail in Section 7.3.1, the national training camps were to provide fertile ground for the rapid and widespread dissemination of typhoid fever. The dimensions of the problem can be seen in Table 7.7; from the first case of the disease at Camp Thomas in mid-May, to the last case at Camp Meade in mid-November, no less than 11,808 typhoid cases (equivalent to a rate of 1,121 cases per 10,000 mean strength) were recorded in the four training camps. This high incidence was to secure the position of Camps Thomas, Alger, Meade, and Cuba Libre as major staging posts for the onwards spread of the epidemic.

SUBSEQUENT MOVEMENTS OF INFECTED REGIMENTS

One important feature of US mobilization in the Spanish–American War was the high degree of spatial mobility of the volunteer commands. So, although the volunteer regiments were initially dispatched to one of the four national training camps listed in Table 7.8, their sojourn of several weeks or months was followed by transfer to other camps. In the absence of an effective quarantine strategy, it may be hypothesized that this mobility played an important role in the spatial development of the epidemic.

Against this background, Figure 7.11 is based on the numerical information included in the Reed–Vaughan–Shakespeare *Report* and charts the implied movements of typhoid fever with the dispersal of regiments from Camps Thomas, Alger, Meade, and Cuba Libre. To form the maps, the documented camp-wise movements of the 89 sample regiments of the First, Second, Third, and Seventh Army Corps were first entered into a set of regiment-specific matrices **M**, where each element, m_{ij}, was set equal to 1 if origin camp i and destination camp j were directly linked by the regiment, and $m_{ij} = 0$ otherwise. For each matrix, the non-zero settings were then examined according to the time

---

[17] Testimony of Colonel John Hoff, Chief Surgeon of the Third Army Corps, cited in Reed *et al.* (1904, i. 266–7).

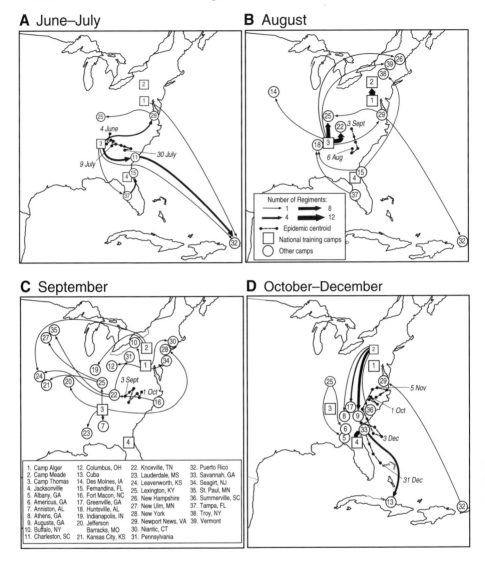

Fig. 7.11. Movements of typhoid-infected regiments of the First, Second, Third, and Seventh US Army Corps, June–December 1898

Notes: The solid vectors trace the camp-wise movements of typhoid-infected regiments in (A) June and July, (B) August, (C) September, and (D) October to December. On each map, the black circles plot the weekly position of the mean geographical centre of typhoid morbidity. Note that the legend and key to the four maps have been positioned in B and C for convenience.

Source: Smallman-Raynor and Cliff (2001*b*, fig. 3, p. 81).

interval t (in days) that elapsed between the date of departure from camp i and the date of the first case of typhoid fever at camp j. With a minimum expected incubation period of eight days for typhoid fever (see App. 1A), and subject to the uncertain role of a long-term (sub-clinical) carrier state in the spread of the 1898 epidemic, values of $t \leq 8$ provide a (conservative) indicator of those regiments that acquired the infection at camp i and carried it to camp j.[18]

On this basis, the solid vectors in Figure 7.11 chart the movements of typhoid-infected regiments in the periods June–July (Fig. 7.11A), August (Fig. 7.11B), September (Fig. 7.11C), and October–December (Fig. 7.11D). In all instances, vector widths are drawn proportional to the number of infected regiments that linked a pair of camps. To assist interpretation, the national training camps from which typhoid fever ultimately spread (Camps Thomas, Alger, Meade, and Cuba Libre) are denoted by squares; all other camps are marked with open circles. Finally, to chart the shifting locus of typhoid activity with regimental movements, the black circles on Figure 7.11A–D plot the weekly position of the mean geographical centre of typhoid morbidity in the entire system of camps (see Sect. 6.5.2); sample dates (coded to the last day of the calendar week) are indicated, while the broken vectors link the position of the morbidity centre in successive weeks.

The solid vectors in Figure 7.11 do not necessarily represent the complete set of diffusion corridors involved in the spread of the typhoid epidemic. Rather, they identify pairs of camps that were linked by the movements of typhoid-infected regiments as deduced from one epidemiologically informed reading of the clinical reports. While the contribution of regimental mobility to the diffusion of the epidemic is examined statistically in Section 7.3.4, Figure 7.11 provides evidence for the role of Camp Thomas (June–Sept.; Figs. 7.11A–C), Camp Alger (Aug.–Sept.; Figs. 7.11B, 7.11C), Camp Meade (Sept.–Dec.; Figs. 7.11C, 7.11D) and Camp Cuba Libre (Oct.–Dec.; Fig. 7.11D) in the dissemination of the epidemic.

Operations associated with the Puerto Rico Campaign (25 July–12 Aug.) were to dominate the early phase of the epidemic (Fig. 7.11A). Beginning in early July, typhoid-infected regiments of the First Division, First Army Corps, began to disperse from an epidemic focus at Camp Thomas, with the coastal transit camps at Newport News (Virginia) and Charleston (South Carolina) as the principal destinations. In the opinion of the regimental surgeon of the Third Wisconsin Volunteer Infantry at least, the Charleston camp was 'not the best from a sanitary point of view'[19] and, from an initial position close to Camp Thomas, the geographical centre of typhoid activity drifted eastwards with

---

[18] The decision to limit the analysis to values of $t \leq 8$ was based on the minimum expected incubation period of typhoid fever and, therefore, a conservative reading of the typhoid reports. In fact, an extension of the analysis to include the entire range of the expected incubation period (i.e. to adopt the criterion of $t \leq 14$) has minimal impact on the patterns depicted in Fig. 7.11.

[19] Report of Maj. and Surgeon John B. Edwards, Third Wisconsin Volunteer Infantry, cited in Reed *et al.* (1904, i. 9).

troop movements to South Carolina. In turn, Charleston formed a staging post for the onwards spread of typhoid fever with US Army transports bound for the Caribbean island of Puerto Rico. The Third Wisconsin, among other regiments, experienced active cases of typhoid fever on the week-long voyage to Puerto Rico,[20] while Captain and Assistant Surgeon T. B. Wright testified to the plight of the Puerto Rico-bound Fourth Ohio: 'We had a batch of cases develop . . . during transit . . . then another apparently distinct lot of cases soon after landing . . . After August 15 we had cases coming on all the time . . . It is certain that we carried the infection with us to Porto Rico . . .'.[21]

As a remedial response to the burgeoning problem of typhoid fever at Camp Thomas and Camp Alger, the month of August was dominated by the exodus of regiments from the two camps. The principal movements are traced by the broad vectors in Figure 7.11B and include: (i) the transfer of infected regiments from Camp Thomas to the newly established camps at Lexington (Kentucky) and Knoxville (Tennessee); and (ii) the transfer of infected regiments from Camp Alger to Camp Meade. One aspect of the latter transfer—an aborted march through Virginia by regiments of the Second Division, Second Army Corps—failed dismally in its aim to rid the commands of typhoid fever, and the completion of the journey by train merely served to hasten the appearance of the disease in Camp Meade.[22] The seeding of Camp Meade was further bolstered by the arrival of regiments from the state assembly camps (see Table 7.8), but most other movements of typhoid-infected regiments were centred on Camp Thomas, Newport News, and Fernandina (Florida) and encompassed the lone transfer of volunteer commands to a variety of state camps, national camps, and Puerto Rico. Overall, the vectors in Figure 7.11B trace a broad northerly movement of regiments and this was accompanied by a northerly drift of the geographical centre of disease activity to North Carolina.

For the remaining time periods in Figure 7.11, the supporting testimony of regimental physicians is largely absent from the *Report* and our knowledge of the movements of typhoid-infected regiments is dependent on the size and direction of the vectors in Figures 7.11C and 7.11D. As Figure 7.11C shows, the month of September was characterized by a set of overlapping transmis-

---

[20] Report of Maj. and Surgeon John B. Edwards, Third Wisconsin Volunteer Infantry, cited in Reed *et al.* (1904, i. 9).

[21] Testimony of Captain and Assistant Surgeon T. B. Wright, Fourth Ohio Volunteer Infantry, cited in Reed *et al.* (1904, i. 23).

[22] In a lengthy consideration of the march of the Second Division, Second Army Corps, the Board on Typhoid Fever noted that: 'it will be plainly seen that this division not only failed to shake off typhoid fever, but even experienced an increase of this disease. We can . . . readily see that this was due to the fact that the division, after marching for six days, went into a more or less permanent camp at Thoroughfare Gap, Va., and as each regiment was already badly infected there was no reason why the disease should not continue to be propagated in increased numbers . . . Indeed, the very object for which this march was begun was effectually defeated by the stay of the division at Thoroughfare Gap . . . From a sanitary point of view the transference of this division by rail from Thoroughfare Gap, Va., to Camp Meade, Pa., was a mistake, since each of the regiments carried the infection with them . . .' (Reed *et al.*, 1904, i. 367).

sion cells, with each cell centred on one of five national camps (Camp Thomas, Camp Alger, Camp Meade, and the camps at Knoxville and Lexington). The cells span much of the northeastern, southern, and midwestern sectors of the United States and reflect the return of some infected regiments to their home states, eventually to be mustered out of the Army. The geographical centre of disease activity remained rooted in the Carolinas during this period.

The final time period in Figure 7.11, relating to the months of October, November, and December (Fig. 7.11D), was associated with three main processes: (i) a wholesale, southerly, relocation of infected regiments from Camp Meade and Lexington to newly established camps in Georgia; (ii) a mass transfer of infected regiments from Camp Cuba Libre to the coastal transit camp at Savannah (Georgia); and (iii) onwards carriage of the disease from Savannah to post-war Cuba. As Figure 7.11D shows, the three processes were to result in a sharp southerly movement of the geographical centre of typhoid activity, eventually to terminate off the coast of Florida.

7.3.4 Diffusion Processes

Although the foregoing analysis provides insights into the camp-wise movements of infected regiments, alternative methods are required to determine the nature of the processes that underpinned the spread of the epidemic. In this section, we use the technique of autocorrelation on graphs (Sect. 6.4.2) to examine the processes by which typhoid spread in (i) the entire system of encampments occupied by regiments of the volunteer army, and (ii) the sub-systems of encampments occupied by the constituent regiments of the individual Army corps.

DIFFUSION PROCESSES AND THE MODEL OF RELOCATION DIFFUSION

Our analysis begins with a brief comment on diffusion processes. As described in Section 6.4.1, accounts of the geographical spread of infectious diseases—based largely on studies of the fixed settlement systems of civil populations—usually recognize two principal types of diffusion process: *contagious diffusion* and *hierarchical diffusion*. It is evident from the foregoing analysis, however, that a further model is required to handle the component of epidemic transmission associated with the inter-camp movements of typhoid-infected regiments. To these ends, we utilize a model of epidemic transmission that is referred to as *relocation diffusion*. As defined in Cliff *et al.* (1981: 6), in relocation diffusion, the objects being diffused leave the areas where they originated as they move to new areas. Such relocation diffusion informed our reconstruction in Figure 7.11; the wholesale relocation of regiments from one encampment to another drove the spatial course of the epidemic—a mechanism that was governed by military diktat and logic.

METHOD: AUTOCORRELATION ON GRAPHS

The method of autocorrelation on graphs is described in Section 6.4.2. The area occupied by each of the five sets of encampments (the entire system of encampments of the volunteer army, and the four subsystems of encampments occupied by the First, Second, Third, and Seventh Army Corps) was reduced to three graphs: (i) a hierarchical graph; (ii) a contagious graph, formed as a minimum spanning tree (MST); and (iii) a relocation graph. Definitions of graphs (i) and (ii) are given in Appendix 6A.1. Graph (iii) was defined by setting each element, w_{ij}, in a matrix W equal to 1 if camps i and j were directly connected by the relocation of a regiment, and $w_{ij} = 0$ otherwise follows. The graph thus defines the area such that each camp is linked to those camps from which a regimental transfer was received.

As outlined in Appendix 6A.1, the goodness-of-fit between each of the graphs and typhoid morbidity was determined by the computation of the spatial autocorrelation coefficient, Moran's I, for each week of the time series of typhoid case rates (per 10,000 mean strength). In this manner, the autocorrelation analysis yielded a total of 15 (5 sets of encampments × 3 diffusion graphs) 35-week time series for I.

RESULTS, I: ALL ENCAMPMENTS

Diffusion Processes

For the entire system of encampments associated with the four sample Army corps, Figure 7.12 plots the weekly values of I for the relocation graph (Fig. 7.12A), the contagious (MST) graph (Fig. 7.12B) and the camp hierarchy graph (Fig. 7.12C). Here, the horizontal axes have been formed by coding the first week of the epidemic (week ending 7 May) as week 1, with subsequent weeks coded sequentially up to, and including, the final week of the year (week 35, ending 31 Dec.). The vertical line, set at week 16 (ending 20 Aug.), marks the week of peak typhoid morbidity; weeks prior to the peak (weeks 1–15) correspond to the build-up phase of the epidemic, while weeks after the peak (weeks 17–35) correspond to the fade-out phase. Finally, the pecked horizontal lines at $z = 1.65$ mark the statistically significant I coefficients at the $p = 0.05$ level in a one-tailed test for positive spatial autocorrelation; values above this level represent periods when the actual diffusion process corresponded significantly with the diffusion graphs.

Figure 7.12A shows that regiment relocation (or transfer) was important during the build-up phase of the epidemic. From the weeks immediately preceding the epidemic peak, however, values dropped to low and negative levels, but with a sharp resurgence in the closing stages of the epidemic. In marked contrast, Figure 7.12B shows that the contagious (MST) graph is of fleeting importance only in the early stages of epidemic fade-out. Finally, and despite isolated spikes of activity in the build-up phase, the camp hierarchy graph (Fig. 7.12C) attains prominence in the later stages of epidemic fade-out.

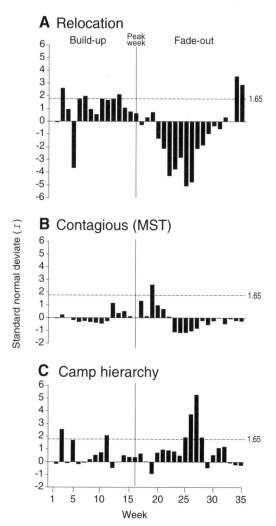

Fig. 7.12. Diffusion of typhoid fever in the system of encampments occupied by the First, Second, Third, and Seventh US Army Corps, May–December 1898

Notes: The bar charts plot weekly values of the spatial autocorrelation coefficient, Moran's *I*, as a standard Normal deviate for different diffusion graphs. (A) Relocation graph. (B) Contagious (MST) graph. (C) Camp hierarchy graph. Horizontal lines at $z = 1.65$ mark the statistically significant *I* coefficients at the $p = 0.05$ level in a one-tailed test for positive spatial autocorrelation. *Source*: Smallman-Raynor and Cliff (2001*b*, fig. 4, p. 84).

Phase Relationships

While Figure 7.12 confirms that each spread process contributed to the overall diffusion of typhoid fever, the results imply that the operation of each process was associated with a discrete stage of the epidemic cycle. Adopting the

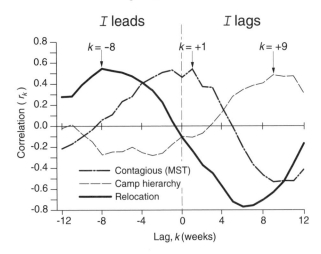

Fig. 7.13. Cross-correlation functions (CCFs) between the weekly typhoid case rate (10,000 mean strength) and the spatial autocorrelation coefficient, I, calculated for three different diffusion graphs: relocation; contagious (MST); and camp hierarchy

Note: For each graph, the lag k at which the maximum CCF value occurs is indicated.
Source: Smallman-Raynor and Cliff (2001*b*, fig. 5, p. 85).

method of cross-correlation analysis (see Sect. 6.7.3), the implied differences in phase relationships can be formally examined by computing the cross-correlation functions (CCFs) between (i) the weekly time series of typhoid case rates and (ii) each of the weekly time series of I as plotted in Figure 7.12.

For each of the diffusion graphs, Figure 7.13 plots the CCFs between I and the typhoid case rate for $-12 \leq k \leq 12$. When examined relative to the $k = 0$ position (epidemic peak), the CCFs identify a temporally ordered sequence of spread processes, with each process waxing and waning in a smooth wave-like manner through the stages of the epidemic cycle. Figure 7.13 confirms that the process of relocation diffusion dominated the early stages of epidemic spread; the maximum CCF value occurs at $k = -8$, implying that the process presaged the epidemic peak by several weeks. Thereafter, relocation diffusion began to weaken, to be replaced by localized spatial contagion (maximum CCF value at $k = 1$) as the dominant spread process around the epidemic peak ($-4 \leq k \leq 4$). Finally, spatial contagion weakened as the epidemic began to wane, to be superseded by hierarchical effects (maximum CCF value at $k = 9$) in the advanced stages of epidemic decay.

Interpretation and Implications

Running through the *Report on the Origin and Spread of Typhoid Fever* is a recognition of the importance of the wholesale movement of regiments in the spatial transfer of typhoid fever. Detailing the disease history of the Second

West Virginia Volunteer Infantry (Second Army Corps), for example, Reed and colleagues pieced together a spatial chain of typhoid infection that spanned three encampments and some 800 miles:

[The] regiment began to suffer to some extent from typhoid fever while in the State camp at Charleston, W. Va. It carried the infection to the national camp in Pennsylvania [Camp Meade] . . . The epidemic continued to drag along through the occurrence of scattering cases . . . until the departure of the regiment from Camp Meade, Pa., for the national camp in the South [Camp Wetherell]. The infection was not altogether extinguished when the command reached Camp Wetherell, near Greenville, S.C., since an attack now and then made its appearance . . .[23]

Although the authors of the *Report* were able to reconstruct similar histories for some other commands, their conclusions focused on the epidemiological implications of the evidence and failed to provide any further insights into the generalized mechanism by which typhoid spread through the camp system.

The evidence in Figures 7.12 and 7.13 confirms the importance of regiment relocation as a mechanism for the spatial transmission of typhoid fever, at least in the formative stages of the epidemic. More particularly, the period for which relocation diffusion operated as the dominant spread mechanism ($-12 \leq k \leq -5$ in Fig. 7.13) corresponds to the main phase of transfer from state assembly camps to national training camps (May and June; see Table 7.8) and suggests that regimental movements were pivotal to the initial seeding of the camp system. Crucially, however, Figures 7.12 and 7.13 identify a phenomenon that was unrecognized by the Board on Typhoid Fever: from the later stages of epidemic build-up, the mechanisms that underpinned the spatial spread of typhoid fever became de-linked from the camp-wise movements of the volunteer regiments, and processes other than regiment relocation began to dominate the geographical transmission of the disease.

In the absence of detailed information regarding the movements of individual members and subgroups of the various Army commands, we can only speculate as to the factors that contributed to the temporal switch in diffusion processes shown in Figure 7.13. However, the findings are consistent with the hypothesis that, following the initial regiment-based seeding of the national training camps in the build-up phase of the epidemic (relocation diffusion), the localized movements of individuals and sub-regimental groups came to dominate the spread process as the disease became geographically more ubiquitous around the epidemic peak (contagious diffusion). In the later stages of the epidemic, localized effects were replaced by transmission down the population size hierarchy (hierarchical diffusion) as the volunteers exited the upper tiers of the camp system. In particular, the period for which hierarchical diffusion operated as the dominant spread mechanism ($5 \leq k \leq 12$ in Fig. 7.13) corresponds to the post-war phase of dispersal from the large national training

---

[23] Consideration by the Board on typhoid fever in the Second West Virginia Volunteer Infantry (Reed *et al.*, 1904, i. 442).

camps (notably Camp Meade, Camp Cuba Libre, and Lexington in Sept., Oct., and early Nov. 1898), variously for (i) geographical realignment in the newly established camps of Georgia and/or (ii) return to the home states for mustering out.

RESULTS, II: ENCAMPMENTS BY ARMY CORPS

Diffusion Processes

One complication of the examination of diffusion processes in the subsystems of encampments associated with the individual Army corps is the issue of multiple-corps occupancy. For example, in the early stages of mobilization, Table 7.8 indicates that Camp Thomas was occupied by regiments of both the First and Third Army Corps. Under such circumstances, two measures of typhoid morbidity in the encampments associated with each corps are apparent: (1) Rate 1, formed as the aggregate typhoid case rate (per 10,000 mean strength) for all regiments in a given camp; (2) Rate 2, formed as the corps-specific typhoid case rate (per 10,000 mean strength) for a given camp. In the context of the technique of autocorrelation on graphs, Rate 1 permits an examination of the overall spread mechanisms in a given subsystem of camps, while Rate 2 permits an examination of the spread mechanisms associated with the corresponding corps.

For each of the three diffusion graphs, the weekly values of Moran's I were computed for (i) Rate 1 (aggregate weekly typhoid cases per 10,000) and (ii) Rate 2 (corps-specific weekly typhoid cases per 10,000) in the sets of encampments associated with each Army corps. The results are summarized by diffusion graph and corps in Figure 7.14A–E; for reasons outlined in Section 7.3.3, the results for the Second Army Corps are examined separately for regiments initially dispatched to Camp Alger (Fig. 7.14B) and Camp Meade (Fig. 7.14C). On each graph, the $\{I\}$ for Rate 1 are plotted as a bar chart, with the $\{I\}$ for Rate 2 superimposed as a line trace; for clarity, only positive values of the I coefficient are shown. To overcome the complication of between-corps variations in the timing of epidemic peaks, the horizontal axes of the graphs have been formed by scaling the series of I to the week of peak typhoid incidence (coded week 0) in the respective corps; weeks before the peak (epidemic build-up) and after the peak (fade-out) have been coded with reference to this origin. Finally, as described for Figure 7.12, the pecked horizontal lines at $z = 1.65$ mark the statistically significant I coefficients at the $p = 0.05$ level in a one-tailed test for positive spatial autocorrelation.

We preface our discussion of Figure 7.14 with a brief note on interpretation. With notable exceptions, the graphs in Figure 7.14 show a broad correspondence between the $\{I\}$ associated with Rate 1 (aggregate rate; bar charts) and Rate 2 (corps-specific rate; line traces). This implies that, for the system of camps occupied by a given corps, the spread processes were directly associated with the commands attached to that corps. In some instances, however, high

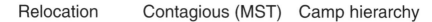

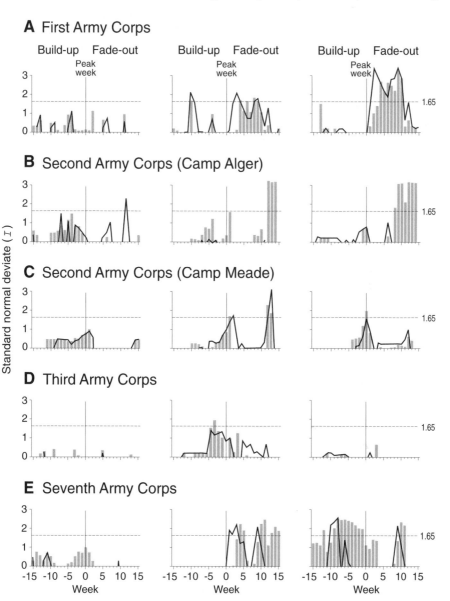

Fig. 7.14. Plots of the weekly values of the spatial autocorrelation coefficient, Moran's *I*, as a standard Normal deviate for the subsystems of camps occupied by the different Army corps

Notes: In all instances, the level of correspondence, *I*, between each of three diffusion graphs and typhoid fever is given for two measures of disease incidence: aggregate case rates per 10,000 mean strength (bar charts) and corps-specific case rates per 10,000 mean strength (line traces). The pecked horizontal lines at $z = 1.65$ mark the statistically significant *I* coefficients at the $p = 0.05$ level in a one-tailed test for positive spatial autocorrelation.

Source: Smallman-Raynor and Cliff (2001*b*, fig. 6, p. 87).

values of the *I* coefficient for Rate 1 (bar charts) occur in conjunction with low values for Rate 2 (line traces). This implies that, for the system of camps occupied by a given corps, the spread processes were contingent on co-occupancy by commands attached to other corps.

Figure 7.14 reveals a complex picture for the transmission of typhoid fever in the subsystems of encampments occupied by the different Army corps. Nevertheless, all corps have one prominent feature in common: the *I* coefficients for the relocation graph (left-hand charts, Fig. 7.14) generally run at very low and statistically insignificant levels. These findings are in marked contrast to the results for the entire system of camps (see Fig. 7.12A) and imply that, at the corps level, the mechanisms that underpinned the spatial transmission of typhoid fever were not conditioned by the between-camp movements of regiments.

Further features of Figure 7.14, which relate to the strength and timing of contagious and hierarchical processes, are also evident:

1. Contagious spread (central charts, Fig. 7.14). All charts reveal some evidence of contagious spread, but with a general tendency for this process to be most important (as judged by the magnitude of the *I* coefficients) in the fade-out stage of the epidemic. For the Second Army Corps (Camp Alger) and the Third Army Corps, however, only the bar charts yield statistically significant values of the *I* coefficient. Although contagious transmission operated in the systems of camps occupied by the two corps, the processes were contingent on co-occupancy by other corps.

2. Hierarchical spread (right-hand charts, Fig. 7.14). With the exception of the Third Army Corps, all charts reveal some evidence of hierarchical spread. There are, however, marked variations in the strength and timing of the process. As judged by the magnitude of the *I* coefficients, hierarchical transmission was most important in the systems of camps occupied by the Seventh Army Corps (epidemic build-up) and the First Army Corps (epidemic fade-out). Although the bar chart for the Second Army Corps (Camp Alger) also identifies the operation of a strong hierarchical component in the later stages of epidemic fade-out, the associated line trace runs at a very low and statistically insignificant level; again, the operation of the transmission process was contingent on the co-occupancy of the camps by other corps.

Interpretation

When the results in Figure 7.14 are examined with reference to the histories of the individual corps, contagious and hierarchical diffusion are found to be most important in the periods of heightened mobility that followed the breaking of camp at Camps Alger, Cuba Libre, Meade, and Thomas (see Table 7.8). So, for the First Army Corps, contagious and hierarchical effects were most pronounced in mid-to-late September, October, and early November ($2 \leq k \leq 10$ in Fig. 7.14A) and occurred in the wake of the exodus of the Second and Third

Divisions from Camp Thomas, variously for (i) realignment in the national camps at Knoxville and Lexington and/or (ii) return to the home states for mustering out. For the Second Army Corps, the main periods of contagious and hierarchical diffusion (Nov. and early Dec.; $8 \le k \le 14$ in Figs. 7.14B, 7.14C) coincided with the movement of commands from Camp Meade to camps in Georgia and the home states, while similar periods of increased mobility correspond to the timing of contagious and hierarchical effects associated with the Third and Seventh Corps (Figs. 7.14D, 7.14E). Given that the periods of mobility in the four Army corps were associated with the geographical relocation of the constituent commands, the lack of evidence for the operation of relocation diffusion in Figure 7.14 is noteworthy and implies that it was the general population flux engendered by the uprooting of regiments rather than the specific process of regiment transfer that underpinned the spread of typhoid fever within the corps.

7.3.5 Summary

The 1898 epidemic of typhoid fever in the newly mustered regiments of the US Volunteer Army highlights the singular impact of a rapid and ill-planned[24] process of military mobilization on the spatial dynamics of an infectious disease. Originating as a multiple-source epidemic in state assembly camps during May and June 1898, the analysis has demonstrated that the spread of typhoid fever in the entire system of assembly and training camps was underpinned by a temporally ordered sequence of diffusion processes. The early seeding of the epidemic was caused by transfer of infected regiments from one camp to another. Such inter-camp transfer was replaced by localized, spatial contagion at the peak of the epidemic, while epidemic fade-out occurred hierarchically across the camps as demobilization proceeded. When examined for the subsystems of encampments associated with the individual corps, however, a more subtle picture emerged. At this level, contagious and hierarchical diffusion effects were found to dominate the spread of the disease. These effects were most important at times of heightened regimental mobility, implying that it was the general population flux associated with the uprooting of regiments, rather than the specific process of regiment transfer, that drove the spread of typhoid fever within the individual corps.

Spurred by the investigations of the Dodge Commission into the conduct of the War Department during the conflict of 1898, the early years of the twentieth century were associated with a major reorganization and strengthening of the Army Medical Department. With a broadened skills and knowledge base, and equipped with developments in vaccination (anti-typhoid vaccination was made compulsory for the Army in 1911; see Fig. 7.15), vector control, and

---

[24] For a summary perspective on the planning, organization, and execution of US mobilization during the Spanish–American War, see Kreidberg and Henry (1975: 141–73).

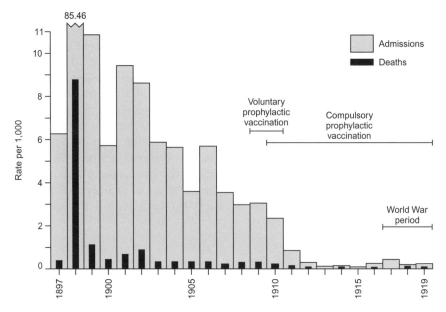

Fig. 7.15. Typhoid fever and anti-typhoid vaccination in the US Army, 1897–1919

Notes: The bar charts plot the annual rate (per 1,000 enlisted men) of admissions and deaths for typhoid fever in the Continental United States (excluding Alaska). The periods of voluntary and compulsory prophylactic vaccination are indicated.

Source: Redrawn from United States Army (1928, chart II, p. 18).

water purification, the Army Medical Department had attained a new level of competence in preventive medicine by World War I (Bayne-Jones, 1968: 149). It is to US mobilization and the world wars that we now turn.

7.4 US Mobilization and the World Wars

7.4.1 *World War I*

In Section 4.4, we examined the spread of one particular infectious disease (measles) associated with the military mobilization of the United States during World War I (1914–18). As described there, differential patterns of measles activity reflected the prior epidemiological experiences of the new recruits. Particularly high disease rates occurred among those from primarily rural (southern and southeastern) areas of the country. As in earlier conflicts, however, measles was one of a number of diseases that accompanied the US mobilization effort of 1917–18 (United States Army, 1928), and so the present section extends our earlier examination of measles to include other infectious diseases which spread with enlistment into the US Army during World War I.

The Mobilization Camps

According to Kreidberg and Henry (1975: 311), US mobilization in World War I was hampered by 'lack of preparation, faulty organization, and failure of military leaders to appreciate the importance of economic mobilization in the early part of the war'. Troop housing lay at the forefront of the logisitic difficulties. At the time of the US declaration of war (6 Apr. 1917), the Army had accommodation for just 124,000 officers and men—for a force that, within a year, would swell to several millions. As a remedial response, 32 National Guard (tent) camps and National Army (wooden) cantonments—with a maximum troop capacity of almost 1.5 million—were hurriedly constructed during the summer and early autumn of 1917. Capacity was further augmented by the establishment of 'special' camps with functions for embarkation, the housing of Coast and Field Artillery, Tank and Signal Corps, and so forth. The locations of the 32 National Guard camps and National Army cantonments, along with seven of the special camps, are plotted in Figure 7.16.

DISEASE PATTERNS

Between April 1917 and November 1918, some 3.7 million recruits passed through the system of US Army cantonments and camps (Bayne-Jones, 1968: 152). To examine the associated patterns of disease activity, we draw on information included in the Surgeon-General's contribution to the US War Department's (1920) *Annual Reports 1919*. For each of the 39 camps in Figure 7.16, volume i (part II) of the *Reports* provides monthly counts of admissions for major infectious conditions, October 1917 to December 1918. From this source, information for eight sample diseases (cerebrospinal meningitis, influenza, measles, mumps, rubella, scarlet fever, tuberculosis, and typhoid fever) was abstracted to form 39 (camps) × 15 (months) matrices of (i) disease counts and (ii) disease rates (per 1,000 enlisted men). Table 7.9 summarizes the number of admissions for each disease and for each of the three classes of camp mapped in Figure 7.16. The aggregate maximum troop capacities of the subsets of encampments are given for reference.

As Table 7.9 shows, the eight sample diseases caused 512,808 admissions during the 15-month observation period. It is evident, however, that the diseases varied widely in their numerical importance. The overall pattern was dominated by influenza (327,480 admissions) accounting for almost two-thirds of the tabled admissions. Other diseases of consequence included mumps (92,388 admissions), measles (60,972), and tuberculosis (16,236). Rubella, cerebrospinal meningitis, and scarlet fever were each associated with less than 10,000 admissions while, compared to the experience of the Spanish–American War (Sect. 7.3), the extremely low incidence of typhoid fever attests to the success of the Army's programme of compulsory vaccination against this disease (Fig. 7.15).

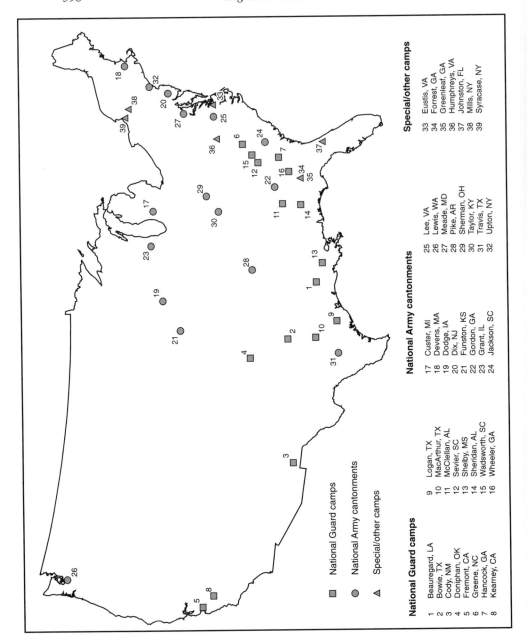

National Guard camps

1   Beauregard, LA
2   Bowie, TX
3   Cody, NM
4   Doniphan, OK
5   Fremont, CA
6   Greene, NC
7   Hancock, GA
8   Kearney, CA
9   Logan, TX
10 MacArthur, TX
11 McClellan, AL
12 Sevier, SC
13 Shelby, MS
14 Sheridan, AL
15 Wadsworth, SC
16 Wheeler, GA

National Army cantonments

17 Custer, MI
18 Devens, MA
19 Dodge, IA
20 Dix, NJ
21 Funston, KS
22 Gordon, GA
23 Jackson, SC
24 Jackson, SC
25 Lee, VA
26 Lewis, WA
27 Meade, MD
28 Pike, AR
29 Sherman, OH
30 Taylor, KY
31 Travis, TX
32 Upton, NY

Special/other camps

33 Eustis, VA
34 Forrest, GA
35 Greenleaf, GA
36 Humphreys, VA
37 Johnston, FL
38 Mills, NY
39 Syracase, NY

■ National Guard camps
● National Army cantonments
▲ Special/other camps

Table 7.9. Admissions for sample infectious diseases among enlisted men in the continental United States, October 1917–December 1918

	National Guard camps	National Army cantonments	Special/other camps[1]	Total
Maximum troop capacity	683,887	769,047	117,156[2]	73,515
Disease				
Cerebrospinal meningitis	693	1,123	75	1,891
Influenza	103,564	201,710	22,206	327,480
Measles	25,774	32,880	2,318	60,972
Mumps	34,472	54,529	3,387	92,388
Rubella	3,914	5,356	126	9,396
Scarlet Fever	1,135	2,965	101	4,201
Tuberculosis	7,314	8,371	551	16,236
Typhoid Fever	112	127	5	244
Total	176,978	307,061	28,769	512,808

Notes: [1] Eustis, Va., Forrest, Ga., Greenleaf, Ga., Humphreys, Va., Johnston, Fla., Mills, NY, and Syracuse, NY. [2] Capacity data not available for two camps (Greenleaf, Ga. and Syracuse, NY).
Source: Data from US War Department (1920, tables 372, 414, 426, 438, 450, 462, 474, 486, 507, pp. 2080–9, 2208–14, 2250–1, 2265, 2278, 2290, 2302, 2314, 2337) and Kreiberg and Henry (1975, tables 41 and 43, pp. 314, 318).

Epidemic Sequences

The temporal pattern of admissions is illustrated by disease in Figure 7.17. On each graph, the heavy line trace plots the median value of the monthly admissions rate (per 1,000 enlisted men) for the 39 Army camps, while the shaded area forms an envelope which delimits the interquartile range of admissions rates in each monthly period. For reference, the broken line traces plot the cumulative monthly count of US Army personnel embarked for Europe.

With the exceptions of influenza (Fig. 7.17B) and typhoid fever (Fig. 7.17H), a notable feature of Figure 7.17 is the tendency for disease activity to peak in the early months of the observation period (Oct. 1917–Mar. 1918). However, within this broad pattern, it is also apparent from Figure 7.17 that the diseases differed in terms of the exact timing and the duration of their main epidemic phases. To examine epidemic duration more closely, the disease-specific monthly admissions rate (per 1,000 enlisted men) for the set of 39 camps was first reduced to standard Normal score (z-score) form. For each disease,

Fig. 7.16. Military camps in the Continental United States, World War I

Notes: The locations of National Guard tent camps (square symbols) and National Army wooden cantonments (circular symbols) are shown, along with certain camps constructed for special and/or other purposes (triangular symbols).
Source: Based on information in Kreidburg and Henry (1975, tables 41 and 43, pp. 314, 318).

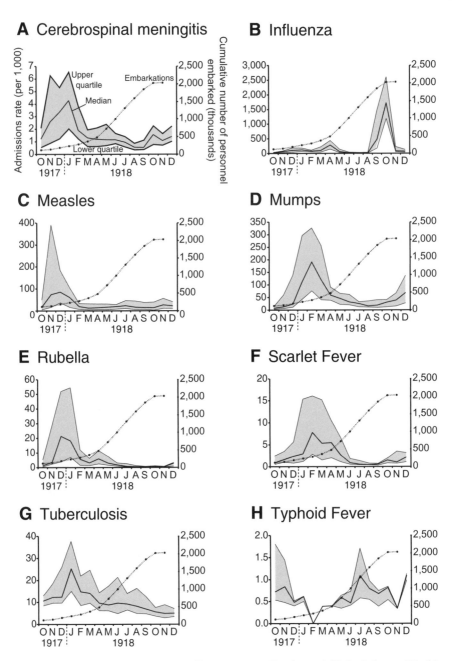

Fig. 7.17. Infectious diseases in military camps, Continental United States, World War I

Notes: Graphs plot, as a heavy line trace, the median value of the monthly admission rate (per 1,000 strength) for sample diseases in 39 military camps. On each graph, the shaded area forms an envelope that delimits the interquartile range of the corresponding admission rates. (A) Cerebrospinal meningitis. (B) Influenza. (C) Measles. (D) Mumps. (E) Rubella. (F) Scarlet fever. (G) Tuberculosis. (H) Typhoid fever. For reference, the broken line trace on each graph plots the cumulative monthly count of Army personnel embarked for Europe. The 39 sample camps on which the graphs are based are mapped in fig. 7.16.

Source: Based on data in US War Department (1920, tables 373, 415, 427, 439, 451, 463, 475, 487, 508, pp. 2090–9, 2215–21, 2252, 2266, 2279, 2291, 2303, 2315, 2338) and Kreidburg and Henry (1975, table 48, p. 335).

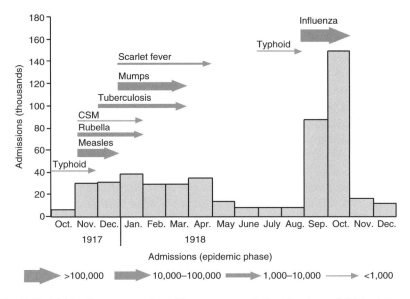

Fig. 7.18. Epidemic sequence in military camps of the Continental United States during World War I, October 1917–December 1918

Notes: The bar chart plots the aggregate monthly count of medical admissions for eight infectious diseases (cerebrospinal meningitis (CSM); influenza; measles; mumps; rubella; scarlet fever; tuberculosis; and typhoid fever) in 39 US military camps. To identify the epidemic phase(s) associated with the constituent diseases, disease-specific monthly admissions rates (per 1,000) were reduced to standard Normal score form; months with scores in excess of 0.5 standard deviations above the mean (defined as 'epidemic months') are indicated by arrows. Arrows have been drawn to indicate the number of admissions associated with the epidemic months for a given disease. The 39 sample camps on which the graph is based are mapped in Fig. 7.16.

Source: Based on data in US War Department (1920, tables 373, 415, 427, 439, 451, 463, 475, 487, 508, pp. 2090–9, 2215–21, 2252, 2266, 2279, 2291, 2303, 2315, 2338).

'epidemic months' with scores more than 0.5 standard deviations above the mean are identified in Figure 7.18 by the vectors. Here, vector widths have been drawn proportional to the associated number of admissions, while the bar chart plots the aggregate monthly count of admissions for the eight sample diseases.

The vectors in Figure 7.18 show an overlapping, time-ordered, sequence of epidemic events of greater or lesser magnitude and duration: (onset: Oct. 1917) typhoid fever ⇒ (onset: Nov. 1917) measles, cerebrospinal meningitis and rubella ⇒ (onset: Dec. 1917) tuberculosis ⇒ (onset: Jan. 1918) mumps and scarlet fever. By May 1918, Figure 7.18 shows that epidemic activity associated with the sample diseases had ceased. Thereafter, a minor upsurge in typhoid fever during July and August 1918 (Figs. 7.17H and 7.18) was followed, in September and October, by the devastating autumn wave of Spanish influenza

(Figs. 7.17B and 7.18). It is to the spread of the latter disease in the camp system that we now turn.

The Spanish influenza pandemic of 1918–19 diffused as three temporally distinct waves of infection: spring and early summer 1918 (Wave I), autumn 1918 (Wave II), and winter 1918–19 (Wave III). Although the source of the virus that caused the pandemic has been the subject of considerable research and debate in recent years (see Sect. 11.3.1), Army training camps in the continental United States provided some of the earliest clinical evidence for the first, and least severe, influenza wave (Soper, 1918; Crosby, 1989). According to Crosby (1989: 19), initial reports of the spring wave can be traced to Camp Funston, Kansas, in early March 1918, with the disease appearing in other camps (including Doniphan, Fremont, Hancock, Kearney, Gordan, Grant, Lewis, Logan, McClellan, Sevier, Shelby, and Sherman) in the days and weeks that followed; see Figure 7.16 for locations. The relatively mild nature of this first influenza wave, however, is reflected in the modest increase in the admissions rate in Figure 7.17B, peaking in April 1918. Thereafter, influenza abated in the Army camps, making a catastrophic reappearance in the autumn of 1918.

Spread of the Autumn 1918 Wave

According to Soper (1918: 1900), Camp Devens, Massachusetts, was the first Army camp to report the occurrence of a severe epidemic of influenza in autumn 1918. On 16 September, the camp surgeon informed the Surgeon-General of the Army that, as part of a general epidemic in Massachusetts and neighbouring states, influenza had now appeared among the troops. In fact, the likely origin of the epidemic in Camp Devens can be dated to Saturday 7 September. On that day, a possible case of influenza (reported as cerebrospinal meningitis) presented in D Company, Forty-Second Infantry.[25] The next day, 12 cases of proven influenza appeared in the same company while, by 12 September, the total number of hospital admissions in the camp had grown to almost 600 (ibid.). The subsequent course of the epidemic in Camp Devens is summarized in Table 7.10. As the table shows, the epidemic spiralled to a peak on 20–1 September, and then declined rapidly to the end of the month. Thereafter, the epidemic continued at a low level, eventually terminating in the latter half of October.

The source of the influenza epidemic at Camp Devens is not known with certainty, although some connection with the civilian epidemic in the nearby city of Boston is generally suspected (Ministry of Health, 1920: 289). Whatever the

---

[25] In his original review of the autumn influenza wave in the Army camps of the continental United States, Soper (1918: 1900) states that the possible case of influenza at Camp Devens on 7 September was a member of D Company, Forty-Second Infantry. Crosby (1989: 5) however, states B Company.

Table 7.10. Progress of the influenza epidemic at Camp Devens, Massachusetts, 12 September–18 October 1918

Epidemic phase	Duration (days)	Influenza cases	Pneumonia cases	Deaths
Rise (12–19 Sept.)	8	3,283	43	16
Peak (20–1 Sept.)	2	2,722	205	43
Rapid decline (22–9 Sept.)	8	3,141	1,495	298
Slow decline (30 Sept.–18 Oct.)	19	571	571	310

Source: Soper (1918, table 1, p. 1900).

source of influenza at Camp Devens, however, other military camps were afflicted by the disease in the remainder of September and early October. The camp-wise sequence of attack is shown in Figure 7.19.[26] To form the map, the putative start of the main phase of the epidemic at Camp Devens (Thur. 12 Sept.; see Soper, 1918: 1901) was coded day 1, with subsequent days coded sequentially thereafter. From these data, the shaded circles in Figure 7.19 identify those camps in which influenza first appeared in week 1 (days 1–7), week 2 (days 8–14), week 3 (days 15–21), and weeks 4–5 (days 22–35) of the epidemic. For reference, Table 7.11 gives the recorded number of influenza cases, pneumonia cases, and total deaths in each camp, 12 September–31 October, along with an estimate of the influenza attack rate (expressed as a percentage proportion of personnel).

Consistent with a postulated introduction of the disease by troopships and other vessels from infected European locations (Soper, 1918: 1907; Ministry of Health, 1920: 284–5),[27] Figure 7.19 shows that the first camps to be attacked by influenza were positioned close to the Atlantic seaboard. So, in addition to the putative index camp (Devens), other camps to be infected in week 1 of the epidemic included Camp Upton (New York) on 13 September, Camp Lee (Virginia) on 17 September, and Camps Dix (New Jersey) and Jackson (South Carolina) on 18 September. From these locations, the disease followed a rapid westward advance, reaching such widely separated camps as Grant (Illinois), Funston (Kansas), and Logan (Texas) by the middle of week 2. At about the same time, on the west coast, Camp Lewis (Washington) was attacked. By the

[26] Information relating to the date of appearance of influenza is unavailable for two of the camps (Doniphan, Okla. and Mills, NY) mapped in Fig. 7.19.

[27] Soper (1918: 1907–8), for example, provides numerous instances of the occurrence of influenza on board vessels arriving in the United States from European locations during the summer of 1918. As early as 22 June, the British steamship *Exeter*, headed from Liverpool, put into Philadelphia with 28 cases of pneumonia aboard. Likewise, in July, the Cunard Liner *Khiva* (operating as a troopship) experienced a probable outbreak of influenza on the voyage from Liverpool to New York (via Halifax, Nova Scotia), while the *Bergensford* arrived in New York on 12 August having registered some 200 influenza cases at sea.

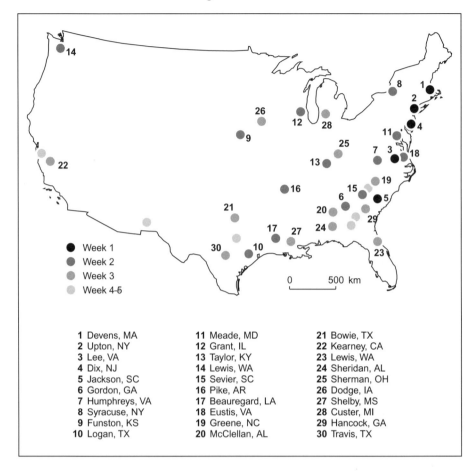

Fig. 7.19. Spread of Wave II of the 'Spanish' influenza pandemic in sample US Army camps, September–October 1918

Notes: Formed relative to the putative start of the main phase of the epidemic at Camp Devens (Thur. 12 Sept., coded day 1), the circles identify those camps in which influenza was first recognized in week 1 (days 1–7), week 2 (days 8–14), week 3 (days 15–21) and weeks 4–5 (days 22–35). Camps infected in weeks 1–3 are identified by numerical code.
Source: Drawn from data in Soper (1918, table 2, p. 1901).

end of week 3, most Army camps of the United States had been infiltrated by the influenza virus.

Military versus civil settlement systems. Table 7.12 is adapted from Soper (1918) and gives, by major geographical division, the week of onset of the influenza epidemic (as judged by a marked increase in deaths from pneumonia) in (i) the military settlement system of Army camps and (ii) the civil settlement system of principal cities. While the table suggests that the disease followed the

Table 7.11. Influenza in sample US Army camps, 12 September–31 October 1918

Camp	Influenza cases	Pneumonia cases	Total deaths	Influenza attack rate (%)
National Guard camps				
Beauregard, La.	5,252	1,007	422	39.6
Bowie, Tex.	4,052	119	104	38.1
Cody, N. Mex.	2,337	252	46	49.8
Doniphan, Okla.	no data	no data	no data	no data
Fremont, Calif.	2,347	392	132	9.8
Greene, NC	4,200	626	258	25.8
Hancock, Ga.	7,715	1,209	462	22.2
Kearney, Calif.	2,450	186	37	13.5
Logan, Tex.	3,137	393	16	24.6
MacArthur, Tex.	6,010	852	188	28.1
McClellan, Ala.	4,718	993	218	16.1
Sevier, SC	4,526	896	319	16.3
Shelby, Miss.	1,761	94	19	18.8
Sheridan, Ala.	4,758	521	132	20.4
Wadsworth, SC	5,505	357	60	38.6
Wheeler, Ga.	70	361	61	0.8
National Army cantonments				
Custer, Mich.	11,626	2,437	669	29.0
Devens, Mass.	13,398	2,288	794	30.1
Dix, NJ	9,283	1,673	829	19.0
Dodge, Ia.	9,398	1,847	570	29.0
Funston, Kan.	13,526	2,328	888	24.9
Gordon, Ga.	4,155	626	192	11.3
Grant, Ill.	10,717	2,335	1,068	25.8
Jackson, SC	7,500	1,114	362	18.9
Lee, Va.	11,298	1,919	672	22.9
Lewis, Wash.	3,141	994	148	9.7
Meade, Md.	11,449	2,013	796	27.8
Pike, Ark.	13,273	1,379	455	26.7
Sherman, Oh.	4,789	1,717	1,058	13.5
Taylor, Ky.	11,587	2,800	830	19.2
Travis, Tex.	8,470	1,742	168	24.7
Upton, NY	5,090	974	343	13.9
Special/other camps				
Eustis, Va.	1,745	67	10	14.8
Forrest, Ga.	2,307	33	22	24.9
Greenleaf, Ga.	4,747	343	263	20.3
Humphreys, Ga.	no data	no data	no data	no data
Johnston, Fla.	2,117	383	161	11.1
Mills, NY	no data	no data	no data	no data
Syracuse, NY	2,031	401	164	18.4
Total	220,485	37,671	12,936	21.6[1]

Note: [1] Estimated attack rate.
Source: Data from Soper (1918, table 10, p. 1904).

Table 7.12. Week of onset of the influenza epidemic (as judged by a marked increase in deaths from pneumonia) in the principal cities and army camps of the United States, 8 September–25 October 1918

Week ending	Atlantic Coast		North Central		Southeastern		Southwestern		Pacific Coast	
	Cities	Camps	Cities	Camps	Cities	Camps	Cities	Camps	Cities	Camps
14 Sept.	Boston	Devens, Mass.								
21 Sept.	Lowell; New York	Dix, NJ								
28 Sept.	Cambridge; Jersey City; Philadelphia; Providence; Washington	Lee, Va.; Upton, NY; Syracuse, NY; Humphreys, Va.	Pittsburgh; Chicago; Minneapolis							
5 Oct.	Baltimore; Buffalo; Fall River; Newark; Syracuse	Meade, Md.; Eustis, Va.	Cincinnati; Indianapolis	Custer, Mich.; Funstan, Kan.; Grant, Ill.; Sherman, Ohio; Taylor, Ky.	Birmingham	Beauregard, La.; Sevier, SC; Logan, Tex.; Hancock, Ga.; Gordon, Ga.	Denver	Pike, Ark.	Los Angeles	
12 Oct.	Albany; Rochester		Kansas City; Louisville; Milwaukee; Omaha; St Paul; St Louis; Cleveland; Columbus; Dayton; Toledo	Dodge	Atlanta; New Orleans	Greene, NC; McClellan, Ala.; Wadsworth, SC; Jackson, SC; Johnston, Fla.; Greenleaf, Ga.; Sheridan, Ala.		Travis, Tex.; Bowie, Tex.	Oakland; Seattle	
19 Oct.	New Haven							MacArthur, Tex.; Cody, N. Mex.	San Francisco; Spokane; Portland	Fremont, Calif.; Lewis, Wash.

Source: Soper (1918, table 12, p. 1908).

same broad spatial course in both types of settlement system (Atlantic Coast ⇒ North Central ⇒ Southeastern/Southwestern ⇒ Pacific Coast), epidemic timings in the two systems differed. For three divisions (Atlantic Coast, North Central, and Pacific Coast), the first entries for the civil settlement system preceded those for the military settlement system by a week or more. Although any interpretation of the evidence must proceed with caution, Soper (1918: 1908) observes that such a lag effect is consistent with the hypothesis that 'the camps derived their infection not from one another but from their immediate [civil] environment'. If this interpretation is correct, we may infer that the rapid, high-level, spread of influenza in the civil population of the United States effectively served to short-circuit any epidemiological integration of the Army camp system in the autumn of 1918 (cf. the spread of smallpox in the Franco-Prussian War, 1870; see Sect. 8.3).

Epidemic severity in camps. Regardless of the source of influenza in the individual camps, available evidence suggests that the epidemic took a more severe course among recruits than their civil counterparts. Writing in the *Journal of the American Medical Association* in early December 1918, Victor G. Heiser summarized the evidence in the following manner:

From the statistics so far available, the death rate in the military camps is higher than among the civil population, even in similar age groups. The mortality in New York and Chicago, for instance, shows that the death rate in the Army is more than double that of the civil population of the same age group. There is also the possibility that when allowances are made for the fact that defectives have been eliminated from the Army, and that these poor 'risks' swell the civil death list, the corrected margin will be still further increased in favour of the civil population. (Heiser, 1918: 1909)

The reason for the difference between camps and cities, Heiser postulated, rested with the living conditions in camps and, in particular, the epidemiological risks afforded by high-density accommodation, sleeping, and messing. The cramped quarters of the barrack camps (National Army cantonments in Fig. 7.16), in contrast to the relatively airy lodgings of the tent camps (National Guard camps in Fig. 7.16), appeared to afford a special danger of pneumonia in influenza patients (Soper, 1918; Heiser, 1918) (Table 7.13). 'It would seem well', Heiser (1918: 1911) recommended, 'to consider plans for "debarracking" aggregations of men throughout the country.' 'As matters stand,' he added, 'those responsible for retaining men in barracks are assuming a heavy responsibility.'

7.4.2 World War II

For US military personnel, both at home and overseas, prophylactic vaccination against diseases such as cholera, plague, smallpox, tetanus, typhoid,

Table 7.13. Severity of influenza in US barrack camps (cantonments) and tent camps, 12 September–31 October 1918

	Barracks (cantonments)	Tent camps
Combined strength	748,632	313,362
Influenza cases	158,104	69,761
Pneumonia cases	30,099	9,740
Total deaths	10,533	2,923
Influenza attack rate[1]	21.1	22.2
Combined influenza and pneumonia attack rate[1]	19.0	13.9
Pneumonia case fatality rate[1]	35.0	30.1

Note: [1] Expressed as a percentage.
Source: Soper (1918, table 3, p. 1902).

typhus, and yellow fever ensured that these conditions were of limited significance in World War II. Thus, during the first year of US military engagement (1942), the Army recorded no cases of cholera or of yellow fever, almost no cases of plague and smallpox, practically no tetanus among inoculated men, and only a few dozen cases of typhus fever. Disease in the US Navy followed a similar pattern (Simmons, 1943).

However, as in previous wars, mobilization entrained a series of epidemics in the military camps of the Continental United States. As early as December 1940—a full year prior to the US declaration of war on Japan—the US Surgeon-General, James C. Magee, reported on the transmission of acute respiratory infections as a consequence of ongoing military preparations. Although the outbreaks were of a mild nature, the spectre of the 1918–19 influenza epidemic still loomed in the minds of the US medical profession. Magee (1941: 512) warned:

As larger numbers of selectees are brought together, the rapid passage of infection from one individual to another will probably cause an increase in prevalence, virulence and fatal complications . . . In fact the possibility cannot be ignored that the Army may again be confronted by another pandemic of influenza of the virulent type which caused such a large proportion of the total deaths among our troops during the last war.

In anticipation, Magee requested authority for the establishment and maintenance of a board for the investigation of the aetiology, epidemiology, prevention, and treatment of influenza and other acute respiratory diseases. Formal approval for the establishment of the Board for the Investigation of Influenza and Other Epidemic Diseases in the Army was granted by the War Office on 11 January 1941.

Table 7.14. Leading infectious and parasitic causes of death in the US Army, continental United States (1942–1945)

	Deaths	Admissions
Tuberculosis (all forms)	390	21,117
Meningococcal (cerebrospinal) meningitis	380	9,702
Pneumonia (bacterial)	252	38,105
Poliomyelitis	84	446
Streptococcal diseases[1]	84	40,094
Hepatitis	81	9,897
Syphilis[2]	34	205,649
Coccidioidomycosis	32	3,399
Measles	27	53,968
Rheumatic fever	24	14,048
All infectious/parasitic diseases	1,592	1,496,241

Notes: [1] Including scarlet fever. [2] Excluding neurosyphilis.
Source: Data from Reister (1976).

OVERVIEW OF EVIDENCE

In the event, there was no repetition of the 1918–19 influenza epidemic in the assembly and training camps of the United States and, although infections of all descriptions accompanied the military build-up, deaths were comparatively few in number. By way of illustration, the lower row in Table 7.14 gives the estimated count of admissions and deaths due to infectious and parasitic diseases in the US Army, continental United States, 1942–5. Although admissions numbered almost 1.5 million, there were just 1,592 recorded deaths. Most of the latter were due to a handful of conditions; the ten leading infectious and parasitic causes of death are defined in rank order of importance in the upper rows of Table 7.14. The monthly incidence of each disease (per 1,000 mean strength per year) is plotted for the period 1942–5 in Figure 7.20. As Table 7.14 indicates, tuberculosis, meningococcal (cerebrospinal) meningitis, and bacterial pneumonia, along with poliomyelitis, streptococcal diseases (including scarlet fever), and hepatitis, ranked as the leading infectious causes of death. Although other diseases included in Table 7.14 accounted for large amounts of sickness in the Army, especially in the early (measles; Fig. 7.20C) and middle (syphilis; Fig. 7.20I) years of the war effort, they yielded relatively few fatalities.

SAMPLE CAMP DISEASES

As evidenced by the entries in the contemporary publication, *Bulletin of War Medicine*, the epidemiological profile of US mobilization in World War II

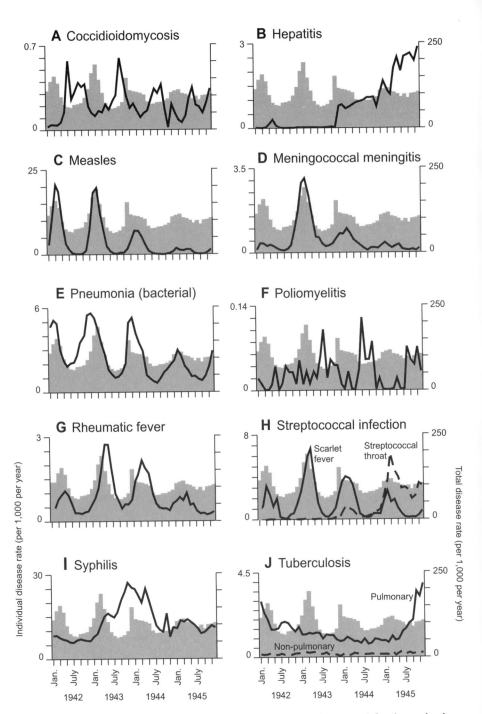

Fig. 7.20. Monthly admissions rate (per 1,000 mean strength per year) for the ten leading infectious/parasitic causes of death among US Army contingents in the Continental United States (1942–1945)

Notes: Line traces plot the monthly admissions rate for the 10 sample diseases. (A) Coccidioidomycosis. (B) Hepatitis. (C) Measles. (D) Meningococcal (cerebrospinal) meningitis. (E) Pneumonia (bacterial). (F) Poliomyelitis. (G) Rheumatic fever. (H) Streptococcal infection (scarlet fever and streptococcal throat). (I) Syphilis (excluding neurosyphilis). (J) Tuberculosis. For reference, the bar chart on each graph plots the monthly admissions rate (per 1,000 average strength per year) for all infectious and parasitic diseases.
Source: Data from Reister (1976).

attracted a substantial literature. In this subsection, we sample from the literature to highlight four diseases of particular military significance and/or interest at the time: meningococcal meningitis, primary atypical pneumonia, Bullis
('Lone Star') fever, and serum hepatitis.

Meningococcal (Cerebrospinal) Meningitis

Among the classic diseases of mobilization, meningococcal meningitis
threatened to reach epidemic proportions in the early months of 1943 (Fig.
7.20D). According to Sartwell and Smith (1944), the majority of cases
occurred in men of three months service or less, with higher disease rates
in large (3.2 cases per 1,000 strength in stations with more than 20,000 men)
compared with small (1.0 case per 1,000 strength in stations with under 10,000
men) camps. Epidemiological investigations further revealed an association
between the level of meningococcal infection and (i) the degree of overcrowding in barracks; (ii) the prevalence of common respiratory diseases; (iii) the
proportion of unseasoned men; and (iv) the rate of turnover of unseasoned
men. The interplay of these various associations was highlighted in Thomas's
(1943) model of multiple disease transmission and mobilization in the Fourth
Service Command:

Among the new troops brought into the army post there is a rate of at least 1 to 2 per
cent meningococcus carriers. If their arrival at camp occurs during the months when
diseases of the upper respiratory tract are prevalent an extremely high rate of such diseases soon develops among the new troops and includes the carriers. The coughing and
sneezing distributes not only the virus responsible for the diseases of the upper respiratory tract but also the meningococci introduced by the carriers. In this way the carrier
rate builds up rapidly. (Thomas, 1943: 265)

Although the prompt implementation of preventive measures, including massive prophylaxis with sulphonamides, succeeded in limiting the total number of
cases of meningococcal meningitis in the Army to less than 10,000 (Table 7.14),
a major epidemic of the disease—possibly originating in the camps—spread in
the civil population of the United States in the spring and summer of 1943
(Anonymous, 1943; Sartwell and Smith, 1944).

Primary Atypical Pneumonia

As part of the more general problem of acute respiratory diseases in military
establishments (Magee, 1941), Army camps in the Continental United States
were the foci for epidemic outbreaks of a disease that had begun to attract the
interest of the medical profession in the mid-1930s—primary atypical pneumonia. Clinically, atypical pneumonia began with fever, headache, malaise,
and dry cough. As the disease progressed, the cough became increasingly

productive, with signs of broncheolar involvement. In more severe cases, secondary bacterial invasion was witnessed. The illness usually lasted for three to eight days. The aetiology was largely unknown and, although airborne droplet transmission was suspected, efforts repeatedly failed to identify a causative agent (see Brown *et al.*, 1943). Today, it is recognized that primary atypical pneumonia is caused by a variety of organisms, of which *Mycoplasma pneumoniae* is one of the most common (Baum, 2000).

The incidence of atypical pneumonia in the US Army followed the broad pattern of undifferentiated respiratory tract infection, with the highest rates of disease activity in new recruits (Anonymous, 1945*a*). Among the local (camp-based) epidemiological studies to be published at the time, Campbell *et al.* (1943) document an outbreak of atypical pneumonia at Camp Eustis, Virginia, in the autumn of 1942. During September and October, 2.2 men per 1,000 at Camp Eustis were incapacitated with the disease. Dingle *et al.* (1943) record 216 admissions for primary atypical pneumonia in an Army camp in Louisiana between February 1941 and March 1942, while van Ravenswaay *et al.* (1944) provide details of 1,862 cases seen at Jefferson Barracks, Missouri, between June 1942 and August 1943. As the latter authors note, slow convalescence ensured that primary atypical pneumonia was one of the chief causes of man-days lost in the US Army during World War II.

Bullis ('Lone Star') Fever

Among the more mysterious diseases to spread as a consequence of mobilization, Woodland *et al.* (1943) and Anigstein and Bader (1943) document the emergence of an apparently new tick-borne disease (variously referred to as 'Bullis fever' or 'Lone Star fever') among US soldiers engaged in field exercises at Camp Bullis, near Houston, Texas, in 1942–3. The first cases of the disease were observed in the spring of 1942, with the number growing to about 1,000 by the summer of the following year. Clinically, the disease was characterized by the abrupt onset of chills and headache, with fever lasting for three to seven days. In more severe attacks, a maculo-papular rash appeared on the trunk, variously resembling the rash seen in typhus fever or German measles. Blood tests revealed no evidence of infection with fevers of the typhus group, undulant fever, tularaemia, typhoid, or paratyphoid. Colorado tick fever was also excluded, as was dengue. On the basis of local studies, Anigstein and Bader (1943) suggest that Bullis fever was a rickettsiosis, for which the tick *Amblyomma americanum* was one of the vectors. As Megaw (1944: 734) notes: 'Hitherto, these fevers, being transmissible only from lower animals to man and not from man to man, have nearly always occurred as sporadic cases. But the war has introduced a new set of conditions in which large outbreaks may be expected.' As such, Bullis fever provides a clear example of the role of war in the process of disease emergence and re-emergence (see Ch. 9).

Serum Hepatitis

Beginning in early March 1942—just three months after the entry of the United States into World War II—a major epidemic of hepatitis began to unfold in US forces at home and overseas. By the start of July, the number of documented cases in the Army had grown to 28,505, the majority of which (24,057) were based in camps of the continental United States (Anonymous, 1942*a*, 1942*b*). Epidemiological investigations related the outbreak to the mass administration of certain batches of yellow fever vaccine (designated 17 D serum-based vaccine) that had been stabilized by 'icterogenic' human serum (Bancroft and Lemon, 1984). Indeed, the possibility that hepatitis may occur some 60 to 120 days after inoculation with contaminated batches of the vaccine had been recognized several years earlier, in 1937 (Anonymous, 1942*b*). In consequence of the severity of the wartime outbreak, large-scale production of a serum-free yellow fever vaccine was initiated in 1942.

7.5 Conclusion

This chapter has examined the spread of infectious diseases with US military mobilization in sample conflicts of the nineteenth (Civil War and Spanish–American War) and twentieth (World Wars I and II) centuries. While each phase of mobilization took on its own distinctive epidemiological profile, the net effect of the coming together of large bodies of unseasoned recruits was essentially the same: the rapid and widespread dissemination of disease agents of all kinds. During the wars of the nineteenth century, diseases such as dysentery, malaria, measles, and typhoid fever spread with great ferocity in the camps of newly enlisted men. The epidemiological pattern, however, began to change in the aftermath of the Spanish–American War. Spurred by the disease experiences of 1898, and assisted by ongoing developments in military hygiene and preventive medicine, some conditions—such as typhoid fever—had largely retreated from the home camps by the time of World War I. Other diseases, however, came to characterize the mobilization efforts of the twentieth century. So, while certain childhood infections (notably measles and mumps) were to prove a continuing nuisance for selectees, particular military significance began to attach to conditions such as respiratory tract infections and meningitis—diseases that had been over-shadowed in earlier periods. At the same time, deaths from infectious causes became relatively rare, thereby paralleling developments in civil life (see Sect. 4.2).

A recurring feature of the present analysis has been the role of military camps in the kindling, acceleration, and spatial transmission of epidemic events. In particular, the example of typhoid fever in the Spanish–American

War has demonstrated how the geographical diffusion of a disease may be structured according to the size and direction of population movements in a camp system. It is the specific issue of the role of military camps as sites and systems for the spatial transmission of diseases that we consider in the next chapter.

8

Europe: Camp Epidemics

This mysterious poison, so subtle as to traverse immeasurable distances
... so gross as to find conveyance in moving battalions, across water,
over hills and valleys, and, if necessary, through climates of opposite characteristics, was at work, and the exhausting flux which it determined, drained off
the manly energies of the soldier, sapped his strength, and rendered him, in
many instances, helpless as a child.

'Cholera—First Epidemic', British Army of the East, 1854–5[1]

8.1 Introduction

One recurring theme of the previous chapter was the role of military assembly
and training camps as sites for explosive outbreaks of infectious diseases

[1] Army Medical Department (1858, ii. 71).

during periods of wartime mobilization. Historically, however, the general problem of *camp epidemics* has extended beyond the initial massing of unseasoned recruits in barrack and tent camps on home soil to include the field camps, siege camps, and bivouacs of deployed armies, as well as temporary and makeshift military settlements such as prisoner of war (POW) and concentration camps. In this chapter, we examine the broader issue of camp epidemics (Theme 2 in Table III.A) with reference to sample wars in the European theatre.

THE SPREAD OF CAMP EPIDEMICS

The social, physical, and environmental conditions that fuelled the spread of diseases in the military encampments of past wars, and which remain a potent threat in modern conflicts, are well known (Prinzing, 1916; Major, 1940; Bayne-Jones, 1968; Cantlie, 1974; Shepherd, 1991). As illustrated in Chapter 7 by the mobilization camps of the United States, military encampments of all kinds—often hastily erected and densely populated—provide a setting for intense population mixing, thereby increasing the likelihood of the transmission of infectious diseases. The epidemiological hazard is exacerbated by the injudicious selection of campsites and by the deleterious consequences of over-crowding, inadequate or non-existent drainage and sewerage systems, poor or contaminated water supplies, and by the failure to institute or to maintain rigid sanitary precautions. As for the occupants, they may be drawn from a variety of epidemiological backgrounds, they may possess different patterns of disease immunity, and their resistance to infection may be compromised by fatigue, trauma, mental and physical stress, exposure to the elements, and poor or inadequate diets. That there is often a high degree of spatial mobility between the constituent units of a camp system adds a powerful geographical component to the spread of camp epidemics.

Against this background, the case studies presented in this chapter have been selected to illustrate different aspects of the geographical spread of camp epidemics. Our examination begins in Section 8.2 with an exploration of cholera transmission in the field and siege camps of one mid-nineteenth-century expeditionary force: the British Army of the East, assembled and deployed in Eastern Europe during the Crimean War of 1853–6. Less than 20 years later, in 1870–1, the Franco-Prussian War sparked an epidemic of smallpox that ran through the military and civil populations of France, Prussia, and the allied states of Germany, killing some 300,000 (Guttstadt, 1873; Prinzing, 1916). In Section 8.3, we examine the manner in which the newly established POW camp system of one belligerent state (Prussia) conditioned the geographical spread of smallpox in the civil settlement system of the country at that time. Finally, Section 8.4 draws on the example of World War II to illustrate the importance of camps in the spread of an apparently new disease of military significance (Q fever) during the first half of the twentieth century. The chapter is concluded in Section 8.5.

Table 8.1. Estimated deaths in the Allied and Austrian forces during the Crimean War, 1853–1856

Army	Effectives	Deaths[1]		
		Killed[2]	Disease	Total
Allied forces				
France	309,268	20,240 (6.5)	75,375 (24.4)	95,615 (30.9)
Great Britain	97,864	4,602 (4.7)	17,580 (18.0)	22,182 (22.7)
Piedmont	21,000	28 (0.1)	2,166 (10.3)	2,194 (10.4)
Turkey	?	?	?	35,000 (?)
Austria[3]	283,000	—	35,000 (12.4)	35,000 (12.4)
Total	711,132[4]	24,870[4] (3.5)	130,121[4] (18.3)	189,991 (26.7)

Notes: [1] Percentages of effectives in parentheses. [2] Includes deaths from wounds. [3] Non-belligerent army of observation. [4] Excluding Turkey.
Source: Smallman-Raynor and Cliff (forthcoming, table 1), based on information in Dumas and Vedel-Petersen (1923: 41–2).

8.2 Crimean War: Cholera in the Field Camps of the British Army, 1854–1855

Many of the factors that contribute to the spread of camp epidemics came together in the military encampments of the Allied Army during the Crimean War of 1853–6. Beginning with the arrival of British and French troops in Turkey and Bulgaria during the spring and early summer of 1854, followed by the allied invasion of the Crimea in the early autumn of the same year, the expeditionary forces of France, Great Britain, Sardinia, and Turkey were plunged into two years of disease turmoil. The dimensions of the resulting population loss can be seen in Table 8.1. Of the estimated 155,000 allied soldiers who perished in the war, 95,000 or more are believed to have succumbed to disease rather than to battle. An additional 35,000 Austrian troops, forming a non-belligerent Army of Observation, were also killed by disease (Dumas and Vedel-Petersen, 1923: 41–2).

Dysentery, malaria, typhus fever, and relapsing fever, among many other infectious diseases, contributed to the death toll recorded in Table 8.1 (Prinzing, 1916; Shepherd, 1991). Especially prominent was an epidemic of Asiatic cholera that spread through the allied ranks as two well-defined waves of infection and claimed upwards of 18,000 lives (Prinzing, 1916: 172). In this section, we examine the manner in which the cholera epidemic diffused in the Bulgarian and Crimean camp systems of one army (Great Britain) during the course of its first—and most severe—wave, from July 1854 to February 1855. Our examination draws on the study of Smallman-Raynor and Cliff (forthcoming).

8.2.1 Background to the Epidemic

Although the Crimean War was fought on two widely separated naval fronts (Baltic and Black Seas)—both of which were to suffer major epidemics of cholera in the years 1854–6—the Black Sea territories of the Russian and Ottoman Empires formed the locus of Allied Army operations throughout the conflict. The site of the Black Sea, along with the territorial divisions of surrounding lands at the time of the war, is shown in the main map of Figure 8.1; inset maps A (Bulgaria) and B (Crimea) identify the locations of British Army encampments referred to in subsequent sections of the text.

THE EPIDEMIOLOGICAL CONTEXT OF THE WAR

The origins and course of the Crimean War have been outlined in a number of authoritative studies.[2] Ultimately rooted in a long-standing policy of Russian expansion towards Constantinople, but prompted by the more immediate claims of Russia as the sole protector of Orthodox Christians within the territories of the Ottoman Empire, Russian troops had moved on the Turkish principalities of Moldavia and Wallachia in July 1853; see Figure 8.1 for locations. While a Turkish declaration of war on Russia followed later that year (23 Oct.),[3] the factors that prompted the subsequent military alliance of Britain and France (and, later, Sardinia) with Turkey have attracted a large historical literature (see e.g. Puryear, 1931; Gooch, 1956, 1969; Goldfrank, 1994) and encompass a series of strategic, commercial, political, and ideological considerations. Whatever the exact reasons for the alliance, an Anglo-French summons for the Russian evacuation of Ottoman territories was issued on 27 February 1854; a month later, on 28 March, Britain and France declared war on Russia. Thereafter, an initial period of assembly of British and French forces in the Near East was followed, in September 1854, by the allied invasion of the Crimean Peninsula and the laying of a year-long siege to the Russian fortress city of Sebastopol. Sebastopol capitulated on 9 September 1855 and, with little enthusiasm among the belligerents for further sustained conflict, peace was finally agreed under the terms of the Treaty of Paris (concluded 30 Mar. 1856).

   Like her French allies, the British response to the declaration of war was marked by the rapid transfer of a sizeable expeditionary force to the vicinity of the Black Sea. Headed by an advance contingent of 10,000 men, and with Malta serving as the principal staging post, successive detachments of the British Army began to mass at Gallipoli and Scutari, Turkey, in April and early May 1854 (see Fig. 8.1 for locations). For the majority of commands, however, a brief and relatively healthful sojourn in Turkey was followed by

---

[2] Classic nineteenth-century studies include: Kinglake (1863); Hamley (1891); and Lysons (1895). For more recent perspectives, see Barker (1970); Curtiss (1979); Conacher (1987); and Palmer (1987).

[3] In fact, the Ottoman war manifesto had been issued almost three weeks earlier, on 4 Oct. 1853.

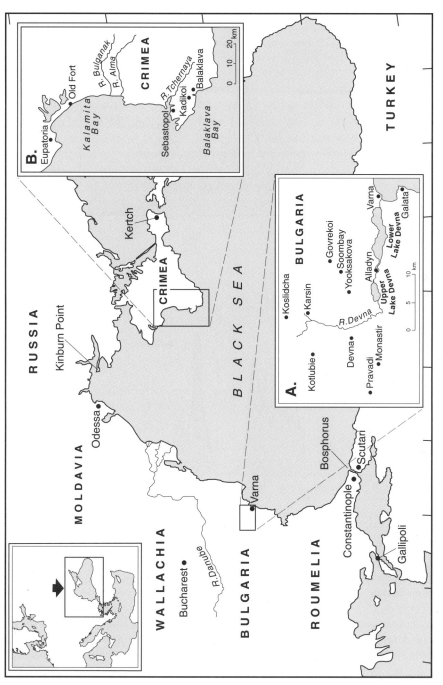

Fig. 8.1. The Black Sea and surrounding lands, c.1853

Source: Smallman-Raynor and Cliff (forthcoming, fig. 1).

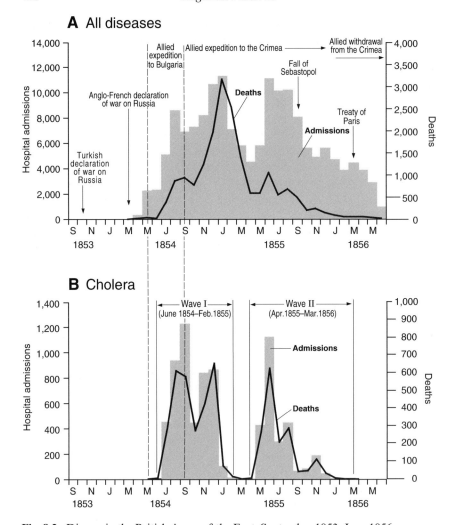

Fig. 8.2. Disease in the British Army of the East, September 1853–June 1856

Notes: Monthly counts of primary hospital admissions (bar charts) and deaths (line traces) are plotted for (A) all diseases and (B) cholera. The principal phases of the Crimean War are shown for reference.

Source: Smallman-Raynor and Cliff (forthcoming, fig. 2), based on data in Army Medical Department (1858, ii, return A, following p. 251).

consecutive—and epidemiologically disastrous—expeditions to Bulgaria (May–Aug. 1854) and the Crimean Peninsula (Sept. 1854–July 1856). To illustrate the magnitude of the disease problem associated with the two expeditions, the graphs in Figure 8.2 are based on information included in the Army Medical Department's (1858) *Medical and Surgical History of the War* and plot the monthly number of hospital admissions and deaths from all diseases

(Fig. 8.2A) and cholera (Fig. 8.2B) in the British Army of the East. For reference, the periods of residence in Bulgaria and the Crimea are indicated on the graphs by the vertical pecked lines.

Bulgaria (May–August 1854)

Towards the end of May 1854, a 28,000-strong British force was transported from its initial bases in Turkey to the vicinity of the Black Sea port of Varna, Bulgaria, where it was to remain inactive for the next three months (Cantlie, 1974, ii. 20–3). The main territory occupied by the British Army in Bulgaria, and which formed the core of the camp system during the summer of 1854, is mapped in Figure 8.1A; the locations of the principal encampments are named for reference. As the map shows, the camp system spanned an 800 square km tract of land, extending some 40 km inland from the Black Sea and encompassing a varied landscape of undulating plains, valleys, lakes, marshes, woods, and heights.[4] Further to the west of the area shown in Figure 8.1A, the village of Yeni-Bazaar formed the site of a peripheral encampment occupied by some regiments of the Cavalry Division. The location of Yeni-Bazaar is marked in Figure 8.4, below.

The conditions that prevailed in the British camp system of Bulgaria, and which were to contribute to the spread of a range of infectious diseases, have been reviewed in detail elsewhere (Army Medical Department, 1858, ii. 2–14; Cantlie, 1974, ii. 21–45; Shepherd, 1991, i. 73–85). From a military perspective, the territory had gained epidemiological notoriety when bubonic plague and assorted fevers had decimated the occupying Russian forces during the Russo-Turkish War of 1828–9 (Prinzing, 1916: 168). Twenty-five years on, the British experience of such an unhealthy place was compounded by the severe logistical difficulties that beset the expedition. In the oppressive heat of an advancing Bulgarian summer, with no Transport Corps and a barely adequate Ambulance Corps, the troops were subject to an irregular and inadequate supply of rations, equipage, and medicines. Local fresh produce soon became exhausted, while boredom, low morale, and drunkenness began to intervene in the daily routine of the men. As for the campsites, some (e.g. Galata, Govrekoi, Koslidcha, and Soombay) were viewed by regimental surgeons as being of generally healthy aspect (Army Medical Department, 1858, ii. 6–9). Others, however, were not. The lower-lying camps, such as those at Alladyn and Devna, were positioned next to malarious lakes and morasses (ibid. ii. 4–5) while the maintenance of a clean and potable water supply represented a more general problem in camp hygiene. Testifying to the deterioration of the water at Devna in July 1854, for example, Assistant-Surgeon William Cattell of the Fifth Dragoon Guards observed that:

There were several excellent springs, and the river was also good when we arrived, but the proximity of the troops did not allow of its continuing so; the horses were watered

---

[4] For a more detailed description of the territory, see Army Medical Department (1858, ii. 2–4).

there, and kept it constantly muddy; the Infantry washed their clothes in it, and to add to the mischief, butchers found it convenient to throw offal into it, while it still formed the chief supply for cooking, and what was of far more consequence, was also drunk by men scorched into excessive and constant thirst from fatiguing duties under an unusually powerful sun. (Cited in ibid. 6)

If such conditions were conducive to the spread of cholera and other water-borne camp diseases, the squalid and insanitary state of native settlements such as Varna (population *c*.15,000 in 1854) and, more particularly, the British military hospital at that place,[5] served to magnify the health risks of the expedition (see ibid. 4–11).

The consequent upsurge in disease activity is depicted in Figure 8.2.[6] During the period of the expedition, the monthly number of disease-related hospital admissions in the British Army increased from little over 2,000 (June) to almost 9,000 (August) while, during the same interval, the monthly count of disease-related deaths increased from less than 20 to almost 900 (Fig. 8.2A). Severe outbreaks of fevers, dysentery, and diarrhoea were to contribute to the recorded morbidity. In terms of mortality, however, these conditions were to pale against the epidemic of cholera that had newly appeared in the ranks (Fig. 8.2B).

Crimea (September 1854–July 1856)

On 7 September 1854, a 57,000-strong allied force embarked near Varna for a week-long voyage and the assault on the Crimean Peninsula. From a landing point near Eupatoria, to the northwest of the Crimea, the combined army marched southwards in mid-September to take up siege positions before Sebastopol by the end of the month. The locations of Eupatoria and Sebastopol, along with auxiliary allied positions at Kadikoi and Balaklava, are plotted in Figure 8.1B.

The severe conditions endured by the British forces before Sebastopol during the winter of 1854–5 are well known and will only be summarized here;[7] graphic accounts are provided by special correspondents to *The Lancet*[8] and,

---

[5] The British military hospital in Varna had been established, alongside the French military hospital, in a disused Turkish barracks. Some impression of the deplorable conditions that prevailed in the British section of the hospital, and which served as a source of cholera and other diseases throughout the expedition to Bulgaria, can be gained from the observations of Dr David Dumbreck, Army Medical Department: 'No words can describe the state of the rooms when they were handed over for the use of the sick; indeed they continued long after, from the utter inability to procure labour, rather to be fitted for the reception of cattle, than sick men. Myriads of rats disputed possession of these dreadful dens, fleas were in such number that sappers employed on fatigue refused to work in the almost vain attempt to clear them . . . [T]he inner walls of the hospital were begrimed and filthy, an aspect of desolation reigned in them, the flooring was rotten, and the air of these miserable chambers was thick and oppressive' (cited in Army Medical Department, 1858, ii. 9).

[6] The data in Fig. 8.2 are abstracted from vol. ii, part I (Return A) of the Army Medical Department's (1858) *Medical and Surgical History* and refer to disease-related primary hospital admissions and deaths in the entire British Army of East, including commands that were not then stationed in Bulgaria.

[7] For an excellent overview, see Shepherd (1991, i. 287–339).

[8] See e.g. *The Lancet* (1855, vol. 1: 22–3, 111–12, 141–2, 199–200).

perhaps more famously, *The Times*,[9] while further insights can be gained from the published correspondence of regimental surgeons[10] and the post-war findings of the Royal Sanitary Commission (Royal Commission, 1858). With long and fatiguing duties in the trenches, little or no shelter from the elements, woefully inadequate dress, an insufficiently nutritious diet, and a dire shortage of fuel—all compounded by a virtual breakdown of the allied supply line to Balaklava—disease was to reach new heights in the British Army. As Figure 8.2A shows, the monthly mortality from disease soared to almost 3,000 (42.1 deaths per 1,000 mean strength) in January 1855, with some 12,000 disease-related hospital admissions during the same month. While fevers, diarrhoea, and dysentery were, as in Bulgaria, to contribute to the morbidity and mortality, Figure 8.2B shows that cholera persisted in the British forces throughout the Crimean winter of 1854–5, for a marked resurgence in the early summer of 1855.

JOHN SNOW, CHOLERA, AND THE CRIMEAN WAR

The nature of classic Asiatic cholera, which spread through the British encampments of Bulgaria and the Crimea during the Crimean War, is described in Appendix 1A. Here, we note that the war came at a time when the waterborne nature of the disease was only just beginning to be unravelled by John Snow. At about the time of appearance of an expanded edition of his *On the Mode of Communication of Cholera* in 1855 (Snow, 1855a), a lesser-known publication highlighted the role of contaminated water supplies as a factor in cholera transmission among the allied forces in the Crimea (Snow, 1855b). However, in the absence of an appropriate remedial response by the Army medical services, and with many of the milder cases of cholera permitted to circulate with the body of their respective commands, the spread of the disease went largely unchecked in the British forces.

8.2.2 The Data

SOURCES OF DATA

In the early months of 1855—just as the epidemiological effects of the disastrous Crimean winter of 1854–5 were beginning to wane—Dr Andrew Smith, Director General of the Army Medical Department (Pl. 8.1), petitioned the British Government for permission to

secure an analysis of the professional documents and returns which might be forwarded to this Office [Army Medical Department], during or immediately after the war, by the Medical Officers of the Army, and so have, at any time, the means of easily ascertaining all that had operated to the prejudice of health, as well as the diseases and

---

[9] Russell (1877). See also Bentley (1966).
[10] See e.g. Bonham-Carter (1968).

wounds from which the troops had suffered, and the treatment that had proved the most beneficial in each affection, in fact, a Medical–Chirurgical History of the War. (Army Medical Department, 1858, i., p. iii)

With the consent of the newly appointed Secretary of State for War, Lord Panmure, a small team of army medical officers (Staff-Surgeons Hanbury and Matthew, Surgeon Laing, and Staff Assistant-Surgeon Fitzgerald) spent the following months and years compiling the medical records of all regiments of the British Army of the East.[11] The resulting two-volume report, published under the full title, *The Medical and Surgical History of the British Army which Served in Turkey and the Crimea during the War against Russia in the Years 1854–55–56*, volumes i and ii, was completed and presented to both Houses of Parliament in 1858 (Pl. 1.2B).

Summary details of the content and scope of *The Medical and Surgical History* are given by Shepherd (1991, ii. 597–600), while the nature and quality of the cholera-related information on which the present analysis draws is outlined by Smallman-Raynor and Cliff (forthcoming). For a 27-month period from April 1854 (the first full calendar month of the allied engagement in the Crimean War) to June 1856 (the last full calendar month of the allied presence in the Crimean Peninsula), the *History* provides:

(a) *Numerical data.* Volume i of the *History* includes consolidated monthly counts of hospital admissions and deaths from cholera in a total of 66 regiments assigned to seven divisions (Light, Cavalry, First, Second, Third, Fourth, and Highland Divisions) of the British Army, along with information on the mean strengths and daily locations of the organizations.

(b) *Textual accounts.* The numerical information included in the *History* is supplemented by textual accounts of the origin and progress of the cholera epidemic in each regiment (vol. i) and the army as a whole (vol. ii).

The distribution of regiments by army division is given in Table 8.2, along with summary information on the number of personnel and recorded levels of disease activity; a full listing of regiments by army division appears in Appendix 8A.

Selection of Time Period

Figure 8.2B shows that the cholera epidemic spread in the British Army as two distinct waves. Summary statistics are given in Table 8.3 while, for reference,

---

[11] In the preface to vol. i of the *History*, Andrew Smith was to pay handsome tribute to the efforts of the staff involved in the production of the report: 'Persons only who, like myself, had an opportunity of observing the exertions that were required while the compilations were in progress, can form a correct notion of what is due to the energy, perseverance, abilities, and circumspection of Staff-Surgeons Matthew and Hanbury, of Surgeon Laing, of the 23rd Regiment, and of Staff-Assistant-Surgeon Fitzgerald' (Army Medical Department, 1858, i., p. iv). For a review of the work of Andrew Smith and the Army Medical Department during the Crimean War, see Cantlie (1974, ii. 1–195).

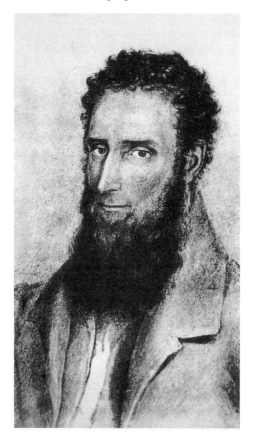

Pl. 8.1. Sir Andrew Smith (1797–1872)

Notes: British physician, explorer, and naturalist. Smith served as Director General of the British Army Medical Department during the Crimean Campaign of 1854–56. His petitions to the British Government were to secure the publication of the two-volume *Medical and Surgical History of the British Army which Served in Turkey and the Crimea during the War against Russia in the Years 1854–55–56*, presented to both Houses of Parliament in 1858. The portrait shows Smith in the early part of 1835.
Source: Original watercolour portrait by George H. Ford, reproduced by kind permission of Iziko Museums of Cape Town.

disaggregated cholera counts are provided by army division and regiment in Tables 8.2 and 8.A1 (App. 8A) respectively.

According to Table 8.3, Wave I began in mid-June 1854 and persisted for nine months, ending in February 1855. It was characterized by a bimodal distribution of cases (peaking in Sept. and Nov./Dec. 1854) and was associated with a recorded 4,630 hospital admissions and 2,717 deaths. The rather less severe Wave II was separated from Wave I by a disease-free interval of some six weeks. It began in mid-April 1855, lasted until March 1856, and is

Table 8.2. Hospital admissions and deaths recorded in military divisions of the British Army during the Crimean War, 1854–1856

Division	n (regiments)	Mean monthly strength	All diseases		Cholera			
					Wave I[1]		Wave II[2]	
			Admissions[3]	Deaths[3]	Admissions[3]	Deaths[3]	Admissions[3]	Deaths[3]
Light	10	6,772	28,156 (415.8)	2,392 (35.3)	1,273 (16.4)	802 (10.3)	416 (6.2)	216 (3.2)
Cavalry	14	3,714	17,777 (478.6)	653 (17.6)	326 (13.6)	192 (8.0)	382 (7.1)	207 (3.9)
First/First & Highland[4]	10	6,138	22,513 (366.8)	1,657 (27.0)	816 (14.9)	540 (9.9)	475 (6.2)	311 (4.1)
Second Division	10	5,524	23,699 (429.0)	1,321 (23.9)	369 (6.5)	227 (4.0)	297 (4.6)	179 (2.9)
Third Division	10	6,247	24,829 (397.5)	1,859 (29.8)	780 (10.3)	514 (6.8)	248 (3.4)	156 (2.2)
Fourth Division	9	5,330	20,482 (384.3)	1,551 (29.1)	1,062 (19.3)	440 (8.0)	248 (4.2)	137 (2.3)
Highland Division	3	1,647	2,714 (164.8)	141 (8.6)	4 (0.6)	2 (0.3)	162 (7.2)	96 (4.3)
Total	66	35,372	140,170 (396.3)	9,574 (27.1)	4,630 (16.4)	2,717 (9.6)	2,228 (5.6)	1,302 (3.3)

Notes: [1] June 1854–Feb. 1855. [2] Apr. 1855–Mar. 1856. [3] Rates per 100 mean monthly strength in parentheses. [4] Includes three regiments later transferred to the Highland Division.

Source: Smallman-Raynor and Cliff (forthcoming, table 2), based on reports included in Army Medical Department (1858).

Table 8.3. Summary details of Waves I and II of the cholera epidemic in 66 regiments of the British Army during the Crimean War, 1853–1856

	Start	End	Admissions[1]	Deaths[1]
Wave I	17 June 1854	Feb. 1855[2]	4,630 (16.4)	2,717 (9.6)
Wave II	12 Apr. 1855[3]	Mar. 1856[2]	2,228 (5.6)	1,302 (3.3)

Notes: [1] Rate per 100 mean monthly strength in parentheses. [2] Exact date not known. [3] Earliest case in Wave II for which the exact date of presentation is known.
Source: Smallman-Raynor and Cliff (forthcoming, table 3), based on regimental reports included in Army Medical Department (1858).

documented to have claimed 1,302 lives. Here we restrict our analysis of the databases to an examination of the more severe Wave I (June 1854–Feb. 1855).

8.2.3 Diffusion of Cholera in the British Camp System of Bulgaria

In this section, we examine the geographical spread of cholera in the British camp system of Bulgaria during the summer of 1854. The basic concepts of epidemiological diffusion on which the analysis draws are outlined in Section 6.4. A standard approach to the diffusion problem, and one that we adopt in the first part of the analysis, is to map the documented sequence of cholera transmission within the conventional geographical space of the camp system. While this approach permits the identification of certain key features of the spread pattern, including the early geographical seed reservoirs of infection, an alternative approach is required to model the complex network of mass population movements by which the spread of *Vibrio cholerae* was mediated through the system. To these ends, the technique of multidimensional scaling (MDS) is used to re-map the camp system into non-Euclidean 'connectivity spaces'. These spaces, which reflect levels of interaction between individual camps (transmission centres) within the system, provide alternative measures of camp separation on which to assess the underpinning processes of disease transmission.

ORIGINS OF THE EPIDEMIC IN BULGARIA

The earliest evidence of Asiatic cholera in the British camp system of Bulgaria—indeed, the first documented evidence of the disease in the entire British Army of the East—can be traced to Saturday 17 June 1854. On that day, two men of the Nineteenth Regiment went down with the disease at the lakeside encampment of Alladyn (Fig. 8.1A), one succumbing within seven hours of onset (Army Medical Department, 1858, i. 192). The visitation, however, was to prove fleeting and, with the exception of a sporadic case in the Ordnance

Corps (ibid. ii. 46), the British Army remained free of the disease for the next three weeks.[12] The epidemiological silence was finally broken when cholera reappeared in the Nineteenth Regiment on 6 July, to be followed by cases in the First Regiment, First Battalion (13 July), the Coldstream Guards (18 July), and, soon thereafter, all British commands on Bulgarian territory.

The ultimate source of *Vibrio cholerae* in Bulgaria, and which sparked the epidemic among the British forces in the summer of 1854, cannot be ascertained with any certainty. As part of the third cholera pandemic of the nineteenth century (1846–63),[13] August Hirsch (1883, i) observes that the disease had spread over a 'great part' of Turkey and the Danubian Principalities several years earlier in 1848–50 (p. 404), only to reappear in the region in 1853 (p. 410). As far as the historical record allows, the disease was absent from Bulgaria on the eve of the Crimean War (Army Medical Department, 1858, ii. 48) and a fresh importation with troops from southern France (where cholera had spread widely in the spring of 1854; see Bourdelais and Raulot, 1978) is generally suspected (Hirsch, 1883, i. 410; Prinzing, 1916: 170–1). So, following the diffusion route depicted by the solid vectors in Figure 8.3, the textual accounts included in the *Medical and Surgical History* relate how the cholera vibrio was conveyed by French army transports from the infected port of Marseilles to stations in Greece (Piraeus) and Turkey (Gallipoli) in early July.[14] As for Bulgaria, the evidence is summarized by Dr William Linton of the Army Medical Department:

> The disease is said to have been imported . . . the circumstances attending its advent are these, the truth of which was corroborated by Colonel Neale, our Consul at Varna. In the early part of June 1854, a French vessel arrived at Varna from Marseilles, bringing troops from Avignon, and, some cases of cholera having occurred on board, the quarantine director wished to place the vessel in quarantine . . . but this was objected to, and the troops were landed. After this, cholera spread progressively through the town and allied forces, attacking the French and Turks simultaneously, and afterwards the English. (Cited in Army Medical Department, 1858, ii. 47)

---

[12] In Turkey, however, two possible cases of Asiatic cholera were recorded among English troops at the General Hospital, Scutari, towards the end of June. According to Staff-Surgeon O'Flaherty, then stationed at the hospital, the men were 'recently arrived from England . . . both cases suffered from vomiting, cramps, collapse, &c., but recovered, and were noticed as instances of "English cholera;" had they died, however, they would have been certainly denominated as Asiatic cholera' (cited in Army Medical Department, 1858, ii. 47).

[13] Hirsch (1883, i. 404–13). There is no general agreement on the exact timing of the third cholera pandemic. For alternative timings, see Pollitzer (1959: 30–1); Cliff and Haggett (1988: 4–11); Barua and Greenough (1992: 11–12).

[14] The importations into Piraeus and Gallipoli were to spark outbreaks of the disease among the British regiments at those stations. At Piraeus, the Ninety-Seventh Regiment was struck down by cholera on 19 July, the disease having been imported by a French steamer from Marseilles earlier that month. Likewise, the Fourth Regiment was assailed by the disease at Gallipoli on 17 July, the disease having appeared a week earlier among a squadron of French troops newly arrived from Marseilles. For further details, see Army Medical Department (1858, i. 148–9, 438); Prinzing (1916: 170–1).

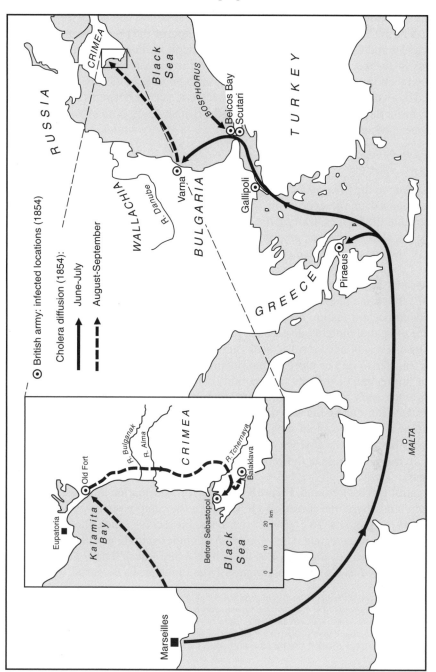

Fig. 8.3. Diffusion of Wave I of the cholera epidemic, Crimean War

Notes: The vectors plot the generalized routes by which cholera spread with the Anglo-French forces, June–September 1854. Sample infected locations for the British Army are identified by the circular symbols.
Source: Smallman-Raynor and Cliff (forthcoming, fig. 3).

While such evidence accords with the timing of the earliest cholera cases in the British Army,[15] the arrival of successive contingents of the French Army from Marseilles and Gallipoli gave rise to a more general seeding of Varna and environs in the weeks that followed. Certainly, the disease had colonized the French section of the military hospital at Varna on or about 3 July, to be followed by an explosive outbreak in the British section of the hospital a fortnight later. From there on, attacks of cholera in the British Army, both at Varna and elsewhere, became commonplace (ibid. 46–7).

SPREAD SEQUENCES

According to the *Medical and Surgical History*, a total of 33 British regiments were engaged in the expedition to Bulgaria. The 33 regiments (variously assigned to the Light, Cavalry, First, Second, and Third Divisions) are listed in Table 8.4, along with summary information relating to the date and camp location of the first documented cholera case in each command. For reference, the table also gives the recorded number of cholera-related hospital admissions and deaths, as well as the associated rates per 100 mean monthly strength, during the Bulgarian phase of the epidemic.

One important feature of the British expedition to Bulgaria was the high degree of spatial mobility displayed by the regiments in Table 8.4. On landing at Varna, a stay of a few days or weeks in the local camp was typically followed by a transfer to one or more of the proximal encampments in Figure 8.1A. Some impression of the resulting mobility can be gained by recognizing that, on average, each of the 33 regiments underwent three wholesale changes of camp location during the expedition, equivalent to a transfer every 28 days. With the advent of cholera serving to increase the frequency of the transfers, such mobility—in the absence of an effective system of quarantine—was to play an important role in the geographical spread of the disease in the camp system.

Against this background, Figure 8.4 is based on information included in the *History* and charts the spread of cholera with the camp-wise movements of the British regiments. To construct the maps, the day on which cholera first appeared in a given regiment (see Table 8.4) was indexed to the putative start of the main outbreak of the disease in the British Army. The first day of the outbreak (specified as 6 July;[16] see 'Origins of the Epidemic in Bulgaria', above)

[15] Commenting on the temporal association, Sir John Hall, Principal Medical Officer of the British Army, noted: 'The history of the disease in the French army is, that a Zouave [an Algerian recruit] who had come direct from Africa, was seized with the disease, and died about the middle of June; and it is a curious coincidence, that a man of the 19th Regiment of the British Army, stationed with the Light Division at Alladyn, was attacked, and died about the same time' (cited in Army Medical Department, 1858, ii. 46).

[16] Despite sporadic cases of cholera in mid-June 1854, our specification of the first case associated with the main outbreak of the disease (6 July) is founded on an epidemiologically informed reading of the available data. First, while the carrier state for classical Asiatic cholera is typically of the order of three to six days, convalescent carriers may shed vibrios for two to three weeks; longer-term, chronic, carriers are

Table 8.4. Cholera in the British Army during the Allied expedition to Bulgaria, May–September 1854, Crimean War

Regiment	Cholera			
	First case		Reported cases/deaths	
	Date	Camp location	Admissions[1]	Deaths[1]
Light Division				
7th Fusiliers	23 July	Devna	43 (4.3)	35 (3.5)
19th Regiment	6 July[2]	Devna	30 (3.0)	13 (1.3)
23rd Regiment	22 July	Devna	46 (5.0)	36 (3.9)
33rd Regiment	23 July	Devna	53 (5.7)	36 (3.9)
77th Regiment	27 July	Monastir	40 (4.1)	24 (2.5)
88th Regiment	23 July	Monastir[3]	71 (9.0)	37 (4.7)
Rifle Brig. (2nd Batt.)	27 July	Monastir	48 (4.3)	30 (2.7)
Cavalry Division				
4th Dragoon Guards	c.28 July	Galata	25 (8.8)	20 (7.0)
5th Dragoon Guards	24 July	Devna	58 (21.8)	35 (13.2)
1st Royal Dragoons	3 Aug.	Karasin	11 (4.1)	9 (3.4)
4th Light Dragoons	c.5 Aug.	Galata	11 (3.4)	5 (1.6)
6th Dragoons	24 July	Galata	56 (19.0)	19 (6.4)
8th Hussars	20 Aug.	Yeni-Bazaar	8 (2.9)	5 (1.8)
11th Hussars	29 July	Yeni-Bazaar	4 (1.3)	2 (0.7)
13th Light Dragoons	c.18 Aug.	Yeni-Bazaar	6 (2.0)	5 (1.7)
17th Lancers[4]	28 July	Devna	7 (2.4)	6 (2.1)
First Division[5]				
Grenadier Guards	24 July	Alladyn	42 (3.9)	36 (3.3)
Coldstream Guards	18 July	Alladyn	31 (3.4)	28 (3.1)
Scots Fusilier Guards	27 July	Alladyn	82 (9.0)	49 (5.4)
42nd Regiment	31 July	Govrekoi	18 (1.8)	12 (1.2)
79th Regiment	27 July	Alladyn	16 (1.7)	8 (0.9)
93rd Regiment	30 July	Govrekoi	23 (1.9)	19 (1.6)
Second Division				
30th Regiment	8 Aug.	Koslidcha	14 (1.7)	9 (1.1)
41st Regiment	7 Aug.	Soombay	6 (0.6)	5 (0.5)
47th Regiment	1 Aug.	Yooksakova	17 (2.0)	11 (1.3)
49th Regiment	Aug.[6]	Soombay	12 (1.3)	9 (1.0)
55th Regiment	30 July	Yooksakova	4 (0.4)	2 (0.2)
95th Regiment	24 July	Yooksakova	26 (2.6)	16 (1.6)
Third Division				
1st Regiment (1st Batt.)	13 July	Varna	26 (3.1)	19 (2.3)
28th Regiment	25 July	Galata	36 (4.2)	26 (3.0)
38th Regiment	23 July	Varna	48 (5.6)	30 (3.5)
44th Regiment	25 July	Galata	20 (2.5)	13 (1.6)
50th Regiment	28 July	Varna	63 (7.1)	36 (4.1)
Total			1,001 (4.0)	645 (2.6)

Notes: [1] Rate per 100 mean monthly strength in parentheses. [2] Excludes two recorded cholera cases in June. [3] First case recorded on the day of transfer from Devna to Monastir; no further details available. [4] First case recorded on the first day of the five-day march from Devna to Yeni-Bazaar. [5] Includes three regiments (42nd, 79th, and 93rd) later assigned to the Highland Division. [6] Exact date of first case not recorded.
Source: Smallman-Raynor and Cliff (forthcoming, table 4), based on regimental reports included in Army Medical Department (1858).

was coded 1, with subsequent days numbered sequentially thereafter. On this basis, the black circles in Figure 8.4 plot the camp locations of newly infected regiments on (Fig. 8.4A) days 1–14 (6–19 July), (Fig. 8.4B) days 15–28 (20 July–2 Aug.), and (Fig. 8.4C) days 29–49 (3–23 Aug.) of the epidemic. The numbers adjacent to the black circles denote the day of the epidemic in which cholera first appeared in the regiment, while the white circles identify regiments included on earlier maps. Finally, the vectors trace the camp-wise movements of regiments (classified by army division). In all instances, vector widths are drawn proportional to the number of regiments that linked a pair of camps.

Days 1–14 (6–19 July; Figure 8.4A)

This phase of the epidemic was associated with the early seeding of cholera in campsites along the rivers and lakes system that linked the settlements of Devna, Alladyn, and Varna. As described above, two sporadic cases of cholera—seemingly unassociated with the main outbreak of the disease in the British Army—had already occurred in the Nineteenth Regiment (Light Division) while encamped at Alladyn in mid-June. Three weeks on, and with the commands of the Light Division now encamped at Devna,[17] the ill-fated Nineteenth Regiment was again attacked by cholera, first on Thursday 6 July (day 1 of the epidemic) and again on the following Sunday (day 4) (Army Medical Department, 1858, ii. 46). While the exact source of the infection in the camp is unknown, and other regiments of the Light Division at Devna were to escape the disease temporarily, Figure 8.4A shows that cholera soon began to appear in encampments elsewhere. At Varna, a drummer boy of the First Regiment, First Battalion (Third Division) was struck down by cholera on 13 July (day 8).[18] Five days later, the disease appeared in the ranks of the Coldstream Guards (First Division) at Alladyn (Army Medical Department, 1858, i. 107).[19]

Days 15–28 (20 July–2 August; Figure 8.4B)

From these early foci of infection, the second fortnight of the epidemic was to witness the rapid and widespread dissemination of cholera in the British camp system. As Figure 8.4B indicates, this main phase of the spread sequence was

generally thought to be rare and are of limited epidemiological importance. Secondly, while uncertainty surrounds the survival times of cholera vibrios in the environment, experimental results suggest a typical survival time of one to three weeks in pools and wells, especially if the pH is high. For the 33 regiments under consideration, therefore, the lag of approximately three weeks between the first two cholera cases (Nineteenth Regiment, 17 June) and the third case (Nineteenth Regiment, 6 July) suggests that the two events were associated with independent introductions of the disease agent.

[17] The regiments of the Light Division had broken camp at Alladyn on 30 June, moving directly to a newly established camp between the village and the right bank of the river at Devna.

[18] The first case of cholera in the First Regiment, First Battalion was a young drummer boy who, incidentally, had no history of fatigue duties in Varna (Army Medical Department, 1858, i. 131 and ii. 51).

[19] It is noteworthy that this early appearance of cholera in the Coldstream Guards at Alladyn was overlooked in the Army Medical Department's summary overview of the epidemic (see Army Medical Department, 1858, ii. 45–85).

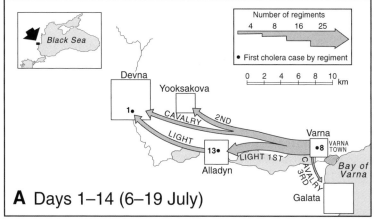

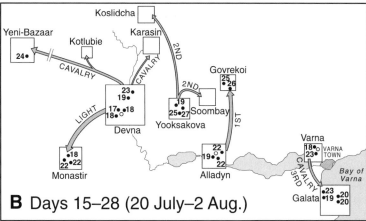

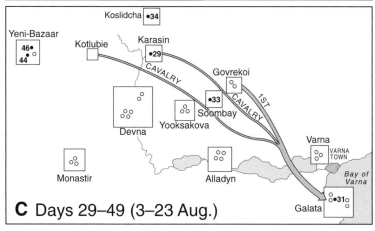

Fig. 8.4. Diffusion of cholera in the camp system of the British Army of the East, Bulgaria, July–August 1854

Notes: The vectors trace the camp-wise movements of regiments of the First, Second, Third, Light, and Cavalry Divisions during the first seven weeks of the epidemic. (A) Days 1–14 (6–19 July). (B) Days 15–28 (20 July–2 Aug.). (C) Days 29–49 (3–23 Aug.). For each regiment, the camp in which the first cholera case was recorded is indicated by a circle. Black circles relate to those regiments in which the first case was recorded during the time period covered by the map. The day of infection (coded relative to the first day of the epidemic, 6 July = day 1) is indicated by numbers. Finally, open circles relate to those regiments that were first infected in prior time periods.
Source: Smallman-Raynor and Cliff (forthcoming, fig. 4).

associated with three interconnected diffusion components: (i) the spread of cholera to previously uninfected commands at Devna (then under the joint occupancy of regiments of the Light Division and a section of the Cavalry Division), Alladyn (First Division), and Varna (Third Division); (ii) the abandonment of these camps in late July on account of the burgeoning cholera problem; and (iii) the consequent establishment of new foci of infection, both on the coast and in the interior of Bulgaria. We consider the sequence of spread from Devna, Alladyn, and Varna in turn.

1. *Devna (Light and Cavalry Divisions).* The circumstances surrounding the spread of cholera with the Light and Cavalry Divisions, initially pitched on opposite sides of the river at Devna, can be traced in the *Medical and Surgical History* with some precision. Notwithstanding the very early appearance of cholera at Devna, most regiments of the Light and Cavalry Divisions had escaped the disease during mid-July. But, with diarrhoea and other complaints now gaining rapidly in incidence and severity (see Army Medical Department, 1858, i. 192, 218, 248, 374, 398), the apparent immunity to cholera finally gave way in the third week of the epidemic. With the disease appearing in rapid succession in commands of the Light Division on days 17 (Twenty-Third Regiment) and 18 (Seventh Fusiliers and Thirty-Third Regiment) of the epidemic, and then across the river in the Cavalry Division on day 19 (Fifth Dragoon Guards), the two divisions immediately broke camp.

The exodus failed to rid the commands of cholera. Regiments of the Light Division, which moved *en masse* to Monastir, continued to be assailed by the disease on the march from Devna.[20] In addition, as Figure 8.4B and Table 8.4 show, cholera spread to previously uninfected regiments at the new encampment.[21] As for the Cavalry Division, the decision to separate the commands and relocate them to several different places (Karasin, Kotlubie, and Yeni-Bazaar) merely served to widen the reach of cholera. The Seventeenth Lancers, headed for Yeni-Bazaar with the rest of the Light Cavalry Brigade, were attacked by cholera on the first day out of Devna (Army Medical Department, 1858, i. 90), while the disease appeared in the accompanying Eleventh Hussars on the evening of its arrival at Yeni-Bazaar (Army Medical Department, 1858, i. 68). At about the same time, the Fifth Dragoon Guards carried cholera to Kotlubie,[22] and the disease appeared in the First Dragoon Guards within a few days of its arrival at Karasin (Army Medical Department, 1858, i. 24).

---

[20] The medical records of the Seventh Fusiliers, for example, document a cholera case with fatal outcome on the road between Devna and Monastir; the duration of the illness (3 days 2½ hours) implies that the infection had been acquired at Devna (Army Medical Department, 1858, i. 157).

[21] In forming Fig. 8.4B, the medical records for one command (Eighty-Eighth Regiment) are insufficient to determine the exact place at which the first cholera case manifested. As noted in Table 8.4, the first case in the regiment is documented to have occurred on the day of transfer from Devna to Monastir (day 18; 23 July) and has been allotted to the latter encampment. Whatever the location, however, acquisition of the infection at Devna must be strongly suspected (Army Medical Department, 1858, i. 398).

[22] Assistant-Surgeon William Cattell, Fifth Dragoon Guards, recorded the circumstances by which cholera appeared at Kotlubie in particular detail: 'The hope that we had removed from the sphere of contagion [Devna] was soon destroyed; two days after our arrival at Kotlubie a case of cholera occurred with

2. *Alladyn (First Division)*. If Devna was to prove a sickly place for the Light and Cavalry Divisions, the First Division fared little better at Alladyn. According to Figure 8.4B and Table 8.4, the majority of commands were infected with cholera before the camp was abandoned in favour of Govrekoi, with the 'more serious' cases of the disease having been left at Alladyn to form a detached Brigade Hospital encampment (Army Medical Department, 1858, i. 107). The latter action had little—if any—discernible containing effect on the spatial transfer of the cholera vibrio. Rapidly fatal cases of cholera accompanied the arrival of the commands at Govrekoi, with the disease spreading in 'a most malignant form' thereafter (Anonymous, 1854a).

At this stage of the spread sequence, the regimental records included in the *Medical and Surgical History* also provide us with the first clear evidence that the divisional networks of campsites were not operating as closed epidemiological systems, but were open to the importation of disease from elsewhere. As a case in point, the circumstances surrounding the initial appearance of cholera in the Forty-Second Regiment, having just arrived at Govrekoi from Alladyn, are recorded in some detail by the regimental surgeon:

On the 29th of July a drummer of the 7th Fusiliers, discharged convalescent (disease not known) from Varna Hospital, where cholera was rife, arrived in the camp: on the morning of the 30th he was seized with cholera, and was treated in the Hospital of the 42nd Regiment, he died the same evening. The next morning, the 31st, the first case of cholera appeared in the Regiment, the subject of which died on the 1st August; the second case occurred on the 4th of August, and the subject of it was a convalescent from Varna Hospital, under the same circumstance as the man of the 7th Fusiliers. (Surgeon John Furlong, cited in Army Medical Department, 1858, i. 281)

The epidemiological significance of the imputed introduction from Varna is uncertain. With the exception of the cases documented above, the Forty-Second Regiment appears to have remained free of cholera until its subsequent transfer to Galata in mid-August (Army Medical Department, 1858, i. 281) (see Fig. 8.4C).

3. *Varna (Third Division)*. The camp at Varna, which had remained the site of the Third Division since its arrival from Gallipoli in late June, was to prove the source of infection for several regiments of the division. The Thirty-Eighth Regiment was attacked on 23 July (day 18 of the epidemic). Two days later, on the abandonment of the camp at Varna, the Twenty-Eighth Regiment was attacked on the march to its new station at Galata (Army Medical Department, 1858, i. 226). Even before the arrival of the infected regiments of the Third Division at Galata, however, cholera had already appeared in the ranks of the Heavy Cavalry Brigade, contingents of which had been posted to the south

the usual cramps and collapse, and proved fatal in thirteen hours. Several cases now intervened, and it was thought the late case had been a solitary one, and that it had been contracted at Devna; for five days we continued to hear with complacency that the pestilence was decreasing at Monaster [*sic*], then another case (also fatal) was admitted simultaneously with one of remittent fever, which latter, after a few days, merged into cholera . . . A general feeling of alarm made all tremble' (cited in Army Medical Department, 1858, ii. 52).

side of Varna Bay a fortnight or so earlier (Army Medical Department, 1858, i. 44).

In addition to Devna, Alladyn, and Varna, Figure 8.4B identifies an additional location (Yooksakova) which also played a central role in the spread of cholera. Despite being occupied by regiments of the Second Division from the first week of July, Yooksakova had escaped the early seeding depicted in Figure 8.4A. The circumstances pertaining to the eventual appearance of cholera in the camp are summarized by the Army Medical Department in the following terms:

cholera broke out on the 24th of July . . . the first case occurred in the person of a recruit who had joined the 95th Regiment about 30 hours previously from Varna, this case proved fatal in about 6 hours. On the 29th July two more cases occurred in the 95th; and on the 30th three other cases were admitted in the same regiment. (Army Medical Department, 1858, ii. 51)

'From this date,' the Department adds, 'the disease extended to all the regiments of the division in succession', appearing in the Forty-Seventh and Fifty-Fifth Regiments while still at Yooksakova (Fig. 8.4B) and subsequently among previously uninfected regiments detached to Koslidcha and Soombay (see Fig. 8.4C).

Days 29–49 (3–23 August; Figure 8.4C)

While cholera continued to intensify among some regiments infected in the previous time periods, this final phase of the spread sequence was associated with two main components: (i) the first appearance of cholera in a disparate set of regiments at established camps (Galata, Karasin, Koslidcha, and Yeni-Bazaar); coupled with (ii) the transfer, in mid-August, of previously infected regiments of the Cavalry and First Divisions to Galata. By the end of the observation period, every regiment and camp of the British Army in Bulgaria had been afflicted—to a greater or lesser extent—by the epidemic of Asiatic cholera.

8.2.4 Camp Spaces: Alternative Spatial Frameworks for Cholera Diffusion

Although the foregoing analysis provides insights into the sequence by which cholera spread in the British camp system of Bulgaria, alternative methods are required to determine the nature of the processes that underpinned the spread patterns. In this section, we use the method of multidimensional scaling (MDS) to model the camp spaces in which cholera diffused. Details of the method are given in Section 6.6.

CAMP CONNECTIVITY SPACES

As described in Section 6.6.1, MDS provides a method by which points (in the present instance, army camps) can be mapped from conventional geographical space into a wide range of different spaces that are significant for our understanding of the geographical occurrence of disease. In the context of the spread of cholera in the British camp system of Bulgaria, for example, an underpinning assumption of Figure 8.4 is that the inter-camp movements of regiments played a fundamental role in the geographical diffusion of the disease. Consequently, we can use MDS to re-map the camp system into a 'connectivity space'. In this connectivity space, camps that are strongly linked by the movements of regiments will appear close together, while camps that are only weakly linked will be widely separated.

Figure 8.5 shows the two-dimensional MDS maps for four different measures of the regiment-based connectivity of the British camp system. Formal definitions of the four measures are given in Appendix 8B and may be summarized as follows:

(i) Figure 8.5A, Camp linkage (first order) defines connectivity according to whether pairs of camps were *directly* linked by the transfer of regiments. The measure is based on the presence or absence of links between camps, irrespective of the number or class of regiments that forged the links;

(ii) Figure 8.5B, Camp linkage (first and second order) defines connectivity in the manner described for measure (i) but, in addition to direct links between camps, it allows for *indirect* links which may arise through the presence of an intermediary camp;

(iii) Figure 8.5C, Regimental occupancy defines connectivity according to the regiment-specific pattern of camp occupancy and transfer. As such, it allows for the differential patterns of connectivity forged by the individual commands;

(iv) Figure 8.5D, Duration of regimental occupancy defines connectivity in the manner described for measure (iii), but weighted by the duration of stay (in days) of regiments at the individual camps.

For the four measures of connectivity defined above, individual camps are represented in Figures 8.5A–D by circles whose areas are drawn proportional to the total number of regiments which were attached to the camps. The vectors on each chart are redrawn from Figure 8.4 and trace the camp-wise movements of regiments; again, vector widths denote the number of regiments transferred between each pair of encampments. Camps have been shaded according to the day of the epidemic in which cholera was first documented in the camp (6 July = day 1).

Figures 8.5A–D yield very different visualizations of the camp system in which cholera diffused. In Figures 8.5A and 8.5B, the four largest camps (Alladyn, Devna, Galata, and Varna) are clustered near the origins of the space

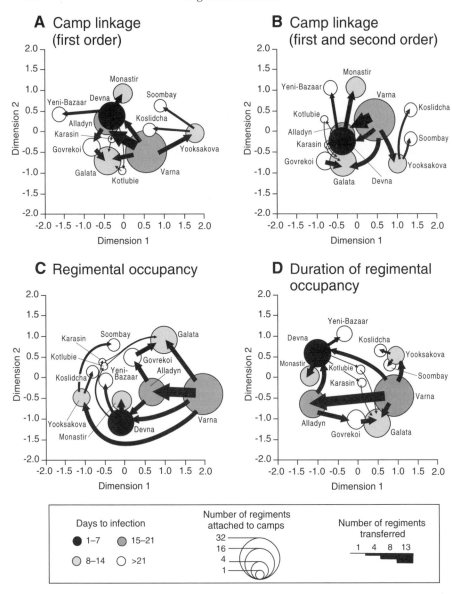

Fig. 8.5. MDS maps of the regiment-based connectivity of British army camps in Bulgaria, May–August 1854

Notes: The maps are based on different measures of interaction between the encampments. (A) First-order camp linkage. (B) First- and second-order camp linkage. (C) Regimental occupancy. (D) Duration of regimental occupancy. Each encampment is represented by a circle whose area is drawn proportional to the total number of regiments that occupied the encampment. Vectors trace the camp-wise movements of regiments during the course of the Bulgarian expedition; vector widths denote the number of regiments transferred between each pair of encampments. Finally, camps have been shaded according to the day of the epidemic in which cholera first appeared in the camp (day 1 = 6 July).

Source: Smallman-Raynor and Cliff (forthcoming, fig. 5).

and form a tightly connected core around which smaller and more loosely connected camps (e.g. Monastir, Soombay, Yeni-Bazaar, and Yooksakova) are situated. In Figures 8.5C and 8.5D, by contrast, the central core of large camps is absent; overall, the data points are more widely separated and the distributions are indicative of a less tightly connected camp system.

CHOLERA DIFFUSION PROCESSES IN MDS SPACE

As described in Section 8.2.3, the first documented cases of cholera associated with the main outbreak of the disease in the British Army can be traced to Devna (day 1) and Varna (day 8). If the spread of the disease from these two putative index locations[23] was mediated by the regiment-based connections between the camps, we would expect the time-ordered sequence of appearance of cholera in the individual units of the camp system (Fig. 8.4) to reflect the separations of camps from Devna and Varna in the connectivity spaces (Fig. 8.5). Thus those camps that were highly connected with Devna and Varna (i.e. camps positioned close to Devna and Varna in the connectivity spaces of Fig. 8.5) would be expected to be infected relatively early in the epidemic. Conversely, those camps that were only weakly connected with the index locations (camps positioned far from Devna and Varna in the connectivity spaces) would be expected to be infected relatively late in the epidemic. As a result, cholera should appear to spread *contagiously* in the connectivity spaces, moving from the index camps to their nearest neighbouring (= most highly connected) camps. These, in their turn, transmit the disease to their nearest neighbouring camps, and so on, until all camps in the system are infected.

To determine which of the four connectivity spaces in Figure 8.5 correspond most closely to this expected process of spatial contagion, the time-ordered sequence of appearance of cholera in the units of the camp system was modelled as a function of their separation from Devna and Varna. Let t_i denote the day t in which cholera was first recorded in camp i. Then the regression model

$$t_i = b_0 + b_1 d_{iD} + b_2 d_{iV} + e_i \tag{8.1}$$

was postulated. Here, d_{iD} is the straight-line separation (or distance) of camp i from Devna in the connectivity space, d_{iV} is the straight-line separation from Varna, and e_i is an error term.

The model in equation (8.1) was fitted by stepwise regression to each of the connectivity spaces of Figure 8.5. The results are summarized as models 1–4 in Table 8.5. For each space, the table gives the order of entry (step) of the independent variables in the stepwise fitting procedure, along with the estimated slope coefficients, $\hat{b}_1$ and $\hat{b}_2$ (with the associated t-statistics in parentheses), the

---

[23] Although the first appearance of cholera in Varna lagged Devna by seven days, the decision to classify Varna as an index location was based on (i) the reputed heavy seeding of Varna by successive contingents of the Allied Army in early July and (ii) the documented role of Varna as the source of infection for the earliest cases of cholera in some encampments.

Table 8.5. Results of stepwise multiple regression analysis to examine the spread of cholera in the camp system of the British Army, Bulgaria, May–September 1854

Model	Space	n (camps)	Independent variable, slope coefficient (t-statistic)		$R^2(F)$	r_{DV}
			Step 1	Step 2		
1	MDS, Camp linkage (first order)	12	No significant regressors			−0.01
2	MDS, Camp linkage (first and second order)	12	No significant regressors			−0.08
3	MDS, Regimental occupancy	12	d_{iV}, 9.46 (4.40*)	d_{iD}, 10.03 (3.63*)	0.73 (12.37*)	−0.33
4	MDS, Duration of regimental occupancy	12	No significant regressors			−0.83*
5	Conventional	12	No significant regressors			−0.01

Independent variables:
d_{iV} = straight-line separation of camp i from Varna
d_{iD} = straight-line separation of camp i from Devna

Notes: * Significant at the $p = 0.01$ level (two-tailed test)
Spread in the camp system is examined for four different MDS connectivity spaces (models 1–4) and conventional geographical space (model 5).
Source: Smallman-Raynor and Cliff (forthcoming, table 5).

coefficient of determination, R^2, and the F-ratio; the degree of correlation, r_{DV}, between the independent variables is also listed. Statistically significant values at the $p = 0.01$ level (two-tailed test) are indicated by an asterisk. For each model, only the statistically significant independent variables are shown.

Table 8.5 shows that the parameters of the models associated with three of the four connectivity spaces (models 1, 2, and 4) are non-significant. In contrast, the model associated with the regimental occupancy space (model 3) records a strong and positive association between the $\{t_i\}$ and the independent variables $\{d_{iD}\}$ and $\{d_{iV}\}$. The relatively greater importance of separation from Varna is indicated by the entry of d_{iV} in step 1 of the model, while the statistically non-significant correlation between the independent variables ($r_{DV} = -0.33$) suggests that the modelling procedure was successful in untangling the effects of separation from the two index locations.

For completeness, model 5 in Table 8.5 gives the results of fitting equation (8.1) to the separations from Devna and Varna in conventional geographical space. The parameters of the model are non-significant and signify the lack of operation of a contagious spread process in the regular space depicted in Figure 8.4.

INTERPRETATION AND IMPLICATIONS

While the authors of the *Medical and Surgical History* were acutely aware of the contribution of regimental movements to the spatial progress of cholera in Bulgaria (Army Medical Department, 1858, ii. 49–54), they were unable to provide detailed insights into the generalized structure of the underpinning contact network by which cholera diffused in the camp system. Through the application of MDS mapping techniques, models 1 and 2 in Table 8.5 demonstrate that the simple existence of linkages between camps—when examined irrespective of the number or class of the regiments that forged those links—contributes little to an understanding of the observed sequence of cholera transmission. Rather, model 3 in Table 8.5 indicates that the spread of cholera was mediated through a series of regiment-based inter-camp connections whose parameters corresponded to the MDS regimental occupancy space in Figure 8.5C. Within this space, similarities in the regimental patterns of camp occupancy with both Devna and Varna were to govern the camp-wise sequence of cholera transmission, but with the overall spread process dominated by the heavily seeded location of Varna. Finally, notwithstanding the epidemiological evidence included in the *History*, the high overall explanation offered by the regiment-level modelling procedure ($R^2 = 0.73$ in model 3) implies that the movements of individual members and subgroups of the various commands had little impact on the primary diffusion of the disease in the camp system. Further research is required to determine the exact role of non-British military contingents and local populations and their specific association with the British forces in the more general diffusion of cholera in Bulgaria during the summer of 1854.

8.2.5 *Cholera in the Crimea, September 1854–February 1855*

Although cholera had begun to abate in the British Army during the latter days of August 1854 (Army Medical Department, 1858, ii. 65), the ensuing invasion of the Crimean Peninsula was to provide Wave I of the epidemic with renewed impetus (see Fig. 8.2B). We begin our consideration of this second phase of the epidemic wave with a brief outline of the route by which cholera spread with the British Army to the Crimea. We then examine the factors that contributed to the continued diffusion of Wave I in the British forces, both on the plateau before Sebastopol and in the Crimean Peninsula more generally. Our analysis of the latter issue is informed by the epidemiological concept of a *virgin soil* population; that is, a population which has no prior immunity—either through natural or artificial exposure—to a particular infection (see Cliff *et al.*, 2000: 119–64). In the context of the present analysis, we relate the general principles of the virgin soil model to newly arrived drafts of soldiers who, through lack of acclimatization in the East, appeared to be particularly prone to infection with cholera and other disease organisms.

SPREAD OF CHOLERA TO THE CRIMEA

The broken vectors in Figure 8.3 trace the route by which cholera spread with the British Army during the allied invasion of the Crimea in September 1854. Details of the invasion are given in Section 8.2.1 but, from the point of embarkation of the allied armada off the coast of Bulgaria in early September, the map traces a chain of cholera infection which, by way of land and sea, stretched some 500 km and linked Varna with the allied offensive positions before Sebastopol. For convenience, the infection chain can be divided into two distinct stages: (1) the sea voyage from Bulgaria (Varna) to the landing point in the Crimea (Old Fort), ending in mid-September; and (2) the onwards march to Sebastopol, ending in late September. We consider each stage in turn.

Stage 1: Varna (Bulgaria) to Old Fort (Crimea) (Main Map, Figure 8.3)

With the Black Sea fleet having scarcely recovered from an explosive outbreak of cholera (Anonymous, 1854*b*; Rees, 1854), and with the disease still not completely extinguished among the British troops in Bulgaria (Army Medical Department, 1858, ii. 65), the decision to crowd the commands aboard many dozens of transport ships was to have a deleterious effect on cholera activity. Although the available evidence is fragmentary, Table 8.6 is based on the regimental reports included in the *History* and summarizes the documented mortality from cholera on British transport ships during the fortnight or so between embarkation at Varna and disembarkation in the Crimea. According to the table, upwards of 100 deaths were recorded in 20 different regiments; further instances of the disease, of unknown outcome, were documented in several other corps. In that the deaths listed in Table 8.6 were distributed throughout the passage to the Crimea, with many more occurring within a few hours or days of disembarkation at Old Fort (see e.g. Army Medical Department, 1854, i. 109, 150, 208, 263, 289), the maintenance of the cholera vibrio across the Black Sea may reasonably be inferred.

Stage 2: Old Fort to Sebastopol (Inset Map, Figure 8.3)

Moving southwards from the epidemic bridgehead near Old Fort, regimental surgeons make frequent reference to the sporadic occurrence of cholera along the route of the 60 km march to Sebastopol. The experience of the Twentieth Regiment, described by Assistant Surgeon Howard, was typical of several corps: 'within 24 hours after our arrival [on 14 September] . . . a case of Cholera presented itself, which speedily advanced into collapse, and during the succeeding days four others terminated fatally at the bivouac, each in a very few hours' (cited in Army Medical Department, 1858, i. 199). No other cases of cholera occurred in the command until the Battle of Alma (20 Sept.), 'after which', Howard continues, 'an increase of Cholera took place . . . five men died at the regimental bivouac. Cases continued to occur along the line of march on the succeeding days, until the army reached and took up its position

Table 8.6. Cholera in regiments of the British Army on the voyage from Bulgaria to the Crimea, August–September 1854

Division/Regiment	Date		Cholera deaths	Vessel(s)
	Embarkation (Varna, Bulgaria)	Disembarkation (Crimea)		
Light Division				
7th Fusiliers	30 Aug.	14 Sept.	7	*Victoria, Emperor, Fury*
23rd Regiment	28 Aug.	14 Sept.	8	*Victoria*
33rd Regiment	29 Aug.	14 Sept.	19	*Andes*
88th Regiment	30 Aug.	14 Sept.	11	Not recorded
Rifle Brigade (2nd Batt.)	29 Aug.	14 Sept.	3	Not recorded
Cavalry Division				
4th Light Dragoons	2 Sept.	16–18 Sept.	?	*Simla*
8th Hussars	31 Aug.–1 Sept.	15–16 Sept.	3	*Himalaya*
17th Lancers	2–3 Sept.	17 Sept.[1]	1	Not recorded
13th Light Dragoons	1 Sept.	18 Sept.	3	*Jason*
First/First & Highland Div.				
Grenadier Guards	29 Aug.	14 Sept.	1	HMS *Simoom*
Coldstream Guards	29 Aug.	14 Sept.	?[2]	HMS *Simoom*
Scots Fusilier Guards	28 Aug.	14 Sept.	8	*Kangaroo*
42nd Regiment	29 Aug.	14 Sept.	?	*Emeu*
93rd Regiment	Early Sept.[3]	14 Sept.	12	Not recorded
Second Division				
47th Regiment	31 Aug.	14 Sept.	8	*Melbourne*
49th Regiment	31 Aug.	14 Sept.	1	*Hydaspes*
95th Regiment	2 Sept.	14 Sept.	2	Not recorded
Third Division				
1st Regiment (1st Batt.)	31 Aug.	14 Sept.	1	*Arthur the Great*
4th Regiment[4]	31 Aug.	14 Sept.	9	*Deva, Asia, William Jackson*
38th Regiment	3 Sept.	14 Sept.	?[2]	*Apollo*
44th Regiment	29 Aug.	14 Sept.	1	*Tynemouth*
50th Regiment	2 Sept.	14 Sept.	3	*Arabia*
Fourth Division				
68th Regiment[4]	1 Sept.	14 Sept.	8	Not recorded

Notes: [1] Date of disembarkation of Head-Quarters. [2] One cholera case reported. [3] Exact date of boarding not specified. [4] Did not tour Bulgaria.
Source: Smallman-Raynor and Cliff (forthcoming, table 6), based on regimental reports included in Army Medical Department (1858).

on the plateau south of Sebastopol' in the latter days of September. While details vary in terms of the number, timing, and severity of cases, the regimental reports indicate that many other commands—of all army divisions—were similarly circumstanced by cholera on the march to Sebastopol (see Army Medical Department, 1858, i. 99, 150, 192, 263, 289, 301, 384).

CHOLERA IN THE BRITISH CAMP BEFORE SEBASTOPOL

From the early days of October 1854, with the British infantry now positioned alongside the French and Turkish contingents on the plateau before Sebastopol, cholera began to spread widely in the newly established siege camp (Pl. 8.2). To illustrate this, the maps in Figure 8.6 plot as proportional circles the monthly cholera case rate (per 100 mean strength) in British regiments before Sebastopol during (Fig. 8.6A) October 1854, (Fig. 8.6B) November 1854, (Fig. 8.6C) December 1854, and (Fig. 8.6D) January–February 1855.[24] The maps are based on a sample of 33 regiments (variously assigned to the Light, Second, Third, and Fourth Divisions) which, from the time of their placement before Sebastopol to the end of the first cholera wave (Feb. 1855), were permanently stationed in the siege camp; for reference, the 33 regiments are identified in Table 8.A1 (App. 8A).

Figure 8.6A shows that cholera was widely distributed in the British camp, albeit at a relatively low level of activity (<10 cases per 100 mean strength), during October. The sharp deterioration in the conditions of service that accompanied the onset of winter resulted in a marked intensification of the epidemic during November (Fig. 8.6B) and December (Fig. 8.6C), especially in the sectors of the camp occupied by the Third and Light Divisions. In the final time period, January–February 1855, Figure 8.6D shows a general collapse in cholera activity, with epidemic fade-out by the end of the observation period. Consistent with the epidemiology of cholera, the January–February collapse corresponded with the onset of the main period of severe cold in the Crimea.[25]

Explanatory Factors

Running through the pages of the *Medical and Surgical History* is a recognition of the role of prior exposure and acclimatization as possible factors in the differential spread of cholera in the British regiments, both before Sebastopol

---

[24] A word of caution must accompany the interpretation of the cholera statistics on which Fig. 8.6 is based. In particular, while the authors of the *Medical and Surgical History* note that a 'vast number' of the cholera cases that define the distributions in Fig. 8.6 were infected in the trenches before Sebastopol (Army Medical Department, 1858, ii. 70), an unknown proportion must be assumed to have acquired their infection in the military hospitals at Balaklava, Scutari, and elsewhere. Unfortunately, the available evidence does not permit a distinction between these various sources of infection; the interpretation of Fig. 8.6 proceeds subject to this data caveat.

[25] According to Dr Bush of the Scots Greys, Second North British Dragoons, for example, 'January [1855] was ushered in by storms of wind and snow, and the cold was also most intense during this month; towards the end of the first week the thermometer in my bell tent, which was lined, stood at 8 A.M. as low as 18 F., and in the single tents it fell as low as 15 [F.]' (cited in Army Medical Department, 1858, ii. 27).

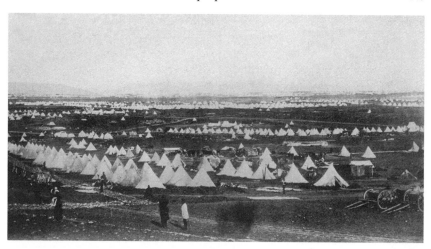

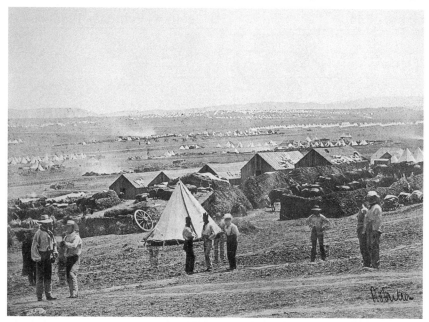

Pl. 8.2. Views of the allied camp on the plain before Sebastopol, Crimean War

Notes: The year-long siege of Sebastopol ended with the Russian withdrawal from the city on 8–9 September 1855. During the course of the siege, the allied encampments were to suffer severe and widespread epidemics of cholera, diarrhoea, dysentery, and fevers.
Sources: (Pl. A) Gernsheim and Gernsheim (1954, pl. 62, between pp. 34–5); (Pl. B) James (1981, pl. 27, p. 89).

A October 1854

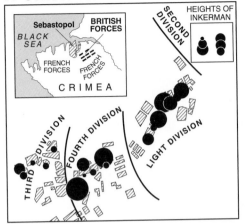

B November 1854

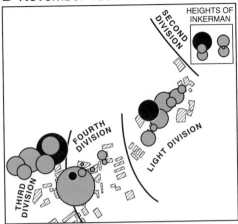

C December 1854

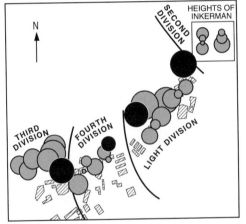

D January–February 1855

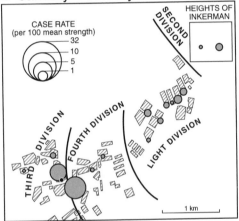

Fig. 8.6. Wave I of the cholera epidemic in the British Army before Sebastopol, Crimea, October 1854–February 1855

Notes: The maps plot, as proportional circles, the cholera case rate (per 100 mean strength) in 33 regiments of the Second, Third, Fourth, and Light Divisions stationed before Sebastopol in (A) October 1854, (B) November 1854, (C) December 1854, and (D) January–February 1855. For the time period under consideration, the black circles identify regiments in which cases of cholera were first reported during the interval covered by the map. Grey circles mark regiments in which cases were first reported in prior time intervals.
Source: Smallman-Raynor and Cliff (forthcoming, fig. 6).

(Fig. 8.6) and in the Crimean Peninsula more generally. By the early winter of 1854, 'it appeared', the authors of the *History* comment, 'as if the choleraic poison had nearly exhausted itself on those who had been some time exposed to its influence, and that it required, as it were, fresh subjects upon whom to develop [*sic*] its effects' (Army Medical Department, 1858, ii. 66). In this context, the reports of regimental surgeons are replete with references to cholera in two such groups of 'fresh subjects': (i) military drafts, consisting largely of raw recruits from Britain and serving as reinforcements for existing regiments in the Crimea; (ii) entire regiments, either newly arrived in the Black Sea theatre or which, like some commands of the Fourth Division, had escaped deployment in Bulgaria on account of the cholera epidemic at that place.

To examine the contribution of these and similar groups to the spread of cholera before Sebastopol, the information included in the *History* was used to form three different measures of prior cholera exposure and acclimatization for each of the 33 regiments included in Figure 8.6. These measures were: (i) the cumulative size of incoming drafts (per 100 mean strength of the receiving regiment) during the observation period, October 1854–February 1855; (ii) whether or not a prior tour of duty had been undertaken in Bulgaria, coded 1 (= yes) or 0 (= no); and (iii) the recorded cholera case rate (per 100 mean strength) in the period prior to arrival before Sebastopol, June–September 1854. To examine the further possibility that the spread of cholera may have been influenced by the relative positions of regiments before Sebastopol, four dichotomous (1/0) measures of residence/non-residence in the sector of the camp occupied by each army division (Light, Second, Third, and Fourth; see Fig. 8.6) were also defined.

Each of the measures was entered as an independent variable in a series of multiple regression models in which two alternative markers of cholera activity in the regiments before Sebastopol formed the dependent variable:

(1) *epidemic magnitude*, defined as the cumulative cholera case rate (per 100 mean strength) in the period October 1854–February 1855. This measure represents the aggregate spatial pattern of cholera activity shown in Figure 8.6;

(2) *epidemic velocity*, defined as the average length of time (in months) that it took a cholera case to become infected in the period October 1854–February 1855. This measure, which is formally defined in Appendix 6A.2, represents the rate at which cholera spread in each regiment to form the spatial patterns plotted in Figure 8.6. A relatively short average time to infection is indicative of a fast moving epidemic; a relatively long average time to infection corresponds with a slow moving epidemic.

As before, all model fitting was by ordinary least squares using a stepwise algorithm.

The results of the regression analysis are summarized in Table 8.7. Following the layout of Table 8.5, the order (step) of entry of the independent variables in the regression procedure is given, along with the slope coefficients, the associated *t*-statistics (in parentheses), the coefficient of determination R^2, and the *F*-ratio. Again, only the statistically significant independent variables are shown. To overcome the potential complication of multicollinearity arising from the inclusion of all four camp residence variables ($x_4 - x_7$ in Table 8.7), the

Table 8.7. Results of stepwise multiple regression analysis to identify factors associated with the magnitude and velocity of cholera transmission in British regiments stationed in the Crimea, October 1854–February 1855

Model	Dependent variable	n	Independent variable, slope coefficient (t-statistic)				$R^2(F)$
			Step 1	Step 2	Step 3	Step 4	
Regiments before Sebastopol							
1	y_1	31[1]	x_1, 0.10 (2.81*)				0.21 (7.89*)
2	y_2	30[2]	x_2, −0.78 (−6.13*)	x_6, −0.80 (−5.50*)	x_1, 0.01 (3.48*)		0.67 (17.84*)
All regiments in Crimea							
3	y_1	49[3]	No significant regressors				
4	y_2	51[4]	x_2, −0.88 (−5.90*)	x_1, 0.01 (3.87*)	x_3, −0.04 (−3.39*)	x_6, −0.82 (−2.80*)	0.64 (20.12*)

Dependent variables

y_1 = epidemic magnitude (cholera case rate per 100 mean strength, Oct. 1854–Feb. 1855)
y_2 = epidemic velocity (average time to infection, Oct. 1854–Feb. 1855)

Independent variables

x_1 = draft size (per 100 mean strength), October 1854–February 1855
x_2 = prior tour of duty in Bulgaria (1 = yes, 0 = no)
x_3 = cholera case rate (per 100 mean strength), June–September 1854
x_4 = residence in the camp of the Second Division before Sebastopol (1 = yes, 0 = no) (regression models 3 and 4 only)
x_5 = residence in the camp of the Third Division before Sebastopol (1 = yes, 0 = no)
x_6 = residence in the camp of the Fourth Division before Sebastopol (1 = yes, 0 = no)
x_7 = residence in the camp of the Light Division before Sebastopol (1 = yes, 0 = no)

Notes: * Significant at the $p = 0.01$ level (two-tailed test). [1] 46th and 63rd Regiments omitted as extreme outliers. [2] 4th, 17th, and 18th Regiments omitted as extreme outliers. [3] 1st (1st Battalion), 20th, 40th, and 68th Regiments omitted as extreme outliers. [4] Grenadier Guards and 46th Regiment omitted as extreme outliers.
Source: Smallman-Raynor and Cliff (forthcoming, table 7).

residence variable associated with one division (Second Division, x_4) was arbitrarily selected for omission from this stage of the analysis. Finally, in preliminary analysis, one or more regiments were identified as extreme outliers that influenced the parameters of the regression model. Consequently, all results relate to models with extreme outliers omitted; these are indicated in Table 8.7.

Models 1 and 2 relate the independent variables to, respectively, the magnitude and velocity of cholera in the regiments before Sebastopol. While model 1 confirms the role of draft size as a determining factor in levels of cholera activity among regiments in the period October 1854–February 1855, the overall explanation offered by the model is low ($100R^2 = 21\%$). That draft size is the only variable included in model 1 suggests that other specified factors (including prior levels of cholera activity and location within the camp) did not account for the regimental variations in levels of disease activity implied by Figure 8.6.

When examined in terms of velocity, model 2 in Table 8.7 yields a more complex set of results. Given the manner in which velocity is specified (a short average time to infection = a fast moving epidemic), the negative associations in model 2 imply that fast moving epidemics were associated with a prior tour of duty in Bulgaria (step 1) and residence in the camp of the Fourth Division (step 2). Conversely, the positive association (step 3) implies that slow moving epidemics were associated with those regiments that received large drafts in the observation period.

Interpretation and Implications

While the results of the analysis are consistent with documentary evidence concerning the apparent predilection of cholera for newly drafted soldiers (Army Medical Department, 1858, ii. 66), model 1 demonstrates that draft size alone explains only a modest amount of the regiment-to-regiment variation in levels of cholera activity in the camp before Sebastopol. Although this finding may reflect the imperfect nature of the draft-related information contained in the regimental reports, it suggests that further explanatory factors—including the possible role of localized patterns of water supply and usage on the plateau (Snow, 1855*b*)—still await identification.

In the absence of more detailed information, we can only speculate as to the nature of the associations identified for epidemic velocity in model 2. According to the model, rapidly moving epidemics were conditioned, in descending order of importance, by: (i) a tour of service in Bulgaria; (ii) residence in the sector of the camp occupied by the Fourth Division; and (iii) a low draft rate. While factor (i) may reflect the detrimental impact of the Bulgarian expedition on the general health of the regiments involved, thereby rendering the men more susceptible to the rapid spread of infections of all kinds, factor (ii) is consistent with the relative lack of acclimatization of the Fourth Division (Army Medical Department, 1858, ii. 66), many regiments of which had arrived in the Near East during August and September 1854. Finally, in interpreting factor (iii), it is important to recognize that the arrival of new drafts was distributed throughout the course of the winter of 1854–5, with the most heavily reinforced regiments receiving men not only in November and December but also in the following January and February.[26] When examined relative to the start of the observation period, the late arrival of large numbers of susceptible troops would give rise to an apparently delayed spread of cholera in these commands.

CHOLERA IN ALL BRITISH COMMANDS IN THE CRIMEA

While the foregoing analysis refers to regiments permanently positioned in the camp before Sebastopol, models 3 and 4 in Table 8.7 extend the analysis to a consideration of all 53 British regiments deployed in the Crimea during the period October 1854–February 1855.[27] The models therefore include commands of the Cavalry, First, and Highland Divisions that were attached to the auxiliary camps at Balaklava and Kadikoi (see Fig. 8.1B for locations). As before, the models were fitted with outliers omitted. Finally, in specifying the independent variables for the modelling procedure, the inclusion of regiments not positioned before Sebastopol has permitted the use of all four residence variables ($x_4 - x_7$ in Table 8.7) for the siege camp.

When models 3 and 4, which relate the independent variables to epidemic magnitude and velocity respectively, are compared with the corresponding models for the camp before Sebastopol, similarities and differences in the models are evident.

1. *Epidemic magnitude (model 3).* In contrast to model 1, which yielded a significant and positive association between epidemic magnitude and draft size for the camp before Sebastopol, no similar association is identified for the entire set of regiments in model 3; as Table 8.7 indicates, statistical non-significance has determined the exclusion of all independent variables from the latter model.

2. *Epidemic velocity (model 4).* Although model 4 yielded results that are broadly similar to those identified in model 2 for the camp before Sebastopol, some between-model differences in the order of entry of the independent variables are evident and these indicate variations in the relative importance of the explanatory factors. Consistent with model 2, the associations in model 4 imply that rapidly moving epidemics were contingent on a prior tour of duty in Bulgaria (step 1), a low draft rate (step 2), and residence in the camp of the Fourth Division (step 4). Additionally, model 4 identifies a negative association with prior cholera case rate (step 3), indicating that high cholera rates in the

---

[26] The experience of the First Regiment, First Battalion (Third Division) is typical. As one of the most heavily reinforced regiments in the period October 1854–February 1855, the corps received 122 new men in November, 65 in December, with a further 178 in the following January and February (Army Medical Department, 1858, i. 132–4).

[27] The 53 regiments include all corps listed in Table 8.A1 (App. 8A), other than those marked 'not in service in East' under Wave I of the epidemic.

period prior to October 1854 were linked with rapidly moving epidemics in the remainder of the epidemic wave. Such a finding is counter-intuitive but may again reflect the impact of a more general deterioration in health on the rate of disease propagation.

Two general findings emerge from this stage of the analysis. First, notwithstanding the evidence included in the *Medical and Surgical History*, the lack of a statistical association between draft size and epidemic magnitude (model 3) once more underscores the need to identify other, possibly localized, factors that may have contributed to the spread of cholera in the British regiments. Secondly, as judged by the order of entry of the independent variables in model 4, a prior tour of duty in Bulgaria again emerges as the most important factor determining the speed with which cholera spread through the British commands in the Crimea.

8.2.6 Summary

In this section, we have used a variety of qualitative and quantitative techniques to isolate the geographical diffusion processes by which cholera spread through the encampments of the British Army during the Bulgarian and Crimean phases of the Crimean War, June 1854–February 1855. In the Bulgarian phase, multidimensional scaling has highlighted the critical role played by regimental occupancy of two camps—primarily Varna and secondarily Devna—in propagating cholera to other camps by a process of regimental transfer. In the Crimea, the factors which influenced cholera transmission on the plateau before Sebastopol were more complex. Multiple regression suggested that rapidly moving cholera outbreaks on the plateau before Sebastopol were associated with regiments which had undertaken a prior tour of duty in Bulgaria, had resided in the camp of the Fourth Division, and which had low draft rates. These findings may reflect the general deterioration of health among troops who had been in the front line for a long time. Only limited statistical evidence has been found to link large epidemics with big drafts (a virgin soil model), and other possibly spatially localized factors so far unidentified may have played a part.

At the time, the Army of the East was one of the largest British expeditionary forces ever to have been assembled. It mainly comprised men who had never been engaged in an extended period of combat, and it was commanded by those whose military understanding and experience harked back to the Napoleonic Wars some 40 years earlier. As for medical knowledge of the specific diseases that plagued the conflict, the Crimean War came at a time when evidence regarding the waterborne nature of cholera was only just accruing. As far as the pages of the *History* allow, general notions of quarantine and isolation—which were to inform the containment and control of later war-related cholera epidemics—were largely absent and, as a consequence, the disease

Regional Patterns

spread apace with the movements of ailing commands. Yet, the cholera epidemic also served as a spur to the work of Florence Nightingale and to the developments in post-Crimea military medicine and hygiene with which her name is usually associated. Within decades, an enduring feature of war history was finally reversed: bombs and bullets supplanted disease as the leading cause of death in the modern mobilized army.

8.3 Prisoner of War Camps: Smallpox Transmission in the Franco-Prussian War, 1870–1871

So far our study of camp epidemics has focused on disease transmission in the field camps of a deployed army. In this section we extend our examination to another type of camp system which has been associated with the spread of war epidemics—prisoner of war (POW) camps. We take as our example the epidemic of smallpox which spread with French soldiers incarcerated in the POW camps of Prussia during the Franco-Prussian War (1870–1). We use the statistical evidence collated in a classic study by Albert Guttstadt (1873) to demonstrate one critical geographical facet of the war–disease association: the role of temporary (POW) settlement systems in the spatial structuring of epidemic transmission in the fixed (urban) settlement systems of civil populations. Our account draws on Smallman-Raynor and Cliff (2002).

8.3.1 Background to the Smallpox Epidemic

THE STUDY SITE

Figure 8.7 shows the state boundaries of Prussia on the eve of the Franco-Prussian War. As the principal member of the North German Confederation, Prussia occupied a *c.*300,000 square km tract of continental Europe extending from France, Belgium, and Holland in the west to the Baltic Sea and Poland in the east. According to the post-war census of 1871, the population of Prussia numbered 24.7 millions (Mitchell, 1998). The capital city, Berlin, was the largest settlement (population 826,341) and dominated the urban system. Only four other cities (Breslau, Cologne, Königsberg, and Magdeburg) recorded populations in excess of 100,000. Next in the urban hierarchy came Danzig,

----

Fig. 8.7. Prussia at the outbreak of war with France, 1870

Notes: The North German Confederation comprises the area contained within the heavy solid line. Prussia is shaded with a dark tint. The South German Confederation is contained within the heavy pecked line and is shaded with a light tint. Other places referred to in the text are named. The inset map locates the study area within Europe.

Source: Smallman-Raynor and Cliff (2002, fig. 1, p. 245).

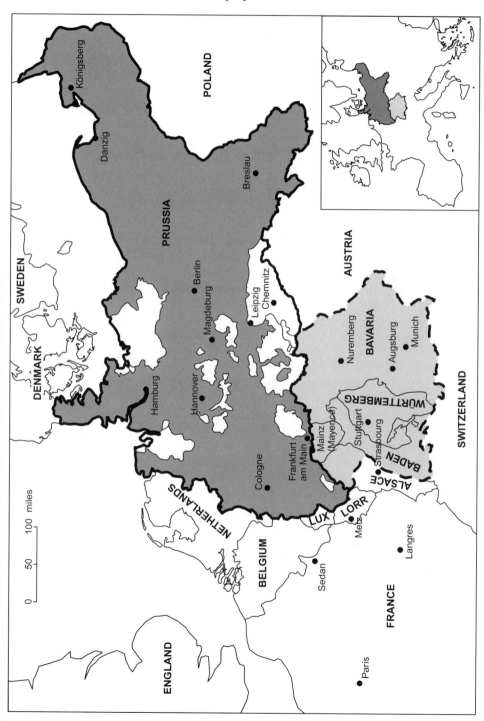

Frankfurt-am-Main, and Hanover with populations of about 90,000 while, elsewhere, urban settlement was typified by smaller cities and towns of less than 75,000 inhabitants (Guttstadt, 1873: 143–4).

The origins and course of the Franco-Prussian War (July 1870–Jan. 1871), and its particular relationship to the changing balance of European power in the wake of the Austro-Prussian War (1866), have been outlined in a number of authoritative studies.[28] Provoked by the diplomatic machinations associated with the Hohenzollern Candidature for the vacant Spanish throne, but with tensions deeply rooted in the political ascendancy of Prussia and its threat to the security of the French Empire, France issued a formal declaration of war on Prussia on 17 July 1870.[29] In fact, France had begun to mobilize on 14 July. The mobilization of Prussia and the other states of the North German Confederation, Baden, Bavaria, and Württemberg took place in the days that followed. See Figure 8.7 for locations. After a brief offensive by the French Army in Saarland, followed by a six-month invasion of France by the allied German forces, an armistice was agreed on 28 January 1871. The Preliminary Peace of Versailles was signed on 26 February and, with the ratification of the Treaty of Frankfurt on 23 May, France ceded Alsace and a sector of Lorraine (Moselle and a part of Meurthe) to the newly formed German Empire.

With deployment of the nascent railway system at the forefront of military strategy, one marked feature of the Franco-Prussian War was the high degree of geographical mobility associated with the fighting forces. So, during the seven-month period of active hostilities, more than 1.5 million soldiers are believed to have crossed the border between France and the states of Germany (Prinzing, 1916: 189, 208–9; Dumas and Vedel-Petersen, 1923: 51). The majority of these were allied German troops engaged in the invasion of France. Pivotal to the appearance of smallpox in Prussia, however, were the large numbers of French soldiers who were transported to Prussia as POWs. Some impression of the number of French prisoners in Prussia can be gained from Table 8.9, below. For a sample of POW camps and related facilities at 56 locations, the table gives the total (maximum) prisoner population as 268,252 officers and men. Other estimates, formed to include the larger states of Germany,

---

[28] The Franco-Prussian War has attracted a very large literature. For the official histories of the war, see France, Armée. État Major, Service Historique (1901–14). *La Guerre de 1870/1, Publiée par la Revue d'Historie, Rédigée à la Section Historique de l'État-Major de l'Armée*, Paris: R. Chapelot; Prussia, Armee, Grosser Generalstab, Kriegsgeschichtliche Abteilung (1872–81). *Der Deutsch-Französische Krieg, 1870–1. Redigirt von der Kriegsgeschichtlichen Abteheilung des Grossen Generalstabes*. Berlin: E. S. Mittler und Sohn (*The Franco-German War 1870–1871*. Translated from the German official account by Capt. F. C. H. Clarke, London: HMSO, 1874–84). Accessible English-language overviews of the origin and course of the war include: Ollivier (1913); Howard (1961); Steefel (1962); Halperin (1973); and Carr (1991).

[29] France had voted war credits on 15 July; the formal declaration of war was issued from Paris on 17 July and presented to the Prussian Prime Minister, Otto von Bismarck, on 19 July.

place the maximum number of French prisoners at almost 373,000. Probably as many as 723,500 French soldiers (including the Paris garrison and Bourbaki's army in Switzerland) were incarcerated at some stage during the war (Prinzing, 1916: 189, 208–9).

SMALLPOX AND THE WAR

The nature of smallpox is outlined in Appendix 1A. Nineteenth-century Europe was no stranger to the ravages of the disease. Despite the introduction of smallpox vaccination in many states of Europe during the early years of the century (Hirsch, 1883, i. 142), continent-wide pandemics (first in 1824–9, and then in 1837–40 and 1870–4) were interspersed with more localized epidemics of greater or lesser intensity (Fenner *et al.*, 1988: p. 231). Although the antecedents of the pandemic events were the subject of contemporary speculation and conjecture (Cornish, 1871), the immediate origins of the epidemic that spread as a consequence of the Franco-Prussian War—an early manifestation of the European pandemic of 1870–4—can be traced with some degree of accuracy to France. As early as New Year's Day 1870, an anonymous report in *The Lancet* warned that smallpox had appeared in Paris.[30] In fact, smallpox had first surfaced in the *départements* of northern and southeastern France in the latter months of 1869 (Rolleston, 1933: 178–9), with the Indian subcontinent as a postulated source of the disease (Cornish, 1871). But, whatever its exact origins, the epidemic continued to escalate in France and, in late May 1870, an emergency conference on smallpox control was convened in Paris (Rolleston, 1933: 179). Two months later, with smallpox still spreading 'fearfully' in the French capital,[31] France declared war on Prussia.

From its putative origins in France, smallpox was to spread in an especially severe (haemorrhagic) form in Prussia and in the other states of Germany.[32] The dimensions of the resulting mortality can be seen in Table 8.8. All told, some 300,000 inhabitants of France, Prussia, and the smaller German states are believed to have succumbed to smallpox during the war period and its immediate aftermath. However, it is also evident from Table 8.8 that the disease did not strike the military and civil populations of the combatant states with equal severity. Low levels of vaccine-acquired immunity were to favour dissemination of the disease in (i) the large contingent of French soldiers transferred to Prussia as prisoners of war and (ii) Prussian civilians.[33] In contrast,

[30] *The Lancet*, 1870, 1: 24.

[31] *The Lancet*, 1870, 2: 183.

[32] With the exception of isolated reports of smallpox in Berlin, and a more severe outbreak of the disease in the city of Chemnitz (Saxony), smallpox was all but absent from Prussia and the allied states of Germany at the start of the Franco-Prussian War. See Guttstadt (1873: 130–8); Prinzing (1916: 199); Rolleston (1933: 186).

[33] For the French Army, a programme of compulsory vaccination of all new recruits had been introduced in 1859. However, the reputedly high failure rate of the Army's (re)vaccination schedule in the years immediately preceding the war with Prussia, coupled with the failure to vaccinate those men who were enlisted after the outbreak of hostilities, ensured that a large sector of the French Army was prone to

Table 8.8. Deaths from smallpox in the military and
civilian populations of France and Germany, 1870–1871

Country	Population size (millions)	Smallpox deaths[1]
France		
Soldiers	1.50[2]	25,077 (167.18)
Civilians	36.01[3]	89,954 (24.98)
Germany		
Soldiers	1.49[2]	297 (1.99)
Civilians	41.06[4]	176,977 (43.10)[5]

Notes: [1] Death rates per 10,000 in parentheses. [2] Estimated total
number deployed. [3] 1872 census. [4] 1871 census. [5] Mortality for
1870–2.
Source: Smallman-Raynor and Cliff (2002, table 1, p. 243), based on
information in Prinzing (1916), Dumas and Vedel-Petersen (1923),
and Mitchell (1998).

with a compulsory programme of smallpox vaccination and revaccination that
dated from 1834, the Prussian Army was to enjoy marked immunity to the
disease (Hirsch, 1883, i. 142; Prinzing, 1916: 198).

8.3.2 The Data

To examine the spread of smallpox in Prussia during the war of 1870–1, we
draw on the epidemiological information collated by a renowned medical
statistician, physician, and veteran of the Franco-Prussian War—Albert
Guttstadt. During the course of his employment with the Prussian Statistical
Office (Berlin) in the early 1870s, Guttstadt undertook a comprehensive review
of reported smallpox activity in the various localities of wartime Prussia.[34] The
results of his historic study, gathered under the title 'Die Pocken-Epidemie in
Preussen, insbesondere in Berlin 1870/72, nebst Beiträgen zur Beurtheilung der
Impffrage' (The smallpox epidemic in Prussia, especially in Berlin 1870/72,
together with contributions for the evaluation of the inoculation question),
were to appear in volume 13 (1873) of the Prussian Statistical Office's publication, *Zeitschrift des königlich Preussischen Statistischen Bureaus* (Guttstadt,
1873); see Plate 1.2G.[35]

smallpox (Rolleston, 1933: 179). For Prussian civilians, a compulsory programme of smallpox vaccination and revaccination awaited the implementation of the post-war Imperial Vaccination Law of 1874
(Prinzing, 1916: 198).

[34] Smallpox had been subject to mandatory notification in the provinces of Prussia since 1835. See
Guttstadt (1873: 129).

[35] For an English-language overview of the contents of Guttstadt's original study, see Prinzing (1916:
214–51 *passim*).

As described in Section 8.3.1, the outbreak of smallpox in wartime Prussia was to spread widely among French POWs and Prussian civilians. Accordingly, Table 8.9 is based on information abstracted from 'Die Pocken-Epidemie in Preussen' and summarizes the progress of the epidemic in the two functionally discrete but geographically concordant settlement systems to which these populations were attached. We consider each settlement system in turn.

1. *Settlement system I: military (POW camps and related facilities)*. For many French soldiers who were captured during the Franco-Prussian War, transfer from the theatre of operations was followed by incarceration in an interconnected system of Prussian POW camps. Although the size and extent of this camp system was to vary over the course of the hostilities, Guttstadt identifies a total of 78 locations which, at some stage during the war, formed the site of POW camps and other POW-related facilities (including military hospitals and lazarets). Unfortunately, however, the demographic and/or disease records for some of these locations are fragmentary. For the present purposes, therefore, we restrict our analysis to POW facilities at a sample of 56 locations for which complete data records are available. These 56 locations are given in Table 8.9, along with information on (i) the maximum strength of the associated POW population and (ii) the time, in weeks, from the start of the war to the first appearance of smallpox in that population.

2. *Settlement system II: civilian (urban centres)*. Each of the 56 locations of POW camps and related facilities was attached to an urban centre (town or city). For these urban centres, Table 8.9 gives (i) the size of the civil population as registered under the post-war census of 1871 and (ii) the time, in weeks, from the start of the war to the first appearance of smallpox in the civil population.

For each settlement system, the time to the first appearance of smallpox at a given location has been formed in Table 8.9 by coding the first week of the war (calendar week ending 23 July 1870) as week 1, with subsequent weeks numbered sequentially up to, and including, the week of the ratification of the Treaty of Frankfurt (coded week 45, ending 27 May 1871). Finally, for reference, Table 8.9 also indicates the calendar month in which smallpox first appeared in the POW and civil populations at a given location. The information in Table 8.9 forms the basis of the analysis in this section.

8.3.3 Diffusion Processes

As described in Section 6.4.1, accounts of the spread of an infectious disease in a settlement system usually recognize two principal types of diffusion process: (i) contagious diffusion; and (ii) hierarchical diffusion. While we have already encountered one method (autocorrelation on graphs) for the identification and analysis of these diffusion processes (see Sects. 6.4.2 and 7.3.4), here we apply an alternative technique (multiple regression analysis) to the data in Table 8.9. We begin with a consideration of the processes by which smallpox spread in the

Table 8.9. Smallpox in Prussia, July 1870–January 1871

Location (town/city)	Settlement system I: Military (POW camps)		Settlement system II: Civilian (urban centres)	
	Maximum Population	Time to first appearance of smallpox (weeks)[1]	Population[2]	Time to first appearance of smallpox (weeks)[1]
Aschersleben	1,618	22 (Dec. 1870)	16,739	22 (Dec. 1870)
Aurich	1,000	28 (Jan. 1871)	4,262	Not known
Bonn	335	16 (Nov. 1870)	26,020	Not known
Coblenz	19,011	10 (Sept. 1870)	33,365	16 (Nov. 1870)
Colberg	5,246	18 (Nov. 1870)	13,130	25 (Jan. 1871)
Cologne	16,774	7 (Sept. 1870)	129,230	9 (Sept. 1870)
Cörlin	798	22 (Dec. 1870)	2,949	Not known
Cosel	5,233	10 (Sept. 1870)	4,517	Not known
Cottbus	142	19 (Nov. 1870)	18,916	Not known
Cüstrin	2,204	5 (Aug. 1870)	10,122	24 (Dec. 1870)
Danzig	9,189	7 (Aug. 1870)[3]	89,121	9 (Sept. 1870)
Düsseldorf	981	5 (Aug. 1870)	69,351	14 (Oct. 1870)
Erfurt	12,400	9 (Sept. 1870)	43,616	22 (Dec. 1870)
Falkenberg	3,983	27 (Jan. 1871)	1,960	Not known
Frankfurt a. O.	756	17 (Nov. 1870)	43,211	27 (Jan. 1871)
Glatz	3,084	17 (Nov. 1870)	11,541	31 (Feb. 1871)
Glogau	13,921	9 (Sept. 1870)	18,265	12 (Oct. 1870)
Görlitz	326	24 (Dec. 1870)	42,224	27 (Jan. 1871)
Graudenz	1,437	7 (Aug. 1870)	15,559	Not known
Halberstadt	619	28 (Jan. 1871)	25,421	31 (Feb. 1871)
Hanover	2,299	14 (Oct. 1870)	87,641	Not known
Jüterbogk	5,002	27 (Jan. 1871)	6,673	Not known
Königsberg	7,324	5 (Aug. 1870)	112,123	7 (Aug. 1870)
Landsberg	133	18 (Nov. 1870)	18,531	19 (Nov. 1870)
Magdeburg	25,450	9 (Sept. 1870)	114,552	18 (Nov. 1870)
Minden	6,171	11 (Oct. 1870)	16,593	16 (Nov. 1870)
Mühlhausen	1,065	21 (Dec. 1870)	19,516	29 (Feb. 1871)
Münster	3,009	29 (Feb. 1871)	24,815	31 (Feb. 1871)
Neisse	17,801	11 (Sept. 1870)	19,376	Not known
Oppeln	1,227	27 (Jan. 1871)	11,879	27 (Jan. 1871)
Papenburg	993	20 (Nov. 1870)	6,077	Not known
Pillau	408	29 (Jan. 1871)	2,909	Not known
Posen	10,303	9 (Sept. 1870)[3]	56,464	9 (Sept. 1870)
Quedlinburg	927	20 (Nov. 1870)	16,402	18 (Nov. 1870)
Ratibor	834	22 (Dec. 1870)	15,323	Not known
Rendsburg	2,592	19 (Nov. 1870)	11,514	24 (Dec. 1870)
Schievelbein	603	28 (Jan. 1871)	5,514	32 (Feb. 1871)
Schleswig	1,571	22 (Dec. 1870)	13,821	24 (Dec. 1870)
Schneidemühl	940[3]	29 (Jan. 1871)	7,536	27 (Jan. 1871)
Schweidnitz	2,621	29 (Feb. 1871)	16,998	35 (Mar. 1871)
Spandau	6,855	10 (Sept. 1870)	19,013	Not known
Stade	2,284	28 (Jan. 1871)	8,693	Not known
Stendal	51	27 (Jan. 1871)	9,938	27 (Jan. 1871)
Stettin	21,000[3]	10 (Sept. 1870)	76,149	22 (Dec. 1870)
Stolp	1,376	29 (Feb. 1871)	16,280	Not known
Stralsund	2,991	21 (Dec. 1870)	26,731	25 (Jan. 1871)
Swinemünde	1,150	25 (Jan. 1871)	6,850	Not known
Tangermünde	798	29 (Jan. 1871)	4,855	Not known
Thorn	2,601	6 (Aug. 1870)	16,620	Not known
Torgau	9,359	12 (Oct. 1870)	10,867	18 (Nov. 1870)
Trier	312	16 (Nov. 1870)	31,842	Not known
Uckermünde	749	28 (Jan. 1871)	3,758	Not known
Weissenfels	148	29 (Feb. 1871)	15,443	31 (Feb. 1871)
Wesel	18,099	10 (Sept. 1870)	18,519	18 (Nov. 1870)
Wittenberg	9,753	8 (Sept. 1870)	11,567	12 (Oct. 1870)
Wohlau	396	28 (Jan. 1871)	2,863	Not known

Notes: [1] Time, in weeks, from the start of the Franco-Prussian War (week ending 23 July 1870, coded week 1) to the first appearance of smallpox. For reference, the calendar month in which smallpox first appeared is given in parentheses. [2] Registered population, 1871 census. [3] Additional data from Prinzing (1916: 215–16).
Source: Smallman-Raynor and Cliff (2002, table 2, pp. 250–1), based on information in Guttstadt (1873).

military system of POW camps and related facilities (settlement system I). We then turn to the spread of smallpox in the civil system of urban centres (settlement system II).

DIFFUSION OF SMALLPOX, I: FRENCH POWS

For the period of the Franco-Prussian War (July 1870–Jan. 1871) and its immediate aftermath, Figure 8.8 is based on the information in Table 8.9 and maps the time-ordered sequence of appearance of smallpox in French POWs detained at 56 locations in Prussia. Shaded circles identify those locations in which smallpox first appeared in the prisoner population in August 1870 (Fig. 8.8A), September 1870 (Fig. 8.8B), October and November 1870 (Fig. 8.8C), and December 1870 to February 1871 (Fig. 8.8D). On each map, the unshaded circles identify camps which were infected in prior time periods. Finally, to assist in the interpretation of Figure 8.8, the area of each circle has been drawn proportional to the (maximum) strength of the POW population.

1. *August 1870 (Figure 8.8A)*. In August 1870, within weeks of the outbreak of war and with France consumed by a severe epidemic of haemorrhagic smallpox, cases of the disease began to appear among French soldiers in the newly established POW camps of Prussia. As Figure 8.8A indicates, this initial phase of the epidemic was centred on eastern Prussia where the earliest transports of French prisoners had begun to arrive on 7 August (Guttstadt, 1873: 140). Eight days later, on 15 August, the first case of smallpox appeared in the POW camp at Königsberg.[36] The disease manifested in the camps at Cüstrin, Danzig, Graudenz, and Thorn in the days and weeks that followed. Elsewhere, to the extreme west of Prussia, the arrival of infected POWs at Düsseldorf can also be traced to mid-August (ibid. 140–2).

2. *September 1870 (Figure 8.8B)*. With the capture of Louis-Napoleon and the 104,000-strong remnants of the Army of Châlons at Sedan in early September, this phase of the epidemic was characterized by the seeding of smallpox in the largest POW camps of Prussia. As Figure 8.8B shows, by the end of the month, smallpox had appeared in a series of camps which spanned the whole of the Prussian state from Coblenz, Cologne, and Wesel in the west to Cosel, Neisse, and Posen in the east.

3. *October 1870 to February 1871 (Figures 8.8C and 8.8D)*. In addition to further large influxes of French prisoners, including those associated with the capitulation of Metz (Oct. 1870) and the battles of Orléans (Dec. 1870) and Le Mans (Jan. 1871), this phase of the epidemic was underpinned by the internal transfer of prisoners from one POW facility to another. The circumstances which gave rise to these transfers are outlined by Guttstadt (1873) but, owing

---

[36] According to Guttstadt (1873: 140–2), one of the first documented cases of smallpox in the POW population was Zuave Hubert, an unvaccinated French soldier who arrived at Königsberg in the second week of August. The patient first presented with smallpox on 15 August; he died seven days later, on 22 August.

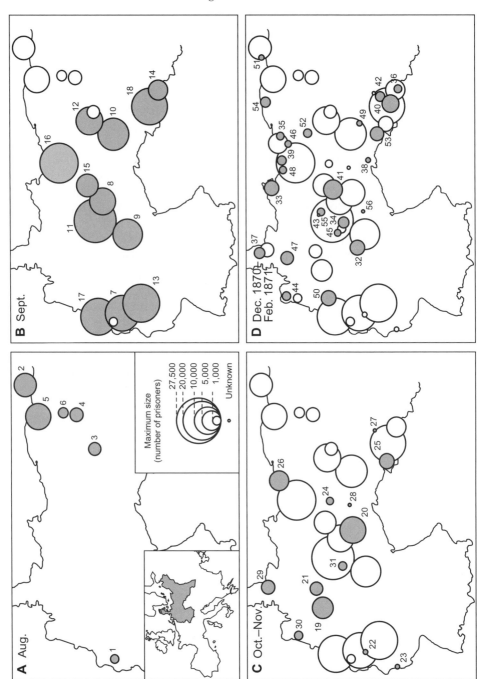

to the poor physical condition of many French soldiers who were captured in the later stages of the war, earlier arrivals were relocated from camps near the French border to other parts of Prussia. This, coupled with numerous other internal transfers of prisoners (Prinzing, 1916: 228, 243), contributed to the broad pattern of spatial 'infill' depicted in Figures 8.8C and 8.8D.

Spread Processes

One important feature of Figure 8.8 is the tendency for the population size of newly infected locations to reduce over the sequence of maps. In general, locations with large POW populations were infected at a relatively early stage of the epidemic (Figs. 8.8A, 8.8B), while locations with small POW populations were infected at a relatively late stage (Figs. 8.8C, 8.8D). Moreover, in some time periods, Figure 8.8 provides some visual evidence for the apparent clustering of newly infected locations in one or more areas of Prussia. These observations, which are suggestive of a mixed contagious–hierarchical diffusion process (see Sect. 6.4.1), can be quantified using multiple regression analysis.

Method. Details of the application of multiple regression techniques to the analysis of diffusion processes are given elsewhere (see e.g. Cliff *et al.*, 1981: 27–32). In the context of the present study, the time-ordered sequence of appearance of smallpox in the system of POW camps and related facilities is modelled as a function of: (1) POW population size, representing the hierarchical component in the spread process; and (2) geographical distance from the location in which smallpox first appeared in the POW population, representing the contagious component. Thus, with reference to the time-based information in Table 8.9, denote the week of the war in which smallpox first appeared in the POW population p at locality i as t_{pi}. Then, the regression model

$$t_{pi} = b_0 + b_1 \log(P_{pi} + 1) + b_2 \log(d_{pi} + 1) + e_i \tag{8.2}$$

Fig. 8.8. Spread of smallpox with French prisoners of war (POWs) in Prussia, 1870–1871

Notes: The maps plot the calendar month in which smallpox first appeared in French prisoners at each of 56 locations. (A) August 1870. (B) September 1870. (C) October and November 1870. (D) December 1870–February 1871. Shaded circles identify locations first infected during the time period covered by the map; unshaded circles mark locations infected in prior time periods. Circles are drawn proportional to the maximum prisoner population at each location. Numbers identify the following locations: 1 Düsseldorf; 2 Königsberg; 3 Cüstrin; 4 Thorn; 5 Danzig; 6 Graudenz; 7 Cologne; 8 Wittenberg; 9 Erfurt; 10 Glogau; 11 Magdeburg; 12 Posen; 13 Coblenz; 14 Cosel; 15 Spandau; 16 Stettin; 17 Wesel; 18 Neisse; 19 Minden; 20 Torgau; 21 Hanover; 22 Bonn; 23 Trier; 24 Frankfurt an der Oder; 25 Glatz; 26 Colberg; 27 Landsberg; 28 Cottbus; 29 Rendsburg; 30 Papenburg; 31 Quedlinburg; 32 Mülhausen; 33 Stralsrund; 34 Aschersleben; 35 Cörlin; 36 Ratibor; 37 Schleswig; 38 Görlitz; 39 Swinemünde; 40 Falkenberg; 41 Jüterbogk; 42 Oppeln; 43 Stendal; 44 Aurich; 45 Halberstadt; 46 Schivelbein; 47 Stade; 48 Uckermünde; 49 Wohlau; 50 Münster; 51 Pillau; 52 Schneidermühl; 53 Schweidnitz; 54 Stolp; 55 Tangermünde; 56 Weissenfels.
Source: Smallman-Raynor and Cliff (2002, fig. 2, pp. 252–3).

was postulated. Here, P_{pi} is the maximum size of the prisoner population at location i, d_{pi} is the straight-line distance (in kilometres) of that location from the location(s) in which smallpox was first reported in the POW population and e_i is an error term. For the epidemic under consideration, the independent variables, P_{pi} and d_{pi}, have a logarithmic relationship with t_{pi}. The logarithmic transformations in equation (8.2) serve to linearize the relationship, while the addition of 1 avoids the computational problem of zero values when taking logarithms.

The model in equation (8.2) was fitted to the 56 locations of POW camps and related facilities in Table 8.9 using stepwise regression. Because the reported origin of the epidemic was at four geographically disparate localities (Berlin,[37] Cüstrin, Düsseldorf, and Königsberg) in week 5 of the war (week ending Sat. 20 Aug. 1870), the distance variable (d_{pi}) in equation (8.2) was taken as the minimum distance between each camp and each of the four index locations. One potential complication in the regression procedure is possible collinearity between population size and distance. In particular, a decrease in POW population size with increasing distance would hinder separation of the contagious and hierarchical components in the model. Consequently, Pearson's r correlation coefficient was used to assess the level of correlation between the independent variables in the regression model.

Results. The application of regression analysis to the diffusion problem is illustrated graphically in Figure 8.9. The white circles in Figure 8.9A plot, on the horizontal axis, the time to infection from the start of the war (week 1) to the appearance of smallpox in French prisoners against, on the vertical axis, the straight-line distance from the nearest index location (Berlin, Cüstrin, Düsseldorf, and Königsberg).[38] Similarly, the white circles in Figure 8.9B plot time to infection against POW population size. Superimposed on each scatter plot is a best fit linear regression line (marked 'prisoners').

A striking feature of Figure 8.9 is the negative association between population size and time to infection (Fig. 8.9B). This implies that large POW populations were infected at an early stage of the epidemic, while small POW populations were infected at a relatively late stage. It is consistent with the hierarchical effect identified in Figure 8.8. However, only weak evidence exists for the operation of a contagious component (Fig. 8.9A). Under this process, a direct (positive) relationship between the distance of camps from the point of initial smallpox introduction and week of outbreak would be expected. The near-horizontal regression line in Figure 8.9A reflects the low association.

[37] According to Guttstadt (1873: 141), smallpox first appeared in the POW population of Berlin on 20 August 1870. Although Berlin has been omitted from Table 8.9 due to lack of demographically related information, the role of this city as an index location is recognized by its inclusion in the computation of d_{pi}.

[38] To assist in the interpretation of Fig. 8.9A, three extreme outliers (the index locations of Cüstrin, Düsseldorf, and Königsberg) have been omitted from the scatter plot.

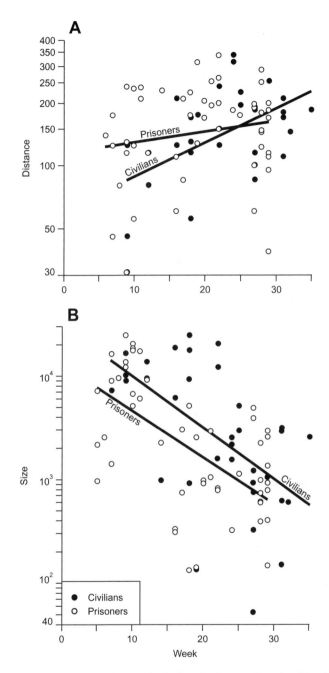

Fig. 8.9. Diffusion of smallpox in Prussia during the Franco-Prussian War, 1870–1871

Notes: Graphs plot the week of the war in which smallpox was first reported in French POWs and Prussian civilians at sample locations in relation to their distance from the points of introduction of smallpox in the POW population (chart A) and POW population sizes (chart B). The horizontal axes have been formed by coding the first calendar week of the war (week ending 23 July 1870) as week 1, with subsequent weeks coded sequentially thereafter. Superimposed on each set of data points is a trend line fitted to the data by ordinary least squares. Note that the vertical axes have been drawn on a logarithmic scale.

Source: Smallman-Raynor and Cliff (2002, fig. 3, p. 256–7).

Models 1 and 2 in Table 8.10 examine the spread process using the framework of the multiple regression model defined in equation (8.2). For each model, the table gives the order of entry (step) of the independent variables in the stepwise procedure, the estimated slope coefficients, $\hat{b}_1$ and $\hat{b}_2$, with the associated t-statistics in parentheses. The coefficient of determination, R^2, the F-ratio, and the degree of correlation, r_{Pd}, between the independent variables are also given. Statistically significant values at the $p = 0.05$ level (one-tailed test) are indicated by an asterisk.

Model 1, which relates to the entire set of 56 locations, shows that time to infection is negatively associated with the population size variable and positively associated with the distance variable. The low and statistically insignificant correlation ($r_{Pd} = -0.12$) between the independent variables implies that the modelling procedure was successful in separating the hierarchical and contagious components. As would be expected from the simple regressions in Figure 8.9, the dominant importance of the population variable is indicated by its entry in step 1 of the model.

Although model 1 implies the operation of a mixed diffusion process with a dominant hierarchical component, three locations (the index locations of Cüstrin, Düsseldorf, and Königsberg) serve as extreme outliers which heavily influence the statistical parameters of the model. Consequently, model 2 repeats the analysis of model 1 but with the three outliers omitted. Modified in this way, the importance of the population variable to the spread process is underscored by its entry in step 1 of model 2. In addition, the distance variable does not make a statistically significant contribution.

Interpretation. When modified for the effects of outliers, the results are consistent with a simple model of geographical transmission in which smallpox spread hierarchically through the system of POW camps and related facilities. It is important to note, however, that the operation of this process was linked closely to the development of the POW population size hierarchy. As the war progressed, the system of POW facilities evolved to include locations with increasingly smaller holdings of prisoners.[39] Some of these smaller holdings are known to have been infected as a result of the internal transfer of prisoners from larger POW populations (Guttstadt, 1873: 140–50; Prinzing, 1916: 214–51) and are therefore consistent with the operation of a strict hierarchical process. However, in the absence of further information, a potential confounding effect (namely, the infection of increasingly smaller POW populations as a result of disease re-importations by later arrivals of prisoners from the French theatre) cannot be excluded.

[39] Based on a sample of 40 locations in Table 8.9, and for which information is provided by Guttstadt (1873), a highly significant and negative association ($r = -0.60$; $t = -4.68$; $p < 0.05$ in a one-tailed test) exists between (i) the time (measured in weeks from the beginning of the war) of arrival of the first POWs and (ii) the maximum size of the POW population.

Table 8.10. Results of stepwise multiple regression analysis to identify diffusion processes for smallpox in Prussia, 1870–1871

Model	Dependent Variable	n	Independent variable, slope coefficient (t-statistic) Step 1	Step 2	$R^2(F)$	r_{pd}	Process
Settlement system I: POW camps							
1	t_{pi}	56	Log(P_{pi}), −7.32 (−5.59*)	Log(d_{pi}), 5.07 (3.69*)	0.49 (25.32*)	−0.12	Mixed (prison system)
2	t_{pi}	53[1]	Log(P_{pi}), −7.60 (−5.66*)	Log(d_{pi}), 2.97 (1.28)	0.42 (18.37*)	−0.15	Hierarchical (prison system)
Settlement system II: urban centres							
3	t_{ci}	34	Log(P_{ci}), −10.41 (−3.22*)	Log(d_{ci}), 2.73 (1.19)	0.33 (7.59*)	−0.29*	Hierarchical (urban system)
4	t_{ci}	31[2]	Log(P_{ci}), −6.74 (−1.70)	Log(d_{ci}), −3.89 (−0.46)	0.12 (1.89)	0.26	None identified (urban system)
5	t_{ci}	34	Log(P_{pi}), −5.82 (−3.90*)	Log(d_{pi}), 4.35 (2.79*)	0.45 (12.62*)	−0.10	Mixed (prison system)

Independent variables
t_{pi} = time (in weeks) from the start of the war to the first appearance of smallpox in French POWs
t_{ci} = time (in weeks) from the start of the war to the first appearance of smallpox in Prussian civilians

Dependent variables
P_{pi} = maximum POW population size
P_{pi} = distance (in km) to location i from the location(s) at which smallpox was first reported in the French POW population
P_{ci} = civilian population size
d_{ci} = distance (in km) to location i from the location(s) at which smallpox was first reported in the Prussian civilian population

Notes: * Significant at the $p = 0.05$ level (one-tailed test). [1] Cüstrin, Düsseldorf, and Königsberg omitted as extreme outliers. [2] Cologne, Danzig, and Königsberg omitted as extreme outliers.
Source: Smallman-Raynor and Cliff (2002, table A1, p. 264).

DIFFUSION OF SMALLPOX, II: PRUSSIAN CIVILIANS

To examine the mechanism by which smallpox spread in the civil system of urban centres, we extend our application of multiple regression to the civilian-based information in Table 8.9. The time-ordered sequence of appearance of smallpox in the civil population is modelled as a function of the structure (population size and geographical position) of settlements in:

(i) the civil system of urban centres. This provides an intra-system examination of diffusion processes for the civil population;

(ii) the military system of POW camps and related facilities. This model represents an inter-system examination of diffusion processes from the POW to the civil population.

The rationale that underpins (i) and (ii) is outlined below. We preface our examination with a brief note on the data analysed. Although Table 8.9 identifies 56 locations for which information on the date of first appearance of smallpox in the POW population is available, the equivalent information for the civil population is limited to 34 locations, and these form the basis of our analysis.

(i) Urban Centres: Intra-system Diffusion Processes

Studies of the spread of infectious diseases in civil populations usually identify a close association between diffusion process and the structure (population size and/or geographical position) of settlements in the urban system. To examine the effect of urban structure on the spread of smallpox in the civil settlement system of wartime Prussia, denote the week of the war in which smallpox first appeared in the civil population c at location i as t_{ci}. Paralleling equation (8.2), we may then set up the regression equation

$$t_{ci} = b_0 + b_1 \log(P_{ci} + 1) + b_2 \log(d_{ci} + 1) + e_i, \tag{8.3}$$

where P_{ci} is the size of the civil population at location i as given in the census of 1871, and d_{ci} is the straight-line distance (in kilometres) of location i from the location in which smallpox was first reported in the civil population. As in equation (8.2), the logarithmic transformation serves to linearize the relationship between the independent variables, P_{ci} and d_{ci}, and the dependent variable, t_{ci}.

The regression model in equation (8.3) was fitted to the 34 civil locations in Table 8.9. As this table shows, the first evidence of smallpox in the civil population can be traced to a single location (Königsberg) in week 7 of the war (week ending 3 Sept. 1870). Accordingly, the distance variable in equation (8.3) was measured as the distance between each locality and Königsberg.

The results are summarized as models 3 and 4 in Table 8.10. Model 3, which relates to the entire set of 34 locations, shows that time to infection is negatively associated with population, while distance fails to make a statistically significant contribution. However, as model 4 shows, the omission of three outliers (Cologne, Danzig, and Königsberg) yields a rather different result. Both independent variables are statistically insignificant, indicating that the spread of smallpox in the civil population was detached from the structural parameters (population size and geographical position) of settlements in the urban system.

(ii) POW Camps: Inter-system Diffusion Processes

When examined with reference to the 34 locations for which complete information is available, one important feature of Table 8.9 is the tendency for the first appearance of smallpox in the civil population to lag the POW population by several weeks or more. So, on average, the time to the first appearance of smallpox in a locality varied from 16.8 weeks for French POWs to 21.7 weeks for Prussian civilians. Here, the (16.8 weeks–21.7 weeks) difference in timing is equivalent to a lag of 34 days, or approximately three generations of the smallpox virus.[40]

This lag effect is consistent with a simple model of epidemic transmission in which, during the Franco-Prussian War and its immediate aftermath, POW camps and related facilities acted as the epidemic seeds from which smallpox spread to the local civil population (Guttstadt, 1873: 140–50). Supported by empirical evidence for the transmission of smallpox from prisoner to civil populations,[41] our model implies that the spread of the disease in the civil settlement system was pinned to the structure of the temporary and makeshift system of POW camps and related facilities.

Graphical analysis. The inter-system diffusion effect is examined graphically in Figure 8.9. Here, the black circles in Figure 8.9A plot, on the horizontal axis, the time to infection from the start of the war (week 1) to the appearance of smallpox among Prussian civilians against, on the vertical axis, the straight-line distance from the location(s) in which smallpox was first reported in French prisoners. Similarly, the black circles in Figure 8.9B plot time to infection against the POW population size.

Figure 8.9B indicates that the negative association shown earlier to exist between POW population size and time to infection (lower regression line) is mimicked by the civil population (upper regression line). Such a pattern accords with the operation of a hierarchical component in the diffusion process for both prisoners and civilians, although the time lag between the first

[40] We define a smallpox virus generation as 12 days. This represents the typical interval between the time at which a case becomes infectious and the onset of clinical symptoms in a contact of that case. See Fenner *et al.* (1988).

[41] For a number of the locations in Table 8.9, Guttstadt traces the earliest cases of smallpox in the civil population to individuals (guards, nurses and sick attendants, clergymen, and laundry workers, among others) who had direct or indirect contact with the French POWs. Writing of the epidemics at Münster and Wittenberg, for example, Guttstadt notes that the first civilian cases of smallpox were clerics who had ministered to the French POWs. Likewise, the earliest civilian cases at Stralsrund and Torgau were employees of the lazarets to which ailing prisoners had been assigned. Similar evidence can also be cited for Frankfurt an der Oder, Minden, and Stettin, among other locations. See Guttstadt (1873: 140–50); Prinzing (1916: 214–51).

appearance of the disease in the two populations (earlier among POWs) is underscored by the relative position of the regression lines. In contrast, Figure 8.9A shows that a positive association between distance and time to infection is more pronounced for civilians than for prisoners. This finding suggests that a spatially contagious component may well have contributed to the diffusion of smallpox in the civil population of Prussia.

Multiple regression analysis. To examine the inter-system diffusion effect, the week of the war in which smallpox first appeared in the civil population, t_{ci}, was substituted as the dependent variable in equation (8.2). The independent variables were unchanged from the original model. The model was fitted using stepwise regression to the 34 locations for which the time of first appearance of smallpox in the civil population is known.

The results obtained are summarized as model 5 in Table 8.10. The model confirms that time to infection for the civil population is negatively associated with POW population size and positively associated with POW distance. The relative importance of the population variable is indicated by its entry in step 1 of the fitting procedure, while the statistically insignificant correlation between the independent variables indicates that the modelling procedure was successful in separating the hierarchical and contagious diffusion components.

Interpretation. Taken together, models 3 to 5 in Table 8.10 indicate that the spread of smallpox in the civil settlement system of Prussia was underpinned by a mixed contagious–hierarchical diffusion process with a dominant hierarchical component. Crucially, however, this process was detached from the basic structure (population size and geographical position) of settlements in the urban system (model 4). Rather, the process was conditioned by the size and geographical arrangement of the temporary and makeshift system of POW camps and related facilities which had been fused onto the urban system (model 5). One plausible interpretation of these findings is that, during the course of the war, the large influx of French POWs was associated with a seeding of the epidemic which was so rapid and widespread that it overrode the processes by which the disease would ordinarily have spread in the civil settlement system of Prussia.

8.3.4 Summary

The enduring historical interest that attaches to the Prussian smallpox epidemic of 1870–2 rests with the intersection of war, disease transmission and demographic loss, the evolution of state legislative responses to smallpox control, and the broader medicalization of the nascent German Empire (Prinzing, 1916: 282–5). The social and political ramifications of the 1870–2 epidemic, including the introduction of compulsory vaccination and revaccination under the German Imperial Vaccination Law of 1874, have been explored elsewhere

(Huerkamp, 1985; Hennock, 1998). The present analysis has added a geographical dimension to historical understanding by examining the processes that underpinned the spread of the epidemic in two functionally discrete settlement systems of Prussia (urban centres and POW camps/facilities) during the Franco-Prussian War, July 1870–May 1871.

Two principal findings have emerged from our analysis. First, we have shown that smallpox spread through the military system of POW camps and related facilities of Prussia as a purely hierarchical diffusion process. Because the number of POW-related facilities expanded during the course of the war to include locations with increasingly smaller holdings of prisoners, the hierarchical spread of smallpox was itself driven by the evolution of the POW settlement system. Secondly, we have shown that smallpox spread through the civil system of urban centres as a mixed diffusion process with a dominant hierarchical component. But contrary to expectation, this process was not structured according to the size and geographical position of settlements in the urban system. Rather, it was determined by the system of POW camps that had developed around the urban system during the course of the war. As such, the results underscore how military populations may influence the propagation of epidemic diseases in civil settlement systems. Additionally, the results highlight the historical importance of inter-linked networks of institutions, such as POW camps, not only in the localized amplification of smallpox outbreaks (Ayers, 1971: 111–15; Fenner *et al.*, 1988: 201–2), but also in the spatial structuring of state-wide epidemics.

8.4 Camp Epidemics in the World Wars

The world wars provide numerous instances of the occurrence of military camp epidemics in the European theatre. Specific examples for the British Army can be found in the medical histories of the wars and campaigns (see e.g. Macpherson *et al.*, 1922–3; Crew, 1956, 1957), while general overviews of the disease experiences of the opposing armies are provided by Major (1940), Councell (1941), and Lancaster (1990). As described by Clara Councell (1941), typhus fever (Polish, Russian, and Serbian Armies), cholera and dysentery (German Army on the Polish front), smallpox (Austro-Hungarian Army), typhoid and paratyphoid fevers (French Army), malaria (British Army in Macedonia), and later, pandemic influenza in all armies, are illustrative of the camp epidemics of World War I. By the onset of World War II, the specific agents of many bacterial diseases, and some viral diseases, had been identified. Epidemiological understanding of the most important infectious conditions had accrued, while advances in vaccination and chemotherapy contributed significantly to disease prevention, treatment, and control (Lancaster, 1990: 338). Indeed, such were the developments that, in his foreword to medical aspects of the British Liberation Army, Field Marshal Montgomery could conclude that 'Modern warfare in a temperate country has proved a healthy thing, and, unlike the Middle East, North African, and Far Eastern Campaigns, medicine has been content to take a second place to surgery' (Field Marshal Sir Bernard Montgomery, foreword to Bulmer, 1945: 873).

Nevertheless, infectious agents of various types still spread within the military camps of the belligerent forces. Dysentery became widely diffused in the German Army during the Polish Campaign of 1939 (Gantenberg, 1939; Wurm, 1940), while infective hepatitis blighted German troops on all fronts (Stuhlfauth, 1941; Dietrich, 1942; Jacobi *et al.*, 1943). As early as January 1940, meningitis appeared in the British Expeditionary Force in France and Belgium (Crew, 1956), and malaria proved particularly problematic for the Allied Eighth Army during the Italian Campaign of 1943–5 (Thompson, 1946). Apparently novel diseases—'Bessarabia fever', 'Russian headache fever', and 'Balkan grippe'—appeared among armies in Eastern Europe (Boehnhardt, 1942; Schulten and Broglie, 1943; Palmer, 1993) while, in other types of camp setting, typhus fever and tuberculosis spread in epidemic form in the concentration camps of Germany (Collis, 1945; Vella, 1984).

8.4.1 World War II: US Camps and Q Fever in Italy

Beginning in the latter months of 1944, the makeshift encampments of US forces in Italy became the sources for explosive outbreaks of an apparently new disease of military significance—Q fever. As Blewitt (1951) notes, prior to World War II, Q fever was regarded as something of a medical curiosity. The disease had gained some recognition in the mid-1930s as a result of studies in Australia and the United States, when the name 'Q(uery) fever' was first coined. During the early 1940s, a widespread epidemic of Q fever (so-called 'Balkan grippe') struck the occupying German forces in Bulgaria, Italy, Crimea, Greece, Ukraine, Corsica, and Yugoslavia, taking a heavy toll on the Axis troops in these locations (Spicer, 1978). However, as military fortunes shifted in favour of the Allies the disease began to attack companies of US troops in Italy, with further sporadic outbreaks in Corsica (US forces) and Greece (British forces) (Robbins and Ragan, 1946; Robbins *et al.*, 1946*a*, 1946*b*; Robbins and Rustigian, 1946; Feinstein *et al.*, 1946).

NATURE OF Q FEVER

Q fever is a febrile, usually acute and self-limiting, zoonosis caused by infection with the rickettsia *Coxiella burnetii*. The causative agent has a worldwide distribution. Natural hosts include many species of mammals, birds, ticks, and other insects, in which the infection is asymptomatic. Transmission to humans may occur through the inhalation of dust contaminated by infected animals and animal products and, occasionally, by tick bites or the consumption of

Table 8.11. Documented epidemics of Q fever among US troops in Italy during World War II

Location	Date	Unit	Cases
Italy/Pagliana	Nov. 1944–Apr. 1945	3840th & 3853rd Q.M. Gas Supply Company	54
Italy/Belvedere	Feb.–Mar. 1945	Reg. Headqtrs. Co., 339th Inf.	53
Italy/Sassaleone	Feb.–Mar. 1945	Company C, 19th Engineers	34
Italy/Pagliana	Mar.–Apr. 1945	3255th Q.M. Service Company	34–47[1]
Italy/Pagliana	Apr. 1945	3rd Batt., 362nd Inf. Reg.	266
Italy/Grottaglie[2]	May–June 1945	449 Bomb Group	368
Italy/Malcesine	June 1945	10th Quartermaster Batt.	34

Notes: [1] The high count (47) includes 13 cases with diagnoses other than atypical pneumonia.
[2] Epidemic broke out *en route* from Italy to America, and continued for several weeks thereafter.
Source: Information from Robbins *et al.* (1946*a*, table 1, p. 24) and Blewitt (1951, table I, p. 380).

unpasteurized milk. *C. burnetii* is relatively insensitive to environmental conditions, and may exist for extended periods (months or years) in dust. As regards the clinical course of acute Q fever, an incubation period of two to four weeks gives way to the abrupt onset of fever, severe headache, retro-orbital pain, photophobia, and malaise. The illness, sometimes manifesting as atypical pneumonia, may last for one to four weeks and is usually associated with a low (<1.0%) case-fatality rate. Manifestations of the chronic form of the disease, presenting months or years after primary exposure, include endocarditis and hepatitis. Asymptomatic infection with *C. burnetii* is common (Palmer, 1993).

US CAMP OUTBREAKS IN ITALY

Table 8.11 is based on information included in Robbins *et al.* (1946*a*) and Blewitt (1951) and summarizes the results of investigations into recorded outbreaks of Q fever among US forces on mainland Italy, November 1944–June 1945. For each outbreak, the table gives the location of the associated campsite, the date of the outbreak, the unit in which the outbreak occurred, and the number of observed cases of Q fever. For reference, campsite locations are mapped in Figure 8.10.

All told, Table 8.11 documents some 850 cases of Q fever in seven well-defined outbreaks. Although the distribution of campsites associated with the outbreaks extended from northern (Malcesine) to southern (Grottaglie) Italy, the majority of outbreaks were linked to three rural North Apennine villages (Belvedere, Pagliana, and Sassaleone) situated between Florence and Bologna (Figure 8.10). At the latter locations, the troops were camped in and around farmhouses, barns, and outhouses, and came into close quarters with pigeons, livestock, and associated ticks (Robbins *et al.*, 1946*a*; Blewitt, 1951).

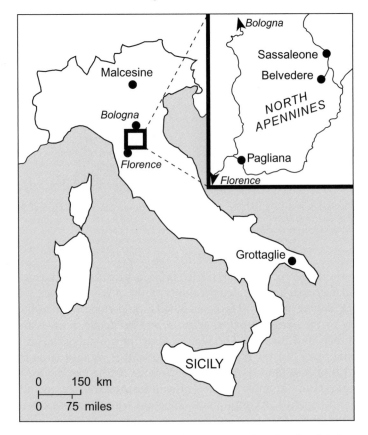

Fig. 8.10. Locations in Italy associated with documented outbreaks of Q fever among US military personnel, November 1944–June 1945

Notes: Seven well-defined outbreaks of Q fever in US military personnel were associated with camps at Malcesine, Belvedere, Pagliana, Sassaleone, and Grottaglie. Details of the outbreaks are provided in Table 8.11.

Q Fever in the US Third Battalion, 362nd Infantry Regiment

To illustrate the circumstances associated with the outbreaks of Q fever in Table 8.11, we draw on an epidemiological investigation of the US Third Battalion, 362nd Infantry Regiment, at Pagliana by Robbins *et al.* (1946*a*: 28–31). The *c.*900-strong battalion had moved into the environs of the small village of Pagliana (Fig. 8.10) on 20 March 1945, with Companies I, K, L, and M forming a tent camp around a requisitioned farmhouse in which Headquarters Company was based. The companies maintained their position until 3 April, when the battalion moved back into line. The course of the ensuing epidemic of Q fever is charted by company in Figure 8.11.

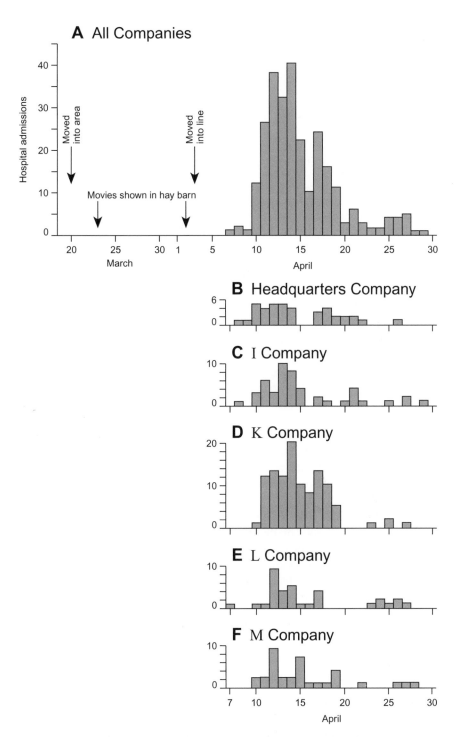

Fig. 8.11. The course of the Q fever epidemic in the US Third Battalion, 362nd Infantry, April 1945

Notes: Daily hospital admissions are plotted for the entire Battalion (A) and each of five companies: (B) Headquarters Company; (C) I Company; (D) K Company; (E) L Company; and (F) M Company.

Source: Redrawn from Robbins *et al.* (1946*a*, figs. 2 and 3, p. 29).

Possible sources of exposure. Among the possible sources of exposure to *C. burnetii* at Pagliana, and which would account for the explosive character of the epidemic in Figure 8.11, epidemiological investigations implicated one particular location—the hay loft of a barn adjacent to the requisitioned farmhouse—in the transmission of the disease agent. The Third Battalion had used the hay loft for the presentation of military training films, with each company attending the screenings in rotation. According to Robbins and co-workers,

The loft was partially filled with old, very dusty hay on which the men sat during the showing of the pictures. In the walls of the barn were numerous holes in which pigeons nested. Some of these communicated directly with the inside of the loft and the wind blew through them carrying dust and debris into the interior of the barn. (Robbins *et al.*, 1946*a*: 28)

A subsequent inspection of the barn revealed abundant evidence of adult and larval ticks in the pigeon nests, while mites of various species were found in the chaff on the loft floor. Perhaps significantly, some men had also used hay from the barn for their bedding.

Course of the epidemic (Figure 8.11). Consistent with an incubation period of two to four weeks, Figure 8.11 shows that the epidemic began in the days immediately following the departure of the Third Battalion from Pagliana. The first patient, a member of L Company, was admitted to hospital on 7 April (Fig. 8.11E), with cases appearing in Headquaters Company and I Company on 8–9 April (Figs. 8.11B, 8.11C) and K and M Companies on 10 April (Figs. 8.11D, 8.11F). Thereafter, the epidemic escalated to a peak on 14 April, for an interrupted decline to the end of the month (Fig. 8.11A). All told, the epidemic was associated with 266 hospital admissions (an attack rate of some 30%), with the largest number of cases occurring in K Company (Fig. 8.11D).

Other Outbreaks among US Personnel

Similar to the experience of the Third Battalion, 362nd Infantry Regiment, many of the other documented outbreaks of Q fever among US personnel in Italy were found to be associated with exposure to animal life and potentially contaminated accumulations of dust in the vicinity of bivouacs. Given that the case totals in Table 8.11 represented some 20–30 per cent of the strength of the individual units involved, the military significance of the disease at this time is apparent (Robbins *et al.*, 1946*a*). As Feinstein *et al.* (1946) observe of 449 Bomb Group, in which Q fever first manifested on transports returning from Italy to the United States in May–June 1945, the disease had the potential to debilitate an entire bomb squadron for several weeks.

CONTINUING MILITARY SIGNIFICANCE OF Q FEVER

Q fever has retained its position as a disease of military significance in the years since World War II. The Greek Army was repeatedly afflicted by the disease in the decade to 1956, while epidemics struck Swiss recruit training camps in 1948 and again in 1950. Subsequent documented outbreaks of Q fever in Europe have included British airmen on the Isle of Man (1958) and British soldiers stationed in the Eastern Sovereign Base Area of Cyprus (1974–5) (Spicer, 1978). As Spicer (1978) notes, a particular epidemiological risk attaches to military activities in goat- and sheep-rearing country, especially when warfare gives rise to large-scale flock migrations, thereby leading to the rapid spread of infection and contamination of the environment.

8.5 Conclusions

In this chapter, we have drawn on sample European conflicts of the nineteenth (Crimean War and Franco-Prussian War) and twentieth (World War II) centuries to examine the role of military camps as sites and systems for the transmission of infectious diseases. The results have highlighted the role of linked networks of encampments such as army field camps and POW camps in the localized amplification of epidemic outbreaks and in the spatial structuring of disease diffusion in both military and civil populations. Two examples illustrate the latter finding:

1. *Military populations: British field camps in Bulgaria (Crimean War)*. Using techniques of multidimensional scaling (MDS), Section 8.2 showed that the spread of cholera in the British camp system of Bulgaria was mediated through a camp *connectivity space*. Within this space, similarities in regimental patterns of occupancy with two camps (Devna and Varna) were to govern the camp-wise sequence of cholera transmission. In contrast, the inter-camp movements of individual members and subgroups of the various commands were found to have little impact on the primary diffusion of the disease in the camp system.

2. *Civil populations: POW camps in Prussia (Franco-Prussian War)*. The analysis in Section 8.3 demonstrated that the spread of smallpox in the civil population of Prussia was underpinned by a diffusion process that involved both geographically localized spread (contagious diffusion), and spread from large to small centres (hierarchical diffusion). This process was detached from the arrangement of settlements in the urban system. Rather, spread was conditioned by the temporary and makeshift system of POW camps which, during the course of the war, had been established in the vicinity of many urban centres.

While the principal focus of the present chapter has been on the spread of old plagues such as cholera and smallpox, the example of Q fever (Section 8.4.1) illustrates the way in which army camps may serve as foci for the emergence of apparently new diseases of military significance. In the next chapter,

Table 8.A1. Cholera cases and deaths recorded in divisions and regiments of the British Army during the Crimean War, 1854–1856

Regiment	Wave I[1]		Wave II[2]	
	Admissions[3]	Deaths[3]	Admissions[3]	Deaths[3]
Light Division	1,273 (16.4)	802 (10.3)	416 (6.2)	216 (3.2)
7th Fusiliers[†,‡]	111 (15.4)	85 (11.8)	41 (6.5)	14 (2.2)
19th Regiment[†,‡]	110 (16.3)	71 (10.5)	27 (4.7)	13 (2.3)
23rd Regiment[†,‡]	190 (27.9)	120 (17.6)	70 (10.8)	20 (3.1)
33rd Regiment[†,‡]	123 (19.8)	83 (13.4)	26 (4.9)	17 (3.2)
34th Regiment[‡]	45 (6.1)	34 (4.6)	76 (10.9)	48 (6.9)
77th Regiment[†,‡]	112 (13.5)	63 (7.6)	28 (3.4)	20 (2.4)
88th Regiment[†,‡]	111 (16.1)	71 (10.3)	30 (4.3)	18 (2.6)
90th Regiment[‡]	55 (7.7)	31 (4.3)	25 (3.9)	16 (2.5)
97th Regiment[‡]	298 (32.0)	177 (19.0)	26 (4.1)	19 (3.0)
Rifle Brigade (2nd Batt.)[†,‡]	118 (14.4)	67 (8.1)	67 (8.5)	31 (3.9)
Cavalry Division	326 (13.6)	192 (8.0)	382 (7.1)	207 (3.9)
1st Dragoon Guards	Not on service in East		55 (17.4)	40 (12.6)
4th Dragoon Guards[†]	33 (13.9)	27 (11.3)	14 (4.2)	5 (1.5)
5th Dragoon Guards[†]	59 (24.6)	36 (15.0)	8 (2.5)	5 (1.6)
6th Dragoon Guards	Not on service in East		18 (6.4)	11 (3.9)
1st Royal Dragoons[†]	25 (10.3)	16 (6.6)	15 (4.2)	6 (1.7)
2nd Dragoons	15 (6.4)	10 (4.2)	16 (4.7)	11 (3.2)
4th Light Dragoons[†]	48 (24.8)	31 (16.0)	44 (12.4)	27 (7.6)
6th Dragoons[†]	68 (27.7)	21 (8.5)	26 (6.9)	9 (2.4)
8th Hussars[†]	15 (6.1)	9 (3.6)	19 (4.9)	12 (3.1)
10th Hussars	Not on service in East		70 (9.5)	33 (4.5)
11th Hussars[†]	27 (12.7)	17 (8.0)	7 (2.4)	7 (2.4)
12th Lancers	Not on service in East		29 (5.2)	13 (2.3)
13th Light Dragoons[†]	21 (9.67)	15 (6.9)	32 (10.1)	14 (4.4)
17th Lancers[†]	15 (7.2)	10 (4.8)	29 (7.6)	14 (3.7)
First/First & Highland Div.	816 (14.9)	540 (9.9)	475 (6.2)	311 (4.1)
Grenadier Guards[†]	133 (19.5)	87 (12.8)	98 (10.6)	63 (6.8)
Coldstream Guards[†]	99 (14.2)	69 (9.9)	35 (5.1)	28 (4.0)
Scots Fusilier Guards[†]	173 (21.1)	118 (14.4)	89 (10.1)	44 (5.0)
9th Regiment	108 (24.8)	78 (17.9)	15 (3.0)	7 (1.4)
13th Regiment	Not on service in East		55 (6.7)	45 (5.5)
31st Regiment	Not on service in East		93 (12.1)	61 (7.9)
42nd Regiment[4†]	97 (11.8)	65 (7.9)	20 (2.4)	13 (1.6)
56th Regiment	Not on service in East		27 (3.3)	19 (2.3)
79th Regiment[4†]	132 (14.4)	66 (7.2)	18 (2.5)	12 (1.7)
93rd Regiment[4†]	74 (8.9)	57 (6.9)	25 (3.5)	19 (2.7)

Regiment	Wave I[1]		Wave II[2]	
	Admissions[3]	Deaths[3]	Admissions[3]	Deaths[3]
Second Division	369 (6.5)	227 (4.0)	297 (4.6)	179 (2.9)
1st Regiment (2nd Batt.)	Not on service in East		28 (4.3)	18 (2.8)
3rd Regiment	Not on service in East		60 (7.8)	30 (3.9)
30th Regiment[†,‡]	58 (9.5)	40 (6.5)	21 (3.9)	13 (2.4)
41st Regiment[†,‡]	34 (4.5)	21 (2.8)	28 (4.2)	14 (2.1)
47th Regiment[†,‡]	78 (10.1)	49 (6.4)	18 (2.5)	15 (2.1)
49th Regiment[†,‡]	56 (7.1)	30 (3.8)	45 (6.7)	23 (3.4)
55th Regiment[†,‡]	51 (7.2)	22 (3.1)	38 (5.3)	25 (3.5)
62nd Regiment[‡]	34 (6.5)	26 (4.9)	22 (5.4)	14 (3.5)
82nd Regiment	Not on service in East		18 (2.3)	12 (1.5)
95th Regiment[†,‡]	58 (8.9)	39 (6.0)	19 (3.6)	15 (2.8)
Third Division	780 (10.3)	514 (6.8)	248 (3.4)	156 (2.2)
1st Regiment (1st Batt.)[†,‡]	151 (20.5)	103 (14.0)	12 (1.6)	9 (1.2)
4th Regiment[‡]	92 (14.1)	61 (9.4)	22 (2.8)	17 (2.2)
14th Regiment	7 (0.9)	3 (0.4)	53 (6.4)	30 (3.6)
18th Regiment[‡]	2 (0.2)	1 (0.1)	22 (3.0)	9 (1.2)
28th Regiment[†,‡]	101 (15.7)	70 (10.9)	29 (4.0)	20 (2.8)
38th Regiment[†,‡]	108 (14.2)	63 (8.3)	17 (2.2)	13 (1.7)
39th Regiment	7 (0.9)	7 (0.9)	46 (5.8)	34 (4.3)
44th Regiment[†,‡]	94 (13.6)	59 (8.5)	30 (4.7)	14 (2.2)
50th Regiment[†,‡]	159 (22.8)	95 (13.6)	6 (1.2)	3 (0.6)
89th Regiment[‡]	59 (8.2)	52 (7.2)	11 (1.6)	7 (1.0)
Fourth Division	1,062 (19.3)	440 (8.0)	248 (4.2)	137 (2.3)
17th Regiment[‡]	20 (2.3)	15 (1.7)	41 (4.8)	25 (2.9)
20th Regiment[‡]	78 (12.3)	30 (4.7)	21 (3.6)	6 (1.0)
21st Regiment[‡]	160 (22.3)	46 (6.4)	21 (3.2)	5 (0.8)
46th Regiment[‡]	359 (90.7)	144 (36.4)	22 (4.6)	12 (2.5)
48th Regiment	Not on service in East		63 (7.8)	42 (5.2)
57th Regiment[‡]	78 (11.3)	47 (6.8)	12 (1.7)	9 (1.3)
63rd Regiment[‡]	172 (35.9)	59 (12.3)	18 (3.6)	5 (1.0)
68th Regiment[‡]	84 (11.7)	43 (6.0)	12 (1.9)	7 (1.1)
Rifle Brigade (1st Batt.)[‡]	111 (15.7)	56 (7.9)	38 (5.4)	26 (3.7)
Highland Division[5]	4 (0.6)	2 (0.3)	162 (7.2)	96 (4.3)
71st Regiment	4 (0.6)	2 (0.3)	33 (3.7)	18 (2.0)
72nd Regiment	Not on service in East		123 (17.8)	74 (10.7)
92nd Regiment	Not on service in East		6 (0.9)	4 (0.6)
Total	4,630 (16.4)	2,717 (9.6)	2,228 (5.6)	1,302 (3.3)

Notes: [†] Engaged in the expedition to Bulgaria. [‡] Encamped on the plain before Sebastopol during the Crimean phase of Wave I. [1] June 1854–Feb 1855. [2] Apr 1855–Mar 1856. [3] Rate per 100 mean monthly strength in parentheses. [4] Later assigned to the Highland Division. [5] See also First Division (42nd, 79th, and 93rd Regiments).
Source: Smallman-Raynor and Cliff (forthcoming, table A1).

we develop the theme of emerging and re-emerging diseases with particular reference to wars in Asia and the Far East.

Appendix 8A

Cholera Counts for British Regiments in the Crimean War

Table 8.A1 lists the 66 regiments of the British Army for which information on cholera is available in the *Medical and Surgical History of the War* (Army Medical Department, 1858). For each regiment, the table gives the number of hospital admissions and deaths from cholera in Waves I and II of the epidemic, along with the associated rate (per 100 mean monthly strength). Regiments that undertook a tour of duty in Bulgaria are indicated ('†'), as are those encamped before Sebastopol during the Crimean phase of Wave I ('‡').

Appendix 8B

MDS and Camp Connectivity Spaces

Computational details of the MDS mapping technique used to form the camp spaces in Figure 8.5 are given in Appendix 6A.4. As described there, the MDS method uses a dissimilarity matrix to define the degree of correspondence between locations in terms of some variable. To construct the spaces in Figure 8.5, four different measures of camp connectivity were used to define (dis)similarity:

(i) *Camp linkage (first order)*. This measure specified connectivity according to whether a given pair of camps was directly linked by the transfer of regiments. Connectivity was formally defined by setting each element, s_{ij}, in a matrix **S** equal to 1 if camps i and j were directly connected by the transfer of one or more regiments, and $s_{ij} = 0$ otherwise.

(ii) *Camp linkage (first and second order)*. This measure specified connectivity according to whether a pair of camps was *directly* or *indirectly* linked by the transfer of regiments. Connectivity was formally defined as in (i), but with the additional criterion that $s_{ij} = 1$ if the transfer between camps i and j was interrupted by residence at a single intervening camp.

(iii) *Regimental occupancy*. This measure defined connectivity according to the regiment-specific pattern of camp occupancy and transfer. To establish the connectivity measure, a 0/1 matrix of presences and absences of regiments at each camp was first constructed. Tanimoto's dichotomy coefficient, $S6$, was then used to compute the degree of similarity of each pair of camps in terms of regiment-specific occupancy (Kotz and Johnson, 1985: 397–405; see App. 6A.4). Connectivity was defined by setting the $\{s_{ij}\}$ in the matrix **S** equal to the corresponding values of the $S6$ coefficient.

(iv) *Duration of regimental occupancy.* This measure specified connectivity according to the regiment-specific pattern of camp occupancy and transfer, weighted by the duration of stay at the camps. A matrix of the length of stay (in days) of a given regiment at each camp was first constructed. Pearson's product-moment correlation coefficient, r, was then used to compute the degree of similarity of each pair of camps in terms of the duration of regiment-specific occupancy. Connectivity was defined by setting the $\{s_{ij}\}$ in the matrix $\mathbf{S}$ equal to the corresponding values of the r coefficient.

The matrices $\mathbf{S}$ are similarity matrices, reflecting the similarity between camps in terms of four alternative measures of regiment-based connectivity. For each of the $\mathbf{S}$, a matrix $\mathbf{D}$ ($= \{\delta_{ij}\}$) of dissimilarities ($\delta_{ij} = K - s_{ij}$ for some constant K) can be obtained. This matrix of dissimilarities served as the basis for the MDS configurations in Figure 8.5.

9

Asia and the Far East: Emerging and Re-emerging Diseases

'The outbreak is in full swing and our death-rate would sicken Napoleon ... Dr M—died last week, and C—on Monday, but some more medicines are coming ... We don't seem to be able to check it at all ... Death is a queer chap to live with for steady company.' *Extract from a private letter from Manchuria.*

Rudyard Kipling, 'The Spies' March' (1913)

9.1 Introduction

In the last chapter, our consideration of camp epidemics ended with an examination of a strange and debilitating illness that, prior to World War II, was hardly known to medical science—Q fever or 'Balkan grippe'.[1] Historically, Q fever is one of many seemingly 'new' diseases that have suddenly and unex-

---

[1] Q fever was first recognized among abattoir workers and dairy farmers in Queensland, Australia, in 1935; the earliest report of the disease was published in the *Medical Journal of Australia* in 1937 (Derrick, 1937).

pectedly erupted into military conciousness. In Chapter 2, for example, we saw how maladies such as the mysterious English sweating sickness, along with venereal syphilis, typhus fever, and yellow fever, appeared—ostensibly for the first time—in association with wars of the fifteenth, sixteenth, and seventeenth centuries. More recently, trench fever (World War I, 1914–18), scrub typhus (World War II, 1939–45) and Korean haemorrhagic fever (Korean War, 1950–3) provide twentieth-century examples of the emergence phenomenon (Macpherson *et al.*, 1922–3; Philip, 1948; Gajdusek, 1956). At the same time, wars have also served to fuel the epidemic re-emergence of many classical diseases, of which human plague (Vietnam War, 1964–73), visceral leishmaniasis (Sudanese Civil War, 1956–), and diphtheria (Tajikistan Civil War, 1992–) are recent instances (Velimirovic, 1972; Seaman *et al.*, 1996; Keshavjee and Becerra, 2000).

In the present chapter, we develop the theme of war and disease emergence and re-emergence, taking selected conflicts and diseases in the Asian and Far Eastern theatres to provide examples. We begin in Sect. 9.2 by locating war within the broader conceptual framework of emerging and re-emerging diseases. Subsequent sections examine the wartime emergence of three zoonoses which, on their novel appearance in deployed western troops, prompted a series of landmark epidemiological investigations into the diseases concerned: scrub typhus among Allied forces in Burma–India during World War II (Sect. 9.3) and Japanese encephalitis and Korean haemorrhagic fever in the UN Command during the Korean War (Sect. 9.4). We then turn to the wartime re-emergence of classical diseases, illustrating the theme with reference to US troops (malaria) and Vietnamese civilians (human plague) during the Vietnam War (Sect. 9.5). The chapter is concluded in Section 9.6.

9.2 Emerging and Re-emerging Diseases

9.2.1 The Concept of Emerging and Re-emerging Diseases

Scientific concern over the global threat of emerging and re-emerging infectious diseases has escalated in recent years (Lederberg *et al.*, 1992; Greenwood and De Cock, 1998; Krause, 1998; Smith *et al.*, 2001) (see Sect. 3.5). Broadly defined by Morse (1995: 7) as infections that have 'newly appeared in the population, or have existed but are rapidly increasing in incidence or geographic range', the present-day list of emerging and re-emerging diseases is headed by such notorious conditions as AIDS, Ebola fever, Hantavirus pulmonary syndrome, Legionnaires' disease, cholera associated with variant *Vibrio cholerae 0139*, malaria, and multidrug-resistant (strain W) tuberculosis (see Table 9.1). As we have already indicated, however, these are only the most recent events in a human history that is studded with instances of disease emergence and

Table 9.1. Examples of emergent and re-emergent diseases and disease agents in the late twentieth and early twenty-first centuries

Disease agent	Related disease/symptoms	Mode of transmission	Cause(s) of Emergence
1. Bacteria, Rickettsiae and Chlamydiae			
Borrelia burgdorferi	Lyme disease: rash, fever, neurologic and cardiac abnormalities, arthritis	Bite of infective *Ixodes* tick	Increase in deer and human populations in wooded areas
Escherichia coli O157:H7	Haemorrhagic colitis; thrombocytopenia; haemolytic uraemic syndrome	Ingestion of contaminated food, especially undercooked beef and raw milk	Probably due to the development of a new pathogen; mass food processing technology allowing contamination of meat
Haemophilus influenzae bio-group *aegyptius*	Brazilian purpuric fever; purulent conjunctivitis, high fever, vomiting and purpura	Contact with discharges of infected persons; eye flies are suspected vectors	Possibly an increase in virulence due to mutation; possibly new strain
Helicobacter pylori	Gastritis, peptic ulcer, possibly stomach cancer	Ingestion of contaminated food or water, especially unpasteurized milk; contact with infected pets	Increased recognition
Legionella pneumophila	Legionnaires' disease: malaise, myalgia, fever, headache, respiratory illness	Air-cooling systems, water supplies	Recognition in an epidemic situation
Mycobacterium tuberculosis	Tuberculosis: cough, weight loss, lung lesions	Exposure to sputum droplets	Immunosuppression; microbial adaptation and development of resistance
Orientia tsutsugamushi	**Scrub typhus: fever, headache, rash, enlargement of the lymph nodes**	**Exposure to infective larval trombiculid mites**	**Ecological changes associated with clearance of agricultural land, hydro-electric and irrigation schemes**
Vibrio cholerae	Cholera; severe diarrhoea, rapid dehydration	Ingestion of water contaminated with the faeces of infected persons; ingestion of food exposed to contaminated water	Poor sanitation/ hygiene; possibly introduced via bilge-water from cargo ships

Table 9.1. (*cont.*)

Disease agent	Related disease/symptoms	Mode of transmission	Cause(s) of Emergence
Yersinia pestis	**Bubonic and pneumonic plague: fever, cough, ischaemic necrosis, haemorrhages, pneumonia, septicaemia**	**Bite of infective rat fleas**	**Breakdown in measures of disease control**
2. Viruses			
Crimean–Congo haemorrhagic fever	Haemorrhagic fever	Bite of an infected adult tick	Ecological changes favouring increased human exposure to ticks on sheep and small wild animals
Dengue	Haemorrhagic fever	Bite of an infected mosquito (primarily *Aedes aegypti*)	Poor mosquito control; increased urbanization in tropics; increased air travel
Filoviruses (Marburg, Ebola)	Fulminant high-mortality haemorrhagic fever	Direct contact with infected blood, organs, secretions and semen	Unknown; in Europe and the USA, virus-infected monkeys shipped from developing countries by air
Hantaan virus	**Korean haemorrhagic fever: abdominal pain, vomiting, haemorrhagic fever**	**Inhalation of aerosolized rodent excreta**	**Human invasion of virus ecologic niche**
Human immunodeficiency viruses (HIV-1 and HIV-2)	HIV disease and AIDS; severe immune system dysfunction, opportunistic infections	Sexual contact with or exposure to blood or tissues of an infected person; perinatal transmission	Urbanization; changes in lifestyles/mores; increased intravenous drug use; international travel; medical technology
Influenza A (pandemic)	Fever, headache, pneumonia	Airborne	Animal-human virus reassortment; antigenic shift
Japanese encephalitis	**Encephalitis**	**Bite of an infective mosquito**	**Changing agricultural practices**
Lassa fever	Fever, headache, sore throat, nausea	Contact with urine or faeces of infected rodents	Urbanization/conditions favouring infestation by rodents
Rift Valley fever	Febrile illness	Bite of an infective mosquito	Importation of infected mosquitoes and/or animals; development (dams, irrigation); possibly

Table 9.1. (*cont.*)

Disease agent	Related disease/symptoms	Mode of transmission	Cause(s) of Emergence
			change in virulence or pathogenicity of virus
Venezuelan equine encephalitis	Encephalitis	Bite of an infective mosquito	Movement of mosquitoes and amplification hosts (horses)
Yellow fever	Fever, headache, muscle pain, nausea, vomiting	Bite of an infective *Aedes aegypti* mosquito	Lack of effective mosquito control and widespread vaccination; urbanization in tropics; increased air travel
3. Protozoans, helminths, and fungi			
Babesia	Babesiosis; fever, fatigue, haemolytic anaemia	Bite of *Ixodes* tick	Reforestation; increase in deer population; changes in outdoor recreational activity
Plasmodium	**Malaria**	**Bite of an infective Anopheles mosquito**	**Urbanization; changing parasite biology; environmental changes; drug resistance; air travel**
Toxoplasma gondii	Toxoplasmosis: fever, lymphadenopathy, lymphocytosis	Exposure to faeces of cats carrying the protozoan; sometimes food-borne	Immunosuppression; increase in cats as pets

Note: Sample diseases and disease agents examined in detail in the present chapter have been emboldened.
Source: Abridged from Lederberg *et al.* (1992, table 2.1, pp. 36–41), with additional information from Morse (1995, table 1, p. 8), Lederberg (1998), and Chanteau *et al.* (1998).

re-emergence. In the first half of the twentieth century, for example, Hans Zinsser (1935: 299) provides a classic account of how typhus fever re-emerged from its 'quiet bourgeois existence' to achieve 'mediaeval ascendancy' in revolutionary Russia (1917). At about the same time, the pandemic of 'Spanish' influenza (1918–19) formed a devastating example of an event associated with the cyclically re-emerging influenza A virus (Oxford, 2000), while, in the years that followed, poliomyelitis was to configure itself as one of the great epidemic diseases of the inter- and post-war periods (Paul, 1971).

FACILITATING FACTORS IN DISEASE EMERGENCE AND RE-EMERGENCE

Specific factors that have facilitated the emergence and re-emergence of infectious diseases in recent times and which inform an epidemiological understanding of past events are reviewed by Lederberg *et al.* (1992), Morse (1995), and Krause (1998) (see Sect. 3.5). As Table 9.2 shows, 'emergence factors' encompass a complex of social, physical, and biological mechanisms, including human demographics and behaviour, technology and industry, economic development and land-use change, international travel and commerce, microbial adaptation and change, and the breakdown of public health measures. These various factors operate at different stages of the emergence/re-emergence process (Fig. 9.1), with several factors often working in combination or sequence to precipitate the (re)appearance of a disease agent in the human population (Table 9.1).

War as a Facilitating Mechanism

War impinges on many of the emergence factors listed in Table 9.2. As Price-Smith (2002: 129) observes, military conflict acts 'as a direct disease "amplifier," creating those physical conditions (poverty, famine, destruction of vital infrastructure, and large population movements) that are particularly conducive to the spread and mutation of disease'. Many of the issues addressed in previous chapters, including high-level population mobility and mixing, differential patterns of disease exposure and susceptibility, the breakdown of public health infrastructure and insanitary living conditions are all pertinent to an understanding of the (re-)emergence complex (Lederberg *et al.*, 1992: 110–12). Additional factors also attain prominence. Within the schema of Figure 9.1, heightened exposure to the 'zoonotic pool' (Morse, 1995: 7) has played a particularly important role in the war-related precipitation of emergent and re-emergent diseases. Historically, ecological changes resulting from warfare, including the burning and firing of forests, the forced abandonment and destruction of agricultural land, and the consequent disruption and alteration of zootic habitats, have served to bring soldiers and civilians into close proximity with disease-bearing wildlife and insects (Gajdusek, 1956; Velimirovic, 1972). For combat troops, the risk is magnified by inadvertent deployment in isolated ecological niches to which humans are ill-adapted (Philip, 1948) while, in the era of military air transport, the rapid deployment and/or evacuation of overseas troops poses an obvious epidemiological threat to the reception country (Neel, 1973).

9.2.2 Selection of Examples

From the list of emergent and re-emergent diseases in Table 9.1, we have selected five diseases (in bold) for examination in the present chapter. The five diseases are given in Table 9.3, along with summary information on the associated

Table 9.2. Factors involved in the emergence and re-emergence of infectious diseases

Emergence factor	Contributory factors	Disease examples
1. Human demographics and behaviour	Immunosuppression; population growth and density; rural–urban migration; sexual activity; substance abuse; urban decay.	HIV (sexual activity, substance abuse); cryptosporidiosis (immunosuppression).
2. Technology and industry	Food processing and handling; globalization of food supply; modern medicine (organ and tissue transplantation, immunosuppressive drugs, nosocomial infections, use of antibiotics); water treatment.	New-variant CJD (contaminated food products); BSE (contaminated cattle feed; hepatitis B and C (blood transfusions).
3. Economic development and land-use change	Agricultural development; climate change/global warming; dam building; deforestation/reforestation; irrigation.	Argentine haemorrhagic fever (agriculture); Rift Valley fever (dams; irrigation); HFRS (agriculture); HPS (weather anomalies); malaria (irrigation).
4. International travel and commerce	Air travel; commerce.	'Airport' malaria; dissemination of O139 *V. cholerae*.
5. Microbial adaptation and change	Natural variation/mutation; selective pressure and resistance.	Multi-drug resistant tuberculosis; vector resistance (malaria, plague).
6. Breakdown of public health measures	Curtailment or reduction of disease prevention programmes; poor sanitation; war.	Multi-drug resistant tuberculosis; louse-borne typhus and cholera among African refugees; diphtheria in former USSR.

Notes: BSE = Bovine spongiform encephalopathy; CJD = Creutzfeldt–Jakob disease; HFRS = Haemorrhagic fever with renal syndrome; HIV = Human immunodeficiency virus; HPS = Hantavirus pulmonary syndrome.
Source: Based on information in Lederberg *et al.* (1992: 49–112) and Morse (1995, table 2, p. 10).

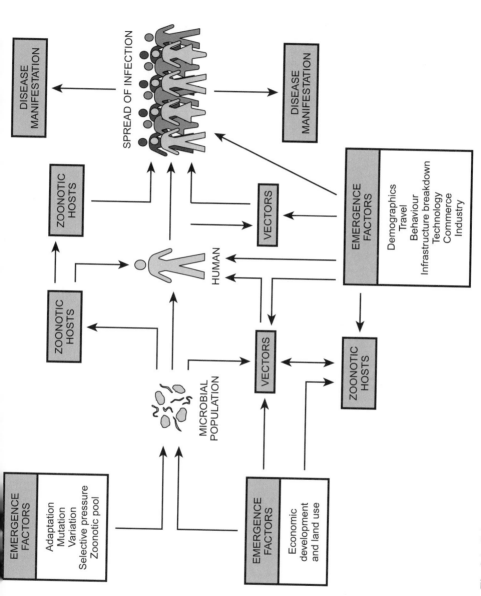

Fig. 9.1. Schematic diagram of infectious disease emergence and re-emergence in human populations

Source: Redrawn from Lederberg *et al.* (1992, fig. 2.1, p. 48).

Table 9.3. Selected examples of disease emergence and re-emergence in Asian and Far Eastern theatres of war

War/conflict	Disease (aetiological agent)	Population	Geographical location	Emergence factor(s)
World War II (1939–45)	Scrub typhus (*Orientia tsutsugamushi*)	Allied Forces	Burma–India	Human invasion of ecological niche of larval trombiculid mite (Philip, 1948)
Korean War (1950–3)	Japanese encephalitis (Japanese encephalitis virus)	UN Command	Korea	Entry of unprotected overseas forces into area of newly recognized clinical infection (Lincoln and Sivertson, 1952)
	Korean haemorrhagic fever (Hantaan virus)	UN Command	Korea	Ecological change associated with abandonment of agricultural land; human invasion of ecological niche of rodent reservoir of Hantaan virus (*Apodemus agrarius*) (Paul and McClure, 1958)
Vietnam War (1964–73)	Malaria (*Plasmodium spp.*)	US forces	Vietnam/USA	Exposure of troops to chloroquine-resistant strains of *P. falciparum*; importation of *P. spp.* to US by Vietnam returnees (Neel, 1973)
	Plague (*Yersinia pestis*)	Vietnamese civilians	Vietnam	War-induced disruption of human and zootic habitats; emergence of resistance to insecticides in principal flea vector (*Xenopsylla cheopis*) (Marshall et al., 1967; Velimirovic, 1972)

wars, afflicted populations, and the emergence factors to be studied. Although a rigid classification into 'emergent' and 're-emergent' diseases is complicated by the length of time for which most of the sample diseases have been known to be circulating,[2] it is convenient to draw a simple distinction between: (1) those diseases that, prior to the twentieth century, were largely or wholly unknown to Western medical science (scrub typhus, Japanese encephalitis, and Korean haemorrhagic fever); and (2) classical diseases that have been known to the West for many centuries or millennia (malaria and plague). Within this simple division, our selection of diseases, wars and populations has been formed to reflect a number of key features relating to the patterns and processes of disease emergence and re-emergence.

(i) *Range of disease agents.* Consistent with the broad range of disease agents represented in Table 9.1, the sample in Table 9.3 includes diseases of bacterial (plague), protozoal (malaria), rickettsial (scrub typhus), and viral (Japanese encephalitis and Korean haemorrhagic fever) aetiologies.

(ii) *Range of afflicted populations.* While the majority of examples in Table 9.3 reflect the particular epidemiological risk for Western troops in the tropical jungle theatres of Asia and the Far East, the example of human plague during the Vietnam War (1964–73) illustrates the danger of emergent and re-emergent diseases for civil populations in war-afflicted countries.

(iii) *Range of emergence factors.* The examples in Table 9.3 highlight a variety of mechanisms in the war-related process of disease emergence and re-emergence including: inadvertent human invasion of the ecological niches of disease-carrying animals and insects; entry into newly recognized areas of disease activity; war-induced ecological change and habitat disruption; exposure to drug-resistant strains of diseases and disease agents; the emergence of insecticide-resistant disease vectors; and disease reintroduction by military returnees.

9.3 Scrub Typhus (Tsutsugamushi Disease) in the Burma–India Theatre, 1942–1945

Epidemiologically, the tropical jungle and mountain terrain of the Burma–India Theatre ranked among the unhealthiest of all battlegrounds in World War II (Leishman and Kelsall, 1944; Marriott *et al.*, 1946; Girdwood, 1950). Writing in *The Lancet* in early June 1945, Brigadier Hugh L. Marriott of the Allied Land Forces, South-East Asia Command (ALFSEA) concluded that

---

[2] The earliest accounts of the most recently described disease in Table 9.3 (Korean haemorrhagic fever) date to the 1930s.

the 'biggest single lesson' of the three years of campaigning in India and Burma had been the 'tremendous importance of disease in wasting manpower' (Marriott, 1945: 679). Marriott's stark testimony—later to be presented before a meeting of the Royal Society of Tropical Medicine and Hygiene[3]—recalled the dire military experience of the period:

In 1943 the admission-rate to [ALFSEA] hospitals and other medical units was just under 1200 per 1000 per annum. In 1944 it was just under 1000 per 1000; this is equivalent to every man in the force being admitted to hospital in the course of a year. Disease has played an enormously greater part in man-power wastage than has enemy action. The ratio of casualties from sickness to casualties from wounds in 1943 was 121 : 1, and in 1944, a heavy year of fighting, it was 19 : 1. (ibid. 679)

Malaria, dysentery and diarrhoeal diseases, sprue, venereal and skin diseases were among the most prevalent conditions to afflict the forces in Southeast Asia (Marriott *et al.*, 1946). Infective hepatitis, of unusual severity, achieved special prominence in the latter months of the Burma Campaigns (Stokes and Miller, 1947), while localized outbreaks of smallpox and cholera were also recorded in the Allied contingent (Leishman, 1944; Marriott *et al.*, 1946). Of particular medical interest, however, was the emergence of a vector-borne disease of apparently new significance to western military forces: *scrub typhus* or *tsutsugamushi disease*, a disease that, some years later, would be re-encountered in the Korean and Vietnam conflicts (Munro-Faure *et al.*, 1951; Hazlett, 1970). In this section, we examine the emergence of scrub typhus in the Burma–India Theatre during World War II; the contemporaneous appearance of the disease among Allied forces in the island environments of the Pacific Theatre is examined in Sect. 11.4.

THE NATURE OF SCRUB TYPHUS

Scrub typhus (tsutsugamushi disease) is an acute febrile disease that occurs when humans are bitten by larval trombiculid (chigger) mites that harbour the rickettsial agent *Orientia tsutsugamushi* (formerly *Rickettsia tsutsugamushi*). As Figure 9.2 shows, the known geographical occurrence of scrub typhus extends across much of southern and eastern Asia, northeastern Australia, and the adjoining islands of the western Pacific. As regards the clinical presentation of the disease, typical symptoms include fever, headache, rash, and enlargement of the lymph nodes. In untreated cases, these may last from three to five days (rash) for up to two weeks (fever). In about one-third of cases, the liver and spleen may also be enlarged and, in serious cases, haemorrhagic signs and loss of consciousness may appear. Prior to the advent of effective antibiotics, mortality from the disease was highly variable. Japanese studies in the 30 years to 1950, for example, revealed case-fatality rates of 3–40 per cent. Since about

---

[3] 'Medical Experiences of the War in the South-East Asia Command', held at Portland Place, London, on 21 Feb. 1946; see Marriott *et al.* (1946).

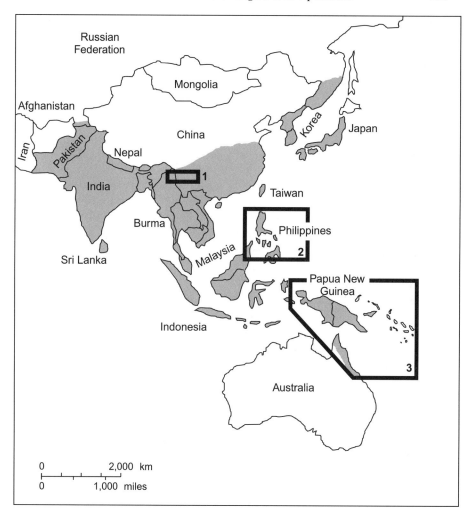

Fig. 9.2. Distribution of scrub typhus (tsutsugamushi disease) in Southeast Asia and the Western Pacific

Notes: The generalized geographical distribution of the disease in the region is shown by the grey shading. For reference, areas in which major episodes of the disease were recorded in US and other Allied forces during World War II are identifed by the numbered boxes: (1) Burma–India and China; (2) Philippine Islands; (3) Southwest Pacific.

Source: Adapted from Kawamura *et al.* (1995, fig. 1, p. 106) and Philip (1964, map 5, p. 276).

1950, however, the development of chloramphenicol and tetracycline antibiotics has provided an effective cure (Kawamura *et al.*, 1995: 3).

Man is an accidental host in the natural cycle of scrub typhus (see Pl. 9.1), and epidemics tend to occur when large numbers of humans (historically,

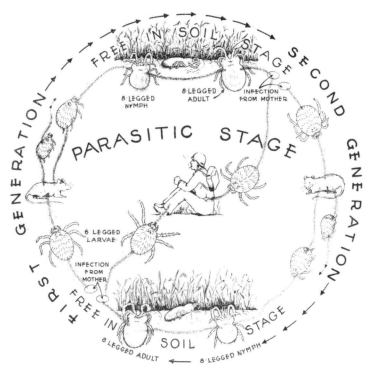

Pl. 9.1. Diagrammatic scheme of theoretical rat–mite–rat cycle of scrub typhus in nature

Note: As Philip (1964: 317) notes, 'The "rickettsial stream" is continuous from generation to generation of chigger mites with new lines started from infected rats. Soldiers were accidental intruders in the cycle.'

Source: Reproduced from Philip (1964, fig. 34, p. 317).

soldiers or labourers) enter environments which harbour the infected chigger mites. The mites are commonly found in the scrub and secondary vegetation of transitional zones between forests and clearings (hence, *scrub* typhus), although endemic areas are known to range from subarctic scree to montane semi-desert locations (Traub and Wisseman, 1968; Saah, 2000*b*). As with some other rickettsial infections, such as the Rocky Mountain spotted fever group, scrub typhus is characterized by the marked localization of disease foci. Among US soldiers in World War II, for example, Philip (1948, 1964) noted sharp variations in levels of disease acquisition over distances of just a few hundred yards. Seasonally, the occurrence of scrub typhus is subject to environmental (temperature and/or rainfall) controls on the time of emergence of the larval mites. In lower-latitude locations, however, conditions are conducive to the year-round occurrence of the disease.

Table 9.4. Reported cases and deaths from scrub typhus in military forces, by theatre and command, 1942–1945

Theatre/command	Total, 1942–5	
	Cases	Deaths
South and Southwest Pacific		
Australia (Army and Navy)	349	11
US (Army)	29	0
New Guinea and adjacent islands		
Australia (Army)	2,839	257
US (Army and Navy)	5,926	258
Philippines		
US (Army and Navy)	382	12
South-East Asia Command		
US (Army)	967	58
China (Army)	349	40
Britain (Army)	5,400	no data
Total	16,241	636

Source: Data from Philip (1948, table 1, p. 178).

9.3.1 The Burma–India Outbreaks

Prior to the outbreak of war with Japan in late 1941, scrub typhus appeared to be of limited epidemiological significance on mainland Southeast Asia. According to Megaw (1945), many of the infected areas were only sparsely inhabited, with the indigenous populations having acquired natural immunity to the infection. But military operations introduced new conditions in the region. From 1942–3, large numbers of Allied troops began to enter infected areas in northeastern India and northern Burma (delimited by box 1 in Fig. 9.2), with a corresponding increase in human exposure to *Orientia tsutsuga-mushi*-carrying larval mites. Some impression of the resulting level of disease activity can be gained from Table 9.4. For Allied British, Chinese, and US troops in South-East Asia Command, the table gives the recorded count of scrub typhus cases and deaths in the period 1942–5; the corresponding information for Allied troops in other infected theatres and commands (South and Southwest Pacific, New Guinea, and Philippines) is given for reference. As Table 9.4 shows, a total of 6,716 cases of scrub typhus were recorded in South-East Asia Command, representing some 42 per cent of the Allied case-load in the Asia–Pacific region.

US AND CHINESE FORCES

The initial results of investigations into the occurrence of scrub typhus among Allied US and Chinese troops in the Burma–India Theatre, undertaken by members of the United States of America Typhus Commission (USATC) Burma team, are reviewed by Mackie (1946); see also Philip (1964). Between 1 November 1943 and 1 September 1945, a total of 1,098 cases of scrub typhus were recorded in the combined US–Chinese forces, with an overall case fatality of 8.9 per cent.[4] Protective measures (including the use of dimethyl phthalate) were not used until the spring of 1945 and so the data allow an analysis of an unmodified epidemiological pattern in non-immune and heavily exposed populations.

Spatial Patterns

Figure 9.3 is based on a sample of 1,041 cases of scrub typhus for which locational information is given by Mackie (1946) and plots, as proportional circles, the assumed place of infection of US and Chinese troops in eastern India and northern Burma, November 1943–September 1945. As the map shows, most infections were acquired along a *c*.500 km stretch of the Stilwell Road, extending southwards from Ledo (Assam, India) in the north, through Burmese territory to the southern limit of US–Chinese penetration in the vicinity of Lashio.[5] Within this broad spatial distribution, several major foci of scrub typhus activity are evident: the area to the east of Ledo; Shingbwiyang; the mountains east of Shaduzup; Myitkyina and the stretch of road southwards to Bhamo and its environs; and the area to the south and southwest of Namhkam. The geographical pattern in Figure 9.3 is consistent with a spatially widespread infection, but with localized pockets or 'islands' of heightened activity, in the combat area (Mackie, 1946; Philip, 1964: 292).

Temporal Patterns

To what extent did operational factors contribute to the spatial pattern of disease activity in Figure 9.3? To examine this question, Figure 9.4 is again based on information in Mackie (1946) and plots the monthly count of documented cases in US (solid line trace) and Chinese (broken line trace) forces, November 1943–July 1945. Five well-defined outbreaks (numbered 1 to 5) are evident, with each outbreak associated with a specific set of field operations. We consider each outbreak in turn.

   (1) *Outbreak 1 (November–December 1943).* The earliest cases of so-called 'CBI' (China–Burma–India) fever, later to be recognized as scrub typhus, were reported to the Base Surgeon, Advance Sect. No. 3, Ledo, India, during December 1943 (Philip, 1964: 297). By this time, however, the first outbreak of the disease was already well-established among the Chinese Twenty-Second Division which was encamped to the east of Ledo (Fig. 9.3) and engaged in combat and jungle training in the sur-

---

[4] Philip (1964: 295) notes that the data relating to early cases of tsutsugamushi disease among the Chinese forces are incomplete owing, in part, to the destruction of records of *c*.300 cases in forward areas.

[5] For a personal account of an attack of scrub typhus acquired by a US Army medical officer in the area depicted in Fig. 9.3, see Jones (1969).

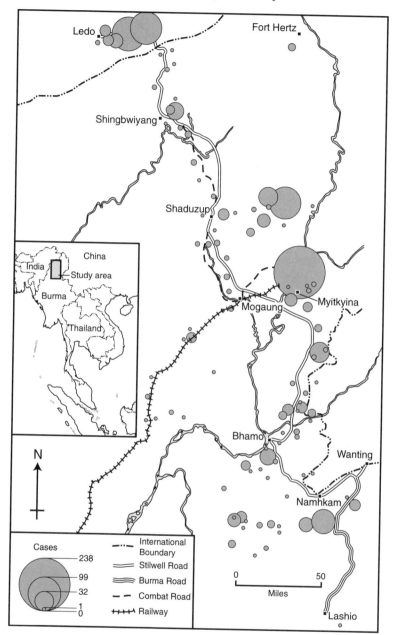

Fig. 9.3. Cases of scrub typhus among US and Chinese troops in northeastern India (Assam) and northern Burma, November 1943–September 1945

Note: Proportional circles plot the probable place of infection of a sample of 1,041 documented cases of scrub typhus, representing 95 per cent of the 1,098 documented cases for which medical records are available.

Source: Based on data in Mackie (1946, fig. 1, parts I and II, pp. 22–5).

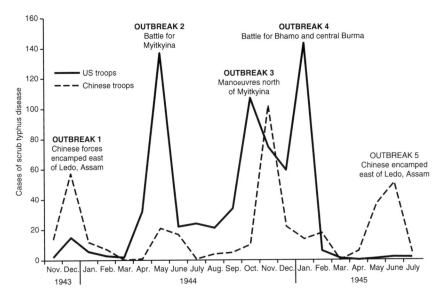

Fig. 9.4. Monthly incidence of scrub typhus among US and Chinese troops in northeastern India (Assam) and northern Burma, November 1943–July 1945

Notes: The line traces are based on a sample of 1,097 cases for which information is available. Military operations associated with five peaks of disease activity are indicated.
Source: Based on Mackie (1946, fig. 2 and table I, pp. 26–7).

rounding countryside. The Twenty-Second Division provided 66 of the 85 Chinese cases associated with the outbreak.

(2) *Outbreak 2 (April–June 1944)*. This outbreak was focused on US troops (Galahad Force) engaged in the operation on Myitkyina (Fig. 9.3). The precipitous drop in disease incidence reflected the static nature of operations from June, being largely restricted to patrols and the extensive air-bombing of Myitkyana.

(3) *Outbreak 3 (October–November 1944)*. Disease activity associated with this outbreak was largely concentrated among US troops of the 5332nd Provisional Brigade (Mars Task Force) who were encamped to the north of Myitkyina and were undertaking combat training and manoeuvres in the surrounding area. The end of the outbreak coincided with the completion of manoeuvres and the movement of troops south, in readiness for the attack on Bhamo (Fig. 9.3).

(4) *Outbreak 4 (January 1945)*. This outbreak represented a resurgence of disease activity in the 5332nd Provisional Brigade which, having moved south from Myitkyina, was now engaged in the operations on Bhamo (Dec. 1944) and central Burma.

(5) *Outbreak 5 (May–June 1945)*. The final outbreak, which was focused on Chinese troops, marked a return to the original locus of disease

activity in the vicinity of Ledo (Outbreak 1). The units were in the process of a return to China and were not engaged in combat training or manoeuvres.

A recurring feature of the foregoing evidence is the role of military training and active operations in the occurrence of scrub typhus. The majority of scrub typhus cases, in both the US and Chinese forces, were combat troops. Very low levels of disease activity were recorded among engineers, signal corps troops, and other non-combat personnel. As Mackie (1946: 30) concludes: 'It appears that the determining factor was the character of the military operations. As would be anticipated, the greatest risk is presented by combat and the training conditions simulating combat in infective terrain.'

BRITISH FORCES

Some 300 km to the west of the area shown in Figure 9.3, British forces on the jungle roads from Imphal, India, to Tiddim and Tamu, Burma, suffered from especially severe outbreaks of scrub typhus during the monsoon season of 1944. As an early observation on the intersection of war, ecological change, and infectious disease emergence, Willcox (1948: 172) provides an informative description of the circumstances that fuelled the transition of scrub typhus from a sporadic to an epidemic disease:

The troops on the central section of the front were scattered throughout the hilly jungle country . . . in many places the undergrowth consisted of secondary vegetation which had arisen on land previously under cultivation by the natives. Indeed, it was often the most dangerous types of scrub on which units were encamped. Troops were patrolling affected country and lying down to rest. Reinforcements were exposed in the same way, fresh units often took over sites used by other units and usually infested with rats. It is thus easy to see that the army was exposed to the bite of larval mites in the most extreme degree, and infection which had hitherto been sporadic became epidemic.

Such were the levels of exposure that, on the Tiddim road, 18 per cent of one British battalion (Second West Yorks) developed scrub typhus in the period August–November 1944, with a full 5 per cent of the unit succumbing to the disease (Philip, 1948: 159). At about the same time, the Fifth Indian Division and the Eleventh East African Division, variously in pursuit of Japanese forces along the Tiddim road and the Kabaw Valley, recorded almost 1,400 cases of scrub typhus (Willcox, 1948: 173).

MILITARY CONTROL OF EMERGENT SCRUB TYPHUS

In the absence of a vaccine, principal strategies for the prevention and control of scrub typhus in infected theatres consisted of (i) the preparation of camp-sites to eliminite mites and (ii) the direct protection of combat troops in hyper-endemic areas. Campsites were cleared of all vegetation by cutting, oiling, and burning; bulldozers were used in the construction of larger sites, while camps were monitored for the presence of mites, rats, and other possible reservoirs of *Orientia tsutsugamushi*. From the spring of 1945, strategies for the direct protection of combat troops became available in the Burma–India Theatre and included the hand treatment or impregnation of uniforms with dimethyl phthalate and other mite repellents. Additional prevention and control strategies, including the promotion of disease awareness and the issuing of local directives to restrict the movements of personnel, were also implemented (Megaw, 1945; Philip, 1964).

9.4 UN Forces, Emergent Viruses, and the Korean War

According to Colonel George W. Hunter, sometime Chief of Parasitology–Entomology in the US Fourth Army Area Medical Laboratory, the Korean War (1950–3) differed 'in many respects' from any war 'heretofore waged by any of the United Nations' (Hunter, 1953: 1408). With a climate that ran from seasonal extremes of tropical summer to arctic winter, a 'forbidding terrain' and 'grossly infested' soil and water, the Korean Peninsula presented the multinational UN Command with medical conditions that were 'without comparison' in the countries from which the bulk of troops originated (Hunter, 1953: 1408). Frostbite, along with other non-battle injuries due to exposure and extreme cold, ranked among the most severe medical problems during the early stages of the war (Anonymous, 1953).[6] Infectious conditions, too, blighted the UN troops. Sexually transmitted diseases (especially gonorrhoea) spread in epidemic form,[7] while malaria due to *Plasmodium vivax*, dysentery and diarrhoeal diseases, respiratory tract infections (including scattered cases of influenza A), intestinal parasites, and infectious hepatitis were encountered at various stages of the conflict (Hunter, 1953; Ingham, 1953). Two emergent viral diseases of the late twentieth century, however, were to achieve particular prominence among the UN troops: Japanese encephalitis and Korean haemorrhagic fever (Lincoln and Sivertson, 1952; McNinch, 1953).

9.4.1 Japanese Encephalitis

Japanese encephalitis is a severe, often fatal, disease of the central nervous system due to infection with Japanese encephalitis virus (JEV). The disease is widespread in southeastern Asia, including China, India, Indonesia, Korea,

---

[6] At an extreme, in January 1951, non-battle injuries reached 352 cases per 1,000 mean strength per annum. Approximately 50 per cent of the case-load was attributable to cold injuries sustained during combat in the Wonju-Suwan area of North Korea (Anonymous, 1953).

[7] Ingham (1953), for example, records a rate of 376 cases per 1,000 strength for sexually transmitted diseases in the British Commonwealth Forces (United Kingdom, Canada, Australia, and New Zealand) during 1952.

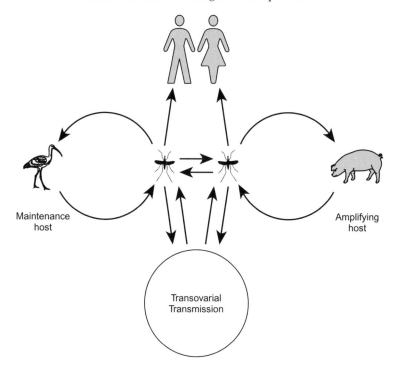

Fig. 9.5. Presumptive natural cycle of Japanese encephalitis virus (JEV)

Notes: Japanese encephalitis virus is maintained in nature by a cycle that includes certain species of mosquito (*Anopheles*, *Culex*, and *Mansonia*) and bird (family *Ardeidae*). Mosquitoes may also serve to maintain the virus by transovarial transmission, while domestic pigs are the main amplifying host for the virus. Transmission to man occurs via the bite of an infected mosquito.
Source: Redrawn from Thongcharoen (1989, fig. 6, p. 30).

and the Western Pacific. The virus is transmitted by a mosquito vector from its reservoir (probably wild birds) to humans and other mammals which, in turn, serve as incidental hosts (see Fig. 9.5). Clinically, an incubation period of five to fifteen days is followed by the acute onset of fever, headache, and prostration, leading to encephalitis, coma, and paralysis within a few days. The fatality rate is 20 to 50 per cent among encephalitis cases, with permanent mental impairment, severe emotional instability, and paralysis being the most common sequelae in survivors (Thongcharoen, 1989; Tsai, 2000).

Descriptions of a disease that is believed to have been Japanese encephalitis can be traced back to 1871, although the importance of the condition was not recognized in South Korea until the 1940s. In 1946, JEV was isolated from a US soldier who was stationed in South Korea (Sabin *et al.*, 1947), while a serologic survey by Deuel and colleagues (1950) confirmed the widespread nature of inapparent JEV infection in the country. In 1949, a major outbreak of the

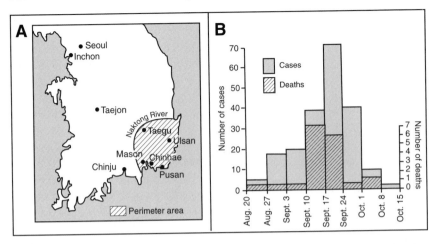

Fig. 9.6. Japanese encephalitis among US troops in the Korean War, August–October 1950

Notes: (A) Location of the 50–100 km radius 'perimeter' area (Pusan Perimeter) of southeastern Korea within which all cases of Japanese encephalitis among US troops occurred. (B) Weekly count of admissions and deaths for a sample of 201 Japanese encephalitis patients admitted to the evacuation hospital at Pusan.
Source: Redrawn from Lincoln and Sivertson (1952, figs. 1 and 2, p. 269).

disease, associated with some 5,616 documented cases and 2,729 deaths (attack rate 27.8 per 100,000), resulted in the addition of Japanese encephalitis to the list of notifiable communicable diseases in South Korea (Thongcharoen, 1989; Sohn, 2000).

THE 1950 EPIDEMIC IN US TROOPS

Epidemic Japanese encephalitis was one of the first severe infectious diseases to strike the UN forces during the Korean War. As described by Lincoln and Sivertson (1952), the start of the epidemic can be traced to the second week of August 1950 when a US soldier died after a short illness (characterized by fever and coma). Autopsy revealed evidence of encephalitis and a virus, identified as JEV, was successfully isolated from the deceased. During the next two months, approximately 300 further cases of Japanese encephalitis were diagnosed in the US contingent of UN Command. Geographically, the epidemic was confined to the 50–100 km radius of the defensive 'perimeter' area (Pusan Perimeter) of southwestern Korea (Fig. 9.6A), with cases occurring both at the front of the perimeter and in the vicinity of the port of Pusan. As judged by a sample of 201 cases admitted to the evacuation hospital at Pusan, the epidemic peaked in the week beginning 17 September, with the last admission on 15 October (Fig 9.6B). Of the sample cases, 17 (8.5%) succumbed to the disease in South Korea, while two further cases died after evacuation to Japan. Yet others, having experienced a mild bout of the disease, were able to return to duty after four or five days of convalescence (Lincoln and Sivertson, 1952).

Following the outbreak of August–October 1950, Japanese encephalitis declined in importance in UN Command. All US troops in Korea, as well as Okinawa and Japan, were vaccinated against the disease and, although the efficacy of the vaccine then remained unproven, subsequent years were to witness little or no disease activity (Hunter, 1953).

9.4.2 Korean Haemorrhagic Fever

The second year of hostilities presented the UN forces with fresh epidemiological challenges. In the spring and early summer of 1951, troops stationed in the vicinity of the Thirty-Eighth Parallel—close to the front line with North Korea—began to present with a severe, frequently fatal, disease characterized by fever, prostration, intense headache behind the eyes, vomiting, and haemorrhages. At first, medical officers suspected the disease to be leptospirosis, acute nephritis, or some other form of renal condition. It soon became apparent, however, that the men of UN Command were suffering from a malady that was previously unknown to western medicine. Variously termed *Korean haemorrhagic fever* (KHF) or *epidemic haemorrhagic fever* (EHF), the disease had, in fact, already been encountered by Russian and Japanese military physicians in the 1930s (Gajdusek, 1956; Paul and McClure, 1958; Trencséni and Keleti, 1971). Today, KHF is recognized as one of several similar, but distinct, emergent viral fevers of global distribution and to which the general term *haemorrhagic fever with renal syndrome* (HFRS) is applied (see Table 9.5).

THE NATURE OF KHF

The specific aetiological agent of KHF is Hantaan virus (Table 9.5),[8] a member of the Hantavirus genus of the virus family *Bunyaviridae*. The natural reservoir of Hantaan virus is the striped field mouse, *Apodemus agrarius* (Pl. 9.2), with incidental transmission of the virus to humans arising from exposure to contaminated rodent excreta—probably aerosolized urine. Major clinical manifestations of KHF include high fever of seven to fourteen days duration, accompanied by prostration, headache, vomiting, and haemorrhaging. Typically, 30 per cent of patients show a mild clinical course, 50 per cent a moderate course, and 20 per cent develop severe disease. The latter usually pass through a series of phases (febrile $\rightarrow$ hypotensive $\rightarrow$ oliguric $\rightarrow$ diuretic $\rightarrow$ convalescent) with death, arising from circulatory shock or renal failure, in 5 to 15 per cent of cases. The incubation period of KHF is of the order of two to three

---

[8] Hantaan virus is named after the Hantaan River, Korea, where the first cases of KHF were identified in UN troops in 1951.

Table 9.5. The haemorrhagic fever with renal syndrome (HFRS) group of diseases

Common appellation	Virus	Principal reservoir	Distribution of virus	Severity of associated disease
KHF[1]	Hantaan	*Apodemus agrarius* (striped field mouse)	China, Korea, Russia	moderate to severe (death rate 1–15%)
Haemorrhagic fever	Dobrava-Belgrade	*Apodemus flavicollis* (yellow-neck mouse)	Balkans	moderate to severe (death rate 1–15%)
Haemorrhagic fever	Seoul	*Rattus norvegicus* (Norway rat)	Global	moderate to severe (death rate 1–15%)
Nephropathia epidemica	Puumala	*Clethrionomys glareolus* (bank vole)	Europe, Russia, Scandinavia	mild (death rate <1%)

Note: [1] Korean haemorrhagic fever.
Source: Based on information in Schmaljohn and Hjelle (1997, tables 1 and 2, pp. 96–8).

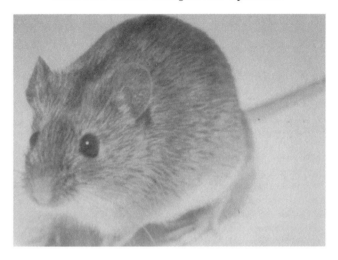

Pl. 9.2. *Apodemus agrarius* (striped field mouse), the rodent reservoir of Hantaan virus in Korea

Source: Reproduced from Lee and Dalrymple (1989, fig. 8, p. 47).

weeks (range one to six weeks) (Lee and Dalrymple, 1989; Nathanson and Nichol, 1998).

Geographical distribution. Figure 9.7 maps those areas of northwest Asia, southeastern Siberia, and Japan in which HFRS is known to occur in endemic form. Within Korea, the zone of KHF activity runs along the Thirty-Eighth parallel of latitude, forming a 160 km (east–west) belt that straddles the border between present-day North and South Korea. Within this predominantly rural zone, outbreaks of KHF occur when human populations invade the micro-environments of *Apodemus agrarius*—especially when, as in the war of 1950–3, the invasion coincides with local ecological changes that promote increases in the density and/or the extent of the rodent population (Nathanson and Nichol, 1998).

Military significance. With hindsight, diseases similar (or identical) to Korean haemorrhagic fever have been of military significance in several Far Eastern wars. As noted above, HFRS was first encountered by the Russians in south-eastern Siberia in the mid-1930s and by the Japanese in the course of the Manchurian Campaigns of 1936. During the Sino-Japanese War (1937–45) and World War II (1939–45), in excess of 12,500 cases occurred among Japanese troops in Manchuria, while several hundred cases were also recorded among Russian soldiers in the Far East (Paul and McClure, 1958; Trencséni and Keleti, 1971; Lee, 1989). In the period to 1950, however, virtually all relevant medical information was confined to the Russian and Japanese languages

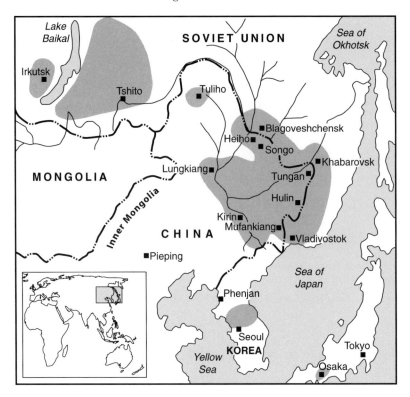

Fig. 9.7. Areas of northwest Asia, southeast Siberia, and Japan in which haemorrhagic fever with renal syndrome (HFRS) is known to occur in endemic form

Note: Areas of endemic HFRS activity are shaded.
Source: Redrawn from Trencséni and Keleti (1971, map 1, p. 16).

and the appearance of KHF among UN forces during the Korean War was unanticipated (Paul and McClure, 1958).

KHF IN THE KOREAN WAR

The known distribution of KHF activity at about the time of the Korean War is mapped in Figure 9.8A, while Plates 9.3A and 9.3B provide views of the infected terrain. According to McNinch (1953), the first UN troops to contract KHF were stationed just north of the Thirty-Eighth Parallel and were admitted to US medical installations in May and June 1951. The subsequent course of reported disease activity in UN forces is plotted on a weekly basis to January 1953 in Figure 9.9. As the graph shows, cases were concentrated in three clearly defined waves of infection, with seasonally based peaks of activity in September–November 1951, April–July, and September–November 1952. As regards mortality, case-fatality rates for KHF declined progressively

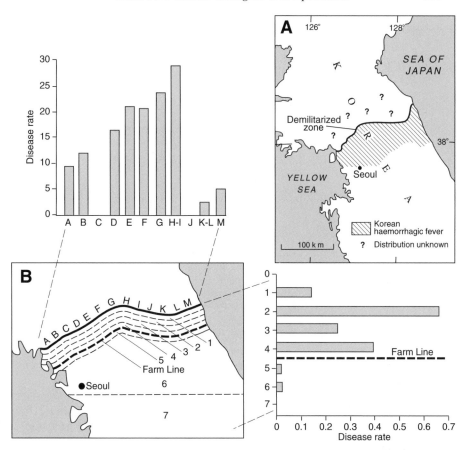

Fig. 9.8. Localized patterns of Korean haemorrhagic fever (KHF) among UN troops fighting on, and near, the front line during the Korean War, April 1952–June 1953

Notes: (A) Map of the known distribution of KHF as defined by Gajdusek (1956). (B) Rates of KHF among UN troops at sample horizontal locations along the front line (coded A–M) and sample vertical locations to the south of the front line (coded 1–7). The position of the 'Farm Line' (dividing vertical locations 4 and 5) marks the northern boundary of continued native agricultural production during the war. Note that disease rates for front-line locations, A–M, are expressed per million man-days of exposure; disease rates for locations south of the front line, 1–7, are expressed per 1,000 estimated population. Disease rates at vertical locations 1–7 relate to the sample period May–June 1953.

Source: Based on Paul and McClure (1958, figs. 1, 3 and 4, and table 2, pp. 128–32, 136).

over the period of the war, falling from 14.6 per cent (Apr.–Aug. 1951) to 5.7 per cent (Sept.–Mar. 1951–2), 5.1 per cent (Apr.–Aug. 1952), and 2.7 per cent (Sept.–Jan. 1952–3) for US personnel. The reason for this documented decline is uncertain, although Pruitt and Cleve (1953) suggest that the under-reporting of mild cases may account for the apparently high case-fatality rate in the spring and summer of 1951.

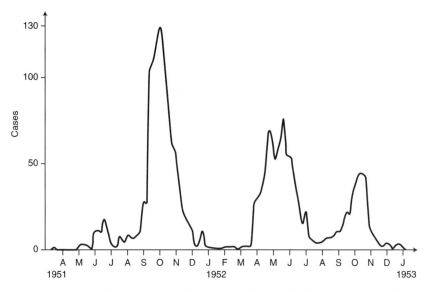

Fig. 9.9. Weekly incidence of Korean haemorrhagic fever (KHF) in UN troops during the Korean War, April 1951–January 1953

Source: Redrawn from Trencséni and Keleti (1971, fig. 34, p. 114), after Marshall (1954).

Spatial Patterns of KHF Activity

The actual locale and circumstances under which UN troops contracted KHF during the period April 1952–July 1953 are examined by Paul and McClure (1958). The study area, along the line of combat to the north of Seoul and the focal point of KHF among UN troops, is mapped in Figure 9.8B; this area forms part of the endemic zone of KHF in Figure 9.8A. The letter codes (A–M) in Figure 9.8B indicate the horizontal positions of 13 UN combat forces during the study period, while the bounded areas running east to west (number coded 1–5) indicate the vertical positions of troops away from the front line. The disease rates associated with the horizontal (A–M) and vertical (1–5) combat positions are plotted on the graphs that accompany Figure 9.8B. We consider the evidence for the horizonal and vertical positions in turn.

Horizontal combat positions. The KHF rates associated with the front-line horizontal positions, expressed per million man-days of exposure, are plotted in the upper graph of Figure 9.8B. As the graph shows, KHF rates varied along the line from 3.2 to 27.9, with the highest rates recorded in the central combat area (sectors D–I). To the extreme west (sectors A–B) and east (K–M), rates varied between 20 and 60 per cent of the central area. The high rates of disease activity in the central area were associated with exposure in war-abandoned agricultural territory, with farms and paddies colonized by underbrush and

A

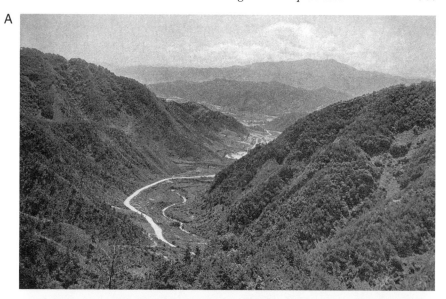

B

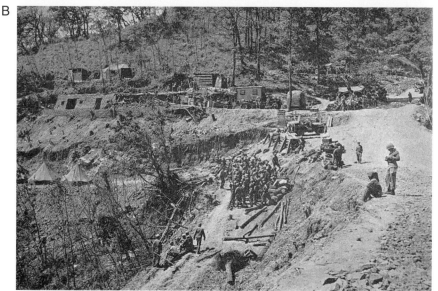

Pl. 9.3. Korean haemorrhagic fever (KHF) in the Korean War, 1950–1953

Notes: (A) Characteristic landscape in the endemic region. (B) Military disruption of natural ecology. (C) American evacuation hospital in the Han River Valley, operating as the Epidemic Hemorrhagic Fever Center. (D) Laboratory of the Field Unit of the US Army's Commission on Epidemic Hemorrhagic Fever, based in the Epidemic Hemorrhagic Fever Center.
Source: Reproduced from Gajdusek (1956, figs. 5, 7, 9 and 11, pp. 34, 36, 38–9).

C

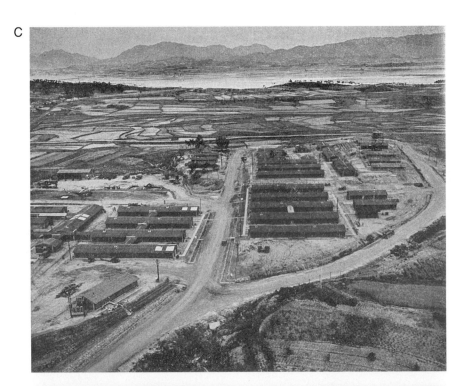

D

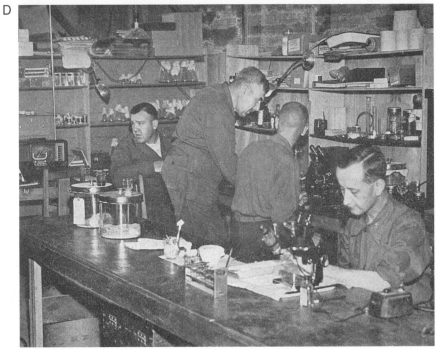

Pl. 9.3. (*cont.*)

weeds. In contrast, the considerably lower rates of disease activity in the eastern sectors, K–M, were associated with a primary, mountainous, and heavily wooded, environment (Paul and McClure, 1958).

Vertical combat positions. From the very first appearance of KHF in UN troops, epidemiological activity had appeared to be more intense in the forward combat area of Figure 9.8B. All land to the north of the front line was under the control of North Korean forces. Away from the front line, vertical cross-sections in Figure 9.8B demarcate the Forward Division (coded 1), the Mid-Division (2), the Rear Division (3), and the Forward Corps Area (4) of UN Command. The latter zone was bordered to the south by the so-called 'Farm Line' (heavy broken line in Fig. 9.8B); between the Farm Line and the Forward Division, all agricultural activity had come to a standstill. The native population had been displaced, villages had been destroyed, secondary invasion of underbrush and weeds had commenced, and the area was studded with military installations of all kinds. Field mice and foxes were in abundance while rodents, in particular, found sustenance in the buried food supplies left by the fleeing Koreans. South of the Farm Line, in the Rear Corps Area (coded 5 in Fig. 9.8B), the native population continued to live and farm.

The KHF rate for troops in vertical zones 1–5 are given in the right-hand graph of Figure 9.8B, along with rates for those positioned to the south of the Rear Corps Area (areas coded 6–7). Owing to insufficient information on mandays of exposure, rates are expressed per 1,000 estimated population. As the graph shows, disease activity was concentrated in the zone north of the Farm Line, reaching 0.67 cases per 1,000 estimated population in the Mid-Division (area 2). South of the Farm Line, rates fell off damatically (Paul and McClure, 1958).

Interpretation. Taken together, the evidence highlights the combined role of war-associated population displacement, ecological change, and patterns of combat exposure in the emergence of an apparently 'new' viral disease. The spatially focused nature of the KHF outbreaks, along and just to the south of the front line, corresponds with the ecological changes that accompanied the abandonment of intensive farming activities and which provided an environment conducive to the rodent reservoir of Hantaan virus, *Apodemus agrarius* (Paul and McClure, 1958). Some 95 per cent of all KHF cases originated from the area between the front line and the line which demarcated the area of civilian evacuation, with the heightened exposure of troops to rodent excreta in trenches, bunkers, and tents. To the south of this zone, native farming practices continued. Ecological changes associated with the war were less marked and the occurrence of KHF was correspondingly low (Trencséni and Keleti, 1971).

KHF Response and Control Activities
In April 1952, an Epidemic Hemorrhagic Fever Center (8228th Mobile Army Surgical Hospital) was established near the focus of KHF activity. Local

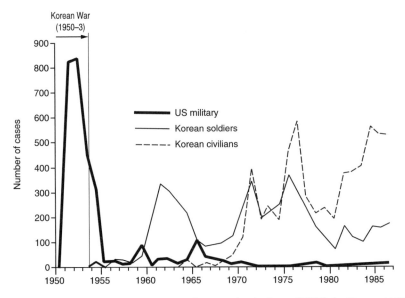

Fig. 9.10. Annual incidence of Korean haemorrhagic fever (KHF) in Korea, 1950–1986

Note: Incidence is based on hospital admissions among US military personnel stationed in Korea, South Korean soldiers and civilians.

Source: Drawn from data in Lee (1989, table 1, p. S865).

investigations were further promoted by the establishment of the US Army's Commission on Epidemic Hemorrhagic Fever in October 1953 (Pls. 9.3C and 9.3D). In the interim, efforts at KHF control included the initiation of an intensive programme of localized rat extermination. Mite-control measures (including the impregnation of clothing, sleeping bags, and tents with miticides) were implemented on the basis of an assumed rat–mite cycle in the natural history of KHF. These responses were accompanied by a considerable reduction in KHF activity (up to 72%) when matched with controls, although the extent to which the reduction was associated with intervention measures or other factors in disease ecology is not known (Pruitt and Cleve, 1953; Gajdusek, 1956).

POST-WAR PATTERNS OF KHF IN MILITARY POPULATIONS

Although an armistice was agreed in July 1953, UN soldiers continued to contract KHF throughout the autumn of 1953 and the spring of 1954. Only in 1955, with the civilian resettlement of the endemic zone and a reversion of the local ecology to its pre-war form, did levels of disease activity begin to reduce among the military population (Trencséni and Keleti, 1971). To illustrate the post-war pattern of KHF activity, the heavy line trace in Figure 9.10 plots the annual count of hospital admissions for KHF in US military personnel stationed in Korea, 1950–86; the remaining line traces plot the equivalent information for South Korean soldiers (full line) and civilians (broken line). As the graph shows, the post-war annual incidence remained very low among US troops, although occasional outbreaks associated with joint US–Korean military training exercises have been described (Pon *et al.*, 1990). However, the disease continued to be of military significance for the South Korean Army, emerging as a more general problem in the civil population in the early 1970s.

9.5 Re-emergent Diseases and the Vietnam War

In a late-twentieth-century survey of the public health consequences of the Vietnam War (1964–73),[9] Myron Allukian and Paul Atwood (1997: 215) furnish the following stark facts of the conflict:

Vietnam suffered 3,000,000 war deaths, millions more wounded or maimed, immense population dislocations, the most massive bombing campaign in the history of warfare, and defoliation of an area the size of Massachusetts. Over 58,000 U.S. military personnel died, 313,616 were wounded, and about 10,000 lost at least one limb—more loss-of-limb injuries to U.S. military personnel than in World War II and Korea combined.

The health impact of a war which resulted in a million widows, 800,000 orphans, 83,000 amputees, more than 10 million evacuees and refugees, and which left the country riddled with up to 600,000 tons of unexploded munitions, was grave indeed (ibid.). By the 1970s, a series of infectious diseases had risen to the status of serious public health problems. Large-scale population dislocation, the decimation of civil health infrastructure, and overcrowding in relief camps all contributed to the epidemic incidence of tuberculosis and intestinal parasites, while haemorrhagic fevers, leprosy, malaria, plague, and rabies—among a raft of diseases—threatened military and civil populations alike. Ecological changes wrought by the military use of Agent Orange and other herbicides, war-induced shifts in the ecosystems of rodents and insects, and the circulation of drug-resistant strains of *Plasmodium falciparum* and *Mycobacterium tuberculosis* further contributed to the disease problems of the Vietnam War (Cowley, 1970; Neel, 1973).

VIETNAM AND THE THEME OF DISEASE RE-EMERGENCE

In the first half of this chapter, our primary concern has been with the *emergence* of exotic infectious diseases that, prior to the twentieth century, were

---

[9] As part of a longer-running civil war between North and South Vietnam (1956–75), the Vietnam War is defined here as the period of hostilities that commenced with large-scale US military involvement after the Gulf of Tonking Incident (Aug. 1964) and ended with the withdrawal of US troops under the the the Paris Peace Accords (Jan. 1973).

largely or wholly unknown to western medical science. In the present section, by contrast, we take the example of the Vietnam War to illustrate the wartime *re-emergence* of two 'classical' infectious diseases: malaria (US forces) and human plague (Vietnamese civilians). Our choice of diseases and populations has been informed by the different mechanisms that drive the process of disease re-emergence (Table 9.2). Framed by the more general theme of microbial resistance and change, our selection of malaria in US forces (Sect. 9.5.1) is founded on the early recognition of chloroquine-resistant strains of the malaria parasite, *Plasmodium falciparum*, acquired by combat units in close promixity to the Viet Cong. On the other hand, our selection of plague in Vietnamese civilians (Sect. 9.5.2) reflects the manner in which war-induced alterations to economies and ecosystems may promote the epidemic transmission of previously low-level, endemic, infections such as *Yersinia pestis*. As Lederberg *et al.* (1992: 111–12) observe, the 'return of US troops from foreign soils offers a unique opportunity for the introduction or reintroduction of infectious diseases into the United States'. In Section 9.5.3, therefore, we conclude our consideration of disease re-emergence with an examination of the role of Vietnam military returnees in the international transfer of classical disease agents such as *Plasmodium spp.* to the North American continent.

9.5.1 US Forces, Tactical Missions, and Malaria

Consistent with the prior experiences of US forces in the Asia–Pacific region, disease operated as the principal drain on US fighting strength in Vietnam. According to Neel (1973: 32), 69 per cent of all Army-based hospital admissions during the main phase of combat activity in Vietnam (1965–9) were attributable to disease. Even so, the overall disease rate (351 admissions per 1,000 mean strength per year) represented a considerable improvement on the epidemiological circumstances of both the Korean War (611 per 1,000 per year) and the Burma–India Theatre in World War II (844 per 1,000 per year). Part of this relative success arose from the timely introduction of a programme of preventive medicine in Vietnam, while innovative methods of disease prediction permitted an assessment of epidemiological risk in the planning of military operations. Levels of incapacity among combat-operative troops were further reduced by the implementation of a standard six-week acclimatization period for draftees. New treatment regimens also had a marked impact on manpower losses from some diseases (Neel, 1973: 33–7).

THE MALARIA PROBLEM

Malaria represented the single most important medico-military problem for US forces stationed in Vietnam. The nature of malaria is outlined in Appendix 1A, but Neel (1973) and Beadle and Hoffman (1993) note that several factors contributed to the particular severity of the disease in the Vietnam War: (i) the relative inexperience of line officers with regard to malaria and malaria discipline in high-risk locations; (ii) the circulation of malignant *P. falciparum* as the predominant species of the malaria parasite; and (iii) the existence of chloroquine-resistant species of *P. falciparum*. Some impression of the extent of malaria in US forces can be gained from Tables 9.6 and 9.7. During the course of the conflict, malaria accounted for no less than 65,000 admissions and 124 deaths in the combined US Army and Naval forces (Table 9.6) while, as an annual average in the sample period 1967–70, the disease ranked second only to the non-specific 'fever of undetermined origin'[10] as a cause of man-days lost from duty in the US Army (Table 9.7).

Tactical Missions, Malaria and Drug-Resistant P. Falciparum

A prominent feature of malaria among US forces in Vietnam was the focus of the disease among combat troops. Some 80 per cent of all malaria cases in the US Army were reported from combat units, with tactical missions in the Central Highlands of South Vietnam forming a primary source of exposure to drug-resistant strains of *P. falciparum* in the early stages of the conflict (Neel, 1973: 109, 170). By way of illustration, Figure 9.11 is based on Nowosiwsky's (1967) study of drug-refractory *P. falciparum* malaria among US combat units in the northern sector of the Central Highlands area. For each of three military units (coded 'A', 'B', and 'C'), the graphs plot the daily incidence of malaria in relation to tactical missions undertaken between October 1965 and June 1966. The periods associated with the missions are identified on the graphs by black horizontal bars, while the bar charts plot the daily occurrence of malaria in the corresponding unit.[11]

Mission-based attack rates. While cases of malaria identified during the tactical missions can be attributed to prior disease exposure, all four graphs in Figure 9.11 are characterized by a marked increase in malaria incidence some 13 to 19 days after the termination of operations. With a median incubation period of *c*.16 days, estimates of mission-based attack rates range from 8.3 cases per 1,000 man-days of exposure (Fig. 9.11D) to approximately 12.0 cases per 1,000 man-days of exposure (Fig. 9.11C). At these rates, and notwithstanding the maintenance of all members of the units on chloroquine-primaquine prophylaxis, a three-month deployment in an endemic area during peak periods of disease transmission would be expected to yield a 90 per cent infection rate among the men.

Prophylactic responses. In response to evidence for the existence of strains of *P. falciparum* for which chloroquine-primaquine prophylaxis was only partially effective, the drug DDS (4,–4′–diamino-diphenylsulfone) was added to the anti-malaria regimen of tactical units in malarious areas. Evaluations

[10] For a consideration of the nature of 'fevers of undetermined origin' among US forces in the Vietnam War, see Reiley and Russell (1969).

[11] Precise details of dates and locations were withheld from the original study for operational reasons.

Table 9.6. Malaria statistics for US military forces during sample wars of the twentieth century

War	Years	Malaria admissions[1]		Number of malaria sick days		Malaria deaths	
		Army	Naval forces[2]	Army	Naval forces[2]	Army	Naval forces[2]
World War I	1917–19	15,555	11,648	194,529	103,257	36	10
World War II	1942–5	492,299	203,251	8–9 million	3,303,543	302	87
Korean War	1950–3	>30,000	4,864	?	50,294	?	0
Vietnam War[3]	1965–73	40,414	24,639	794,500	391,965	78	46

Notes: [1] Includes re-admissions. [2] Includes Marine Corps. [3] For US Army personnel, the data variously relate to the periods 1965–70 (malaria admissions and deaths) and 1967–70 (malaria sick-days).
Source: Beadle and Hoffman (1993, table 6, p. 327).

Table 9.7. Average annual admissions rate and average annual number of man-days lost from duty, US Army in Vietnam, 1967–1970

Disease/condition	Admissions rate[1]	Man-days lost from duty
Malaria	24.6	198,625
Acute respiratory infections	34.3	71,078
Skin diseases[2]	25.8	65,541
Neuropsychiatric conditions	16.2	119,408
Viral hepatitis	7.3	92,495
Venereal disease[3]	1.8	5,293
Fever of undetermined origin	60.7	225,600

Notes: [1] Rate expressed per 1,000 mean strength. [2] Including dermatophytosis. [3] Excluding cases 'carded for record only'.
Source: Based on information in Neel (1973, tables 2 and 3, pp. 34, 36).

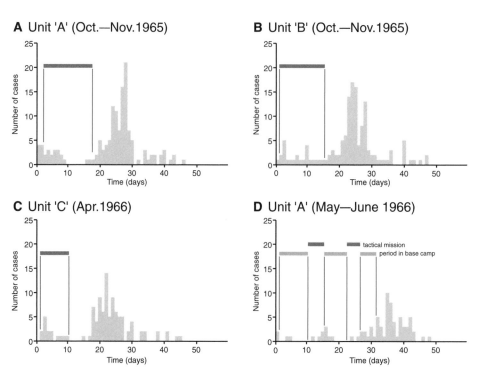

Fig. 9.11. Daily incidence of *Plasmodium falciparum* malaria in sample US military units, Republic of Vietnam, 1965–1966

Notes: Graphs plot the daily number of malaria cases in relation to the timing of tactical missions undertaken by units in the north-central highlands of South Vietnam. Tactical missions are marked by the black horizontal bars. (A) Unit 'A', October–November 1965 (16-day tactical mission). (B) Unit 'B', October–November 1965 (14-day tactical mission). (C) Unit 'C', April 1966 (9-day tactical mission). (D) Unit 'A', May–June 1966 (5-day and 4-day tactical missions). Graphs A and B are based on the day of onset of symptoms; Graphs C and D are based on the day of admission to hospital.
Source: Redrawn from Nowosiwsky (1967, figs. 1–3, pp. 464–5).

Table 9.8. Malaria rates (per 1,000 strength) in the Fifth and Seventh US Marine Regiments, Que Son Mountains, Vietnam, during the malaria seasons of 1969 and 1970

Month	Malaria rate (per 1,000 strength)	
	1969	1970
September	136	58
October	72	39
November	87	21
December	28	15
Total	81	33

Source: Bridges (1973, table III, p. 414).

indicated that a daily 25 milligram dose of DDS served to reduce the incidence of malaria among the troops by some 50 per cent, with evidence of further benefits in terms of reduced incidence of relapse and length of hospitalization for malaria patients (Neel, 1973: 170–1).

P. falciparum Malaria and Level of Enemy Contact

In an epidemiological investigation of malaria in the Fifth and Seventh US Marine Regiments, operative in the Que Son Mountains of north-central Vietnam in 1969–70, Bridges (1973) correlates the level of disease activity with the estimated size of the local Viet Cong/North Vietnamese (VC/NVA) forces. Between the malaria seasons (Sept.–Dec.) of 1969 and 1970, the disease rate in the Marine regiments fell from 81 per 1,000 strength to 33 per 1,000 strength (Table 9.8). Such a marked decrease, Bridges argues, could not be attributed to changes in vector density or improved malaria discipline alone. Rather, given that the only persons in the foothills and mountain areas were US Marines and VC/NVA soldiers, and that Marines were evacuated on presentation with symptoms of malaria, enemy troops served as the principal reservoir of the disease in the Que Son Mountains. During the study period, the estimated strength of the VC/NVA force reduced from a high of 16,800 (May 1969) to 8,560 (Dec. 1970), with a corresponding reduction in the reported level of *P. falciparum* malaria in US troops.

9.5.2 *Vietnamese Civilians and the Re-emergence of Plague*

In 1962, an epidemic of bubonic plague, accompanied by outbreaks of plague pneumonia, began to spread across the war-torn Republic of Vietnam (Marshall *et al.*, 1967; Cavanaugh *et al.*, 1968; Velimirovic, 1972). Originating as a persistent low-level infection associated with just a handful of recorded human

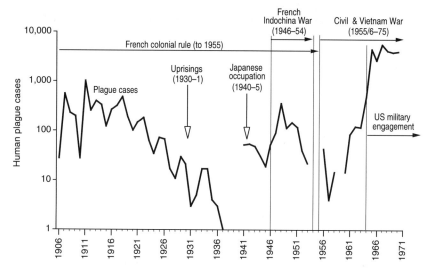

Fig. 9.12. Annual incidence of human plague in the Republic of Vietnam, 1906–1970

Notes: Note that the vertical axis is drawn on a logarithmic scale. No data are available for the years 1954–5.

Source: Data from Velimirovic (1972, table X, p. 496).

cases each year, the plague epidemic continued for more than a decade, extending to virtually every province of the country and resulting in an estimated 100,000 to 250,000 cases in the native population (Kohn, 1998: 353). The capacity of plague to re-emerge from localized disease foci in such dramatic fashion, Velimirovic (1972) observes, serves to underscore the profound epidemiological dangers associated with war-induced disturbances to both human and zootic habitats.

THE PATTERN OF RE-EMERGENCE IN HISTORICAL PERSPECTIVE

Vietnam has been regarded as a permanent reservoir of the aetiological agent of plague, *Yersinia pestis*, since the introduction of the disease to Saigon in 1906 (Cavanaugh *et al.*, 1968; Velimirovic, 1972). From this putative beginning, Figure 9.12 is based on information included in Velimirovic (1972) and traces the reported pattern of human plague in the Republic of Vietnam over the seven decades to 1970. The vertical axis has been plotted on a logarithmic scale to allow for widely varying case totals. Although the available evidence is fragmentary, and under-reporting of cases must be suspected, the relative success of French colonial efforts at plague control (including quarantine, vaccination, disinfection, and general measures of rodent and flea control) is clearly reflected in the progressive reduction of disease activity to near-zero levels by the mid-1930s. Thereafter, Japanese occupation (1940–5) was associated with a modest resurgence in human plague, to a peak (335 cases) in the early years of the French Indochina War (1946–54). However, with the onset of civil war in 1956 and, more particularly, with the escalation of hostilities from 1964, Figure 9.12 shows that the reported number of cases spiralled from an annual average of below 60 (1956–63) to over 3,600 (1964–70).[12]

Factors in Re-emergence

The nature of plague is outlined in Appendix 1A. The upsurge in plague activity in Vietnam during the 1960s was intimately associated with factors that increased the level of contact between human beings, plague-carrying rodents (preliminary studies implicated *R. norvegicus*, *R. rattus*, and the house shrew, *Suncus murinus*, in the spread of the epidemic) and their associated fleas. From late 1964, large-scale US bombing and firing resulted in the destruction of an estimated 50 per cent of forest cover and 20 per cent of agricultural land, thereby forcing rodents and humans into close proximity in towns, cities, and relief camps (Velimirovic, 1973). The profound disruption of Vietnam's agricultural economy resulted in a reversal of the regular lines of food shipment and the associated patterns of human–rodent contact. Neel (1973: 171) explains:

Plague in the Vietnamese civilian population pointed up . . . the shifting of disease patterns when the normal way of life of any peoples whose structure, economically or environmentally, is altered. Vietnam is a rice-producing and rice-exporting country. Normally, the grain flowed from the rice bowls of the interior to the few major ports of the country. The rodents which infest the areas followed the path of the rice to the ports. There they were controlled; thus, the danger of a serious outbreak of plague was averted. During the war when, for economic reasons, the South Vietnamese began to import grain, a reverse situation was created. The rice was shipped from the ports into the countryside; the rodents followed the flow of the grain inland and created havoc in the form of increased incidence of plague among the native population in areas which had hithertofore been relatively free of the disease.

However, changes in human and rodent habitats formed only part of the re-emergence complex. High resistance to DDT (dichloro-diphenyl-trichloroethane), probably arising from prolonged exposure under the local mosquito-malaria eradication programme, was recognized in the principal flea vector, *Xenopsylla cheopis*, from 1965. Vector resistance to a further insecticide (Dieldrin) emerged in some localities from about 1970. With efforts at plague control hindered by the development of vector resistance and with any possibility of the implementation of a comprehensive programme of plague eradication stultified by the ongoing hostilities, the epidemic continued to spread apace in the late 1960s and early 1970s (Marshall *et al.*, 1967; Velimirovic, 1972).

---

[12] As Marshall *et al.* (1967) note, however, part of the explosive rise in reported plague activity from the mid-1960s may be attributable to improved systems of disease surveillance that accompanied the arrival of US and third country personnel.

SPATIAL DIFFUSION

Figures 9.13 and 9.14 trace the spatial extension of human plague in Vietnam during the decade to 1970. The annual map sequence in Figure 9.13 shades those provinces in which cases of plague were reported in the period 1962–70, while aggregate evidence for a ten-year period prior to epidemic onset (1951–60) is shown for reference. To assist interpretation of the main phase of spatial transmission in Figure 9.13, the graphs in Figure 9.14 plot the monthly incidence of reported plague cases in ten sample cities, 1962–7.

From a primary focus of plague activity in south-central Vietnam in 1962, the map sequence in Figure 9.13 traces a progressive north-eastwards extension of the disease in 1963–4. Coincidental with the escalation of hostilities, rapid colonization of more northerly provinces occurred in 1965–6. As judged by the city-level evidence in Figure 9.14, this phase of rapid northerly transmission approximated a wave-like (contagious) transmission process with the disease pushing out of the central settlements (Ban Me Thuot, Dalat, and Nha Trang) for more distant localities at increasingly later dates: Quinhon (Feb. 1965) → Pleiku and Quang Ngai → Da Nang → Hue (Dec. 1965). According to Marshall *et al.* (1967), this northwards drift of the disease was associated with the transportation of foodstuffs. In Da Nang, for example, the appearance of human plague in September 1965 followed a major rat die-off which was consequent on the arrival of a rice shipment from the endemic focus of Saigon. With the road from Da Nang to Hue also open to food shipments, the disease appeared in the latter place in December 1965. The subsequent spread of the disease in Hue, based on evidence for 60 documented cases in the period 2 January–6 March 1966, is shown in Figure 9.15. As the map indicates, early cases of plague were focused in the central area, with transmission along the waterways of the city as the epidemic developed (Marshall *et al.*, 1967).

Following the period of rapid geographical expansion in 1965–6, inspection of Figure 9.13 reveals that the overall spatial distribution of plague remained relatively static in the years 1967–70. Plague continued to be reported from virtually all the provinces of central and northern Vietnam at this time, but with an apparent absence from many of the more southerly localities. Spatial contraction of the epidemic followed the US military withdrawal from Vietnam in the early 1970s (Kohn, 1998: 353).

9.5.3 Vietnam Returnees and Re-emergent Disease Threats in the Continental USA

As shown in Table 9.2, the risk of disease importation as a consequence of international travel represents one of the principal factors in the modern-day emergence and re-emergence of infectious diseases. The particular risk is magnified when many tens of thousands of deployed troops, potentially exposed to one or more of a long list of infectious diseases, begin to return to their

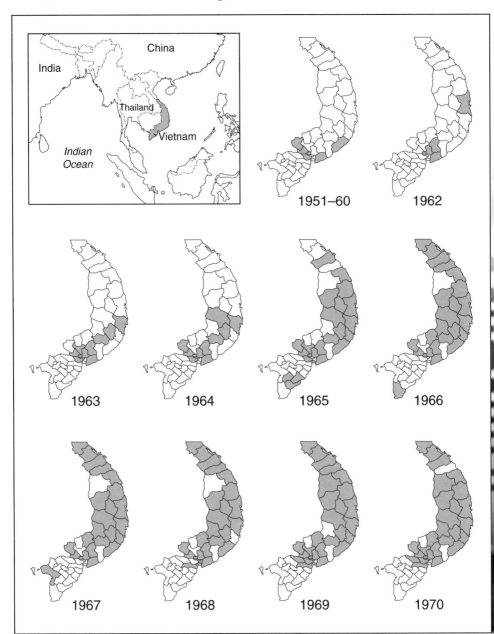

Fig. 9.13. War and the spread of human plague in the Republic of Vietnam, 1951–1970

Note: Provinces in which cases of human plague were reported in a given time period have been shaded.

Source: Redrawn from Velimirovic (1972, fig. 9, p. 500).

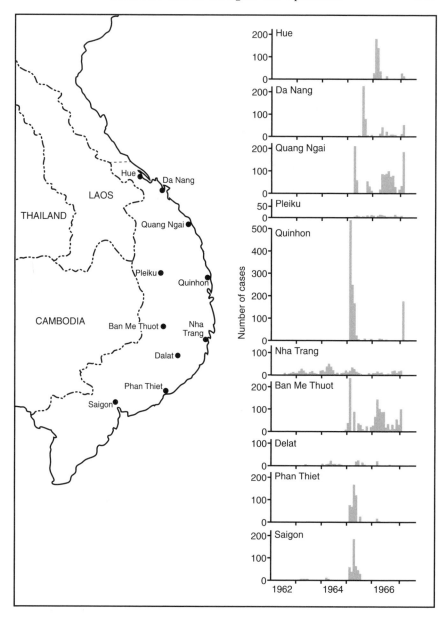

Fig. 9.14. Major outbreaks of human plague reported in the Republic of Vietnam, 1962–1967

Notes: For the period associated with the rapid geographical extension of human plague (see Fig. 9.13), the graphs plot the monthly incidence of documented cases of human plague at selected locations. As judged by the timing of the first documented cases at each location, wave-like spread from a central focus of infection in 1965 is evident.

Source: Redrawn from Cavanaugh *et al.* (1968, fig. 3, p. 745).

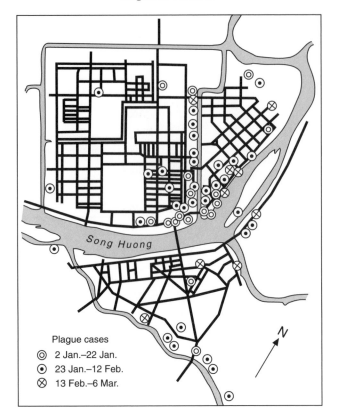

Fig. 9.15. Spread of human plague in Hue City, Republic of Vietnam, 1966

Notes: Hue City is located in Thua Thien Province, to the north of the Republic of Vietnam (see Fig. 9.14). The map shows the location of a sample of 60 human plague cases recorded in Hue City, 2 January–6 March 1966.
Source: Redrawn from Marshall *et al.* (1967, map 5, p. 611).

homeland (Lederberg *et al.*, 1992: 111–12). The spread of the 'Spanish' influenza pandemic of 1918–19 with the demobilization of troops in the wake of World War I represents a classic example of the problem (see Sect. 11.3). But the Vietnam War heralded a new era in the mass transfer of US soldiers: for the first time ever, air transport (rather than sea transport) formed the principal means for the return of overseas forces to the continental United States. The profound epidemiological implications of this development were succinctly expressed by Col. Jerome H. Greenberg (1969: 697):

In 1968 alone, over 290,000 US Army personnel are expected to return from Vietnam. It takes less than 24 hours to return from Vietnam to the United States, which makes it possible to arrive back in the preclinical stages of almost every infectious disease. One of the concerns of the US Army Medical Service, of the Public Health Service (PHS),

Table 9.9. Health problems associated with US military personnel stationed in Vietnam and among Vietnam returnees (status: late 1960s)

Disease	Documented occurrence	
	US personnel in Vietnam	US returnees
Group 1: potential threats		
Tuberculosis	Few cases	Few cases
Plague	5 cases	1 case
Cholera	No cases	No cases
Japanese encephalitis	Few cases	No cases
Filariasis	No clinical cases	—
Helminthiasis	Localized outbreaks	—
Leptospirosis	Few cases	No cases
Melioidosis	72 cases	10 cases
Group 2: actual disease problems		
Respiratory tract disease	Significant	—
Diarrhoeal disease[1]	Severe local outbreaks	Some cases
Skin disease	Serious problem	—
STDs	Moderate incidence	Few cases
Dengue	Few cases	—
Scrub typhus	Few cases	3 cases
Malaria	Serious problem	2,700 cases (1967)

Note: [1] Dysentery, infectious hepatitis, paratyphoid and typhoid fevers.
Source: Based on information in Greenberg (1969).

of state and local public health personnel, and of the medical profession generally is the possibility that diseases introduced from Vietnam may gain a foothold in the United States.

DISEASES AMONG VIETNAM RETURNEES

In the event, relatively few cases of many of the anticipated disease threats were identified among Vietnam returnees (Gilbert *et al.*, 1968; Greenberg, 1969). By way of illustration, Table 9.9 relates to the period prior to January 1969 and summarizes the status of selected infectious diseases among (i) US military personnel in Vietnam and (ii) Vietnam returnees in the conterminous United States. Of the diseases that were generally regarded as potential threats to US forces in Vietnam (Group 1 in Table 9.9), vaccination and other methods of disease prevention and control ensured that very few (or no cases) of cholera, plague, or Japanese encephalitis, among other conditions, were identified in returnees. Likewise, many of the actual disease problems among US forces in Vietnam (Group 2 in Table 9.9) yielded few cases on return to the United States.

Table 9.10. Cases of malaria treated in US Army facilities in the Continental United States, 1965–1970

Year	Cases
1965	62
1966	303
1967	2,021
1968	1,598
1969	1,969
1970	2,222

Source: Neel (1973: 40).

Malaria

One disease listed in Table 9.9 did, however, gain particular prominence in contemporary discussions of disease re-emergence in the United States—malaria. Malaria had been the subject of an intensive elimination programme prior to the war, with a correspondingly low incidence in the civil population of the United States. Under these circumstances, the danger of increased transmission as a result of importation with military returnees was widely recognized (Gilbert *et al.*, 1968; Greenberg, 1969; Cowley, 1970). The concern was well founded. Between 1965 and 1970, the annual count of malaria cases treated in domestic US Army medical facilities grew from 62 to 2,222 (Table 9.10), with a corresponding surge in the national malaria curve (Fig. 9.16). In contrast to Vietnam, where the majority of malaria cases in US troops (>90%) were attributable to *P. falciparum*, most cases in returnees (>80%) were due to *P. vivax*—probably arising from partial failure of the Army's terminal prophylaxis programme (Barrett *et al.*, 1969; Neel, 1973). Notwithstanding sporadic reports of mosquito-transmitted *P. vivax* malaria as a consequence of exposure to returnees (Luby *et al.*, 1967), lack of evidence for the general re-establishment of malaria in the United States is signalled in Figure 9.16 by the precipitous fall in disease activity at the end of the Vietnam War (Gibson *et al.*, 1974).

9.6 Conclusion

In this chapter, we have examined the role of war as a mechanism in the emergence and re-emergence of infectious diseases. Drawing on sample conflicts, diseases, and populations in Asia and the Far East during the three decades to 1973, a range of facilitating factors have been identified as contributing to the (re-)emergence complex. Foremost among the factors examined, heightened exposure to the 'zoonotic pool' has regularly promoted the wartime transmis-

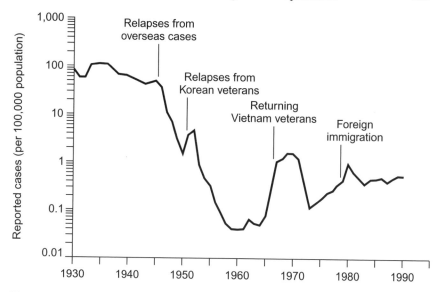

Fig. 9.16. Annual incidence (per 100,000 population) of malaria in the continental United States

Source: Redrawn from Lederberg *et al.* (1992, fig. 2.5, p. 80).

sion of animal- and insect-borne diseases for which human beings are incidental and potentially highly susceptible hosts. The military invasion of isolated ecological niches, the disruption of human and zootic habitats and the promotion of local conditions favourable to the wildlife reservoirs of disease agents all add to the wartime risk of disease emergence and re-emergence. The evolution of drug-resistant pathogens and insecticide-resistant vectors has further contributed to the (re-)emergence complex while, in the era of mass air transport, the rapid de-deployment of troops has threatened the reintroduction of pathogens into disease-free areas.

For military populations, a prominent feature of the present chapter has been the role of front-line combat troops in both the emergence of apparently 'new' diseases and in the re-emergence of old plagues. For example, during World War II, the focal outbreaks of scrub typhus in Allied British, Chinese, and US troops were concentrated in field combat units deployed in the isolated jungle habitats of northern Burma and northeastern India. In the Korean War, outbreaks of KHF were focused on UN combat troops who were bivouacked in the environs of the Thirty-Eighth Parallel. During the Vietnam War, the occurrence of chlorquine-resistant *P. falciparum* malaria was associated with tactical missions which brought US troops into contact with Viet Cong forces. Such examples underscore the importance of active military operations and enemy engagement as factors in the wartime emergence and re-emergence of infectious diseases.

As for other diseases and theatres of war, military investigators made an outstanding contribution to the scientific understanding of many of the emergent and re-emergent diseases examined in the present chapter. The pioneering studies of scrub typhus by the United States Typhus Commission (USATC) Burma team during World War II (Mackie, 1946), and of KHF by researchers at the Epidemic Hemorrhagic Fever Center during the Korean War (Gajdusek, 1956), provide two mid-twentieth-century examples. Likewise, in Vietnam, a series of seminal studies of disease transmission in militarily hostile localities, including investigations of malaria and plague, were undertaken by the US Army Special Forces–Walter Reed Army Institute of Research Field Epidemiologic Survey Team (Airborne) (WRAIR–FEST) between 1966 and 1968 (Fuenfer, 1991). As Philip (1948) reminds us, however, such pioneering studies of emergent and re-emergent diseases were not without occasionally tragic consequences for the field and laboratory workers involved.

10

Africa: Soldiers, Sexually Transmitted Diseases, and War

A terrible plague destroys our armies. It is the flock of women and girls who follow it . . . The barracks and cantonments are choked with them and the destruction of morals is complete. They enervate the troops, and through the serious diseases which they transmit, they destroy ten times more men than the enemy.

Lazare Carnot, 1793[1]

10.1 Introduction

As we observed in Chapter 4, from time immemorial, sexually transmitted diseases (STDs) have been a scourge of military personnel and of the wars in which they were deployed. So, in her excellent historical review, *Venereal Diseases in the Major Armies and Navies of the World*, Josephine Hinrichsen (1944, 1945a, 1945b) traces the military problem of female prostitution—and, by implication, the associated spread of STDs—to the great army camps of classical Greece and Rome. In more recent times, the Italian War of Charles VIII

[1] Cited in Hinrichsen (1944: 741).

(1494–5) provides one of the most dramatic instances of the intersection of armies, STDs, and war—the pan-European dissemination of venereal syphilis by the disbanded mercenary troops of France, Germany, and Italy (see Sect. 2.3.3). Thereafter, epidemics of syphilis and other venereal diseases followed wave-like on wars in Europe and elsewhere (Prinzing, 1916: 18). In Sweden, the syphilis epidemics of 1762 and 1792 were sparked by military returnees from the Seven Years' (1756–63) and the Russo-Swedish (1788–90) Wars. In the nineteenth century, the Russo-Turkish Wars (1806–12, 1828–9) contributed materially to the spread of the disease in the Balkans (Hinrichsen, 1944). Elsewhere, in World War II (1939–45), the high-level transmission of gonor-rhoea, chancroid, and syphilis among Allied personnel in the Burma–India, Africa–Middle East, and Mediterranean Theatres provides a twentieth-century example of the war-related problem of STDs (Sternberg *et al.*, 1960).

MILITARY POPULATIONS

As Berg (1984: 90) notes, the historical concern of the military wth STDs was eminently a practical one. Prior to the era of antibiotics (penicillin was first used in the military treatment of syphilis and gonorrhoea in 1943), STDs were associated with extended periods of hospital treatment with correspondingly high economic and medical manpower costs to the armed forces. Some impres-sion of the dimensions of the STD problem for one army (US Army) and war (World War I) can be gained from Table 10.1. During a 21-month period of military engagement, April 1917–December 1918, three STDs (chancroid, gonorrhoea, and syphilis) accounted for over 6.8 million days of lost service in the US Army. Over 10 per cent of all disease-related admissions were associ-ated with STDs, with the absolute count of STD admissions (357,969) exceed-ing the number of killed and wounded by a full 10,000. Total expenditure on treatment amounted to US$45 million while, in terms of the burden on the medical services, the treatment and care of STD patients occupied the

Table 10.1. Burden of sexually transmitted diseases (STDs) in the US Army during World War I, April 1917–December 1918

Parameter	Count/estimate
STD admissions	357,969 admissions
STD-related days lost	6,804,818 days
STDs as percentage of all disease admissions	10.2%
Total cost of STD treatment	US$45 million
Medical manpower lost to STD treatment/care	3,000 medical department troops + 200 MOs

Note: Counts/estimates are based on evidence for three diseases: gonorrhoea, chancroid, and syphilis.
Source: Data from Pappas (1943: 173–4).

equivalent of 3,000 medical department troops and 200 medical officers (Pappas, 1943: 173–4).

A broad range of social, physical, and psychological factors contributed to the high rate of spread of STDs in past military populations, and they remain a significant threat today (Hinrichsen, 1944; Carson and Johnson, 1973; Berg, 1984). At one level, emotional factors such as loneliness, boredom, peer pressure, and, under conditions of war, a fatalistic attitude, have all been identified as contributing to the acquisition of STDs among military personnel. The presence of female prostitutes in the vicinity of military installations, often in the absence of adequate regulation or control by local civil authorities, further added to the disease risk while, historically, voluntary exposure to STDs has been cited as a means of escaping active service. Additional studies have correlated inflated levels of venereal disease in military populations with such factors as deployment overseas, specific demographic and personality traits (including young age, heavy alcohol use, and low educational attainment), the lack of alternative recreational outlets, and race (Carson and Johnson, 1973; Berg, 1984).

CIVIL POPULATIONS

The onwards transmission of STDs from military personnel to the civil population at large is a recurring theme in the epidemic history of war (Prinzing, 1916; Major, 1940). Wartime atrocities of sexual violence and rape provide an obvious means of STD transmission to (and within) a civil population (Ashford and Huet-Vaughn, 1997), while military returnees may serve as a source of infection for the civil population of their homeland (Hinrichsen, 1944). Commenting on the longer-term ramifications of the latter problem, Hinrichsen (ibid. 770–1) draws attention to the dire experience of France in the wake of the 1914–18 war:

Touraine, in 1933, estimated the disaster which syphilis had created in France, in addition to all the other disasters of war. He estimated that as a result of 500,000 cases of syphilis contracted during the war, there were lost 2 million lives, 641,000 years of work, 5 military classes between 1915 and 1940, and that there had been produced 112,000 cases of general paresis and tabes, 45,000 cases of syphilitic involvement of the brain or cord or other than paresis and tabes, 16,000 aneurysms of the aorta, and 45,000 cases of heart disease.

CHAPTER OUTLINE

Against this background, the present chapter examines the theme of soldiers, STDs, and war, taking Africa as the geographical frame of reference. We begin, in Section 10.2, by exploring the occurrence of three STDs (gonorrhoea, chancroid, and syphilis) in the French Army in Algeria and Tunisia, North Africa, during an historic period of French colonial expansion and consolidation,

1875–1929. For the same three diseases, Section 10.3 examines patterns of
STD activity in (free) US troops and (incarcerated) Axis troops in Africa and
related commands of the Mediterranean and Africa–Middle East Theatres
during World War II. In the latter decades of the twentieth century, an apparently new STD—HIV (Human immunodeficiency virus)/AIDS (acquired
immunodeficiency syndrome)—began to spread widely in the states of East
and Central Africa (Smallman-Raynor *et al.*, 1992). In Section 10.4, we assess
the role of civil war as a possible factor in the historical spread of HIV/AIDS
in one country of the region—Uganda. The chapter is concluded in Section
10.5.

10.2 Historical Patterns: French Troops in Algeria–Tunisia, 1875–1929

To examine the historical occurrence of STDs in the French Army overseas, we
draw on the sanitary returns collated by the Ministère de la Guerre and published in the summary report *Aperçu Statistique sur l'Évolution de la Morbidité
et de la Mortalité Générales dans l'Armée* (Ministère de la Guerre, 1932). For
a 55-year period, 1875–1929,[2] the report provides annual morbidity rates
(per 1,000 effectives) for three STDs (gonorrhoea, chancroid, and syphilis)
in French forces stationed in the North African colonies of Algeria and
Tunisia, along with the corresponding rates for troops in the French Interior.
A description of the three diseases is provided in Appendix 10A while, for
reference, Figure 10.1 maps the geographical expansion of French interests in
Algeria, Tunisia, and proximal lands of North Africa during the observation
period. A general overview of mortality trends in the French Army in Algeria
during the late nineteenth and early twentieth centuries has already been given
in Section 4.2.

10.2.1 Long-Term Trends

TRENDS IN ALGERIA–TUNISIA

The graphs in Figure 10.2 plot, as heavy line traces, the annual series of morbidity rates (per 1,000 effectives) for STDs in the combined French forces of
Algeria–Tunisia, 1875–1929. Figure 10.2A shows the aggregate series for gonorrhoea, chancroid, and syphilis, while Figures 10.2B–D show the individual
series for the three sample diseases. For reference, Table 10.2 gives the average
annual morbidity rate for each disease over the 55 years.

---

[2] Although regular (annual) reports for the French Army began in 1862, categories of venereal disease
(gonorrhoea, chancroid, and syphilis) were not differentiated in the published statistics until 1875
(Hinrichsen, 1944: 768; Curtin, 1989: 5–6).

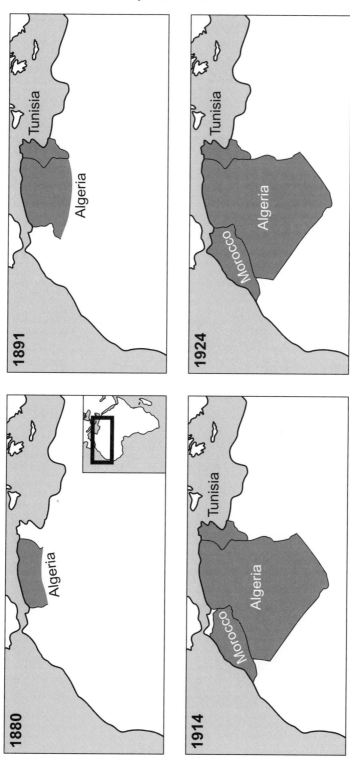

Fig. 10.1. Geographical expansion of French territories in North Africa, 1880–1924

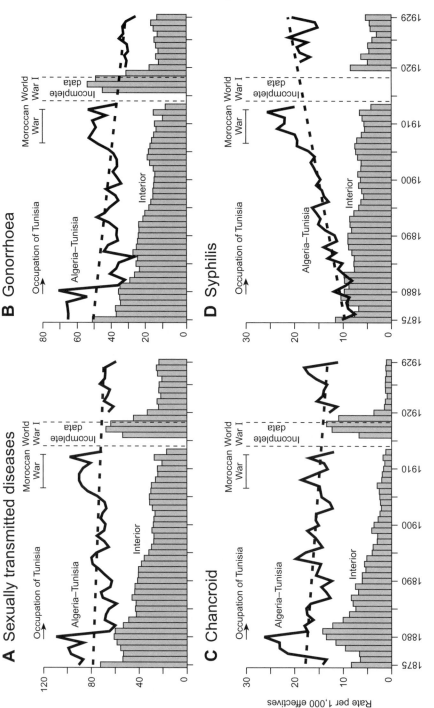

Fig. 10.2. Annual rate of sexually transmitted diseases (per 1,000 effectives) for French troops in Algeria–Tunisia, 1875–1929.

Notes: The heavy line traces plot the annual morbidity rate for French troops in Algeria–Tunisia. The 55-year linear trends are shown by pecked lines. For reference, the histograms plot the annual morbidity rate for troops in the French Interior. (A) Aggregate series for three sexually transmitted diseases (gonorrhoea, chancroid, and syphilis). (B) Gonorrhoea. (C) Chancroid. (D) Syphilis.

Source: Drawn from data in Ministère de la Guerre (1932, graphiques 78, 79, pp. 97, 100).

Table 10.2. Average annual morbidity rate (per 1,000 effectives) for three sexually transmitted diseases in French troops, 1875–1929

Disease	Mobidity rate (per 1,000 effectives)	
	France (Interior)	Algeria–Tunisia
Gonorrhoea	25.1	43.3
Chancroid	5.1	15.7
Syphilis	6.9	15.1
Total	37.1	74.1

Source: Based on data from Ministère de la Guerre (1932).

Aggregate series (Figure 10.2A). The solid line trace in Figure 10.2A depicts a relatively high (average annual rate = 74.1 cases per 1,000 effectives; see Table 10.2) and fluctuating rate of STD activity. From an early peak (109.0 cases per 1,000) at about the time of the French occupation of Tunisia (1880–1), the morbidity curve falls sharply. This is followed by a steady and progressive rise to a secondary peak (97.1 cases per 1,000) with the military activity that accompanied the Moroccan War (1907–12). While information for World War I and its immediate aftermath is lacking, the post-war period was associated with a reversion to the aggregate disease levels of the 1880s (60–70 cases per 1,000). The 55-year linear trend (pecked line) is slightly downwards.

Individual diseases (Figures 10.2B–D). As judged by the average annual morbidity rates in Table 10.2, gonorrhoea (43.3 cases per 1,000) was the most prevalent of the sample STDs to afflict French troops in Algeria–Tunisia. Rates for chancroid (15.7 cases per 1,000) and syphilis (15.1 cases per 1,000) were substantially lower and roughly equal. However, the line traces in Figures 10.2B–D show marked variations in the long-term trends of the three diseases. While gonorrhoea (Fig. 10.2B) followed the broad pattern of the aggregate series (Fig. 10.2A), chancroid (Fig. 10.2C) displayed a gradual reduction in the underlying level of reported activity in the 30 years to World War I. In contrast, syphilis (Fig. 10.2D) displayed a progressive rise from relatively low rates (<10 cases per 1,000) in the 1870s to relatively high rates (>20 cases per 1,000) in the period of the Moroccan War (1907–12). Thereafter, annual syphilis rates fell back to 15 to 20 cases per 1,000 in the wake of World War I.

COMPARISONS WITH THE FRENCH INTERIOR

One prominent feature of the historical pattern of STDs in European armies was the generally higher incidence of disease in overseas troops as compared with their counterparts in the interior (Hinrichsen, 1944, 1945*a*, 1945*b*; Curtin,

1989). For the French Army, some impression of this intrinsically geographical phenomenon can be gained from Figure 10.2 by comparing the STD rates for Algeria–Tunisia (line traces) with the corresponding rates for the French Interior (histograms). On all four graphs, STDs rates are universally higher in Algeria–Tunisia than in the French Interior, with visual evidence of a growing disparity over the observation period.

To examine this latter feature, Figure 10.3 invokes the principles of Curtin's (1989) concept of *relocation costs* by plotting, for each disease category in Figure 10.2, the annual series of STD morbidity rates (per 1,000 effectives) for Algeria–Tunisia (R_O) and the French Interior (R_E) as the ratio

$$R_O/R_E. \tag{10.1}$$

In the interpretation of Figure 10.3, ratio values in excess of 1.0 (marked by the horizontal line) indicate a higher morbidity rate in Algeria–Tunisia than the French Interior, while values less than 1.0 indicate a lower morbidity rate.

Figure 10.3 illustrates a secular increase in the ratios of STD rates, thereby confirming the long-term temporal divergence of disease levels in Algeria–Tunisia and the French Interior. The pattern is most striking for chancroid, with an inexorable rise of the ratio from approximately 2 : 1 in the 1880s to 11 : 1 in the period immediately preceding World War I, on to a peak of 17 : 1 during the Rif War (1919–26). The remaining curves in Figure 10.3 are characterized by more modest increases in the period to World War I, with variable experiences thereafter. When read in conjunction with Figure 10.2, the overall pattern in Figure 10.3 implies that STD control efforts were singularly more successful in the French Interior than in the commands of Algeria–Tunisia during the half century from 1875 (Hinrichsen, 1944).

BIPROPORTIONATE SCORES

An alternative way to examine temporal patterns of STD activity in Algeria–Tunisia and the French Interior is to analyse the 55 (year) × 3 (disease) matrices of annual morbidity rates by the method of biproportionate scores. The method is described in Appendix 5A but, for a given geographical location, biproportionate scores permit an assessment of *relative* changes in levels of each disease over time. The results of the computational procedure are summarized in Figure 10.4 for Algeria–Tunisia (line traces) and the French Interior (histograms). Here, the scores have been scaled to a base of 100; scores above 100 mark a relative excess of gonorrhoea (Fig. 10.4A), chancroid (Fig. 10.4B) and syphilis (Fig. 10.4C) in time while scores below 100 mark a relative deficit.

Notwithstanding the differential patterns of disease activity implied by Figure 10.3, Figure 10.4 depicts common trends in the changing relative importance of sample STDs in Algeria–Tunisia and the French Interior: (i) the progressive reduction in chancroid in the 30 years to World War I (Fig. 10.4B);

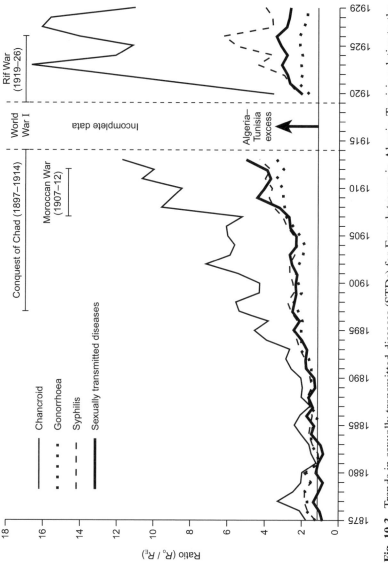

Fig. 10.3. Trends in sexually transmitted diseases (STDs) for French troops in Algeria–Tunisia relative to the French Interior, 1875–1929

Notes: For each of four disease categories (gonorrhoea, chancroid, syphilis, and the three diseases combined), the line traces plot the annual morbidity rates (per 1,000 effectives) for Algeria–Tunisia (R_o) and the French Interior (R_E) as a ratio, R_o/R_E. Ratio values in excess of 1.0 indicate a higher morbidity rate in Algeria–Tunisia than the French Interior, while values less than 1.0 indicate a lower morbidity rate. Periods of conflict that involved French troops stationed in Algeria–Tunisia are marked for reference.

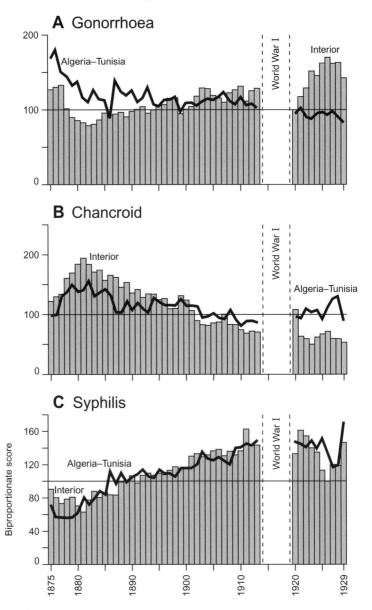

Fig. 10.4. Biproportionate scores for sexually transmitted diseases in French troops stationed in Algeria–Tunisia and the French Interior, 1875–1929

Notes: The charts plot, on an annual basis, the temporal concentration of sample diseases among French troops in Algeria–Tunisia (line traces) and the French Interior (bar charts). For a given geographical location, scores > 100 (indicated by the horizontal lines) mark a relative excess of the corresponding disease in time, while scores < 100 mark a relative deficit. (A) Gonorrhoea. (B) Chancroid. (C) Syphilis.

and (ii) the progressive increase in syphilis during the 50 years to 1929 (Fig. 10.4C). In contrast, opposing trends of increasing (French Interior) and decreasing (Algeria–Tunisia) relative importance are identified for gonorrhoea (Fig. 10.4A).

10.2.2 Summary

Our examination of patterns of STD activity in the French Army in Algeria–Tunisia, 1875–1929, has shown that:

(1) in the aggregate, reported rates of STDs increased steadily and progressively between the occupation of Tunisia (1880–1) and the Moroccan War (1907–12), but reduced in the period following World War I;

(2) while gonorrhoea followed the aggregate pattern (1), other sample STDs were characterized by a marginal reduction (chancroid) and a progressive increase (syphilis) over the observation period;

(3) consistent with the study of Curtin (1989), levels of STD activity were considerably higher for troops in Algeria–Tunisia than for their counterparts in the French Interior. The between-location differences widened over the observation period, implying that ongoing military efforts at STD control were singularly more successful in the French Interior than in the sample commands of North Africa (Hinrichsen, 1945*b*: 229–30);

(4) notwithstanding findings (1)–(3), Algeria–Tunisia and the French Interior shared a common trend in the changing relative importance of chancroid (decreasing importance) and syphilis (increasing importance). Opposing trends of decreasing (Algeria–Tunisia) and increasing (French Interior) relative importance were identified for gonorrhoea.

10.3 Sexually Transmitted Diseases in World War II

Initiated by Mussolini's strike on Anglo-Egyptian Sudan in July 1940, followed swiftly by Italian incursions in Kenya, the occupation of British Somaliland and, in the latter months of the same year, the Axis advance on Egypt, Africa was drawn piecemeal into World War II (Keegan, 1989: 320). The loci of subsequent military engagements on the continent extended across two vast battlegrounds (East Africa and North Africa), with additional duties of the Allied Army formed to include parts of Central, West, and Southern Africa. In this section, we examine the occurrence of STDs among deployed forces in Africa and related commands during the course of the hostilities. We begin, in Section 10.3.1, with an examination of gonococcal infections, chancroid, and syphilis in the US contingent of the Allied Army stationed in the Mediterranean and Africa–Middle East Theatres, 1942–5. Throughout the period of the war, delegates of the International Committee of the Red Cross (ICRC) submitted reports of the health and living conditions that prevailed in prisoner-of-war (POW) camps around the world. Drawing on the evidence of the ICRC delegates, Section 10.3.2 briefly reviews the occurrence of STDs among Axis prisoners held in the POW camps of North and East/Southern Africa.

10.3.1 US Soldiers in the Mediterranean and Africa–Middle East Theatres

We preface our examination of STDs among US soldiers with a note on the data available for geographical analysis. For the purposes of US military activities in World War II, Africa fell within two theatres of operations (Mediterranean and Africa–Middle East Theatres), both of which extended to include non-African localities. As the theatre of operations forms the basic spatial unit for which disease data are collated for the US Army (Medical Department, United States Army, 1960; Reister, 1976), the Mediterranean and Africa–Middle East Theatres are taken as the geographical points of reference in the following analysis.

HISTORICAL CONTEXT: STDS IN THE US ARMY

Trends to World War II

Reported rates of venereal disease in the US Army had fallen to an historic low in the period immediately preceding World War II (Fig. 10.5). After a century of towering wartime peaks in STD activity, set against a high and fluctuating background disease rate, early twentieth-century measures of STD control began to pay dividends. Between 1912 and 1914, a series of General Orders decreed that periods of service lost on account of diseases arising from drugs, alcohol, or 'misconduct' would result in the forfeiture of pay of the officers and enlisted men concerned. Compulsory prophylaxis following illicit sexual intercourse, with penalty of trial under court martial for failure to comply, was instituted under the same set of orders, while a physical examination was also introduced into the monthly regimen of the Army. With the issuing of further articles and regulations for venereal disease control in the aftermath of World War I,[3] the recorded annual STD rate in the US Army began to decline in the 1920s to an unprecedented low of 29.6 cases per 1,000 strength by 1939 (Pappas, 1943; Hinrichsen, 1944).

The Impact of World War II

The onset of World War II was associated with a marked resurgence of STD activity in the Army. For the period of US military engagement in the war,

---

[3] Relevant regulations and Articles of War are reviewed by Pappas (1943) and included: the making up of 'bad time' on account of disease acquired through the misconduct of enlisted men (article *A. W. 107*); forfeiture of pay by STD patients (regulation *A. R. 35-1440*); physical inspections (regulation *A. R. 615-250*); and the implementation of general and special preventive measures for STDs (including prophylaxis, the suppression of prostitution, and cooperation with civil agencies) (regulation *A. R. 40-210*).

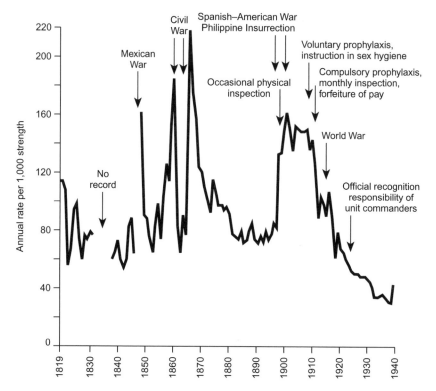

Fig. 10.5. Annual rate (per 1,000 strength) of sexually transmitted diseases in the US Army to World War II, 1819–1940

Notes: Periods of military engagement are indicated, along with major developments in the US Army's response to sexually transmitted diseases and their control.
Source: Redrawn from Pappas (1943, fig. 1, p. 174).

1942–5, the left-hand columns of Table 10.3 give the ten leading disease-related causes of hospital admissions in the entire US Army (all stations). All told, the US Army recorded a fraction under 3 million disease-related admissions, of which gonococcal infections (rank 1; 844,872 admissions), syphilis (rank 3; 288,735 admissions), and chancroid (rank 10; 94,049 admissions) accounted for over 41 per cent of the disease burden. To these recorded cases of STDs can be added many tens of thousands who, through means of concealment or otherwise, were never admitted to hospital or carded for record (Medical Department, United States Army, 1960: 469).

WORLD WAR II: US TROOPS IN AFRICA AND RELATED COMMANDS

Venereal disease proved an especial problem among US troops stationed in Africa and related commands. As described by Sternberg *et al.* (1960) and Wiltse (1965), part of the problem rested with the very high background levels

Table 10.3. Leading causes of disease-related admissions in the US Army, 1942–1945

Rank	All stations[1]		Mediterranean		Africa–Middle East	
	Disease	Admissions[2]	Disease	Admissions[2]	Disease	Admissions[2]
1	**Gonococcal infections**	844,872 (28.47)	**Gonococcal infections**	93,424 (30.33)	Malaria	10,255 (31.28)
2	Malaria	403,689 (13.60)	Malaria	75,337 (24.46)	Dysentery	4,322 (13.18)
3	**Syphilis**	288,735 (9.73)	**Chancroid**	31,260 (10.16)	**Gonococcal infections**	3,721 (11.35)
4	Influenza	188,225 (6.34)	**Syphilis**	20,227 (6.56)	Virus infections[3]	3,513 (10.71)
5	German measles	134,159 (4.52)	Hepatitis	18,400 (5.96)	**Chancroid**	2,727 (8.32)
6	Hepatitis	109,695 (3.70)	Influenza	15,367 (4.96)	**Syphilis**	1,837 (5.60)
7	Mumps	101,854 (3.43)	Dysentery	10,819 (3.56)	Influenza	1,047 (3.19)
8	Spirochetal infections[3]	101,194 (3.41)	Scabies	8,195 (2.66)	Sandfly fever	970 (2.96)
9	Scabies	99,954 (3.37)	Sandfly fever	7,255 (2.36)	Hepatitis	659 (2.01)
10	**Chancroid**	94,049 (3.17)	Virus infections[3]	4,551 (1.46)	Food poisoning	520 (1.59)
	Total disease admissions	2,967,461	Total disease admissions	308,050	Total disease admissions	32,788

Notes: [1] Continental United States, Europe, Mediterranean, Africa–Middle East, China–Burma–India, Southwest Pacific, Pacific Ocean Areas, North America, and Latin America. [2] Disease as a percentage proportion of all disease-related admissions is given in parentheses. [3] Uncategorized.
Source: Data from Reister (1976).

of STDs in the native populations. In some areas of the Africa–Middle East Theatre, for example, Army medical officers estimated that approximately 100 per cent of women with whom soldiers came into contact had at least one STD (Wiltse, 1965: 92). Factors other than the high background level of STDs, however, also contributed to the military problem of venereal disease in the region. So, in addition to the more general issue of the 'moral laxness' of troops in overseas stations (Wiltse, 1965: 92), Sternberg *et al.* (1960) highlight both (i) the initial failure of commands to comprehend the scientific principles of STD control and (ii) the associated difficulties of coordinating effective STD programmes at the military–civilian interface.

Patterns, I: Inter-theatre Comparisons

To examine patterns of STD activity among US soldiers in Africa and related commands, we draw on the monthly estimates of US Army hospital admissions, January 1942–December 1945, for gonococcal infections, chancroid, and syphilis included in Reister's *Medical Statistics in World War II* (1976). Of the nine global divisions (eight theatres of operations[4] and the Continental United States) for which the US Army disease counts are available, two have been selected for analysis:

(1) *Mediterranean Theatre*, embracing North Africa (Algeria, Morocco, and Tunisia) in the period prior to the Sicilian Campaign (June–Aug. 1943), thereafter extending to include Austria, the Balkan States, and Italy;

(2) *Africa–Middle East Theatre*, embracing Central Africa, West Africa (including Gold Coast, Nigeria, Liberia, Senegal), and East Africa (including Egypt, Anglo-Egyptian Sudan, Libya), along with Iran and the Persian Gulf.

The locations of the Mediterranean and Africa–Middle East Theatres within the global division of US military operations are mapped in Figure 10.6, while Table 10.3 gives the ten leading causes of hospital admissions in the two sample theatres. Here, we note that caution must be exercised in the interpretation of the available STD statistics. In particular, the US Army Medical Department emphasizes that, owing to clandestine medical treatment within or beyond military facilities, many cases of STDs were never included in the official disease records of the Army (Medical Department, United States Army, 1960: 469). Our analysis proceeds subject to this data caveat.

Box and whisker plots. Figure 10.7 shows box and whisker plots (Tukey, 1977) for each of the three sample STDs (gonococcal infections, chancroid, and syphilis) in the Mediterranean and Africa–Middle East Theatres (dark-shaded boxes). For the purposes of comparison, the equivalent plots for the six other

---

[4] Europe, Mediterranean, Africa–Middle East, China–Burma–India, Southwest Pacific, Pacific Ocean, North America, and Latin America.

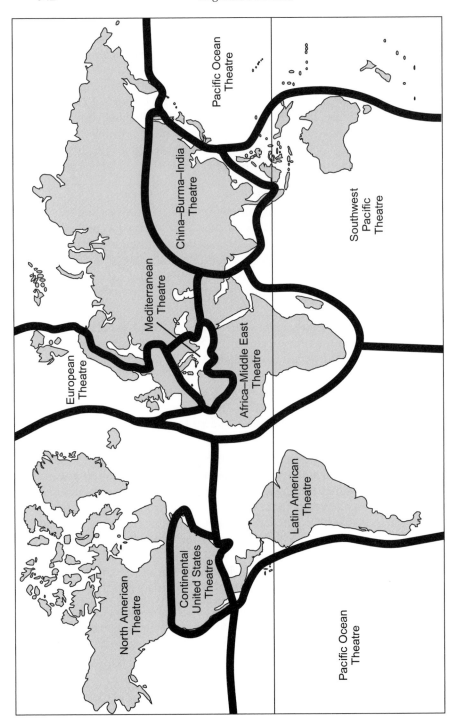

Fig. 10.6. Theatres of operations of the US Army, 1942–1945

Source: Based on information in Reister (1976: 57).

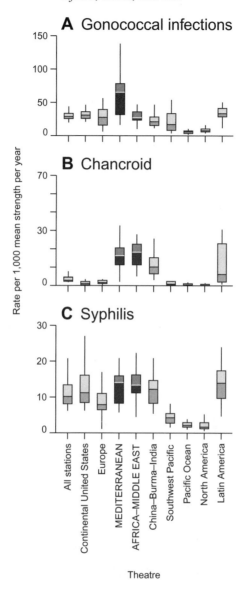

Fig. 10.7. Geographical variations in sexually transmitted disease (STD) rates in the US Army, 1942–1945

Notes: Box and whisker plots show the monthly distribution of admissions rates (per 1,000 mean strength per year) for the US Army as a whole, for the Continental United States, and for eight theatres of operations (Europe, Mediterranean, Africa–Middle East, China–Burma–India, Southwest Pacific, Pacific Ocean, North America, and Latin America). Theatres are mapped in Fig. 10.6. (A) Gonococcal infections. (B) Chancroid. (C) Syphilis. Plotting conventions for box and whisker plots are given in the text. The plots relating to the Mediterranean and Africa–Middle East Theatres have been highlighted by the darker shading categories.

theatres of operations (Europe, China–Burma–India, Southwest Pacific, Pacific Ocean, North America, and Latin America), the Continental United States, and all US Army stations are also given (light-shaded boxes). Each plot has been formed to show the distribution of monthly hospital admission rates (expressed per 1,000 mean strength per year) for a given disease and geographical unit in the period, January 1942–December 1945. The horizontal line in each box gives the median monthly admissions rate over the four-year observation period. The variability in the monthly values is shown by plotting, as the outer limits of the shaded box, the first and third quartiles, Q_1 and Q_3, of the values. The whiskers extend from the box edges to encompass all monthly values that satisfy the following limits:

Lower limit: $Q_1 - 1.5(Q_3 - Q_1)$;
Upper limit: $Q_3 + 1.5(Q_3 - Q_1)$.

Finally, the open circles denote outliers beyond these limits.

One striking feature of Figure 10.7 is the prominence of STDs in the Mediterranean and Africa–Middle East Theatres relative to other geographical divisions. The evidence is especially marked for gonococcal infections in the Mediterranean Theatre (Fig. 10.7A) and chancroid in the Mediterranean and Africa–Middle East Theatres (Fig. 10.7B), with the patterns highlighted by (i) the inflated values of the median rates (horizontal lines) and (ii) the raised positions of the interquartile ranges (boxes). The evidence is less striking for syphilis where, with the notable exceptions of the Southwest Pacific, Pacific Ocean, and North American Theatres, a more equable pattern is identified across the set of units. Two further features of Figure 10.7 are also noteworthy:

(1) the interquartile ranges, denoted by the upper and lower edges of the boxes, are indicative of a relatively high degree of variability in the monthly rates of gonococcal infections (Europe, Mediterranean, and Southwest Pacific), chancroid (Mediterranean, Africa–Middle East, China–Burma–India, and Latin America), and syphilis (Continental United States, Europe, Mediterranean, Africa–Middle East, China–Burma–India, Latin America). In accounting for such variability, we note here the historical tendency for STD rates in deployed armies to vary inversely with levels of combat and field activity (Berg, 1984);

(2) the Pacific Ocean and North American Theatres are characterized by very low levels of activity for all three STDs, with similarly low rates for two diseases (chancroid and syphilis) in the Southwest Pacific.

Patterns, II: Trends in Time

The dark-shaded box and whisker plots in Figure 10.8 show, by disease and year, the distribution of monthly STD admissions rates for the US Army in the Mediterranean (Figs. 10.8A–C) and Africa–Middle East (Figs. 10.8D–F) Theatres, 1942–5. For reference, the light-shaded boxes on each chart give the

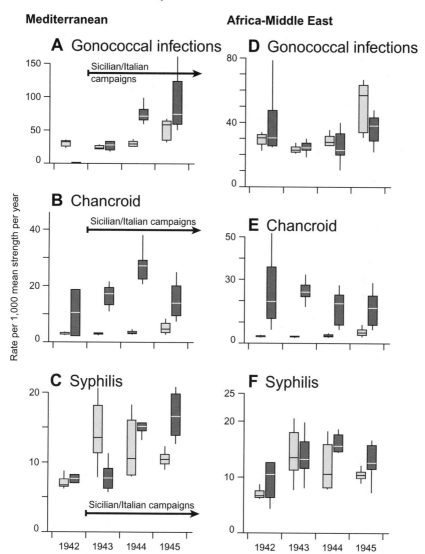

Fig. 10.8. Time trends in sexually transmitted disease (STD) rates for US Army forces stationed in the Mediterranean and Africa–Middle East Theatres, 1942–1945

Notes: For each year, the dark-shaded box and whisker plots show the monthly distribution of admissions rates (per 1,000 mean strength per year) for sample diseases (gonococcal infections, chancroid, and syphilis) in the Mediterranean Theatre (charts A–C) and the Africa–Middle East Theatre (charts D–F). For reference, the light-shaded box and whisker plots on each chart show the corresponding information for the entire US Army (all stations). Plotting conventions for box and whisker plots are given in the text.

corresponding information for the entire US Army. We consider the evidence for the Mediterranean and Africa–Middle East Theatres in turn.

Mediterranean (Figures 10.8A–C). As judged by the median disease rates (horizontal bars), one marked feature of Figures 10.8A–C is the general tendency for STD rates in the Mediterranean Theatre to increase over the years 1942–4. This period of increasing disease activity corresponds broadly with a geographical extension of the locus of campaigns from North Africa (Nov. 1942–May 1943) to Sicily (May–Aug. 1943) and Italy (Aug. 1943–May 1945). With the end of the Italian Campaign and the cessation of hostilities, the latter months of 1945 were accompanied by a surge in STD activity (especially gonococcal infections) and this is reflected in the large variability of monthly rates (boxes) for 1945 as compared with preceding years.

Africa–Middle East (Figures 10.8D–F). A rather more complex pattern emerges for the Africa–Middle East Theatre in Figures 10.8E–F. As compared with the Mediterranean Theatre, the median disease rates (horizontal bars) for gonococcal infections (Fig. 10.8D) and chancroid (Fig. 10.8E) were characterized by relative stability over the observation period. In contrast, syphilis (Fig. 10.8F) displayed an increase over the years 1942–4, but fell modestly in the final year of the series.

While between-theatre differences in patterns of STD activity are apparent from Figure 10.8, a common feature also emerges: the importance of chancroid in the Mediterranean and Africa–Middle East Theatres *vis-à-vis* the US Army as a whole (Figs. 10.8B, 10.8E).

Conclusion. Commenting on the occurrence of STDs in the US Army during World War II, the Army Medical Department summarized the evidence in the following manner: 'it can be stated very simply that the lowest venereal disease rates in the US Army occurred during 1943 and that the rates began to rise in 1944, further increased in 1945, and showed marked increases after the cessation of hostilites' (Medical Department, United States Army, 1960: 470). While Figure 10.8 confirms that the Mediterranean Theatre followed this Army-wide pattern, the Africa–Middle East Theatre displayed a relative stability in the year-to-year incidence of two (gonococcal infections and chancroid) of the three sample diseases. Such varying experiences in the Mediterranean and Africa–Middle East Theatres underscore the role of theatre-level factors—including campaigns, exposures, and disease-control efforts—in the observed pattern of STD incidence (Carson and Johnson, 1973).

STD TREATMENT AND CONTROL

In overseas commands such as the Mediterranean and Africa–Middle East Theatres, control of STDs in the US Army was largely dependent on a series of internal mechanisms including: the education of officers and men; the provision of sports, recreational, and 'morale-building' activities; the provision of prophylaxis and treatment; disciplinary action (including forfeiture of pay[5]); and the delegation of responsibility for STD control on commanding officers (Pappas, 1943; Sternberg *et al.*, 1960). Alongside these internal mechanisms, external mechanisms of prostitute control were also implemented. In Casablanca, North Africa, for example, the native quarters of Medinas (which included all the established houses of prostitution) were placed off limits to military personnel for most of the period of US occupation (Sternberg *et al.*, 1960: 208). Elsewhere, in Oran and Algiers, Algeria, US troops were directed to selected brothels in which prophylactic stations were established (Sternberg *et al.*, 1960: 210) while, in Liberia, West Africa, 'tolerated women's villages' were established near US barracks (Wiltse, 1965: 64). But it was the advent of antibiotic therapy (penicillin was first used in the military treatment of gonorrhoea and syphilis in 1943) which had the most dramatic implications for the military management of STDs. By 1945, the average time lost for a hospital admission in the US Army had fallen to six days (gonorrhoea) and 18 days (syphilis), with a corresponding increase in the outpatient treatment of the two diseases (Medical Department, United States Army, 1960: 470; Berg, 1984).

10.3.2 Axis Prisoners

The military problem of STDs in Africa extended beyond the free fighting forces to include detainees in prisoner of war (POW) camps. Table 10.4, which is based on information gathered by delegates of the International Committee of the Red Cross (ICRC), summarizes evidence regarding the occurrence of STDs among Axis prisoners in POW camps of North and East/Southern Africa, 1940–6 (ICRC, 1950; see Pl. 1.2L). Although the information is fragmentary, an extract from ICRC evidence relating to Axis (primarily Italian) POWs in Rhodesia, 1942–4, is illustrative of the general situation:

In 1942: 70 gonorrhoea and 300 syphilis . . .

In 1943: 20 gonorrhoea and about 150 syphilis . . . In August, Fort Victoria Camp still had over 110 cases of chronic syphilis (one retinitis) . . .

In 1944, 71 gonorrhoeas were treated in hospital (anti-gonococcal serum), of whom 3 were fresh. Records showed 900 syphilitics, including 208 primary, 213 secondary, 4 tertiary and 1 inguinal adenitis . . . (ICRC, 1950: 31)

Table 10.4 suggests that the Rhodesian experience was replicated in POW camps across East, Southern, and North Africa during the course of World War II.

---

[5] The pay stoppage law was rescinded by Congress in September 1944. See Berg (1984: 96).

Table 10.4. Sexually transmitted diseases among Axis prisoners of war in Africa, 1940–1946, based on sample evidence from the International Committee of the Red Cross (ICRC)

Location/country	Date	Group	Notes
North Africa			
Algeria	1942–6	German and Italian POWs	Five cases of blenorrhagia; no reported syphilis
Libya	?	Italian POWs attached to 72nd Pioneer Group	32 cases of STDs
Libya	1944	Camp for Italian POWs	51 cases of syphilis
Morocco	?	Italian POWs in French camp	10 of 16 patients had STDs
East/Southern Africa			
Eritrea	1944	Camp for Italian POWs	12 cases of syphilis
Kenya	1942	Camp for Italian POWs	30–5% of sick were syphilitic (few primary cases)
Kenya	1943	Italian (and German?) POWs	3,500 cases of STDs in six camps and one hospital
Kenya	?	Camp No. 365	20–5% of men were syphilitic
Rhodesia	1940	POWs from Abyssinia	70 cases of gonorrhoea, 300 cases of syphilis
Rhodesia	1943	POW camp	20 cases of gonorrhoea, 150 cases of syphilis
Sudan (Anglo-Egyptian)	1944	POW camp hospital	350 cases of STDs
Tanganyika	1943	Camp for Italians	400 cases of syphilis treated

Source: Information abstracted from International Committee of the Red Cross (ICRC, 1950: 29–32).

10.4 Civil War and the Spread of HIV/AIDS in Central Africa

In Section 4.6, we noted that there was compelling evidence for the role of late-twentieth-century civil wars—and the deployed forces of national, liberation, and rebel armies—in the epidemic transmission of HIV/AIDS in Sub-Saharan Africa (Hankins *et al.*, 2002). For example, in the embattled states of Angola and Mozambique, serological studies from the late 1980s revealed inflated levels of HIV infection in military personnel and war-displaced civilian populations (Palha de Souza *et al.*, 1989; Santos-Ferreira *et al.*, 1990). Similarly, McCarthy *et al.* (1989) link the occurrence of HIV in Sudanese soildiers to military deployment in and around the rebel lands of southern Sudan while, in neighbouring Uganda, de Lalla *et al.* (1988) identify raised levels of HIV infection among soldiers in rural northern districts of the country.

The present section examines the role of civil war as a mechanism for the historical diffusion of HIV/AIDS in Uganda, Central Africa, during the decade that followed the overthrow of President Idi Amin in 1979 (Smallman-Raynor and Cliff, 1991; Smallman-Raynor *et al.*, 1992: 287–305). Our consideration begins, in Section 10.4.1, with a brief overview of the nature of HIV/AIDS. Both the conveyors responsible for the evolving geographical patterns of AIDS in Central Africa and the associated corridors of virus spread have been the subject of considerable speculation and research during the last 20 years (Smallman-Raynor *et al.*, 1992: 151–5). Framed by the existing evidence, Section 10.4.2 undertakes an analysis of three alternative hypotheses (*truck town hypothesis*, *migrant labour hypothesis*, and *civil war hypothesis*) advanced to account for the spatial distribution of reported AIDS cases in Uganda. Of the alternative hypotheses, it is shown that the spread of HIV infection in the 1980s, and the subsequent development of AIDS to its 1990 spatial pattern, were significantly and positively correlated with ethnic patterns of recruitment into the Ugandan Liberation Army (UNLA) in the immediate post-Amin period.

10.4.1 The Nature of HIV/AIDS

AIDS (ICD–10 B20–24), described in Appendix 10B, is one of the great emergent diseases of the late twentieth century. The Joint United Nations Programme on HIV/AIDS (UNAIDS) estimates that some 40 million people globally are infected by the causative agent, HIV (UNAIDS, 2002: 8). Yet it was only in 1979 that the first cases of AIDS were officially notified and it was not until the mid-1980s that the two principal strains of HIV (HIV-1 and HIV-2)[6] had been isolated. Since that time, the starkest impact of HIV/AIDS has

---

[6] While HIV-1 is recognized as the virus associated with the global AIDS pandemic, the geographical distribution of HIV-2 is primarily restricted to parts of West and South Central Africa (see Smallman-Raynor *et al.*, 1992: 174–82).

been witnessed in Sub-Saharan Africa. The pioneering studies by Piot *et al.* (1984) and Van de Perre *et al.* (1984) were among the first to indicate the severity of the problem. Since then, the steady accumulation of epidemiological evidence has confirmed that parts of Southern and Central Africa rank among the most severely affected regions of the world. Although data from the continent are notoriously patchy, UNAIDS (2002) suggests that almost three-quarters of the world's 40 million cases of HIV/AIDS are located in Sub-Saharan Africa, with adult HIV infection rates of 25 per cent or more in the most severely affected countries.

THE NATURE OF AIDS AND HIV

First described in the United States in 1981 (Gottlieb *et al.*, 1981; Hymes *et al.*, 1981; Masur *et al.*, 1981; Siegal *et al.*, 1981), AIDS is a strictly defined and advanced stage of disease due to infection with HIV (Pl. 10.1). The condition arises as a result of the ability of HIV to target and destroy one central actor in the human immune system, the *CD*4 white blood cell. The immune system usually serves to safeguard the body against the invasion of disease-causing microorganisms such as bacteria, protozoa, and viruses. In AIDS, however, the immune system collapses and leaves the body open to potentially life-threatening opportunistic infections, the development of rare and unusually aggressive cancers, dementia, wasting, and other severe conditions. HIV itself is spread in three main ways: (i) by intimate hetero- or homosexual contact; (ii) parenterally; (iii) perinatally.

The relative importance of these three modes of HIV transmission varies by world region. Full details are given in Mann *et al.* (1988) and Piot *et al.* (1988) but, for the purposes of the present discussion, heterosexual and perinatal exposure form the predominant routes of HIV transmission in Sub-Saharan Africa. Parenteral exposure in both medical and cultural settings may also have played a part in the development of the HIV/AIDS epidemic in some parts of the region; see Appendix 10B.

10.4.2 AIDS and Civil War in Uganda

From 1982, the attention of medical personnel was drawn to the increasingly frequent reports of an apparently new disease afflicting residents of Rakai district in the rural southwest of Uganda (see Fig. 10.9 for location). The new illness was known colloquially as *slim* on account of the characteristic weight loss and wasting seen in the patients. But it was not until the latter months of 1984 when physicians, equipped with the newly developed HIV antibody test, confirmed that slim disease was a clinical manifestation of advanced HIV-1 infection (Serwadda *et al.*, 1985; Ankrah, 1989).

By the end of the 1980s, Uganda displayed the reported impact of AIDS in its most extreme form. Official estimates placed the number of HIV infections

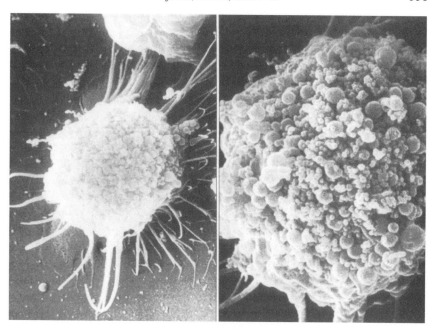

Pl. 10.1. Scanning electron microscopy of HIV-infected H9 cells

Notes: (Left) Overview of a virus producing cell at *c*.11,000 magnification. (Right) The same cell, *c*.22,000 magnification, shows virus particles on the cell surface.

Source: Reproduced from Cliff and Haggett (1988: 218); micrographs originally supplied by Dr Muhsin Özel, Robert Koch Institut, Berlin.

at 1 million (6% of the population) in February 1990 (AIDS Control Programme, Ugandan Ministry of Health, 1990), while the 12,444 reported AIDS cases at the same date probably under-represented the true clinical AIDS burden by an order of magnitude. Documented AIDS cases were approximately equally distributed between the sexes, with the predominant routes of HIV exposure in the country (heterosexual and perinatal transmission) giving rise to a bimodal distribution of disease activity in young adults (aged 20–39 years) and infants (aged <4 years).

SPATIAL PATTERNS TO 1990

Figure 10.9 is based on surveillance data collated by the AIDS Control Programme, Ugandan Ministry of Health (1990), and plots the cumulative reported AIDS case incidence rates per 100,000 for each district of Uganda by the end of 1989. The rates have been calculated by scaling the crude AIDS case levels (Table 10.5) by 1989 mid-point population estimates for each district generated from the 1980 Ugandan Census (Census Office, Uganda, 1982).

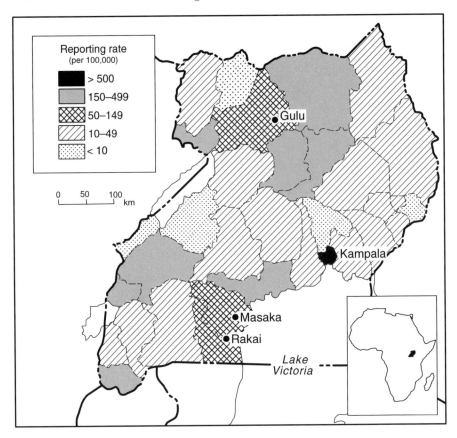

Fig. 10.9. Reported cumulative AIDS incidence rates (per 100,000 population) to February 1990 for 34 districts of residence of Ugandan AIDS cases

Source: Redrawn from Smallman-Raynor *et al.* (1992, fig. 8.2(G), p. 291).

Figure 10.9 shows that a distinct bipolar pattern underlay the Ugandan AIDS epidemic in the 1980s. The southern districts of Rakai, Masaka, and Kampala, situated along the shore of Lake Victoria, represented a primary focus of reported AIDS cases. In these districts, cumulative rates ranged between 167 and 517 per 100,000 population as compared with the national rate of 75 per 100,000. In the north of Uganda, a secondary focus of high AIDS incidence (255 per 100,000) was centred on Gulu and neighbouring districts. In most other districts, incidence rates fell below 50 per 100,000.

Data Quality

We recognize that the disease pattern observed in Figure 10.9 partly reflects geographical variations in AIDS case reporting completeness in Uganda.

Table 10.5. Reported Ugandan AIDS cases to 28 February 1989 by district of residence

District	Cases	District	Cases
Apac	231	Lira	295
Arua	172	Luwero	178
Bundibugyo	9	Masaka	2,433
Bushenyi	112	Masindi	36
Gulu	822	Mbale	136
Hoima	19	Mbarara	341
Iganga	117	Moroto	98
Jinja	267	Moyo	9
Kabale	170	Mpigi	599
Kabarole	435	Mubende	158
Kalangala	7	Mukono	357
Kampala	3,335	Nebbi	251
Kamuli	29	Rakai	677
Kapchorwa	3	Rukungiri	55
Kasese	232	Soroti	84
Kitgum	216	Tororo	147
Kotido	39	Other	293
Kumi	82		

Source: Smallman-Raynor and Cliff (1991, table 1, p. 71), based on AIDS Control Programme, Ugandan Ministry of Health (1990).

Although the passive nature of the country's AIDS surveillance system precludes a systematic assessment of disease under-reporting (Berkley *et al.*, 1989), we note that geographical variations in the quality of AIDS data may arise from the spatially uneven provision of health-care services. In particular, reporting completeness is likely to be higher in major towns, such as Kampala, which have been foci of AIDS research. In addition, the place of residence of an AIDS cases is not necessarily the place of infection, especially given the long incubation period between primary HIV infection and the development of AIDS. However, despite these caveats, restricted analysis of HIV prevalence in healthy adult cohorts in different parts of the country broadly accords with the reported AIDS case distribution shown in Figure 10.9 (Carswell *et al.*, 1986; Carswell, 1987; de Lalla *et al.*, 1990; Wawer *et al.*, 1991).

EXPLANATORY HYPOTHESES

Three principal hypotheses have been proposed to explain how the distinctive AIDS pattern in Figure 10.9 may have evolved:

   (1) The *truck town hypothesis* (Wood, 1988). This hypothesis proposes that the geographical distibution of HIV and AIDS reflects a diffusion

process in which major roads have acted as the principal corridors of virus spread between urban areas and other proximal settlements.

(2) The *migrant labour hypothesis* (Hunt, 1989; Larson, 1990). Here, HIV is hypothesized to have diffused through a process of return migration from areas of labour demand in urban areas to areas of labour supply in rural districts.

(3) The *civil war hypothesis* (Smallman-Raynor and Cliff, 1991). Relatively little attention has been paid to the implications of the historical association between soldiers, prostitute contact, and the spread of sexually transmitted diseases for the diffusion of HIV in Central African countries such as Uganda which have experienced protracted periods of civil war (Willcox, 1946; Ongom, 1970; Berg, 1984). This association may be particularly important in a region where heterosexual intercourse is the predominant route of HIV exposure and where high HIV prevalences have been documented in female prostitutes (Quinn *et al.*, 1986; Fleming, 1988; N'Galy and Ryder, 1988). Accordingly, the civil war hypothesis proposes that the Ugandan military has been instrumental in the historical development of the AIDS pattern in Figure 10.9. In particular, given the long mean incubation period of eight to ten years for HIV (Costagliola *et al.*, 1990), it is hypothesized that the patterns of clinical disease to their 1990 distribution reflect an earlier historical diffusion of HIV associated with six years of civil war that followed the overthrow of Idi Amin in 1979.

REGRESSION ANALYSIS OF DIFFUSION HYPOTHESES

To test each hypothesis as an explanation of the disease pattern shown in Figure 10.9, variables have been assessed as follows.

Truck Town Hypothesis

Measures of the degree of urbanization of each district (absolute urban population levels, urban populations as a percentage proportion of total population, district population densities and growth rates) have been taken from the 1980 Census (Census Office, Uganda, 1982). Two of these measures are mapped in Figure 10.10. The vertical bars indicate the absolute size of the urban population of each district; the four-category choropleth shading shows this population as a percentage of the total district population.

It is evident from Figure 10.10 that, with the notable exception of Kampala district in the south, most districts have substantially fewer than 30,000 urban residents. The overwhelmingly rural nature of Uganda in 1980 is underscored by the fact that urban residents comprised 10 per cent or more of the population in only three districts.

The second component of the truck town hypothesis, the proximity of district urban populations to principal routeways, is illustrated in Figure 10.11.

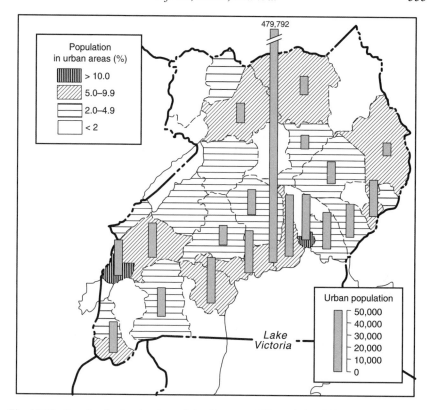

Fig. 10.10. Levels of urbanization of the districts of Uganda in 1980

Notes: Vertical bars indicate the absolute size of the urban population of each district. The four-category choropleth shading shows the absolute urban population size as a percentage proportion of the total district population.

Source: Redrawn from Smallman-Raynor *et al.* (1992, fig. 8.2(I), p. 294).

Here, the Ugandan road network is shown against a backcloth of district population densities per square mile. Four principal trade routeways can be defined (Herrick *et al.*, 1969) and these are indicated by the captial letters A, B, C, and D in the inset map to Figure 10.11:

(1) Road A: the west–east truck route linking the countries of Zaire, Rwanda, and Tanzania with the districts of southern Uganda and the Kenyan port of Mombassa. This road skirts the southern border of Uganda. It runs from Kabale to Masaka, follows the perimeter of Lake Victoria, and then continues east into Kenya for Mombasa;

(2) Road B: the truck route linking southeastern Uganda (Mbale) with the central and northern districts of Soroti, Lira, and Gulu;

(3) Road C: the road linking Kampala with Gulu via Masindi;

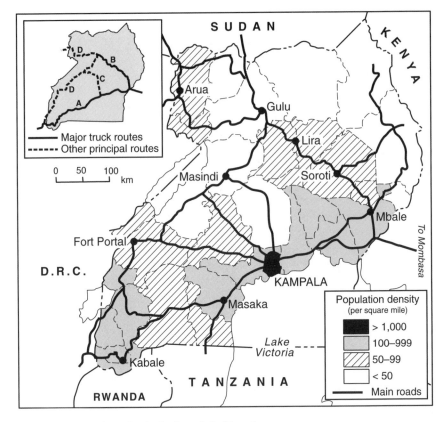

Fig. 10.11. Location of principal roads in Uganda

Notes: District population densities per square mile are indicated by the choropleth shading.
Source: Redrawn from Smallman-Raynor *et al.* (1992, Figure 8.2(J), p. 294).

(4) Road D: the road linking the Democratic Republic of Congo (Zaire)
with southwest Uganda, running via the western border of Uganda
from Arua in the northwest to Gulu, Masindi, Fort Portal, and on to
Kabale.

For the purposes of analysis, the proximity of a district to each of these major
roads was defined as the shortest distance from the geographical centroid of a
district to the highway.

Migrant Labour Hypothesis

Figure 10.12 shows principal labour source (labour reserve) and reception
(labour concentration) regions in Uganda as defined in the original formulation of the migrant labour hypothesis (Hunt, 1989). Labour source regions
include much of northern and southwestern Uganda, while principal labour

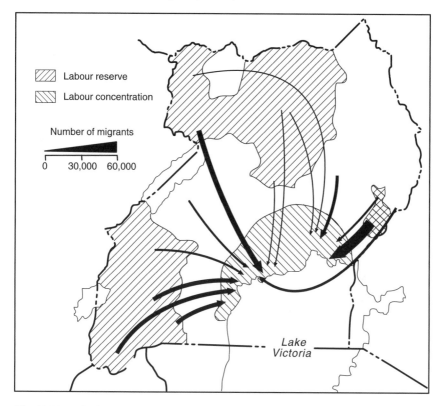

Fig. 10.12. Principal areas of labour supply and labour demand in Uganda

Notes: Vectors show inter-censal migration flows, 1959–69, upon which the original formulation of the hypothesis for migrant labour and the spread of AIDS in Uganda was based.
Source: Redrawn from Smallman-Raynor *et al.* (1992, fig. 8.2(K), p. 295).

reception regions encompass the southern districts situated along the shore of Lake Victoria. Based upon the migration data sources used by Hunt (1989), the vectors plot migration patterns over the 1960s.

In the regression analysis described below, source and reception districts were delimited by projecting Figure 10.12 onto a district base map of Uganda. Dummy variable techniques were then used to separate source and reception districts from other districts by coding such districts with a value of 1; all other districts were allocated a value of 0.

Civil War Hypothesis

To assess the hypothesis that the Uganda military has been instrumental in the development of the geographical pattern of AIDS in Figure 10.9, November

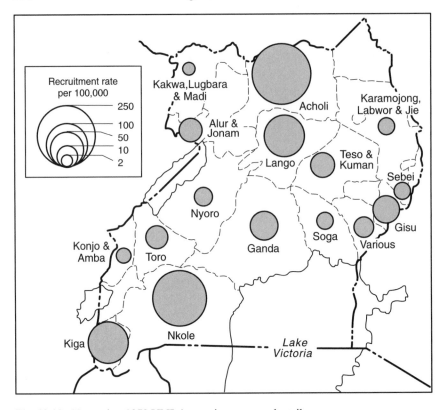

Fig. 10.13. November 1979 UNLA recruitment rates by tribe

Source: Redrawn from Smallman-Raynor *et al.* (1992, fig. 8.2(L), p. 295).

1979 ethnic recruitment levels into the Ugandan National Liberation Army (UNLA), taken as a measure of the ethnic composition of the army shortly after the overthrow of Idi Amin in March 1979, were extracted from Omara-Otunnu (1987). Recruitment rates per 100,000 population by major tribal groupings appear in Figure 10.13. As this indicates, UNLA recruitment rates varied greatly between tribes, ranging from 2.3 per 100,000 among the Kakwa, Lugabara, and Madi in the extreme northwest of the country to 250 per 100,000 among the neighbouring Acholi. High recruitment rates were also found among the Lango (77.7 per 100,000) in central Uganda and the Nkole (182.3) and Kiga (71.2) in the southwest. For all other tribes, recruitment rates fall below 30 per 100,000.

To estimate UNLA recruitment rates by district, the tribal rates shown in Figure 10.13 were projected onto a district base map and proportionally distributed into districts on the basis of district population size.

Regression Models

Each of the variables outlined above was entered as an explanatory (x) variable in a series of simple and multiple regression models in which AIDS case incidence rates formed the dependent (y) variable. Model fitting was by ordinary least squares; the sample size consisted of $n = 34$ districts. Because Kampala district (incidence rate 517 per 100,000) acted as an extreme outlier which heavily influenced model fitting, following Tukey (1962), the district was omitted from the analysis.

The main regression results are summarized in Table 10.6. The intercept and slope coefficients of each model are given, along with their associated t-statistics in parentheses. The coefficients of determination, R^2, and their F-ratios also appear. Statistically significant t and F values, using the $p = 0.05$ level (one-tailed test), are indicated by an asterisk.

Regression models 1 to 6 in Table 10.6 relate the truck town hypothesis to the disease pattern; models 1 to 4 examine the impact of urbanization while models 5 to 6 explore the association between AIDS reporting rates and district accessibility to the main highways. All these models were statistically insignificant as judged by the F-ratios. Table 10.6 confirms a similar result for regression model 7 which relates AIDS incidence to the migrant labour component.

In contrast, models 8 and 9 in Table 10.6, which relate UNLA ethnic recruitment rates to AIDS rates, display a markedly different picture. In model 8 there is a highly significant positive relationship between the two variables; 43.0 per cent of the variability in AIDS incidence rates is accounted for by recruitment patterns. In model 9, the two northern districts of Gulu and Kitgum which, with high levels of Acholi recruitment, served as outliers influencing parameter estimation in model 8, were omitted. As Table 10.6 shows, however, their omission had little impact and a highly significant overall explanation was maintained ($R^2 = 0.41$).

Regression Residuals

The residuals from model 8 in Table 10.6 have been plotted in Figure 10.14. Districts with AIDS rates underestimated by the fitted model (positive residuals) have been shaded black; districts with overestimated AIDS rates (negative residuals) have been left unshaded. Since positive autocorrelation in regression models will inflate the statistical parameters (t, F, and R^2) of a regression model, the residual pattern in Figure 10.14 was tested for spatial autocorrelation (Cliff and Ord, 1981; see App. 6A.1) to yield a standard Normal score (z score) of −0.26; this is non-significant at conventional levels. The test yielded a similar result for the residuals from regression model 9 ($z = −0.32$).

The spatially random patterns formed by the residuals from these regressions imply that the recruitment rate variable accounts for all the systematic spatial variation in AIDS incidence rates at the district level, despite the

Table 10.6. Regression results for tests of hypotheses to explain geographical patterns of AIDS in Uganda

Model	Intercept[1]	Slope coefficients for independent variables[1]											R^2 (F-ratio)
		x_1	x_2	x_3	x_4	x_5	x_6	x_7	x_8	x_9	x_{10}	x_{11}	
1	31.80 (1.71)	4.80 (1.43)											0.063 (2.03)
2	48.60 (19.94)*		0.04 (1.10)										0.002 (0.77)
3	30.60 (1.62)			0.001 (1.56)									0.075 (2.44)
4	59.40 (1.79)*				−2.50 (−0.23)								0.002 (0.05)
5	50.30 (1.72)*					−0.02 (−0.12)	0.02 (0.25)						0.004 (0.06)
6	10.30 (0.15)					4.63 (0.28)	0.17 (0.77)	0.08 (0.51)	−0.33 (−1.80)*				0.174 (1.09)
7	31.40 (1.46)									23.80 (0.84)	42.30 (1.31)		0.057 (0.88)
8	21.90 (1.96)*											0.60 (4.79)*	0.430 (22.95)*
9[2]	19.90 (1.94)*											0.68 (4.39)*	0.410 (19.29)*

Independent variables:
x_1 = Percentage of district population living in urban centres (Fig. 10.10)
x_2 = 1980 population density per square m. (Fig. 10.11)
x_3 = Absolute urban population size (Fig. 10.10)
x_4 = 1969–80 annual percentage population growth rate
x_5 = Distance from road A (see text and Fig. 10.11)
x_6 = Distance from road B (see text and Fig. 10.11)
x_7 = Distance from road C (see text and Fig. 10.11)
x_8 = Distance from road D (see text and Fig. 10.11)
x_9 = Regions of labour out-migration (see Fig. 10.12)
x_{10} = Regions of labour in-migration (see Fig. 10.12)
x_{11} = Nov. 1979 UNLA recruitment rates per 100,000 population (see Fig. 10.13).

Notes: * Significant at $p = 0.05$ level (one-tailed test). [1] Student's t-statistics in parentheses. [2] Gulu and Kitgum omitted.
Source: Smallman-Raynor *et al.* (1992, table 8.2.1, p. 297).

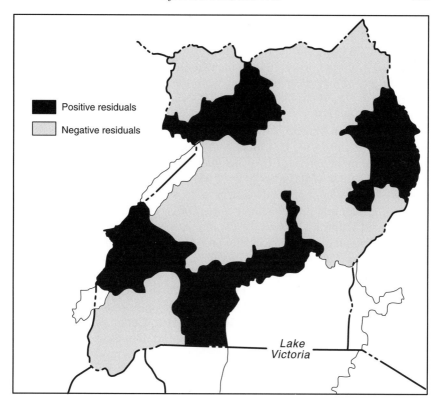

Fig. 10.14. Pattern of regression residuals associated with model 8 in Table 10.6
Source: Redrawn from Smallman-Raynor *et al.* (1992, fig. 8.2(M), p. 296).

relatively modest values for R^2. The outstanding variability may reflect as yet unreported factors that have influenced the evolution of the AIDS pattern in Uganda. However, since omission of a significant explanatory variable in a regression using geographically located data usually gives rise to spatially auto-correlated regression residuals (Cliff and Ord, 1981: 197–228), the lack of autocorrelation in the residuals of model 8 may imply that the residual vari-ability in AIDS rates is associated with data quality factors rather than unknown causal mechanisms.

DISCUSSION: UNLA, WAR, AND AIDS

The analysis presented in Table 10.6 suggests that both the truck town hypoth-esis and the migrant labour hypothesis fail to explain the district-to-district variability in AIDS incidence in Uganda. This may be a function of the quality of Ugandan AIDS surveillance data. For example, serological studies from the late 1980s indicated that major roads were acting as principal corridors for the spread of HIV in Central Africa in general (Mohammed Ali *et al.*, 1990) and Uganda in particular (Carswell, 1987; Carswell *et al.*, 1989; Wawer *et al.*, 1991). But given the observed long incubation period between primary HIV infection and the development of clinical disease, geographical patterns of AIDS seen in Uganda to the start of the 1990s will partly reflect the earlier historical spread of HIV.

The association between UNLA and the spatial distribution of reported AIDS cases is supported by observations regarding soldiers, prostitute contact, and war in the spread of HIV in Sudan, the country abutting the northern border of Uganda (McCarthy *et al.*, 1989). The findings also accord with reports of high rates of HIV infection in soldiers in Angola (Santos-Ferreira *et al.*, 1990), Mozambique (Newman *et al.*, 2001), and Zimbabwe (Bureau of Hygiene and Tropical Diseases, 1990), and with the correlation between war-associated population displacement and HIV infection in parts of Sub-Saharan Africa (Palha de Sousa *et al.*, 1989). Also noteworthy is the impact of recent hostilities on the spread of HIV in Central America (Chelala, 1990; Low *et al.*, 1990), the evidence of HIV infection in former European soldiers deployed during the wars of Portuguese Africa (Saimot *et al.*, 1987; Bryceson *et al.*, 1988; Botas *et al.*, 1989) and HIV infection in Cuban soldiers returning from Angola (Bureau of Hygiene and Tropical Diseases, 1989). Within Uganda itself, the findings are supported both by formal reports of high HIV prevalences among northern soldiers (de Lalla *et al.*, 1988) and by anecdotal evidence (Hooper, 1990).

Thus it appears that the reported geographical pattern of clinical AIDS in Uganda partly reflects the diffusion of HIV associated with civil war during the first six years of the post-Amin period. In particular, the association between 1979 UNLA recruitment patterns and the spatial distribution of documented AIDS cases in the mid-to-late 1980s accords with the estimated mean incubation period of eight to ten years for HIV-1 (Costagliola *et al.*, 1990). The twin foci of high rates of reported clinical AIDS cases mapped in Figure 10.9 may be explained by the deployment of soldiers, predominantly of northern origin, in southern districts of the country where HIV was spreading unnoticed in the late 1970s and early 1980s. Carriage of HIV from the south to the north both accords with evidence regarding the time of appearance of HIV in north and south Uganda (Serwadda *et al.*, 1985; de Lalla *et al.*, 1988) and explains why other regions of Uganda remained apparently relatively unaffected by the disease during the 1980s.

10.5 Conclusion

In this chapter, we have explored aspects of the military-related spread of STDs in Africa over 125 years from 1875. Our consideration began with an examination of long-term disease trends in the French Army in Algeria–Tunisia for a half-century period to the 1920s. While each of the three diseases examined (gonorrhoea, chancroid, and syphilis) displayed a marked increase in incidence during the periodic wars that punctuated the observation period, the longer-term underlying trends in disease activity were found to vary from one disease to another. When compared to the experience of troops in the French Interior, however, a common pattern emerged: a secular increase in the relative incidence of all sample STDs in Algeria–Tunisia. Such a finding implies that late nineteenth and early twentieth century efforts at STD control in the military were singularly more successful in the French Interior than in the overseas commands of North Africa.

As a window on disease activity in World War II, we focused on data relating to US Army admissions for STDs in Africa and related commands of the Mediterranean and Africa–Middle East Theatres, 1942–5. The sample theatres displayed inflated levels of gonococcal infections (Mediterranean) and chancroid (Mediterranean and Africa–Middle East) relative to virtually all other theatres of US Army operations, although a more equable pattern was identified for syphilis. As regards time trends in STD activity, the Mediterranean Theatre mimicked the Army-wide pattern of increasing disease incidence in the years to 1945. Although the Africa–Middle East Theatre displayed a more complex pattern, the dominant tendency was for a relative stability in STD levels over the course of the war. Such between-theatre variations underscore the role of regional factors—including campaigns, exposures, and disease-control efforts—in the observed patterns of STD incidence during World War II.

Turning to the late twentieth century, we demonstrated that the classic association of war and disease substantially accounted for the observed geographical distribution of reported clinical AIDS cases in Uganda, Central Africa, during the first decade of the recognized HIV/AIDS pandemic. Both the spread of HIV infection in the 1980s and the subsequent development of AIDS to its 1990 spatial pattern were shown to be significantly positively correlated with ethnic patterns of recruitment into the Ugandan National Liberation Army following the overthrow of Idi Amin some ten years earlier in 1979. This correlation reflects the estimated mean incubation period of HIV-1 and underlines the need for cognizance of historical factors which may have influenced the observed patterns of AIDS in Central Africa and elsewhere.

In this and the preceding three chapters, our regional–thematic examination of the intersection of war and disease has concentrated on the continental mainland areas of the Americas, Europe, Asia, and Africa. Oceanic islands, with their own distinctive disease environments (Cliff *et al.*, 2000), provide an alternative setting for war epidemics, and it is to the theme of island epidemics—with special reference to the Pacific region—that we now turn.

Appendix 10A

Gonorrhoea, Chancroid, and Syphilis
(Sections 10.2 and 10.3)

This appendix provides a brief profile of the three STDs examined in Sections 10.2 and 10.3.

Gonorrhoea and Gonococcal Infections

Gonococcal infections (ICD-10 A54) are a range of inflammatory conditions caused by the bacterium *Neisseria gonorrhoeae*. The bacterium is transmitted by sexual contact and perinatally from mother to child, with presence in the lower genital tract—the most common site of infection—defining the condition 'gonorrhoea'. In symptomatic males, gonorrhoea manifests as a purulent discharge from the penile opening, often with discomfort or pain on urination. In symptomatic females, mild urethritis, cervicitis, and/or an endocervical discharge may be observed. Potential complications of infection with *N. gonorrhoeae* include pelvic inflammatory disease, arthritis, endocarditis, meningitis, and septicaemia. *N. gonorrhoeae* is susceptible to a variety of antibiotics (DeMaio and Zenilman, 1998; Sparling and Handsfield, 2000).

Chancroid

Chancroid (soft chancre) (ICD-10 A57) is an ulcerative disease of the male and female genitals caused by infection with the bacillus *Haemophilus ducreyi*. Although the disease has a worldwide distribution, it is most commonly encountered in tropical and subtropical locations. Transmission is by direct sexual contact with discharges from the sores of an infected person. Clinically, a typical incubation period of three to five days (range one to fourteen days) is followed by the development of lesions that, in turn, become pustular and erode to cause painful ulcers. Superinfection of the ulcers may result in irreparable damage to tissues and extensive destruction of the external genitalia. Oral administration of antibiotics (erythromycin) generally provides an effective means of patient therapy (Schmid, 1998; Hand, 2000).

Syphilis

Venereal syphilis (ICD-10 A50–53) is a potentially severe disease caused by the bacterium *Treponema pallidum*. The disease has a worldwide distribution. Sexual contact is the primary mode of transmission, although non-sexual transmission may occur as a consequence of contact with an exposed lesion, by blood transfusion, or *in utero*. The natural course of syphilis is characterized by three clinical stages (primary, secondary, and tertiary syphilis), with each stage separated by a latent period. In *primary syphilis*, a typical incubation period of three weeks (range ten days to ten weeks) is followed by the development of a painless chancre on the genitals or other site(s) of initial entry. The chancre spontaneously heals after two to six weeks. After a further six to eight weeks, the skin lesions and constitutional symptoms (including fever, malaise, and bone aches) of *secondary syphilis* appear. While the secondary manifestations resolve after weeks to months, a long and variable latent period (one to 20 years, or more) may eventually give way to the appearance of the destructive skin lesions and late disabling manifestations (including central nervous system and cardiovascular dysfunction) of *tertiary syphilis*. Antibiotic therapy is effective in the management of primary and secondary syphilis; higher dosages, for longer periods, are indicated for tertiary disease (Arrizabalaga, 1993; Cates, 1998).

Appendix 10B

AIDS and HIV (Section 10.4)

As noted in Section 10.4.1, AIDS (acquired immunodeficiency syndrome) is a strictly defined and advanced stage of disease due to infection with HIV (human immunodeficiency virus). Most bodily fluids and some tissues have been shown to harbour HIV. However, only blood, semen, cervico-vaginal secretions, and possibly breast milk have been consistently implicated in HIV transmission.

Three major corridors of virus transfer are usually identified:

1. *Sexual transmission.* HIV is carried in both semen and cervico-vaginal secretions, so both homosexual and heterosexual contact with an HIV carrier can result in virus transmission.
2. *Parenteral transmission.* Intravenous inoculation with contaminated blood is probably the most efficient route for the transfer of HIV. Prominent groups in this transmission category include (i) recipients of blood and blood products and (ii) intravenous drug users who share injecting equipment.
3. *Perinatal transmission.* Transmission of HIV from an infected mother to a child may occur *in utero* and possibly during or after birth. In the absence of antiretroviral therapy, which appears to reduce the likelihood of perinatal transmission, current evidence suggests that 25 to 35 per cent of children born to HIV-infected mothers will themselves be infected.

AIDS arises as a result of destruction of *CD*4 white blood cells by HIV. These cells are central to the body's immune system. Their destruction causes the immune system to collapse and leaves the body open to potentially life-threatening opportunistic infections, the development of rare and unusually aggressive cancers, dementia, wasting, and other severe conditions. The immune dysfunction that eventually gives rise to AIDS is a continuous process over a variable, but usually protracted, period of several years or more. During this time, an HIV-infected person will typically pass through a series of stages ranging from an acute retroviral syndrome (a short-lived glandular fever-type disease) in the very early stages of infection with HIV, through a prolonged period of asymptomatic infection associated with a progressive sub-clinical immune dysfunction, an early symptomatic stage (sometimes referred to as AIDS-related complex or ARC), eventually progressing to advanced or late stage disease (AIDS).

11

Oceania: War Epidemics in South Pacific Islands

Thou art slave to Fate, Chance, kings and desperate men,
And dost with poyson, warre, and sickness dwell . . .

John Donne, *Holy Sonnets*, X (extract, *c.*1617)

11.1 Introduction

So far, the geographical foci of our regional–thematic examination of the linkages between war and disease have been the great continental land masses of the Americas, Europe, Asia, and Africa. We now turn our attention to a different stage for the geographical spread of war epidemics—oceanic islands. As well as the particular interest which attaches to islands as natural laboratories for the study of epidemiological processes (Cliff *et al.*, 1981, 2000), island epidemics also hold a special place in war history. For example, we saw in Chapter 2 how the islands of the Caribbean became staging posts for the spread of wave upon wave of Old World 'eruptive fevers' (especially measles, plague, smallpox, and typhus) brought by the Spanish conquistadores to the Americas during the sixteenth century. Much later, the mysterious fever that broke out on the island of Walcheren in 1809 ranks as one of the greatest medical disasters to have befallen the British Army.

In this chapter, we examine the theme of island epidemics with special reference to the military engagements of Australia, New Zealand, and the neighbouring islands of the South Pacific since 1850. Figure 11.1 serves as a location map for the discussion, while sample conflicts—exclusive of tribal feuds, skirmishes, and other minor events for which little or no documentary evidence exists—are listed in Table 11.1.[1]

Our analysis begins in Section 11.2. There we provide a brief review of the initial introduction and spread of some of the Old World diseases which occurred in association with South Pacific colonization and conflicts during the last half of the nineteenth century. In Sections 11.3 and 11.4, we move on to the twentieth century. In the Great War, Australia and New Zealand made a relatively larger contribution to military manpower than any other allied country. At the end of the conflict, the return of many tens of thousands of antipodean troops from the battlefields of Europe fuelled the extension of the 1918–19 'Spanish' influenza pandemic into the South Pacific region (Cumpston, 1919). In Section 11.3, we examine the spread of influenza on board returning troopships and subsequently within Australia, New Zealand, and the neighbouring islands of the region. Finally, Section 11.4 analyses the spread of infectious diseases among US forces stationed in the Pacific Theatre during World War II. The chapter is concluded in Section 11.5.

As we shall see, many of the war–disease themes apparent in continental areas repeat in island locations. In continental settings, we have examined the links between mobilization and disease (the Americas), camp epidemics (Europe), the way in which war can cause the emergence of new and the re-emergence of old infections (Asia), and the role of soldiers in the propagation of STDs (Africa). The epidemics of mobilization in the Americas are echoed on islands by the nineteenth-century civil wars in the kingdom of Samoa (Sect. 11.2). These wars were associated with virgin soil epidemics of whooping cough, mumps, and measles. Just as Cumpston used quarantine to control the spread of influenza in Australia (Sect. 11.3), so quarantine was routinely used to control epidemics of war-related plague in the Asian continent throughout the twentieth century. Similarly, the camp epidemics of Europe described in Chapter 8 were mirrored during World War II on the South Pacific islands. Malaria, filariasis, dengue, and scrub typhus sapped the US Army, Navy, and Marine Corps, threatening the success of General MacArthur's island campaigns (Sect. 11.4). The Pacific Theatre also witnessed a sharp rise in the incidence of sexually transmitted diseases once military operations ceased, a classic association explored for Africa in Chapter 10.

---

[1] Our inclusion of World War I in Table 11.1 is merited by the large deployment of antipodean troops in the Northern Hemisphere between 1914 and 1918.

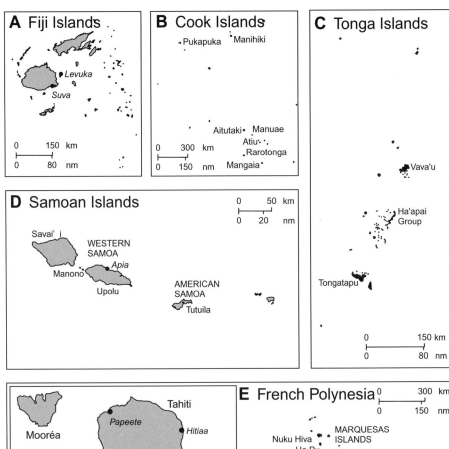

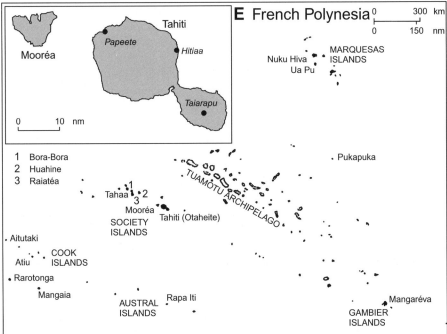

Fig. 11.1. Islands of the Pacific Ocean

Note: Map of the Pacific Ocean showing the main island groups and settlements discussed by McArthur (1968) in her *Island Populations of the Pacific*.

Source: Cliff *et al.* (2000, fig. 4.5, pp. 132–3).

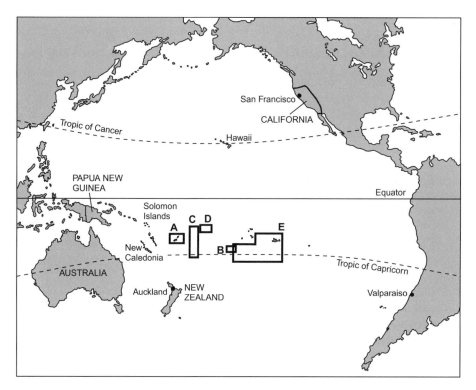

Fig. 11.1. (*cont.*)

Table 11.1. Sample conflicts in the South Pacific region, 1850–2000

War	Date	Participants	Estimated mortality (000s)[1]
Samoan Civil War	1848–53	Samoa	~0.4
Leeward Islands[2] (French Polynesia) Civil War	1852–4	Leeward Islands	'little loss of life'[3]
First Taranaki War	1860–1	Britain, New Zealand Maoris	⎫
Second Taranaki War	1863–4	Britain, New Zealand Maoris	⎬ 50
Third Taranaki War	1864–72	Britain, New Zealand Maoris	⎭
Samoan Civil War	1880–1	Samoa	?
Samoan Civil War	1887–9	Germany, Samoa	'several hundred'[4]
Samoan Civil War	1893–4	Britain, Germany, Samoa	?
Samoan Civil War	1898–9	Britain, Germany, Samoa, USA	<1?
World War I	1914–18	Allied and Central Powers	9,000–15,000[5]
World War II	1939–45	Allied and Axis Powers	15,000–20,000[5]
New Caledonian Uprising	1984–5	France, New Caledonia	?
Papua New Guinea Civil War	1988–98	Papua New Guinea	~20

Notes: [1] All mortality figures should be interpreted as broad estimates of the losses sustained. [2] Including the islands of Huahine, Raiatéa, and Tahaa (see Fig. 11.1). [3] Cited in McArthur (1968: 267). [4] Cited in McArthur (1968: 109). [5] Global mortality estimates.
Source: Based on information in Dumas and Vedel-Petersen (1923), Richardson (1960), McArthur (1968), Singer and Small (1972), Brogan (1992), and Kohn (1999).

11.2 Old World Diseases and South Pacific Wars, 1850–1900

Prior to European contact in the latter half of the eighteenth century, many of the great infectious diseases of the Old World were entirely unknown to the islanders of the South Pacific (Cliff *et al.*, 1993, 2000). The sequence by which the diseases were eventually introduced to several major island groups of the region has been traced by the Australian demographer, Norma McArthur (McArthur, 1968). In this section, we first look at McArthur's evidence for the sequence of disease introduction (Sect. 11.2.1) before examining the spread of the newly introduced diseases in association with conflicts in the South Pacific between 1850 and 1900 (Sect. 11.2.2). Our account draws in part upon Cliff *et al.* (2000: 127–48).

11.2.1 The Old World Diseases Introduced

Within the huge canvas of the Pacific (the Pacific Ocean covers nearly half of the planet's surface area), McArthur (1968) chose five island groups with good historical records for detailed study: Fiji, Cook Islands, Tonga, Samoa, and French Polynesia (Fig. 11.1A–E). Together, these extend over 25 degrees of latitude and 35 degrees of longitude and encompass a geographical area comparable to that of the conterminous United States.

EUROPEAN CONTACT AND DISEASE INTRODUCTION

Where the indigenous populations of the South Pacific islands came from has been a source of scholarly controversy between archaeologists and anthropologists (see Terrell, 1986). The balance of opinion is that the islands were populated over a period of some 3,000 years by peoples originating from the Indonesian archipelago. The process of indigenous island colonization was probably completed half a millennium before the first European explorations of the Pacific brought modern continental colonization (and continental diseases) into play. Figure 11.2 maps the main lines of European colonization in

→

Fig. 11.2. Main lines of European exploration and contact in the Pacific before 1800

Notes: 1: Roggeveen, 1721–2 discovered Easter Island and some of the Samoan group. Circumnavigation. 2: Wallis, 1766–8 discovered the Society Islands (Tahiti), encouraged hope of a habitable southern continent. Circumnavigation. 3: Cook–Clarke, 1776–80 discovered Sandwich Islands (Hawaii), explored northwest coast of North America from Vancouver Island to Unimak Pass, sailed through Bering Strait to edge of pack ice, ending hope of navigable passage through the Arctic to the Atlantic. 4: Bering, 1728, sailed from Kamchatka, discovered the strait bearing his name separating Northeast Asia from Northwest America. 5: Cook, 1772–5, made circuit of southern oceans in high latitude, discovered many islands and ended hope of habitable southern continent. Circumnavigation. 6: Cook, 1768–71 charted coasts of New Zealand. Explored east coast of Australia, confirmed existence of Torres Strait. Circumnavigation.
Source: Cliff *et al.* (2000, fig. 4.7, p. 136), originally from *The Times Atlas of World History* (London: Times Books Ltd., 1978: 157).

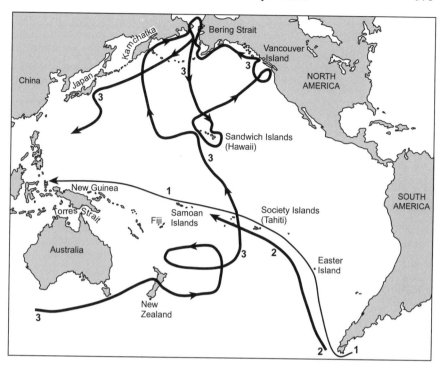

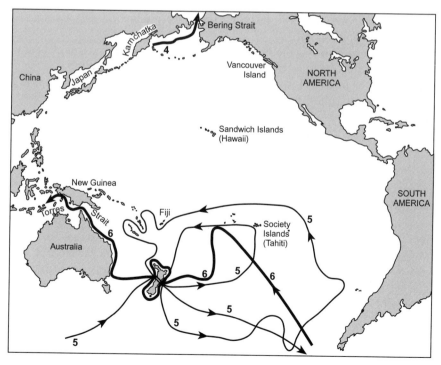

the eighteenth century. However important these early voyages were, they were but tips of an iceberg compared with the ever closer contacts which came from nineteenth-century missionary activities, from whalers, from the exploitation of sandalwood and *bêche-de-mer*, from military occupation and slaving, and later from immigration to sugar-cane plantations. The whole history of occupation has been brilliantly surveyed by the Australian geographer, Oskar Spate, in his three-volume history of Pacific occupation, *The Pacific since Magellan* (Spate, 1979, 1983, 1989).

The Main Diseases Introduced, 1770–1920

The period covered by McArthur extends from the first major European contacts in the late eighteenth century through to the start of modern demographic and epidemiological records after World War I. We can date this roughly as the 150-year period from 1770 to 1920. For this window of time, McArthur has analysed the records available—both the unofficial records of ships' surgeons, missionaries, and other visitors which span the first 100 years and official reports from *c.*1870; official records wait till the European occupation of the islands (France from 1842, Britain from 1875, Germany from 1884, the United States from 1898). Her record of disease introduction does not claim to be complete or exhaustive, but it does capture many of the major epidemic episodes of the period.[2] All told, 58 episodes are recognizable between 1770 and 1920, and these are plotted in Figure 11.3. Fig. 11.3A shows episodes of all diseases; the five smaller graphs, Figures 11.3B–F, chart the episodes for five of the major Old World infections (dysentery, influenza, measles, smallpox, and whooping cough).

As Figure 11.3 shows, the first episodes of influenza can be traced to the 1770s, to be followed in later decades by dysentery (1790s), smallpox (1830s), whooping cough (1840s), and measles (1850s). To these diseases can be added early reports of tuberculosis (1840s), scarlet fever (1840s), mumps (1850s), and dengue fever (1880s). We note here that the same diseases had, for the most part, also reached Australia and New Zealand by the dates given (Table 11.2).

DEMOGRAPHIC CONSEQUENCES OF THE EPIDEMICS

Before any estimate can be made of the impact of infectious diseases upon the mortality of the Pacific islands, we need some benchmark for the population at risk. Even for well-recorded countries (perhaps, Sweden apart) an accurate population estimate for 1790 is difficult to obtain; for the Pacific islands, the task is wellnigh impossible. Estimates made by earlier explorers had a very wide margin of error. McArthur cites two guesses made for the population of Tahiti in 1792: 50,000 by the missionaries made on their first tour of the island

---

[2] We define an 'epidemic episode' as a recorded outbreak of an identified disease in an identified island group at a particular time.

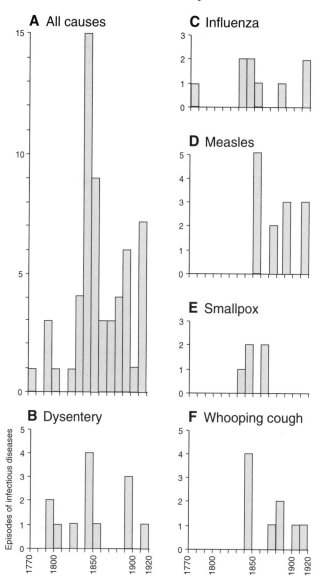

Fig. 11.3. Infectious diseases on Pacific islands

Note: Number of episodes by decade, 1770–1920, of infectious diseases introduced into the five main island groups studied by McArthur (1968).
Source: Cliff *et al.* (2000, fig. 4.8, p. 138).

Table 11.2. Decade in which cases of sample diseases were first recorded in Australia and New Zealand

Disease	Australia	New Zealand[1]
Dengue fever	1870s	?
Dysentery	1780s	1790s
Influenza	1820s	1790s
Measles	1850s	1800s
Mumps	1820s (or before)	1850s
Plague	1900s	c.1900s
Scarlet fever	1830s	1850s
Smallpox	1790s	1910s
Tuberculosis	1820s (or before)	?
Typhoid/enteric fever	1780s	1860s
Typhus	1780s	1860s?
Whooping cough	1820s	1820s

Note: [1] First documented epidemic among the native Maori population.
Source: Based on information in Pool (1977, tables 5.1, 5.2, pp. 117, 120–1) and Cumpston and Lewis (1989, *passim*).

and 16,050 made by Wilson a few days later using a tally of houses and average occupation (McArthur, 1968: 346). But, by 1850, some reasonable estimates can be made and some comparison with 1900 is possible (see Table 11.3). The most striking aspect of the table is the very low numbers. The total population of this huge area was less than a quarter of a million people for the whole of the period, 1770–1920. If we also note that this tiny population total was hugely fragmented by the island geography, then we realize that none of the individual islands in McArthur's sample had populations capable of maintaining the agents responsible for the most common infectious diseases (see Cliff *et al.*, 2000: 85–117). The diseases recorded were essentially epidemic and introduced, rather than endemic and home-grown.

This fact is reinforced by the population changes observed in Table 11.3. If we set aside the uncertain values for French Polynesia, McArthur suggests that 1800 totals would not have been very different from those of 1850, if anything slightly smaller. The change in the second half of the century was generally downwards, with an overall loss of some 20,000 largely due to deaths from the newly introduced infectious diseases. From 1900, notwithstanding the major influenza pandemic of 1918, came a period of population growth which nearly tripled the total population of the islands over the next half-century.

Given these very low population totals, it is not surprising that estimates of the number of deaths believed to have arisen from the introduced diseases were also low. For the 58 incidents of infectious diseases recorded in Figure 11.3, only seven had a death toll estimated at more than 100 in any year. As Table

Table 11.3. Pacific islands, 1790–1920: McArthur's estimates of population totals for the five major island groups

Location	1800	1850	1900	1950
Cooks	?	11,000	8,000	17,000
Fiji	?	135,000	120,000	346,000
French Polynesia	16–50,000	38,000	29,000	72,000
Samoa	?	34,000	40,000	117,000
Tonga	20,000	20,000	21,000	57,000
Total	?	238,000	218,000	609,000
Change			−20,000	+391,000

Source: Cliff *et al*. (2000, table 4.1, p. 146), based on data from McArthur (1968: 345–6).

Table 11.4. Pacific Islands, 1790–1920: McArthur's estimates of major epidemic incidents by deaths

Location	Disease	Date	Estimated deaths
Fiji	Measles	1875	>10,000
Tonga	Influenza	1918	1,595
Moorea	Measles	1854	800
Tahiti	Measles	1854	700
Tahiti	Smallpox	1848	200
Samoa	Whooping cough	1849	150
Rarotonga	Dysentery	1843	130

Source: Cliff *et al*. (2000, table 4.2, p. 146), McArthur (1968, *passim*).

11.4 shows, leaving to one side the exceptional Fijian measles outbreak of 1875, the roll of deaths is small; 50 of the outbreaks resulted in deaths of less than 100.

However, if mortality is measured as a rate (deaths per resident population from a given episode occurring within a year), then a somewhat different picture emerges. Estimates are available for approaching a quarter of all the episodes. As Table 11.5 shows, seven of the 15 episodes refer to measles followed by influenza (four episodes). It should be emphasized that the 'rates' are not based on exact demographic calculations but, particularly for the first half of the period, upon more-or-less educated guesses by the local missionary or the editor of a local newspaper such as the *Samoa Times*. Phrases such as '. . . introduced by a trading schooner in 1865 and allegedly decimating the infant population on all the Leeward islands' (McArthur, 1968: 313) has been recorded as a '10 per cent' mortality rate in Table 11.5.

Table 11.5. Pacific islands, 1790–1920: McArthur's estimates of major epidemic incidents by mortality rate

Location	Disease	Date	Estimated mortality rate (%)
Leeward	Dysentery	1865	33
Fiji	Measles	1875	25
Samoa	Influenza	1918	25
Leeward	Influenza	1918	25
Tahiti	Smallpox	1848	10
Tahiti	Measles	1854	10
Samoa	Measles	1893	10
Tonga	Influenza	1918	10
Samoa	Whooping cough	1849	5
Tonga	Measles	1893	5
Samoa	Measles	1911	5
Bora-Bora	Dysentery	1843	3
Leeward	Measles	1843	3
Bora-Bora	Measles	1854	3
Cooks	Influenza	1839	2.5

Source: Cliff *et al.* (2000, table 4.3, p. 147), based on data from McArthur (1968, *passim*).

11.2.2 Epidemics and War, 1850–1900

The foregoing evidence indicates that many of the main epidemic diseases of the Old World had reached the larger islands and island groups of the South Pacific by the mid-nineteenth century. In this subsection, we examine evidence for the spread of the introduced diseases in association with local wars that began and/or ended in the 50 years to 1900 (Table 11.1). As noted above, this half-century period broadly coincides with the onset of European occupation of many of the island groups.

THE SAMOAN CIVIL WARS

While tribal warfare had long been a feature of the independent kingdom of Samoa (Fig. 11.1D), leadership struggles—variously fuelled by the commercial interests of Britain, Germany, and the United States—underpinned a series of civil wars in the decades to 1900 (Table 11.1). In 1899, with the Samoan monarchy finally abolished, the islands were divided up between Germany (western islands) and the United States (eastern islands). Britain, in turn, gained rights to Tonga and the Solomons. From an epidemiological perspective, a particularly noteworthy feature of the periodic hostilities was their association with the first-time introduction of several infectious diseases, namely whooping cough and mumps in the Civil War of 1848–53 and measles in the Civil War of 1893–4.

Civil War of 1848–1853

McArthur (1968: 102–3) records that Manono, part of Savai'i and the greater part of Upolu were involved in a tribal conflict which, although claiming its largest number of casualties in the first year of fighting, continued sporadically until 1853.[3] On Upolu, the 'bulk' of the people were crowded in camps, leading to a neglect of cultivation. In 1849, there was much sickness due to 'the [w]hooping cough, said to have been imported in a vessel from Tahiti, [which] made its appearance for the first time, causing, in conjunction with the war, but in larger proportion, a calculated reduction of five per cent of the population in a period of eighteen months' (J. E. Erskine, 1853, cited in McArthur, 1968: 103). 'Many children' are said to have died as a result of whooping cough on Upolu while, on the north coast of Savai'i, no less than 150 persons are believed to have succumbed in a few months (McArthur, 1968: 103).

Civil War of 1893–1894

While the civil wars of the 1880s (Table 11.1) were occasionally associated with severe hardships, they were apparently free from major epidemic events. The Civil War of 1893–4 was a different matter. In September and October 1893, within months of the onset of hostilities between the rival factions of Chief Mata'afa (d. after 1899) and King Malietoa Laupepa (d. 1898), measles made its first appearance on the islands. Although the disease—spreading in an apparently virgin soil population—is said to have 'prostrated the whole group' of islands (A. H. Carne, 1893, cited in McArthur, 1968: 109), evidence regarding the severity of the epidemic is contradictory. On the one hand, the *Samoa Times* pointed to the relative mildness of the disease, estimating the total number of deaths at 300 by the termination of the epidemic in February 1894 (McArthur, 1968: 109–10). On the other hand, the Methodist Mission Society's *Savai'i Circuit Report* for 1893 noted that the epidemic was 'the first experience of measles the Samoans have had and it is an exceedingly bitter one. All are being, or have been, attacked, and many have been carried off. The death-rate is very high notwithstanding all the precautions which have been taken to keep it down' (J. W. Collier, 1893, cited in McArthur, 1968: 100).

Another Methodist missionary, C. Bleazard, placed the number of measles deaths at 1,600 (approximately 5% of the Samoan population) although, owing to the lack of a civil registration system at this time, the actual mortality may never be known with certainty (McArthur, 1968: 110). Whatever the death toll, however, the compound effects of war and disease were to have a severe and lasting effect on the islanders:

Epidemic upon epidemic, and the long-continued war, have been followed by a severe famine in the greater part of the Group. Plantations, which of necessity, had been much neglected during the measles, were left to ruin during the excitement of the war,

---

[3] According to McArthur (1968: 104), the total number of war-related casualties probably numbered between 350 and 400.

consequently the scarcity of food became very great. (C. Bleazard, 1894, cited in McArthur, 1968: 110)

The epidemiological legacy varied from one island to another. Thus, while the island of Savai'i is reported to have experienced drought, famine, and an epidemic of dysentery in 1896, McArthur (1968: 111) gauges the relative peace and prosperity of the people of Upolu and Manono by their interest in the construction of big churches rather than war canoes.

OTHER CONFLICTS

Leeward Islands (French Polynesia) Civil War (1852–1854)

Civil war broke out on the Leeward Islands (Huahine, Raiatéa, and Tahaa) of French Polynesia (Fig. 11.1E) in October 1852. Rebel forces were soon vanquished and, for a time, some of the rebels were banished to Raiatéa. By January 1853, Raiatéa is said to have been 'lying under a scourge of [a febrile] sickness' (G. Platt, 1853, cited in McArthur, 1968: 267), with the same fever having reached Huahine by April 1853. The unidentified disease 'proved severe in most cases and was followed by prostration of strength yet it proved fatal in some few cases only of children and old people' (J. Barff, 1853, cited in McArthur, 1968: 267–8). The following year, measles—generally of a mild form—was introduced into the islands. Most deaths occurred among the elderly and infirm. On Huahine, 12 of the 194 church members are said to have died of measles, with 34 deaths from other causes (McArthur, 1968: 268).

New Zealand: The Taranaki Wars (1860–1872)

Characterized by sporadic fighting between native Maori tribes and British forces in the North Island of New Zealand, the Taranaki Wars of 1860–72 (Table 11.1) were a series of conflicts which severely disrupted the underpinning structures of Maori society. They resulted in such massive social and geographical dislocation of the indigenous population that demographic recovery of the Maori awaited the twentieth century (see Pool, 1977).

Maori. According to Cowan, cited in Pool (1977: 134–5), an estimated 2,000 'hostile' and 200 'friendly' Maori died as a direct consequence of the hostilities. As for indirect mortality, the Maori population was enumerated at 47,300 in the post-war period (1874), having fallen from as high as 65,000 before the outbreak of the fighting (1858). But interpretive caution must be exercised because the rapid wartime decline was set against a continuing long-term downward trend in the Maori population. As for the spread of infectious diseases, Pool (1977: 119) notes that typhoid and measles attained a regional prevalence in the war years, although direct evidence for epidemic transmission in association with the conflict is scanty. However, in 1860 influenza is reported to have spread in the rebellious region of Wakaito, attacking men, women, and children and resulting in a general prostration of the Maori population (ibid. 126).

Table 11.6. Continent-level mortality estimates for Wave
II of the influenza pandemic, 1918–1919

Continent	Deaths (millions)	Death rate (per 1,000)
Africa	1.9–2.3	14.2–17.7
Asia	19.0–33.0	19.7–34.2
Europe	c.2.3	c.4.8
Latin America	0.8–1.0	8.4–10.6
North America	0.6	5.3
Oceania	<0.1	—
Total	24.7–39.3	13.6–21.7

Source: Data from Patterson and Pyle (1991, table 1, pp. 14–15).

British forces. According to Hirsch (1883, i. 633), typhoid fever was 'the commonest and most malignant kind of camp sickness in the campaign of 1864–65' (corresponding to the opening years of the Third Taranaki War) in the colony of New Zealand. Overall, however, it seems that the temperate climate of New Zealand's North Island was generally healthful for the British contingent. As an anonymous contributor to *The Lancet* commented in November 1867:

It is probable that the British army engaged during the late war in New Zealand enjoyed better health, and sustained fewer losses, than any previous campaign. Dr. Mackinnon attributes this to the very beautiful and salubrious climate; and he adds, that the change which it effected in the men of the regiments arriving from India was most marked. Sickly and sallow-complexioned on arrival, they soon lost the marks of ill-health engendered by tropical service, and regained health and strength while undergoing arduous service in the field. (Anonymous, 1867: 651)

11.3 World War I, Demobilization, and the Spread of Influenza in Australasia

The influenza pandemic of 1918–19 ranks as one of the greatest demographic shocks the human race has ever experienced. From uncertain origins in the spring of 1918, an apparently new variant of influenza A virus rolled around the world as three successive waves of infection, infecting over half a billion people and killing an estimated 20–40 million (Jordan, 1927; Oxford, 2000; Johnson and Mueller, 2002); see Table 11.6.[4] In India, as many as 12.5 million

---

[4] Estimates of the global mortality associated with the 1918–19 pandemic vary widely. E. O. Jordan places the death toll at 21.6 million (Jordon, 1927: 229–30). A revised estimate by Patterson and Pyle (1991: 19) places the mortality at 30 million while, more recently, Oxford *et al.* (1999) and Oxford (2000) place the mortality at 40 million. Other, more extreme, estimates have ranged up to a high of 100 million (see e.g. Burnet, 1979: 203).

are believed to have succumbed to influenza and its sequelae (Jordon, 1927). In the United States, the death toll is said to have exceeded 500,000 (Collins, 1930) while, in England and Wales, almost 200,000 are thought to have died (Ministry of Health, 1920, p. iv).

The influenza pandemic of 1918–19 spread in the closing stages and immediate aftermath of World War I (1914–18)—a war which had enveloped much of continental Europe and the Near East and which, through the combined agencies of battle, famine, and disease, had claimed over 20 million lives (Dumas and Vedel-Petersen, 1923). As described by Patterson and Pyle (1991), the heightened population mixing engendered by the war was to provide ideal conditions for the rapid dissemination of the influenza virus. Not least, the continuous flux of troops in the European theatre—where the new, albeit mild, influenza had reputedly arrived with US contingents in April 1918—ensured the early and widespread transmission of the disease on the European continent. In mid-November, however, with the disease having taken a much more severe turn, military demobilization served to spread the influenza virus far beyond its autumnal European focus to the rest of the world.

LAYOUT OF SECTION

Case studies of the spread of the 1918–19 influenza pandemic in military (United States, Sect. 7.4.1) and civil (England and Wales, Sect. 12.5.3) settlement systems are undertaken elsewhere in this book. Here we examine the spread of the pandemic to and within the South Pacific region. In so doing, we illustrate how a disease agent, first appearing among the military on one side of the world, may spark a civilian epidemic some 12,000 miles away. We first look at the global transmission routes of the pandemic (Sect. 11.3.1), before examining how the maritime quarantine of troopships and other vessels was used by one island state—Australia—to protect its population from the worst ravages of the disease (Sect. 11.3.2). We then review the impact of the pandemic on the indigenous population of New Zealand (Sect. 11.3.3) before tracing the onwards spread of the disease to other islands of the South Pacific (Sect. 11.3.4). The nature of influenza is outlined in Appendix 1A.[5]

[5] While uncertainty surrounds the precise nature of the virus responsible for the influenza pandemic of 1918–19, the causative agent appears to have been characterized by a virulence of unusual magnitude (Stuart-Harris *et al.*, 1985: 119–21; Kilbourne, 1987: 16). So, while the first wave (spring and early summer 1918) of the pandemic took a typically mild course, the second (autumn 1918) and third (winter 1918–19) waves were distinguished by an exceptionally high mortality from pulmonary and septicaemic conditions. Young adults in the 15–35-year age bracket were unusually prone to the development of these complications (Ministry of Health, 1920: 69; Langford, 2002). Factors which may have contributed to the exceptionally high levels of influenza-related mortality among young adults in 1918–19 remain the subject of considerable speculation (Crosby, 1993; Langford, 2002). Biological explanations have tended to favour the circulation of a virulent new strain of influenza A virus with a particular propensity for the respiratory systems of younger people (Stuart-Harris *et al.*, 1985: 121). However, such explanations cannot be divorced from the broader social and epidemiological circumstances of the war (Kilbourne, 1987: 16). The clustering of large numbers of young people in barracks, factories, and elsewhere, with all the privations and strains of war, may well have contributed to the peculiar epidemiological circumstances of the

11.3.1 Global Dispersals

As we have already noted, the influenza pandemic of 1918–19 occurred in three waves: spring and early summer 1918 (Wave I); autumn 1918 (Wave II); and winter 1918–19 (Wave III). Here, we provide a brief overview of the global dispersal of the three influenza waves. Our account draws on the study of Patterson and Pyle (1991).

Wave I (Spring and Early Summer 1918)

Wave I of the influenza pandemic was attributed at the time to Spain by France and vice versa, and to Eastern Europe by the Americans. But, whatever the truth, the disease acquired its popular name of *Spanish influenza* at this stage. As described in Section 7.4.1, some of the first records of influenza activity can be traced to US Army recruits at Camp Funston, Kansas, where an epidemic of influenza first manifested in early March 1918. By the end of the month, influenza had appeared in a number of military camps in the midwestern and southeastern United States, with the disease becoming widely diffused in April. The global spread of influenza from this putative beginning[6] is traced in Figure 11.4A. Transatlantic spread of the disease occurred with American troopships which reached France in April, with subsequent spread across the European continent. At about the same time, the map depicts the trans-Pacific spread of influenza from North America to Southeast Asia in April and May. The Caribbean Basin and Latin America were attacked in June. The disease finally reached the South Pacific in July (Patterson and Pyle, 1991).

Wave II (Autumn 1918)

Wave I of the pandemic was comparatively mild. During the summer of 1918, the virus mutated into a more lethal strain and a second, more severe, form of the disease emerged. Pneumonia often developed quickly, with death usually coming two days after the first indications of the influenza. The global dispersal of the new, more severe, Wave II is traced in Figure 11.4B. As with Wave I, the exact origins of Wave II are also unknown, although western France is

---

pandemic (Ministry of Health, 1920: xiv–xv), while the chance synergy of concurrent viral and bacterial infections cannot be excluded (Kilbourne, 1987: 16; Crosby, 1993: 810).

[6] The origin of the 1918–19 influenza pandemic cannot be ascertained with any certainty. As far as the historical record allows, outbreaks of influenza—generally assumed to be associated with the first wave of the pandemic—were first recognized in military training camps of the United States in March 1918 (Soper, 1918; Patterson and Pyle, 1991), with the disease appearing among US and other troops on the Western Front during April (Stuart-Harris *et al.*, 1985; Patterson and Pyle, 1991). Contemporary commentators, however, have pointed to the sporadic outbreaks of an unusually severe respiratory disease ('purulent bronchitis'), resembling Spanish influenza, among troops in France and troops and civilians in Britain as early as the mid-winter of 1916 (Ministry of Health, 1920: 69; Macpherson *et al.*, 1922–3, i. 212–14). The implication that the germs of the pandemic wave may have been circulating in Europe for up to two years prior to the massive outbreaks of 1918–19 is consistent with the suggestion that the ancestor virus entered the human species around 1912–15 (Oxford *et al.*, 1999; Oxford, 2000; Reid *et al.*, 1999; Webster, 1999), although caution must be exercised in the interpretation of the evidence (Shortridge, 1999; Webster, 1999).

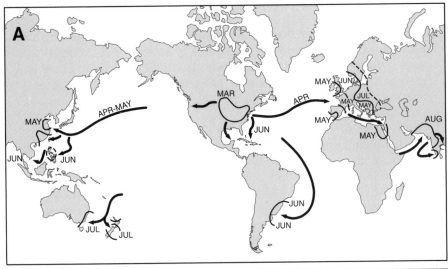

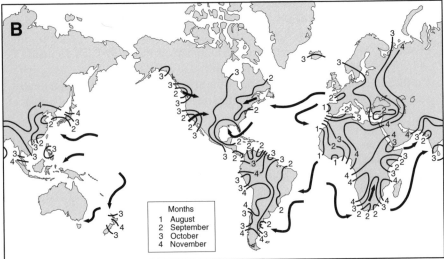

Fig. 11.4. Global diffusion of pandemic influenza, March–November 1918

Notes: The transmission routes of influenza Waves I (spring and early summer 1918) and II (autumn 1918) are plotted in maps A and B, respectively.
Source: Redrawn from Patterson and Pyle (1991, fig. 1, 5, pp. 6, 12).

generally viewed as the source of the disease; the first reports can be traced to the French Atlantic port of Brest, a landing point for American troops, in late August. From here, ships appear to have carried the disease to coastal locations of North America, Africa, Latin America, South Asia, and the Far East by September. New Zealand was infected in October by ships from the United

States while, as described in Section 11.3.2, Australia remained largely free of the disease until January 1919 (Patterson and Pyle, 1991).

Wave III (Winter 1918–1919)

In the aftermath of Wave II, a third influenza wave—of intermediate severity to the preceding waves—appeared in the winter of 1918–19. While relatively little is known of the origin and spread of this tertiary wave, the influenza pandemic appears to have finally run its course by the spring of 1919.

11.3.2 Australia, Pandemic Influenza, and Maritime Quarantine

Australia's involvement in World War I was on a massive scale in relation to its small size (Sect. 4.4.1). From a population of some 5 million, over 300,000 troops served in Europe, and the problems of bringing the survivors home in the autumn and winter of 1918—at the very height of the influenza pandemic—was on a similarly massive scale. In the early part of October 1918, with the health authorities of Australia cognizant that a virulent form of influenza was within striking distance of the country, instructions were issued for the quarantining of all vessels with cases of influenza aboard (Cumpston, 1919: 7). So began Australia's six-month maritime defence against the great influenza pandemic. The medical officer who successfully led the strategy was J. H. L. Cumpston (Pl. 11.1), Director of Quarantine and later Australia's first Commonwealth Director-General of Health.

THE QUARANTINE RECORD

Records have survived for 228 vessels arriving in Australia between October 1918 and April 1919, of which 79 document cases of influenza (Table 11.7). Figure 11.5 plots, by week of arrival in Australia, the distribution of the 79 infected vessels according to the inferred place of virus acquisition: Pacific Rim (Fig. 11.5A); Europe (Fig. 11.5B); and other (Fig. 11.5C). Vessels on which cases of influenza were documented after arrival in Australia and which, in the absence of quarantine, would have served as potential sources of infection for the population of Australia, are indicated by the black shading. Figure 11.5 suggests a temporal shift in the geographical source of maritime influenza, from the Pacific Rim in October–December 1918 (Fig. 11.5A) to Europe in January–April 1919 (Fig. 11.5B). This temporal shift was associated with the arrival of generally larger, and more heavily crowded, troopships from Europe (via Suez) in the latter period.

Evidence from Infected Troopships

The influenza records for four troopships (*Devon*, *Medic*, *Boonah*, and *Ceramic*), arriving at Australian ports between November 1918 and March 1919, are shown in Figure 11.6; the vessels involved are illustrated in Plate 11.2.

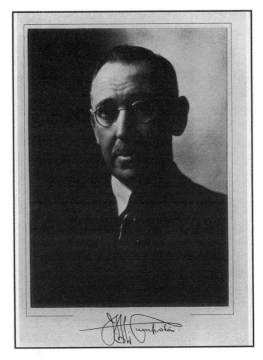

Pl. 11.1. J. H. L. Cumpston (1880–1954)

Notes: Australia's first Commonwealth Director-General of Health, 1921–45. Cumpston oversaw the health of Australia and the troops she put in arms in two world wars. He produced a number of service handbooks on diseases in Australia from 1788 to 1920. The findings were summarized in a book, *Health and Disease in Australia*, completed in 1928. This was not published until 1989, when the work was edited and introduced by Milton Lewis as part of Australia's bicentennial celebrations.

Source: Cliff *et al.* (2000, pl. 5.4, p, 193), from Cumpston and Lewis (1989, frontispiece).

Table 11.7. Vessels arriving at Australian ports during the 'Spanish' influenza outbreak, October 1918–April 1919

Value	Vessels (number)	Susceptibles (crew and passengers)	Average susceptibles per vessel
Total	228	73,482	322
Uninfected	149	15,016	101
Infected[1]	79	57,741	731[2]
Influenza cases		2,795	
Influenza deaths		99	

Notes: [1] Quarantined. [2] Including troopships.
Source: Cliff *et al.* (2000, table 5.3, p. 195).

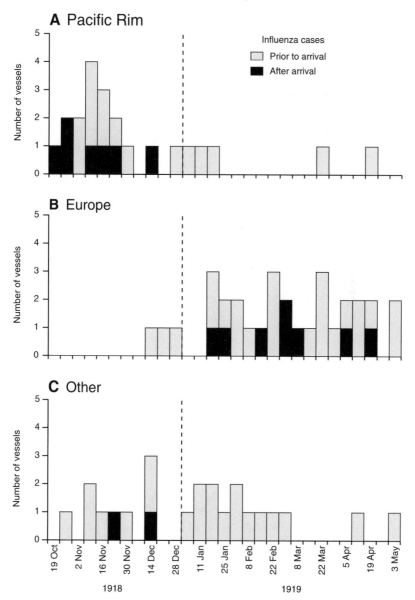

Fig. 11.5. Maritime quarantine and 'Spanish influenza', Australia, 1918–1919

Notes: Graphs plot, by overseas source of infection, the weekly count of vessels infected with influenza and quarantined on arrival at Australian ports, October 1918–May 1919. (A) Pacific Rim. (B) Europe. (C) Other. Vessels on which cases of influenza were recorded after arrival in Australia, and which may therefore be assumed to have maintained an unbroken chain of infection aboard ship, are indicated on each graph by the black shading.

Source: Based on information in Cumpston (1919, table C, pp. 38–9).

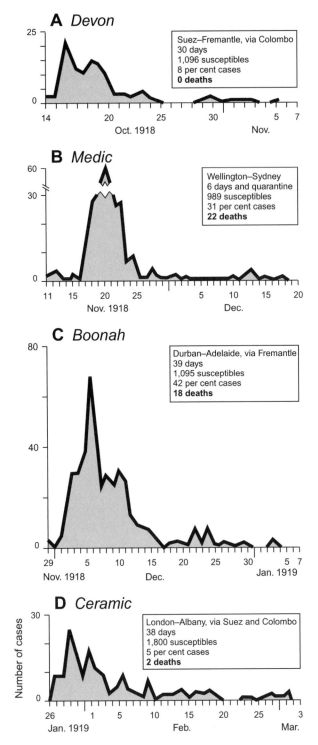

Fig. 11.6. The role of ships in dispersing 'Spanish' influenza, 1918–19

Notes: Number of cases of influenza reported daily on four troopships repatriating troops from Europe to Australia in the aftermath of the Great War. (A) *Devon*. (B) *Medic*. (C) *Boonah*. (D) *Ceramic*.

Source: Cliff *et al.* (2000, fig. 5.9, p. 194).

A

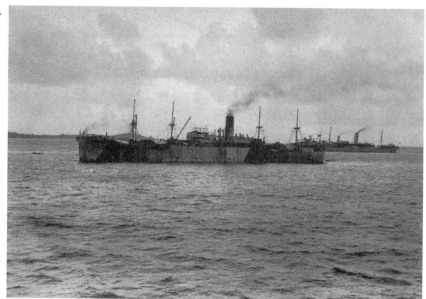

B

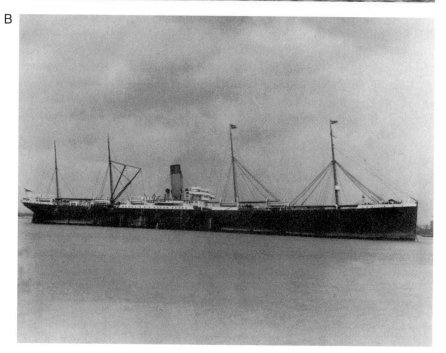

Pl. 11.2. Australia and the influenza pandemic of 1918–1919

Notes: Four troopships which carried 'Spanish' influenza from the European Theatre to Australia in the aftermath of the Great War. (A) *Devon* (foreground) in World War I camouflage with troops aboard, 1915. (B) *Medic* off Tilbury, 8 May 1907. (C) *Boonah* ex-Melbourne, late 1914. (D) *Ceramic* in Cape Town harbour *c.* August 1914.

Sources: Reproduced from Cliff *et al.* (2000, pl. 5.5, pp. 196–7). (Pl. 11.2A–C) National Maritime Museum, Greenwich; (Pl. 11.2D) World Ship Photograph Library, Carlisle.

C

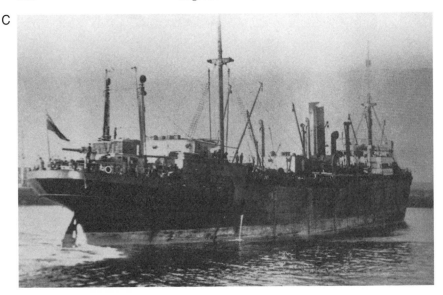

D

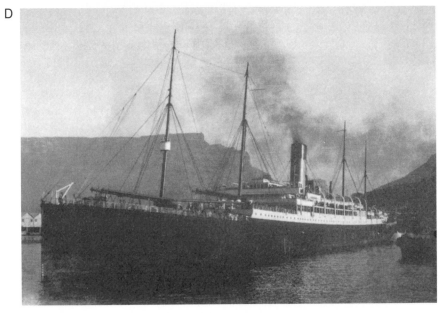

Pl. 11.2. (*cont.*)

Some impression of the conditions that prevailed on the ships can be gained from the eyewitness accounts of senior officers. According to one anonymous officer aboard the *Medic* (Fig. 11.6B and Pl. 11.2B), the scene

. . . was remarkable. A score or more of stalwart young men lay helpless about the after well-deck, awaiting transport to the improvised and overflowing hospitals in the troop-

Table 11.8. 'Spanish' influenza, 1918–1919: international maximum weekly death rates

Location	Rate
USA (Philadelphia)	261
USA (San Francisco)	135
South Africa[1]	$>103^2$
New Zealand	$>65^2$
Australia (New South Wales)	34
Australia (Victoria)	19
Australia (Rest)	$<20^2$

Notes: [1] Europeans only. [2] Averaged from monthly values.
Source: Cliff *et al.* (2000, table 5.4, p. 195).

decks. That they lay there was not due to any neglect or delay on the part of the busy stretcher-bearers, but to the extraordinarily sudden and disabling onset of the disease. One smart, well set-up young soldier came up a companion-ladder close to where I stood, held on for a few seconds to a rail, and then sagged slowly down till he assumed the characteristic flattened sprawl on the deck. There was no pretence or 'old-soldiering' about it. The men were literally being knocked down by a profound systematic intoxication of extraordinarily rapid onset. (Anonymous, cited in Cumpston, 1919: 53)

As Figure 11.6 shows, the influenza curve for the *Medic* followed a broadly similar course to other troopships, with two marked features of the frequency distribution of cases:

(1) a generally lognormal nature. Cases peaked within three to ten days of start of voyage, with a long positive tail to the distribution;

(2) recurring secondary cycles of cases within general lognormal shape. Statistical analysis using the autocorrelation function (ACF) suggests that there is a periodicity in the time series of about four days, roughly corresponding with the known serial interval of the disease.

The long journey from Europe gave Cumpston time to organize a quarantine system. Boats reporting influenza were isolated in harbour, and troops were not allowed ashore until they were free of the disease. Once soldiers were landed and returned to their homes, they found that interstate travel was also restricted to inhibit transmission—by armed guards in the case of the land border between Queensland and New South Wales. The effect of these measures is seen in Table 11.8. Peak death rates in Australia were about an eighth of those in the United States, and a quarter of those in South Africa and New Zealand.

DIFFUSION OF INFLUENZA IN AUSTRALIA

Such was the success of the influenza control measures, concluded Cumpston, that during the last three months of 1918, maritime quarantine had the effect of holding at the sea frontiers an intensely virulent and intensely infective form of influenza, which not only caused disastrous epidemics in New Zealand and South Africa, but actually arrived at the maritime frontiers of Australia, and caused alarming epidemics amongst the personnel of vessels detained in quarantine. (Cumpston and Lewis, 1989: 318–19)

Although the effectiveness of the quarantine measures of late 1918 has been questioned (McQueen, 1975), epidemiological evidence does point to a delay of several months in the spread of virulent influenza in Australia. So, on the basis of recorded mortality, Cumpston traces the start of the Australian epidemic to early 1919. The first influenza deaths were reported in the state of Victoria (January), to be followed thereafter by New South Wales (February), South Australia (March), Queensland (April), Western Australia (June), and Tasmania (August). In explaining the timing of the epidemic sequence, Cumpston notes that: 'Western Australia and Tasmania are the two States having the least human contact with the two [earliest] infected States, New South Wales and Victoria; they were the two States which most vigorously applied inter-State quarantine restrictions; and they were the States latest infected in the series' (Cumpston and Lewis, 1989: 119).

11.3.3 New Zealand Indigenes

Unlike Australia, where the spread of virulent influenza was delayed until early 1919, the second—and most deadly—wave of the influenza pandemic reached New Zealand in October 1918. Acording to Pool (1973), the wave first appeared among native (Maori and Pacific Islander) troops who were stationed at Narrow Neck Camp, Auckland (Fig. 11.1). From this location, the disease spread across the whole of North and South Island in the remainder of October and November (Fig. 11.4B).

MAORI MORTALITY

Between October and December 1918, Pool (1973) notes that 1,160 registered deaths from respiratory diseases occurred among the Maori population (a crude death rate of 22.6 per 1,000), compared with just 27 deaths in the equivalent period of 1917. The death rate for males (27.7 per 1,000) was considerably higher than that for females (16.3 per 1,000). As in other locations, young adults (20–49 years) suffered the heaviest mortality rates, with the gender differential being most marked in this age bracket (Fig. 11.7).

Comparative Rates

The mortality rate for respiratory diseases in the period October–December 1918 was five times higher for the Maori (22.6 per 1,000) than for the non-Maori (predominantly British) population of New Zealand (4.5 per 1,000). According to Pool (1973), factors which may have contributed to the inflated

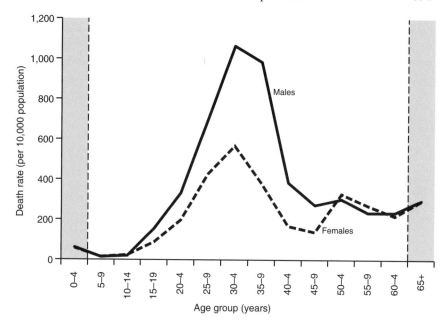

Fig. 11.7. Estimated age- and sex-specific death rates (per 10,000 population) for influenza in New Zealand Maoris, October–December 1918

Note: Age categories associated with the highest mortality rates in a 'typical' influenza year are identified by the shading.
Source: Drawn from data in Pool (1973, table 3, p. 277).

levels of influenza mortality among the Maori included: (i) a relative lack of medical care; (ii) lower levels of acquired immunity among isolated rural populations; and (iii) the high background level of morbidity from all causes, thereby rendering the indigenes less resistant to a particularly virulent disease agent.

11.3.4 Diffusion to Other South Pacific Islands

In the latter months of 1918 and the early months of 1919, influenza was reported from many of the smaller islands of the South Pacific. As described by Norma McArthur, the main vector of spread appears to have been from New Zealand and was linked to the voyage of a single freighter:

New Zealand was in the throes of an epidemic when the S.S. *Talune* left Auckland early in November [1918], with a captain who did not know that influenza was an infectious disease and Suva [Fiji] as her first port of call. There she discharged and loaded cargo under quarantine and, as was then customary, about 90 Fijians stayed on board to perform the same service in each port. Passengers destined for Fiji were landed after medical inspection, and though none of the crew was allowed ashore in Suva, there was

Table 11.9. Recent estimates of mortality associated with the 1918–1919 influenza pandemic in the South Pacific

Location	Published death toll[1]
Australia	14,528 (2.7–2.8)
Fiji	9,000 (52.0–54.9)
Guam	858 (?)
Nauru	? (160.0)
New Zealand	? (<20.0)
Tonga	? (42.0–84.0)
Western Samoa	8,500 (220.0–236.1)
Regional estimate	~85,000 (?)

Note: [1] Mortality rate per 1,000 population in parentheses.
Source: Data from Johnson and Mueller (2002, table 5, p. 114).

no restriction on the movements of either the remaining passengers or the crew when the ship called at Levuka [in the northeast corner of the main island, Viti Levu] before proceeding to Samoa. Their quarantine in Suva was not mentioned when the ship arrived at Apia on 7 November, and passengers were allowed to disembark. The *Talune* left Apia two days later for Vava'u, and within two days about 70 of the Fijians were ill, so presumably local labour was used to discharge and load cargo there and at Ha'apai and Tongatapu where she called before returning to Suva, twelve momentous days after she had left it.

All of the Fijians were placed in quarantine on their return, but the epidemic had already begun and though the first known cases occurred in Suva, there was probably some spread of infection from Levuka as well. The dispersal of Fijians from Suva as the incidence increased may have been repeated by the Samoans in and around Apia, or perhaps the arrival of a ship was sufficiently novel in 1918 to attract numbers of people from a wide radius up and down the coast. The disease spread rapidly in both Upolu and Savai'i and soon practically all the Natives were down with influenza or fright, and they either could or would not do anything to help themselves or others. (McArthur, 1968: 352–3).

Several commentators refer to the speed of spread once an island had been reached. Within seven days of the arrival of the *Talune* from Auckland via Fiji, 'pneumonic influenza was epidemic in Upolu; . . . it spread with amazing rapidity throughout Upolu, and later throughout Savai'i' (cited in ibid. 125).

DEMOGRAPHIC IMPACT

The demographic impact of the pandemic varied greatly from island to island (Table 11.9). In some instances, mortality was very high. Lambert (1934) claimed that 1,595 Tongans died in the epidemic, although Wood (1938: 64) states that 'the influenza epidemic of 1919 caused 1,000 deaths'. The general consensus is that the Samoans and Tongans probably suffered the most devastating epidemic in their modern history; one-tenth or more of the populations probably died on some islands.[7] But, in contrast to the situation at the times of main nineteenth-century epidemics reviewed in Section 11.2, by 1918 most island governments had provided health services of a sort, even if these were meagre and more often than not limited either to the main island or to the administrative centre of the island group. In compensation, McArthur (1968: 352–4) notes that most overseas shipping used only the principal port where quarantine regulations might be imposed with some hope of their being enforced.

11.4 The United States and the Pacific War, 1942–1945

The US move to counter Japanese expansion in the Pacific Basin during World War II—triggered by the infamous air strikes on US bases at Pearl Harbour (Hawaii) and Manila (Philippines) on 7–8 December 1941—ranks as one of the largest and most complex operations in American military history (Dear and Foot, 1995: 855). The task necessitated the occupation of numerous, widely scattered, tropical, and subtropical islands, many of which were known to be endemic foci for dengue, dysentery, filariasis, malaria, and yaws. The epidemiological risk was heightened by the haste with which the plans were implemented, the lack of familiarity of many medical officers with the diseases to which the men were potentially exposed, and, in some instances, the mysterious nature of the disease agents encountered. As a consequence, most—if not all—US troops involved in the early stages of the Pacific War were exposed to one or more epidemic diseases. Only as the war progressed and familiarity with the epidemiological hazards of the area grew did the disease problem come under control.

11.4.1 Disease Patterns in the Pacific Theatre

To examine patterns of disease activity among US forces in the Pacific Theatre, we draw on information included in Reister's *Medical Statistics in World War II* (1976). Details of the data source are given in Section 10.3.1. The volume includes monthly estimates of US Army hospital admissions from infectious and parasitic diseases, January 1942–December 1945, for two divisions of the Pacific region:

(1) *Southwest Pacific*, including the Admiralty Islands, Australia, New Britain, New Guinea, and the Philippine Islands;
(2) *Pacific Ocean Areas*, including Fiji, New Hebrides, New Zealand, Samoa, and the Solomon Islands in the Southern Hemisphere and

---

[7] On the influenza pandemic in Western Samoa, see Tomkins (1992).

Hawaii, Japan, the Marianas, and Marshall Islands in the Northern Hemisphere.

Figure 10.6 gives the position of the Southwest Pacific and Pacific Ocean Areas within the global division of US military operations during World War II, while Figure 11.8 serves as a location map for the present section. Infectious and parasitic diseases for which more than 1,000 admissions were listed by Reister for the Southwest Pacific (1), the Pacific Ocean Areas (2), and the Pacific Theatre as a whole (1) + (2), 1942–5, are given in Table 11.10.

PATTERNS IN TIME: CLUSTER ANALYSIS

As the right-hand columns of Table 11.10 show, a total of 24 diseases were associated with over 1,000 hospital admissions in the combined divisions of the Pacific. To classify the 24 diseases in terms of their temporal activity, the monthly time series of admissions, 1942–5, were subjected to complete linkage cluster analysis as described in Section 3.3.2. The dendrogram plotted in Figure 11.9 reveals four well-defined groups of diseases, labelled Groups A to D. The aggregate time series of admissions that comprise each disease group are plotted on a monthly basis in Figure 11.10; the sequence of occupation of sample islands by US forces is indicated on the graph for reference.

One striking feature of Figure 11.10 is the high level of activity associated with disease Group A (comprising the vector-borne diseases: malaria, filariasis, dengue, and scrub typhus), as compared with disease Groups B to D, during the main period of island-based military operations, 1942–4. As the graph indicates, a sharp increase in Group A admissions was associated with the Guadalcanal offensive (Aug. 1942–Feb. 1943), with high levels of activity accompanying the subsequent occupation of such islands as New Georgia and Bougainville in 1943, and New Guinea and the Philippines in 1944. Thereafter, Group A admissions began to decline in late 1944, to be superseded by admissions associated with disease Groups B and C towards the end of the war. The latter groups include gonococcal infections (Group B), and chancroid, lymphogranuloma, and syphilis (Group C) and partly reflect the classic rise of sexually transmitted diseases with the cessation of military operations (see Sect. 10.3.1). Finally, with the exception of a minor increase in hospital admissions during 1942, activity associated with disease Group D (influenza, German measles, mumps, and Weil spirochetosis) remained at a relatively low level throughout the conflict.

11.4.2 Diseases of Military Significance

In addition to the geographically ubiquitous problem of dysentery, Sapero and Butler (1945) rank the four vector-borne diseases comprising Group A of Figure 11.9 (malaria, filariasis, dengue, and scrub typhus) as the principal

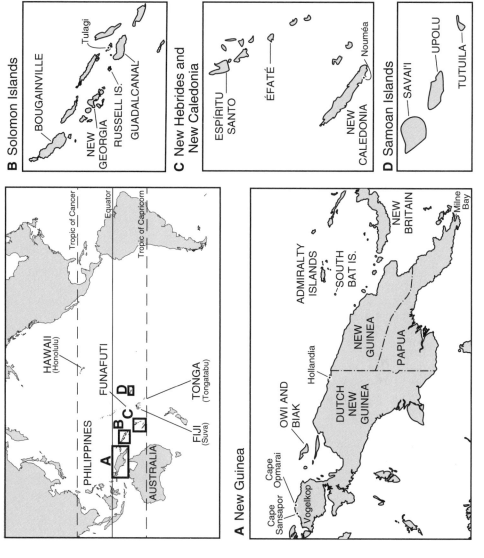

B Solomon Islands

BOUGAINVILLE

Tulagi

NEW GEORGIA

RUSSELL IS.

GUADALCANAL

C New Hebrides and New Caledonia

ESPÍRITU SANTO

ÉFATÉ

Nouméa

NEW CALEDONIA

D Samoan Islands

SAVAI'I

UPOLU

TUTUILA

Tropic of Cancer

Equator

Tropic of Capricorn

PHILIPPINES

HAWAII (Honolulu)

FUNAFUTI

TONGA (Tongatabu)

FIJI (Suva)

AUSTRALIA

A New Guinea

ADMIRALTY ISLANDS

SOUTH BAT IS.

NEW BRITAIN

Milne Bay

Cape Sansapor

Cape Opmarai

Vogelkop

OWI AND BIAK

Hollandia

DUTCH NEW GUINEA

NEW GUINEA

PAPUA

Fig. 11.8. Location map for Section 11.4

Table 11.10. Infectious and parasitic diseases resulting in more than 1,000 hospital admissions in the US Army, Pacific War, 1942–1945

Rank	Southwest Pacific (1)		Pacific Ocean Areas (2)		Pacific Theatre (1) + (2)	
	Disease	Admissions	Disease	Admissions	Disease	Admissions
1	Malaria	97,794	Malaria	81,036	Malaria	178,830
2	Dengue	50,025	Dengue	29,864	Dengue	79,889
3	Gonococcal infections	41,459	Gonococcal infections	12,567	Gonococcal infections	54,026
4	Hepatitis	41,102	Dysentery	9,387	Hepatitis	45,532
5	Dysentery	28,081	Influenza	4,857	Dysentery	37,468
6	Chancroid	12,149	Hepatitis	4,430	Chancroid	14,350
7	Hookworm	8,409	Spirochetosis, Weil	3,618	Hookworm	11,643
8	Syphilis	7,154	Syphilis	3,234	Syphilis	10,388
9	Scrub typhus	4,243	Hookworm	3,234	Influenza	8,186
10	Influenza	3,329	Chancroid	2,201	Scabies	4,864
11	Helminths	3,201	Scabies	1,788	Helminths	4,603
12	Scabies	3,076	Food poisoning	1,640	Spirochetosis, Weil	4,352
13	Pneumonia	2,137	Helminths	1,402	Scrub typhus	4,333
14	Mumps	1,906	Mumps	1,397	Food poisoning	3,345
15	Food poisoning	1,705	Filariasis	1,392	Mumps	3,303
16	Schistosomiasis	1,261	Streptococcal infections	1,201	Pneumonia	3,059
17	Tuberculosis	1,189	Tuberculosis	1,059	Tuberculosis	2,248
18	Protozoal infections	1,099			Streptococcal infections	2,194
19					Measles	1,727
20					German measles	1,653
21					Filariasis	1,627
22					Protozoal infections	1,603
23					Schistosomiasis	1,358
24					Lymphogranuloma	1,230

Source: Data from Reister (1976).

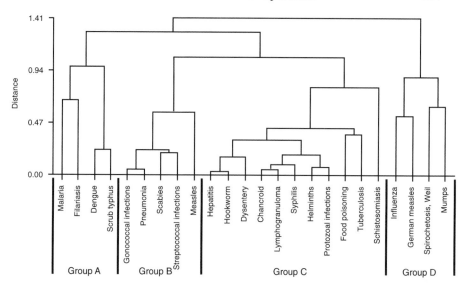

Fig. 11.9. Classification of 24 disease-related causes of hospital admission in terms of their time-series behaviour, US Army, Pacific Theatre, 1942–1945

Note: For each cause, the input data consisted of the combined monthly count of admissions for the US Army in the Southwest Pacific and Pacific Ocean Areas. The total number of admissions for each of the 24 causes, selected on the basis of >1,000 recorded admissions over the observation period, is given in Table 11.10.
Source: Data from Reister (1976).

diseases of military significance to US forces in the Pacific War. For each of the four diseases, Figures 11.11A–D in plot the monthly series of admission rates (per 1,000 average strength per year) for the US Army in the Southwest Pacific (full line trace) and Pacific Ocean Areas (broken line trace). Periods of epidemic activity associated with each disease and geographical area are summarized in Table 11.11.[8]

Of the diseases included in Figures 11.11A–D, malaria (Fig. 11.11A) and dengue (Fig. 11.11C) were widely distributed in the theatre of operations, but with the latter characterized by focal outbreaks. Bancroftian filariasis (Fig. 11.11B) was largely confined to the Samoan group and adjacent islands of the Pacific Ocean Areas, while scrub typhus (Fig. 11.11D) was prevalent on Bougainville, New Georgia, New Guinea, the Philippines, and proximal islands of the Southwest Pacific (Sapero and Butler, 1945). In the remainder of this section, we examine the wartime ocurrence of each of the sample diseases

---

[8] To define the epidemic periods in Table 11.11, the monthly series of rates (per 1,000 average strength per year) for each disease and geographical area was first reworked as standard scores. A score in excess of 0.5 standard deviations above the zero mean was then used to define an epidemic month.

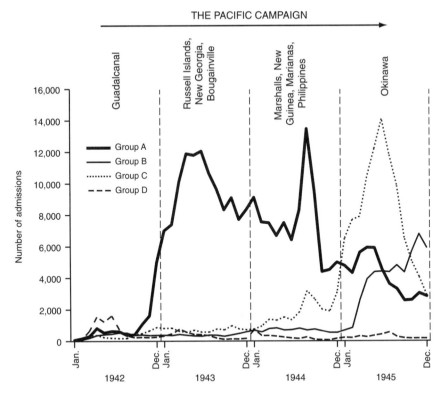

Fig. 11.10. US Army, Pacific Theatre, 1942–1945: monthly series of hospital admissions for each group of diseases in Fig. 11.9

Notes: The sequence of occupation of sample islands by US forces is indicated for reference. Island locations are given in Fig. 11.8.

with special reference to Pacific islands south of the equator. Figure 11.8 serves as a location map for the discussion.

MALARIA

The initial entry of the United States into the Pacific Theatre was associated with the occurrence of malaria epidemics of crippling proportions among the forces, serving to incapacitate whole units and severely limiting the operational effectiveness of island campaigns (Harper *et al*., 1963; Hart and Hardenburgh, 1963). As Joy (1999) notes, malaria was endemic to hyperendemic in the South and Southwest Pacific, but it took the epidemiologically disastrous campaigns in New Guinea (Aug. 1942–Jan. 1943) and Guadalcanal (Aug. 1942–Feb. 1943) for combat commanders to acknowledge fully the military threat of malaria and to provide unstinting support in the control of the disease (Pl. 11.3).

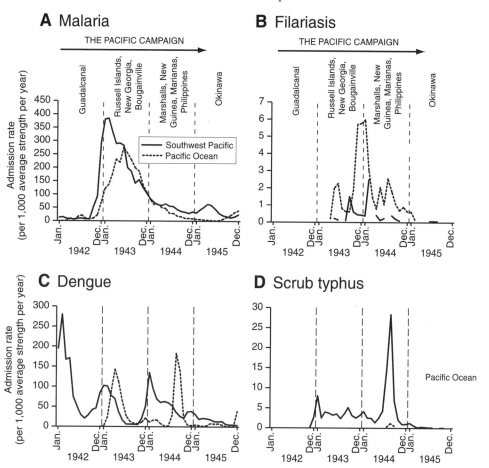

Fig. 11.11. Monthly series of hospital admission rates (per 1,000 average strength per year) for sample diseases of military importance, US Army, Pacific Theatre, 1942–1945

Notes: Rates are plotted for the Southwest Pacific (full line trace) and Pacific Ocean Areas (broken line trace). (A) Malaria. (B) Filariasis. (C) Dengue. (D) Scrub typhus. The sequence of occupation of sample islands by US forces is indicated for reference. Island locations are given in Fig. 11.8. *Source*: Data from Reister (1976).

Malaria Attack Rates, 1942–1943

As illustrated for the US Army in Figure 11.11A, malaria attack rates were especially high in the early phases of the Pacific War. For example, writing of the initial advances in the New Hebrides and the Solomon Islands, Beadle and Hoffman (1993: 322) note that:

On the island of Éfaté [New Hebrides], the primary attack rate of malaria . . . peaked at 2,632 cases per 1,000 average strength per year for all U.S. and Allied forces in April

Table 11.11. Epidemic periods for sample diseases of military significance to the US Army in the Pacific War, 1942–1945

Disease	Southwest Pacific					Pacific Ocean Areas				
	Start	End	Duration (months)	Admissions	Deaths	Start	End	Duration (months)	Admissions	Deaths
Malaria	Dec. 1942	Oct. 1943	11	37,130	17	Jan. 1943	Dec. 1943	12	54,819	28
Filariasis	Sept. 1943	Sept. 1943	1	29	0	Nov. 1943	Feb. 1944	4	649	0
	Feb. 1944	Feb. 1943	1	70	0	July 1944	July 1944	1	95	0
Dengue	Jan. 1942	Apr. 1942	4	1,200	0	Mar. 1943	June 1943	4	8,756	0
	Dec. 1942	Feb. 1943	3	2,669	1	Aug. 1944	Sept. 1944	2	12,400	0
	Jan. 1944	Feb. 1944	2	6,255	0					
Scrub typhus	Jan. 1943	Jan. 1943	1	74	4					
	July 1944	Sept. 1944	3	2,510	74					

Source: Based on information in Reister (1976).

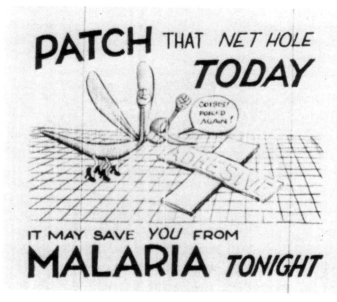

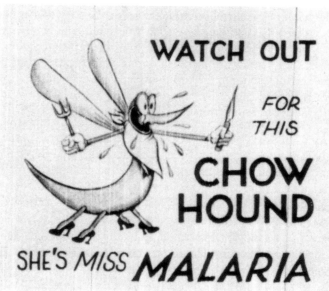

Pl. 11.3. US Army: cartoons for the control of malaria in the Southwest Pacific, World War II

Source: Reproduced from Hart and Hardenbergh (1963, fig. 62, 63, p. 566).

1942. Troops landed on Espíritu Santo [New Hebrides] in May 1942, but no cases of malaria were reported until September 1942. The peak rates on that island occurred in January 1943 when the primary attack rates experienced by the marines, navy forces, and all Allied forces were 442 per 1,000 per year, 85 per 1,000 per year, and 219 per 1,000 per year, respectively. On Guadalcanal [Solomon Islands], the next island that was occupied, 'almost every man who served . . . during the period of 7 August 1942 to 9 February 1943 fell victim to the disease.' . . . it is known that the total malarial attack rate (which includes all relapses) among all U.S. and Allied forces on the island was as high as 1,781 per 1,000 per year in November 1942.

Elsewhere, Hart and Hardenbergh (1963: 568) note that malaria rendered the First and Second US Marine Divisions, along with the US Army Thirty-Second Division, non-effective for up to six months after their withdrawal from the Pacific combat area. No less than two-thirds of the Thirty-Second Division developed symptoms of malaria in the ten months after leaving New Guinea while, within nine months of the onset of the Guadalcanal offensive (Aug. 1942), four-fifths of the First Marine Division had been admitted to hospital with malaria.

Malaria Discipline and Control in the South Pacific
Such high rates of disease activity reflected a series of errors relating to malaria discipline in the early stages of the Pacific War. Unit commanders generally disregarded the importance of protection from malarial mosquitoes, while many men had lost head and bed nets during landing operations. Natives, employed as manual labour by the US and Allied forces, provided a ready reservoir of the malaria parasite, while suppressive drugs were either unavailable (as on Éfaté) or failed on account of lack of supervision in their administration (as on Guadalcanal). Finally, veterans of the New Guinea and Guadalcanal campaigns carried the malaria parasite to other stations and, in the absence of local reservoirs, served as sources for the onwards transmission of the disease to their comrades (Beadle and Hoffman, 1993).

Malaria control. By mid-1943, senior commanders had begun to issue orders for appropriate malaria control. Malariologists, survey and control units were drafted into the Pacific Theatre, while draining, ditching, and oiling were undertaken to remove mosquito breeding sites in non-combat zones. Base and airfield sites were distanced from native settlements, new developments in insecticides (DDT) and insect repellents (DEET) were applied, and malaria discipline was intensified. Atabrine was introduced as a prophylactic/suppressive drug. As Figure 11.11A illustrates for the US Army, the various control measures were accompanied by a progressive reduction in malaria activity from July 1943 and, although subsequent phases of combat were typically associated with a modest rise in malaria activity, disease rates never returned to the earlier high levels (Harper *et al.*, 1963; Hart and Hadenbergh, 1963; Joy, 1999).

FILARIASIS

'Of all the diseases which were encountered in the South Pacific,' Sapero and Butler (1945: 505) observe, 'the appearance of filariasis in epidemic form excited by far the most interest. It was the first epidemic of the disease in the history of American or other military forces.' The earliest cases of the disease—a parasitic condition that is transmitted from human to human by a mosquito vector[9]—followed the initial deployment of US personnel to Samoa in 1942. By 1943, significant numbers of men had begun to develop swellings of the extremeties, with evidence of painful involvement of the scrotum and spermatic chord (Goodman *et al.*, 1945; Savitt, 1993). Subsequent surveys revealed that the disease was occurring on the Samoan islands of Tutuila and Upolu, along with Wallis, Funafuti, Fiji, Tonga, and adjacent islands of the central South Pacific (Goodman *et al.*, 1945; Swartzwelder, 1964; Savitt, 1993). As regards the distribution of cases by branch of service, the *c.*1,600 cases documented in the US Army (Table 11.10) were overshadowed by the *c.*12,000 cases recorded in the US Navy and Marine Corps. The difference in disease incidence reflected the larger numbers of Navy and Marine Corps personnel who were stationed on filarial islands (Swartzwelder, 1964).

Manpower Implications

As one of the leading causes of medical evacuation from the South Pacific, filariasis occasionally resulted in the loss from service of entire military units. For example, Swartzwelder (1964) relates the experience of two US Army organizations (134th Field Artillery Battalion and 404th Combat Engineer Company) which had been stationed at Tongabatu, Tonga, between May 1942 and May 1943. After several months of declining health, filariasis surveys of the two organizations revealed infection rates of 65 per cent (134th Field) and 55 per cent (404th Combat). The organizations were medically evacuated *in toto* in July 1944, having never been in combat and having spent some seven months in hospital.

Epidemiological Investigations: Camp Locality and Native Contact

In a wartime study of an undisclosed island, Englehorn and Wellman (1945) correlated the incidence of filariasis among US troops with (i) the proximity of army camps and other military installations to native villages and (ii) the

---

[9] Filariasis is the name given to a group of diseases caused by infection with parasitic filarial worms, including *Wuchereria bancrofti*. Bancroftian filariasis is transmitted by a mosquito, forming an intermediate host between human blood meals. Adult *W. bancrofti* lie in the human lymphatic vessels and lymph glands and produce larvae (microfiliae) that enter the peripheral blood and lymph channels of the human host. Obstruction of the lymph channels ultimately causes an abnormal swelling and enlargement (elephantiasis) of the scrotum, labia, breasts, legs, and/or arms. Elephantiasis, however, is usually only seen in those repeatedly exposed to the parasite over many years. Previously unexposed adults in endemic areas typically show an inflammatory response to infection. Such a response may immediately kill the worm but, in some instances, massive disruption of the lymphatic system may give rise to the early development of elephantiasis (Savitt, 1993).

frequency of the mingling of soldiers and natives. In one military unit, located close to a native village and with whom the troops had daily contact, the annual infection rate was estimated at 28 per cent. In contrast, in another unit, located some five miles from the nearest native village, the annual infection rate was estimated at just 6 per cent (ibid.). Such findings were consistent with evidence that levels of infection of the mosquito vector fell off rapidly with distance from native villages (Swartzwelder, 1964), and implied that transmission to US forces was intimately related to the geographical propinquity of soldiers and civilians. Unfortunately, in the early stages of the Pacific War at least, US personnel had arrived on infected islands (first and foremost, Samoa) in such numbers that it was not possible to separate the men from the natives, and some troops were actively billeted in native villages. Under such circumstances, high levels of infection rapidly accrued among exposed contingents of the occupying forces (Sapero and Butler, 1945; Swartzwelder, 1964).

Military Control: Spatial Segregation

Spatial segregation formed a central platform for the military control of filariasis. Military camps were (re)located as far as possible from native villages, personnel were prohibited from visiting the villages, while natives were barred from military facilities. Troops were removed from the islands as soon as the tactical situation allowed, while a system of rotation of personnel to non-filarial islands was recommended. As for the mosquito vector, malarial control units were diverted to filariasis control and the use of insect repellants, bed nets, and full-length clothing was promoted among the men (Swartzwelder, 1964).

DENGUE

Dengue is an acute viral disease[10] transmitted to humans by mosquitoes of the *Aedes* genus (Tsai, 2000). Long before US military operations in the South Pacific, several urban centres of the region—including Suva (Fiji), Nouméa (New Caledonia), and Tulagi (Solomon Islands)—were recognized as endemic foci of the disease. As the Americans moved into the Pacific, military camps (occasionally strewn with tin cans and other potential sources of standing water) provided new breeding grounds for *Aedes spp.* (Sapero and Butler, 1945; McCoy and Sabin, 1964). With camp conditions ripe for the high-level transmission of dengue, and with little or no acquired immunity among US personnel, major epidemics of the disease spread in the overseas forces (Table 11.12). Indeed, such was the magnitude of the problem that dengue ranked second

[10] In adults, dengue usually follows a well-defined clinical course. A typical incubation period of four to five days is followed by the abrupt onset of fever with headache and retro-orbital pain, backache, musculoskeletal pain, rash, and prostration. Acute illness terminates after eight to ten days in uncomplicated cases, with recovery characterized by an extended period of listlessness and fatigue. Complications, often resulting in death, include haemorrhagic manifestations (haemorrhagic dengue) and circulatory collapse (dengue shock syndrome) (McSherry, 1993; Tsai, 2000).

Table 11.12. Sample epidemics of dengue among US forces in South Pacific islands, Pacific War, 1942–1945

Island	Epidemic		Notes
	Start	End	
Australia	Mar. 1942	May 1942	Epidemic in Northern Territory and Queensland (80% attack rate).
Australia	Jan. 1943	Mar. 1943	Epidemic in the vicinity of Rockhampton and Brisbane, Queensland.
New Hebrides	Feb. 1943	Aug. 1943	Epidemic in military base at Espíritu Santo, resulting in the infection of *c.*5,000 personnel (25% attack rate).
New Caledonia	Feb. 1943	Aug. 1943	Occurring in conjunction with the New Hebrides epidemic (above), but with a less severe course.
Dutch New Guinea	1944		Epidemic in units stationed in the Hollandia and Biak areas.

Source: Based on information in McCoy and Sabin (1964: 32–40).

only to malaria as a cause of US Army hospital admissions in the Pacific Theatre (Table 11.10).

Inter-island Transmission and Control

A series of factors contributed to the inter-island transmission of dengue. At one level, the evacuation of patients from such endemic foci as New Caledonia, New Hebrides, and Fiji appears to have underpinned an eastwards drift of the disease to Wallis Island, Funafuti, and eventually Honolulu (Sapero and Butler, 1945; McCoy and Sabin, 1964). At another level, US aviation personnel contributed to the more localized inter-island transmission of the disease (Carson, 1944).

Control of inter-island transmission. Zeligs *et al.* (1944) provide a case study of the manner in which a major epidemic of introduced dengue was avoided in an undisclosed US combat area ('Island X') during 1943. Between 22 and 24 July, seven servicemen—newly arrived from an epidemic focus of dengue some 450 miles distant ('Island Y')—reported sick with the disease. A few days later, with an indigenously acquired case having now been recognized on Island X, rigorous methods of disease control were invoked. Patients were segregated in mosquito-free areas, daily checks were undertaken of all personnel in the infected zone, while an intensive mosquito control campaign was implemented. Although 27 people on Island X contracted dengue between 26 July and 7 August, and despite the arrival of more disease-carriers from Island Y between

9 and 31 August, only two further people stationed on Island X were attacked by the disease (Zeligs *et al.*, 1944).

SCRUB TYPHUS

In Section 9.3, we observed how Allied combat troops were blighted by scrub typhus (tsutsugamushi disease) in the Burma–India Theatre during World War II. The endemic focus of scrub typhus was, however, by no means restricted to the continental mainland of South and Southeast Asia. As Figure 9.2 shows, the area of endemic activity extended across the Indonesian archipelago, into New Guinea and proximal islands of the Southwest Pacific. Within this latter zone, delimited by Box 3 in Figure 9.2, some 6,000 US Army and Navy personnel contracted scrub typhus, and over 250 died as a consequence of the disease (Table 9.4).

Outbreaks in Dutch New Guinea and Adjacent Islands, 1944

During 1944, the Vogelkop Peninsula and adjacent islands (Owi and Biak) of Dutch New Guinea were the sites for explosive epidemics of scrub typhus among US forces (Griffiths, 1945; Irons and Armstrong, 1947). Together, the epidemics—associated with some 2,200 reported cases and 40 deaths—constituted the most serious episodes of this disease in US forces during World War II (Philip, 1964). Figure 11.8 gives the locations of the places named, while Figure 11.12 plots the weekly series of disease counts associated with the epidemics. We consider the Vogelkop and Owi–Biak outbreaks in turn.

Vogelkop outbreak (Griffiths, 1945). On Sunday 30 July 1944, elements of a US infantry division landed on the enemy-held coastline between Cape Sansapor and Cape Opmarai, Vogelkop Peninsula. The first case of scrub typhus presented in the force a week later, on 6 August, to be followed by an explosive rise in cases in the fortnight that followed (Fig. 11.12). At the peak, in mid-August, over 60 cases of scrub typhus were admitted to hospital each day, with a total of 931 cases and 34 deaths recorded during the entire seven-week course of the epidemic. For the majority of patients, it was possible to determine the specific geographical source of infection and, hence, the several types of environment associated with the disease: (i) abandoned native village and garden areas (>500 cases); (ii) beach and forest margins (90 cases); and (iii) overgrown coconut groves (26 cases). No infection could be attributed to climax rainforest—the primary environment of the Sansapor–Opmarai base.

Owi–Biak outbreak (Irons and Armstrong, 1947). As Figure 11.12 shows, the epidemic of scrub typhus on the neighbouring islands of Owi and Biak presaged the outbreak on the Vogelkop Peninsula by some six weeks. Operations had begun on the islands in early June 1944, with the first cases of scrub typhus appearing in the latter part of the month. Disease incidence was higher on Owi than on Biak, with the Air Force being particularly afflicted on the former

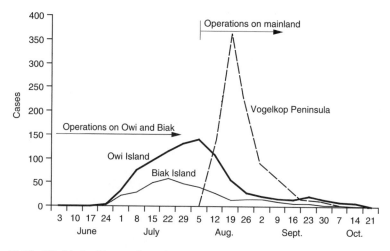

Fig. 11.12. Weekly incidence of scrub typhus among US military personnel stationed in Dutch New Guinea, 1944

Note: Line traces plot the weekly incidences for separate outbreaks among personnel on the Vogelkop Peninsula and on adjacent islands of Owi and Biak, June–October 1944. See Fig. 11.8 for locations.

Source: Redrawn from Griffiths (1945, fig. 1, p. 342) and Irons and Armstrong (1947, chart 1, p. 202).

island. Although the long tail of the outbreak continued until October, the implementation of control activites (including the clearing of undergrowth and the application of mite repellants) resulted in a significant reduction in cases from August (Pl. 11.4).

Epidemiological Observations

Drawing on evidence from the Vogelkop and Owi–Biak outbreaks, among many other episodes in New Guinea and elsewhere, Philip (1948) identified a series of key epidemiological features relating to the military occurrence of scrub typhus in the Southwest Pacific: (1) small island foci; (2) grass associations; and (3) seasonal occurrence.

1. *Small island foci.* A number of outbreaks of scrub typhus could be traced to small, palm-covered, Pacific islands. Rats—a reservoir of *Orientia tsutsugamushi*—often heavily colonized the islands and this may have served to exaggerate the focal occurrence of the disease. On Bunamu Island (200 × 400 yards),[11] a tiny coralline island with heavy vegetational cover and a place for the feeding, roosting, and nesting of South Sea Island pigeons, the dense population of brown rats was heavily infested with trombiculid mites. South Bat

[11] Located to the north of Bougainville, Solomon Islands.

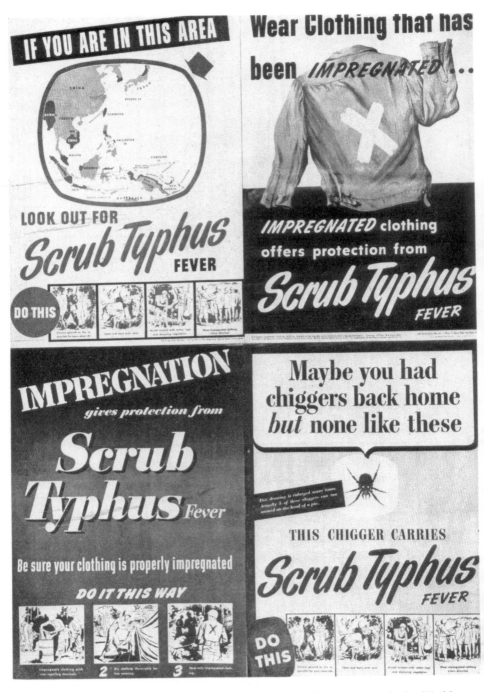

Pl. 11.4. Educational posters developed for the control of scrub typhus during World War II

Notes: (A) Posters developed in the Office of the US Surgeon General for field distribution. (B) Poster used in the Southwest Pacific Area.

Source: Reproduced from Philip (1964, fig. 64, 65, pp. 342–3).

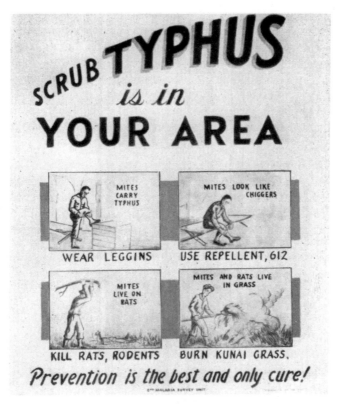

Pl. 11.4. (*cont.*)

Island (46 acres), on which the Australians and Americans had established observation posts, is reported to have been saturated with rats; the island was soon abandoned on account of scrub typhus. Likewise, ideal rat cover was provided in the undergrowth of the neglected coconut groves of Owi and Biak Islands. Within these small island foci, local case fatality rates for scrub typhus varied widely, from 0.6 to 35.5 per cent (Philip, 1948: 182–3).

2. *Grass associations.* During the early phases of fighting in Papua and British New Guinea and later Dutch New Guinea, many scrub typhus cases were associated with units which came into contact with a tall, rank, grass (kunai). The grassed areas occurred either as primitive fields or as secondary invaders in man-cleared sites. Abandoned villages, gardens, and neglected plantations provided the basis for colonization by grass and subsequently invasion by rodent and mite populations. As illustrated by the Vogelkop outbreak, these areas of abandoned and neglected land formed the focus for potentially explosive outbreaks of scrub typhus (Philip, 1948: 183–4).

3. *Seasonal occurrence.* A seasonal dimension to the occurrence of scrub typhus was generally lacking in the Southwest Pacific. Rather, peaks of disease activity were contingent on exposure during combat and military exercises. Outbreaks tended to occur among troops during the initial development of an infected area, with continuing sporadic cases after the establishment of a base. Mites appeared to be sensitive to lowered humidity in cleared areas, and did not remain long after the area had been settled. Subsequent, sporadic, cases were usually associated with exposure during combat operations (Philip, 1948: 184–5).

11.5 Conclusion

In this chapter, we have examined the spread of war epidemics with special reference to the islands of the South Pacific. Our consideration has been framed both by the particular interest which attaches to islands as laboratories for the study of epidemiological processes (Cliff *et al.*, 1981, 2000), and by the prominence of island epidemics as a theme in war history (Smallman-Raynor and Cliff 1998*a*, 1999). For the nineteenth century, we have shown how European contact occasionally resulted in the first-time introduction of Old World infections to warring states of the South Pacific. For example, nineteenth-century civil wars in the kingdom of Samoa were associated with virgin soil epidemics of whooping cough, mumps, and measles while, in French Polynesia, measles spread with mid-century unrest in the Leeward Islands (Huahine, Raiatéa, and Tahaa). Although evidence for mortality arising from the epidemics is fragmentary, information is sufficient to infer that the classical association of war, disease, and famine had a severe impact on the peoples involved (McArthur, 1968).

Turning to the twentieth century, the example of the Spanish influenza pandemic of 1918–19 illustrates how one island (Australia) exploited its isolation to afford protection from the disease. Between October 1918 and April 1919, wave upon wave of troopships from the battlefields of northern Europe— many having experienced outbreaks of influenza on board—arrived at Australian ports, only for the crew and passengers to be placed in quarantine. In this manner, Australia succeeded in delaying the introduction of severe influenza by several months (Cumpston, 1919). In New Zealand, by contrast, the civil population acquired the disease early on (Pool, 1973), with rapid spread by way of commercial vessels to other islands of the South Pacific (McArthur, 1968).

During World War II, a series of diseases endemic to the South Pacific islands—malaria, filariasis, dengue, and scrub typhus—served as a major drain on the fighting strength of the US Army, Navy, and Marine Corps, thereby threatening the success of General MacArthur's island campaigns.

Deployment in unfamiliar epidemiological environments, lack of acquired immunity to prevalent diseases, inadequate discipline, poor camp hygiene, the geographical propinquity of natives and military personnel, and the difficulties of infection control during active combat missions all contributed to the disease problem. But, as familiarity with the epidemiological environment of the South Pacific grew, so infectious diseases came increasingly under control. Indeed, as Sapero and Butler (1945: 502) note, in the course of time 'Allied successes in disease control so greatly exceeded those of the Japanese that a major advantage in the war was thereby gained'.

12

Further Regional Studies

We've got the cholerer in camp—it's worse than forty fights;
We're dyin' in the wilderness the same as Isrulites.
It's before us, an' be'ind us, an' we cannot get away,
An' the doctor's just reported we've ten more today!

Since August, when it started, it's been stickin' to our tail,
Though they've 'ad us out by marches an' they've 'ad us back by rail;
But it runs as fast as troop trains, and we cannot get away,
An' the sick-list to the Colonel makes ten more today.

Rudyard Kipling, 'Cholera Camp' (1896)

12.1 Introduction

In Chapters 7 to 11, we have examined a series of recurring themes in the geography of war and disease since 1850 through regional lenses. In this chapter, we conclude our regional–thematic survey by illustrating further prominent themes which, either because of their subject-matter or because of their geographical location, were beyond the immediate scope of the foregoing chapters. In selecting regional case studies for this chapter, we concentrate on wars which have not been examined in depth to this point (the South African War and the Cuban Insurrection) or which, on account of their magnitude and extent, merit examination beyond that afforded in previous sections (World War I and World War II). Four principal issues are addressed:

(1) *Africa: population reconcentration and disease (Section 12.2)*, illustrated with reference to civilian concentration camps in the South African War, 1899–1902;

(2) *Americas: peace, war, and epidemiological integration (Section 12.3)*, illustrated with reference to the civil settlement system of Cuba, 1888–1902;

(3) *Asia: prisoners of war, forced labour, and disease (Section 12.4)*, illustrated with reference to Allied prisoners on the line of the Burma–Thailand Railway, 1942–4;

(4) *Europe: civilian epidemics and the world wars (Section 12.5)*, illustrated with reference to the spread of a series of diseases in the civil population of Europe during, and after, the hostilities of 1914–18 and 1939–45.

As before, the study sites in (1) to (4) span a broad range of epidemiological environments, from the cool temperate latitudes of northern Europe, through the tropical island and jungle environments of the Caribbean and Southeast Asia, to the warm temperate and subtropical savannah lands of the South African Veld. Diseases have been sampled to reflect this epidemiological range.

12.2 Africa: Population Reconcentration and Disease in the South African War[1]

The South African War (1899–1902)[2] has been described as the last of the 'typhoid campaigns' (Curtin, 1998)—a closing chapter on the predominance of disease over battle as a cause of death among soldiers (Pakenham, 1979:

---

[1] The material included in this section has been prepared in association with Dr Daniel Low-Beer, Department of Geography, University of Cambridge. Under the direction of one of the authors (ADC), the original research was conducted by Dr Low-Beer during his employment as Postdoctoral Research Associate on Leverhulme Trust Grant No. F/753/D.

[2] Our use of the term *South African War*, rather than (*Second* or *Great*) *Boer War*, follows recent thought by historians on appropriate nomenclature for the conflict (see Smith, 1996).

382). From the military perspective, typhoid was indeed the major health issue of the war, accounting for a reported 8,020 deaths in the British Army (Simpson, 1911: 57).[3] There is, however, a second disease history to the South African War associated with the health impacts of concentration camps on civil populations. As a tactic of modern warfare, population reconcentration had first been employed by the Spanish to quash support for rural guerrilla forces during the Cuban Insurrection of 1895–8 (Sect. 12.3). A few years later, during the South African War, the British employed similar tactics by herding many tens of thousands of Boer and Black civilians into tented camps in Natal, Orange Free State, and the Transvaal. As had happened in Cuba, the crowding together of so many people was to result in the explosive spread of all manner of infectious diseases. In this section, we examine the disease history of the South African War with particular reference to patterns of mortality in the concentration camps that housed Boer and Black civilians. Our discussion is based on Low-Beer *et al.* (forthcoming).

ESTABLISHMENT OF THE CONCENTRATION CAMPS

The South African War formally began with the declaration of war on Britain by the South African Republic (Transvaal) and her ally, Orange Free State, in October 1899. Within a year, the major military engagements of the conflict appeared to be over; the Boer Army had scattered, and the Transvaal was formally annexed. However, a new stage of the hostilities was now initiated. The Boer citizen army of commando units, fighting on and for their homelands, continued increasingly diffused hostilities across the Veld. The long tail of the war extended to May 1902, with the British uncertain at first how to deal with Boer 'guerrilla'[4] tactics or, indeed, the civilians involved. Eventually, the British undertook great military sweeps across the land, constructing over 3,700 miles of wire mesh that linked some 8,000 blockhouses. Homesteads and crops were destroyed while, from January 1901,[5] the civil population was increasingly concentrated in a system of camps that extended across Natal, Orange Free State,

---

[3] There is some difficulty in distinguishing typhoid from continued fevers, but this does not have a substantial impact on the documented death rate. Simpson (1911: 58) suggests that the diagnosis of enteric fever was 'probably approximate to the true incidence', better than previous campaigns and consistent with previous experience in South Africa.

[4] The contemporary characterization of Boer resistance as guerrilla and illegitimate was rejected by the British Intelligence Division: 'While it is true that the Boers have adopted guerilla tactics, it is none the less true that their method . . . is very different from that which is understood by the term "guerilla war". Though their forces are distributed in small commandos over an immense stretch of territory . . . they are capable of organised concentration and their continued resistance can hardly be termed illegitimate' (cited in Spies, 1977: 11).

[5] There is some disagreement as to when the first concentration camps were established. Brodrick states that the first concentration camp was erected in January 1901, before Lord Roberts left South Africa for London. Emily Hobhouse, on the other hand, states that the camp at Mafeking existed from July 1900. See Spies (1977: 114).

and the Transvaal (see Fig. 12.1 and Pl. 12.1). Undoubtedly this was the most determinant and elusive stage of the war, leaving enduring legacies in the Boer memory and colonial enthusiasm in Britain (Spies, 1977; Pakenham, 1979).

12.2.1 Nature of the Data

To examine patterns of mortality in the concentration camps of South Africa, two principal sources of secondary data were accessed:

1. *The British Parliamentary Sessional Papers.* Mortality data were compiled from the thicket of tables and reports which appear in volume lxviii (1902) of the British Parliamentary *Sessional Papers* (especially Cd. 793, 819, 853, 893, 902, 924, 934, 936, 939, 942, 1161). The *Sessional Papers* include the monthly statistical returns for Boer concentration camps in Natal, Orange Free State, and the Transvaal, supplemented by the reports of camp superintendents on local conditions and the prevailing causes of death. In addition, the *Papers* include background information on death rates in South Africa, 1896–1900, along with statistical excerpts from the *Transvaal Government Gazette.*

2. *Other major secondary sources.* To provide a broader perspective on war-associated mortality, information was drawn from a variety of other secondary sources. These include the Fawcett Commission's 'Report on the Concentration Camps' (1901) and Simpson's *Medical History of the War in South Africa* (1911) among other contemporary (Hobhouse, 1901, 1902) and modern (Warwick, 1983; Fetter and Kessler, 1996) sources.

A general overview of the quality of the data contained in sources (1) and (2) is provided by Low-Beer *et al.* (forthcoming). However, we note here that an inspection of the sources and their associated commentaries reveals the existence of a 'data gradient' between soldiers and civilians and, for the latter, between Boers and Blacks. Thus, relatively systematic reporting of mortality for British soldiers (21,942 documented deaths) gives way to widening mortality estimates for Boer (25,000–34,000 deaths) and Black (7,000–20,000 deaths) civilians (see Simpson, 1911; Pakenham, 1979; and Warwick, 1983).

12.2.2 Concentration Camps and Mortality in Wartime Perspective

The charts in Figure 12.2 are based on an integrated analysis of the secondary data sources described above and summarize the overall pattern of mortality in the South African War.[6] While the distributions are based on higher estimates

---

[6] Estimates are taken for British soldiers (Simpson, 1911), Boer soldiers (Pakenham, 1979), Boer camps (Spies, 1977; Curtin, 1998), and Black camps (Kessler 1999a, 1999b). The Black camp mortality includes deaths of Blacks when they were under White camp administration, for which over 17,000 deaths have been verified. Mortality in the Boer and Black camps is probably underestimated.

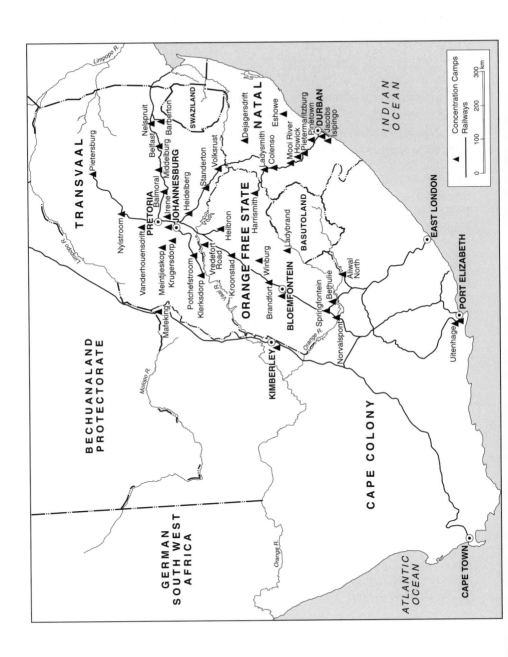

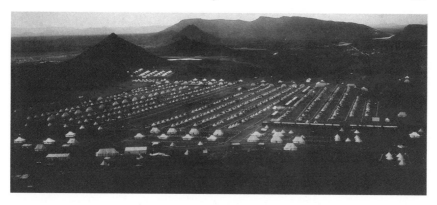

Pl. 12.1. Concentration camp at Norvalspont, South Africa, during the war of 1899–1902

Note: The location of Norvalspont is given in Fig. 12.1.
Source: Jackson (1999: 148–9).

of mortality in the civil concentration camps than previously used (Warwick, 1983), the data for the Black and Boer camps may well underestimate the true mortality totals for these institutions.

Distribution of wartime mortality (Figure 12.2A). According to Figure 12.2A, an estimated 77,000 soldiers and civilians died as a consequence of the war. Of these, internees in the Boer and Black concentration camps accounted for the majority of deaths (42,000), with women and children dominating the civilian mortality profile. For example, in the Boer camps, 81 per cent of the deaths were among children, 13 per cent among women, and only 6 per cent among men. In these camps alone, female and child mortality (~26,000 deaths) approached the male mortality in the combined British and Boer Armies (~29,000 deaths).

Comparative patterns (Figure 12.2B). Figure 12.2B provides estimates of the overall mortality rate (expressed per 1,000 population per annum) for the civil populations of the Black and Boer camps, along with parallel estimates for the British Army at various stations during the war. The mortality rates for both the Black and Boer camps exceeded 180 per 1,000 per annum, well in excess of the mortality rates for the British Army at the famous siege of Ladysmith (110), at Bloemfontein (84) and during the entire period of the war (38).

Fig. 12.1. Map of Boer concentration camps in the South African War, 1899–1902
Source: Low-Beer *et al.* (forthcoming).

A

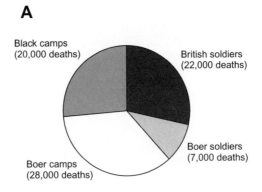

B

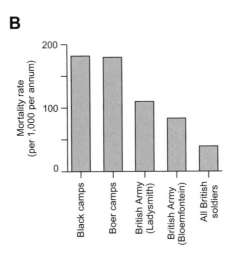

Fig. 12.2. Military and civilian deaths in the South African War, 1899–1902

Notes: (A) Distribution of an estimated 77,000 deaths by population group. (B) Estimated mortality rate (per 1,000 per annum) for Black camps, Boer camps, and British soldiers. The mortality rates for British soldiers are shown for the entire British Army in South Africa, and for those at Ladysmith and Bloemfontein.

Source: Low-Beer *et al.* (forthcoming).

12.2.3 Time Series of Mortality in the Concentration Camps

Figure 12.3A relates to the main phase of population concentration, April 1901–April 1902, and plots the monthly series of mortality rates (expressed per 1,000 deaths per annum) for the Boer and Black concentration camps. An additional mortality series, formed for a subset of 25 Boer camps located in the Transvaal (Fig. 12.1), is plotted for reference. While Figure 12.3A serves to underscore the high levels of mortality in the camps, three features of the timing of mortality are also noteworthy:

(1) high levels of mortality were recorded in the early phases of population concentration. For example, in the set of Transvaal Boer camps a mortality rate of over 100 per 1,000 per annum was recorded at the beginning of the time series in Figure 12.3A. Similarly high rates were registered in the early months of the series for both the entire set of Boer camps and the Black camps;

(2) the decline in mortality in the Boer camps (beginning in Nov. 1901) appears to coincide with the publication of the Fawcett Commission's (1901) 'Report on the Concentration Camps' and the associated shift from military to civil administration of the camps. Such a finding is consistent with the observations of historians such as Spies (1977) and Pakenham (1979);

(3) the mortality peak in the Black camps (Dec. 1901) lagged the Boer camps (Oct. 1901) by several months, with a consequently lagged decline. Set against observation (2), the reputedly 'magical effect' on camp mortality of the Fawcett Commission (Pakenham, 1979: 518) does not appear to have extended to the Black camps in 1901.

DISAGGREGATING MORTALITY: BOER CAMPS IN THE TRANSVAAL

To explore local patterns of mortality in the concentration camps, we draw on the detailed information relating to a sample of 25 Boer camps in the Transvaal. The monthly time series of mortality in the 25 camps is plotted in Figure 12.3A. Together the camps had a peak population of 65,500, with a total of 10,618 recorded deaths in the 13-month period April 1901–April 1902.

Timing of Mortality by Camp

Figure 12.3B plots the time series of monthly mortality rates, April 1901–April 1902, for the five Boer camps of the Transvaal with the largest reported mortality counts: Middelburg (1,367 deaths); Klerksdorp (1,094); Mafeking (1,002); Potchefstroom (904); and Irene (829). The locations of the five camps are given in Figure 12.1. When compared to the aggregate pattern in Figure 12.3A, Figure 12.3B reveals a very different picture of the timing of mortality in the camps. Four features of 12.3B merit comment:

(1) the very high mortality rates in all five camps, peaking at 1,020 deaths per 1,000 population per annum at Mafeking;

(2) the marked differences in the timing of mortality peaks, ranging from June 1901 (Potchefstroom) to October 1901 (Mafeking);

(3) the existence of two periods of heightened mortality for some camps (Irene, Klerksdorp, and Middelburg) in June–July and October–December 1901;

(4) consistent with observation (3), between-camp variations in the duration of periods of heightened mortality, ranging from the temporally

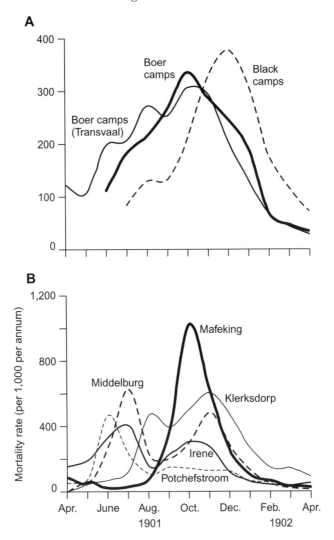

Fig. 12.3. Monthly mortality rates in Black and Boer camps during the South African War, April 1901–April 1902

Notes: (A) Mortality rate (per 1,000 population per annum) in the Boer camps (all camps and the Transvaal camps) and Black camps. (B) Mortality rate (per 1,000 population per annum) in the five Boer camps of the Transvaal with the largest reported mortality counts.
Source: Low-Beer *et al.* (forthcoming).

concentrated mortality of Mafeking to the temporally extended mortality of Klerksdorp and Middelburg.

Taken together, these observations are consistent with the occurrence of single-source epidemics in the camps, with very rapid, intense periods of infection and high mortality.

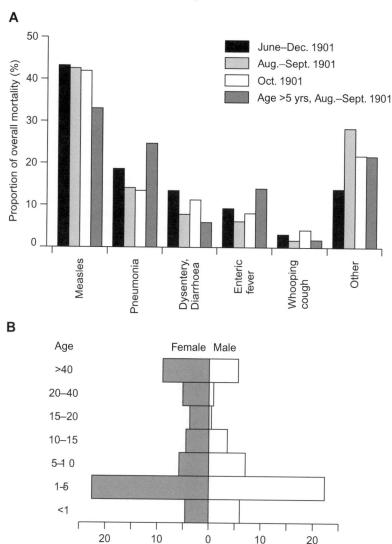

Fig. 12.4. Mortality in Boer concentration camps of the Transvaal, 1901

Notes: (A) Percentage distribution of mortality by disease for sample time periods, June–December 1901. (B) Percentage distribution of deaths by age group and sex, Bloemfontein camp, May–June 1901.

Source: Low-Beer *et al.* (forthcoming).

Analysis by Disease

Figure 12.4A relates to the 25 Boer camps in the Transvaal and plots the percentage contribution of six categories of mortality (measles, pneumonia, dysentery/diarrhoea, enteric fever, whooping cough, and all other causes) to overall mortality in the camps.[7] The information is given for (i) the entire population of the camps in three sample time periods (June–December 1901; August–September 1901; and October 1901) and (ii) the population aged over 5 years (Aug.–Sept. 1901).

(i) *Entire population of the camps.* Measles consistently appears as the leading single cause of mortality in Figure 12.4A, accounting for over 40 per cent of deaths in the entire population of the Boer camps during the period June–December 1901. The next largest cause of death is pneumonia, followed by dysentery/diarrhoea, enteric fever, and whooping cough.

(ii) *Population aged over 5 years.* As Figure 12.4A indicates, measles was by no means restricted to young children aged 5 years and under. Measles was also the leading cause of mortality in older populations, accounting for some 33 per cent of deaths in those aged over 5 years in August–September 1901. Such a finding implies that large numbers of Boers had not been exposed to measles on the Veld for at least five years previously, and probably considerably longer. The issue of the age distribution of measles cases in the Boer concentration camps is examined further below.

Correlation Analysis

To what extent did measles account for camp-to-camp variations in overall levels of mortality? In the two camps with the highest mortality rates, measles accounted for 68 per cent (Mafeking) and 71 per cent (Standerton) of all recorded deaths. By contrast, in the camp at Nylstroom diarrhoeal disease (diarrhoea, dysentery, and enteric fever) was the leading cause of death and accounted for 50 per cent of recorded mortality. Across the set of camps, however, computation of Pearson's correlation coefficient reveals that overall mortality rates are (i) strongly and positively correlated ($r = +0.77$) with the proportion of deaths attributable to measles, and (ii) weakly and negatively correlated ($r = -0.11$) with the proportion of deaths attributable to diarrhoeal disease. Thus, notwithstanding the existence of several disease-related causes of death, we infer that measles was a prominent factor in the overall pattern of extreme mortality in the sample set of Boer concentration camps.

12.2.4 Epidemiological Determinants of Severe Measles

Factors which may have contributed to the severity of measles in the concentration camps of South Africa include a series of macro- and micro-level determinants. We examine each set of determinants in turn.

---

[7] Balmoral camp has been omitted from the analysis in Fig. 12.4A on account of the lack of disease-specific information.

MACRO-LEVEL DETERMINANTS

At one level, the severity of measles reflected the lack of acquired immunity to the disease in the civil population of South Africa. The general epidemiological relations between population size and periodic measles outbreaks are outlined in Cliff *et al.* (1981: 40) but we note here that, in the period prior to the war, the highly dispersed population of the Veld was unable to maintain measles in endemic form. Geographical isolation may have afforded some defence against the disease and, notwithstanding the occasional appearance of measles in pre-war South Africa, overall levels of herd immunity may be assumed to have declined over an extended period of time. Evidence for this phenomenon is provided by the age distribution of recorded deaths in the concentration camps. Figure 12.4B relates to the Boer camp at Bloemfontein and shows the age category of measles deaths in the months of May and June 1901. The pyramid identifies a primary concentration of mortality in the age group 1 to 5 years, with a secondary peak in the age group of over 40 years. Such a finding implies that certain sectors of the population were so isolated that they had not been exposed to measles for over 40 years. As would be expected under conditions of low herd immunity, the concentration of increasingly large numbers of people gave rise to measles epidemics of almost virgin soil-like intensity in the concentration camps.

MICRO-LEVEL DETERMINANTS

Micro-level factors which contributed to the occurrence and severity of measles in the concentration camps are particularly important as they are closely linked to evaluations of medical neglect, deliberate or otherwise.

Introduction of Measles to the Camps

Rather than a synchronous mortality curve which rose to an aggregate peak in late 1901 and then declined with improved conditions (Fig. 12.3A), the differential mortality peaks in Figure 12.3B imply that the timings of epidemics varied from one camp to another. By way of analogy with the army camp epidemics in Sections 7.3 and 8.2, the patterns in Figure 12.3B are consistent with the occurrence of separate single-source epidemics, suggesting that the movement and transfer of infected people to and between camps may have played a significant role in the spatial dynamics of measles. In this context, we note that camp officials clearly failed to control the entry of measles-infected refugees into their camps. 'There is barely language too strong', the Fawcett Commission commented at the time, 'to express our opinion of the sending of a mass of disease to a healthy camp' (cited in Pakenham, 1979: 516).

Overcrowding

Epidemiological studies have revealed the role of overcrowding as a factor in measles mortality (Chalmers, 1930), with a possible dose effect influencing the severity of disease (Aaby *et al.*, 1986). In this respect, overcrowding in the South African concentration camps was acute, and measles cases—numbering up to four at a time in a family tent—were often concealed from the British authorities. As Emily Hobhouse, who provided the first reports on the conditions in the camps, observed: 'When the 8, 10 or 12 persons who occupied the bell-tent were all packed into it . . . there was no room to move, and the atmosphere was indescribable' (cited in Pakenham, 1979: 506). In the light of modern epidemiological knowledge, it seems likely that such gross overcrowding would have had a deleterious impact on the course and severity of measles in the camps.

Malnutrition

Given the established role of malnutrition in the development of severe measles (Cliff *et al.*, 1993: 27), it may be conjectured that the severity of measles was related both to the malnutrition of civilians entering the concentration camps and to the limited rations they received while under guard.

12.2.5 Conclusions

The South African War highlights the epidemiologically divisive nature of population concentration as a strategy of modern warfare. In the South African context, the gathering together of large numbers of susceptible civilians, often in crowded conditions, with few rations and with little medical assistance, fuelled measles epidemics of unusual (almost virgin soil-like) severity. The experience of Emily Hobhouse, working in the midst of one such camp epidemic, reflects the dawning realization of the true magnitude of the associated mortality on contemporary observers: 'I began to compare a parish I had known at home of 2,000 people where a funeral was an event . . . here some twenty to twenty-five were carried away daily . . . The full realization of the position dawned upon me—it was a death-rate such as had never been except in the times of the Great Plagues' (cited in Pakenham, 1979: 507). The post mortem on the concentration camps reveals much about the British military and civil administrations and the changing nature of war at the turn of the century. Once conditions in the camps were exposed, it was difficult to use the same moral, political, and financial arguments to generate enthusiasm for the British imperial project. The estimated loss of 77,000 soldiers and civilians remained in the imperial memory of both Britain and South Africa. In terms of war, a step function in the financial costs was apparent. Previous imperial subjects were incorporated into the British Empire at a cost of 15 pence. The Boers, however, cost £1,000 each to subdue (Smith, 1996: 4).

12.3 Americas: Peace, War, and the Epidemiological Integration of Cuba, 1888–1902

In this section, we take the example of late-nineteenth-century Cuba to examine a fundamental geographical issue in the historical association of conflict and disease: how does the epidemiological integration of a settlement system differ as between war and peace? To address the issue, we focus on the spread of three of the most prominent infectious diseases (yellow fever, smallpox, and enteric fever) to diffuse across Cuba during a 38-month period of hostilities associated with the Cuban Insurrection against Spain, February 1895–March 1898.[8] As a benchmark against which to assess the affects of war, we compare our 38-month 'window' on the Cuban Insurrection with the period of relative epidemiological calm which preceded the hostilities. Our examination draws on the study of Smallman-Raynor and Cliff (1999), where details of the course of the insurrection and its reconfiguration as an arm of the Spanish–American War discussed in Section 7.3 are given.

THE STUDY SITE

Figure 12.5 shows the location of Cuba and names the principal places referred to in the text. On the eve of the insurrection, in February 1895, the US War Department (1900: 10) estimated the population of the island to be approximately 1.8 million. However, for detailed information on the settlement of late-nineteenth-century Cuba, we are largely reliant on the post-war census of October 1899. By this date, the hostilities had reduced the population to approximately 1.57 million. Almost half were resident in 96 settlements of 1,000 inhabitants or more. The port city of Habana, situated on the northwest coast of the island, was the largest (population 235,981) and dominated a markedly primate urban system; only five other cities (Cardenas, Cienfuegos, Matanzas, Puerto Príncipe, and Santiago de Cuba) recorded populations in excess of 15,000. Elsewhere, the settlement pattern was characterized by scattered towns and villages of less than 4,000 inhabitants (US War Department, 1900).

Impact of the Insurrection on Mortality

As Figure 12.6 shows, the war period was associated with an enormous increase in mortality. The bar chart plots the monthly mortality rate (per 10,000 population) for seven of the most populous settlements of Cuba, 1888–1902; for reference, the average mortality rate for each calendar month

---

[8] Although the Cuban insurrection against Spain continued until August 1898, our selection of time period (which ends with the month preceding US military engagement in Cuba) was dictated by the cessation of prospective disease surveillance that accompanied the onset of the Spanish–American War (Apr.–Aug. 1898).

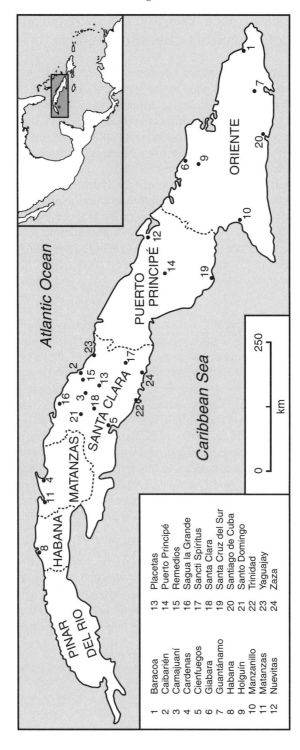

Fig. 12.5. Location map of Cuba, c.1900

Note: Place names and spellings are in accordance with the *Census of Cuba* (US War Department, 1900).
Source: Smallman-Raynor and Cliff (1999, fig. 1, p. 333).

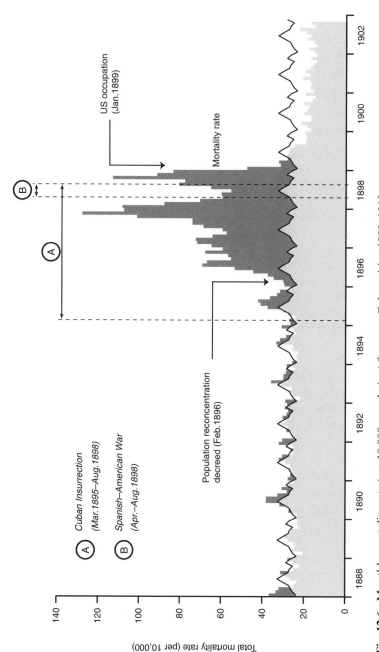

Fig. 12.6. Monthly mortality rate (per 10,000 population) for seven Cuban cities, 1888–1902.

Notes: The mortality rate, which relates to deaths from all causes, is plotted as a bar chart. The line trace plots the monthly mortality rate as a seasonal average over the 15 annual periods; months of above-average mortality are identified by the dense shading. The period of the Cuban Insurrection and the Spanish–American War is indicated.

Source: Smallman-Raynor and Cliff (1999, fig. 2, p. 335).

(formed by averaging the rates across corresponding months in the 13 annual periods) is superimposed as a line trace. From a steady background rate of 20 to 30 deaths per 10,000 in the years that preceded the insurrection, the mortality soared to levels in excess of 100 per 10,000 in the latter months of 1897. High death rates were to continue throughout the period of the Spanish–American War and, only with the US annexation of the island in 1899, did the death rate fall to, and eventually below, its pre-war level.

DISEASES AND DATA

For the 38-month period of the Cuban Insurrection prior to US military engagement, February 1895–March 1898, Smallman-Raynor and Cliff (1999) describe how severe epidemics of three infectious diseases (yellow fever, smallpox, and enteric fever) spread in the two largest populations of the island: Cuban civilians and Spanish soldiers. To analyse patterns of activity associated with the three diseases, 1888 was selected as the initial year of a 15-year time 'window' which straddled the Cuban Insurrection and the Spanish–American War (Feb. 1895–Aug. 1898) and ended with the establishment of the Cuban Republic in 1902. For this 180-month period, mortality counts for seven sample cities of Cuba (Cardenas, Cienfuegos, Habana, Matanzas, Puerto Principé, Sagua la Grande, and Santiago) were abstracted from the international disease surveillance section of the contemporary US *Public Health Reports* (Pl. 1.2H) for (i) all causes, (ii) yellow fever, (iii) smallpox, and (iv) enteric fever. In addition, a fifth matrix of mortality for 'infectious diseases' was formed by summing the separate matrices relating to yellow fever, smallpox, and enteric fever. The epidemiological information was supplemented by demographic information from the *Public Health Reports* and the Cuban censuses of 1899 (US War Department, 1900) and 1907 (Oficino del Censo de los Estados Unidos, 1908).

Differential Susceptibility and Disease

The three sample diseases did not strike the Cuban (civil) and Spanish (military) populations with equal severity. Epidemiological details are given in Appendix 12A but, for the purpose of the analysis to follow, we note here that differential patterns of susceptibility to infection were to favour the spread of yellow fever among Spanish soldiers, smallpox among Cuban civilians, and enteric fever in both populations.

12.3.1 The War Epidemics

The graphs in Figure 12.7 have been produced by combining the mortality counts for the seven cities. They plot, as a heavy line trace, the monthly mortality rate (per 10,000) for yellow fever (Fig. 12.7A), smallpox (Fig. 12.7B) and

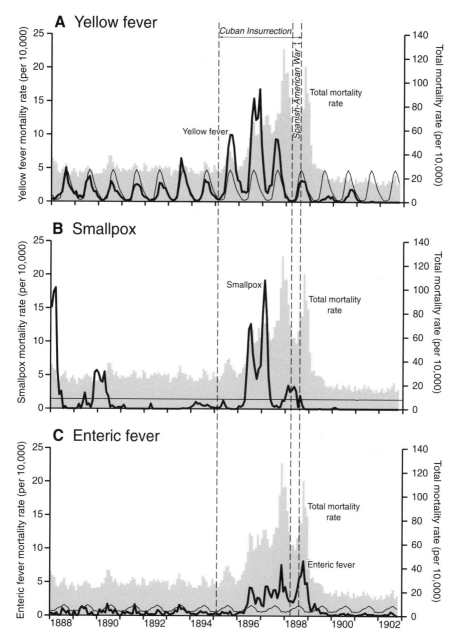

Fig. 12.7. Mortality from infectious diseases in seven Cuban cities, 1888–1902

Notes: The monthly mortality rate (per 10,000) for a given disease (heavy line trace) is superimposed on the mortality rate (per 10,000) for all causes (bar chart) replotted from Fig. 12.6. (A) Yellow fever. (B) Smallpox. (C) Enteric fever. For each disease, the fine line trace provides a measure of the average monthly mortality rate over the 15 annual periods. The period of the Cuban Insurrection and the Spanish–American War is indicated.

Source: Smallman-Raynor and Cliff (1999, fig. 3, p. 339).

Table 12.1. Periods of epidemic activity in the Cuban Insurrection, February 1895–March 1898

Cause of death	Epidemic period[1]		Duration (months)	Deaths
	Start	End		
All causes	May 1895	March 1898	35	76,096
Infectious diseases[2]	May 1895	March 1898	23	14,059
Yellow fever	March 1895	November 1897	33	7,211
Smallpox	May 1896	April 1897	12	4,207
Enteric fever	May 1896	March 1898	23	2,641

Notes: [1] Defined as the phase of above-average mortality in the period February 1895–March 1898.
[2] Combined mortality from yellow fever, smallpox, and enteric fever.
Source: Smallman-Raynor and Cliff (1999, table III, p. 340).

enteric fever (Fig. 12.7C), 1888–1902. For reference, the fine line traces plot a measure of the mean monthly rate for each disease which was calculated as follows:

(i) for yellow fever and enteric fever, which display evidence of a recurrent annual (seasonal) swing in mortality, the mean rate for a given calendar month (January, February, . . . , December) has been calculated by averaging over the corresponding months in the 15 annual time periods;

(ii) for smallpox, which displays no evidence of a seasonal swing in mortality, the horizontal line at 1.46 marks the average rate over the 180 monthly periods.

Finally, on each graph, the mortality rate (per 10,000) for all causes has been replotted from Figure 12.6 as a bar graph.

The epidemic waves which accompanied the Cuban Insurrection (Feb. 1895–Mar. 1898) appear as peaks of mortality in Figure 12.7. Summary details of each epidemic phase, as defined by periods of activity above the monthly mean, appear in Table 12.1; the corresponding information for mortality from all causes (Fig. 12.6) is also given. Together, Figure 12.7 and Table 12.1 reveal distinctive features of the three epidemic events:

(1) Yellow fever (Fig. 12.7A). From an onset in the second month of the insurrection (Mar. 1895), the epidemic phase continued for an unbroken period of 33 months to November 1897. During this period, the epidemic was characterized by three waves which correspond to the yellow fever seasons (June–Dec.) of 1895, 1896, and 1897;

(2) Smallpox (Fig. 12.7B). The epidemic phase began in May 1896, within months of General Weyler's initial order for the reconcentration of rural civilians. It followed a distinctive course with two sharp peaks of activity (July 1896 and Jan. 1897), to end abruptly in May 1897. Thereafter,

the virus continued to circulate at a low (sub-epidemic) level, with a minor resurgence in the early months of 1898;

(3) Enteric fever (Fig. 12.7C). As for smallpox, the epidemic phase began in May 1896. From thereon, mortality tracked the death rate from all causes (bar chart) rising to a peak in the latter months of 1897. The epidemic continued throughout the Spanish–American War (Apr.–Aug. 1898), reaching a second peak in the immediate aftermath of the conflict.

12.3.2 Disease Centroids

For each month of the Cuban Insurrection to US intervention, February 1895–March 1898, geographical centroids of disease activity (see Sect. 6.5.2) were computed for the combined series of mortality rates from yellow fever, smallpox, and enteric fever. The results are summarized for the period of above-average mortality (May 1895–Mar. 1898; see Table 12.1) in Figure 12.8A. Here, the location of the disease centre in each of the 35 monthly periods is indicated by a circle. Vectors link the position of the mortality centre in successive months.

The most striking feature of Figure 12.8 is the drift of the centre of infectious disease mortality (Fig. 12.8A) with the shifting locus of Cuban guerrilla activity (Fig. 12.8B). During the early months of the war (May 1895–Mar. 1896), the mortality centre was focused on the southeastern provinces of Oriente and Puerto Príncipe (see Fig. 12.5 for locations). However, coincidental with the invasion of the west by the Cuban *insurrectos* in 1896 (Fig. 12.8B) and the introduction of population reconcentration by the Spanish administration (late Feb. 1896), the mortality centre moved rapidly to the central and northern provinces of Matanzas and Santa Clara. The mortality centre was to remain in these provinces until the end of the observation period (Mar. 1898).

Although not shown in Figure 12.8, a parallel analysis of the combined mortality series for the pre-war period (Jan. 1890–Jan. 1895) yielded a mortality centre that was firmly rooted in the northwestern and central sectors of Cuba. When compared with the findings for the war period, these results imply that the events of the insurrection were associated with a fundamental change in the spatial course and geographical extent of disease activity in the island.

12.3.3 Spatial Associations

While the preceding analysis provides information on the broad spatial course of the wartime epidemics, other techniques are required to determine whether the war was associated with a fundamental shift in the epidemiological integration of urban centres. To address this issue, we employed cross-correlation analysis (see Sect. 6.7.3).

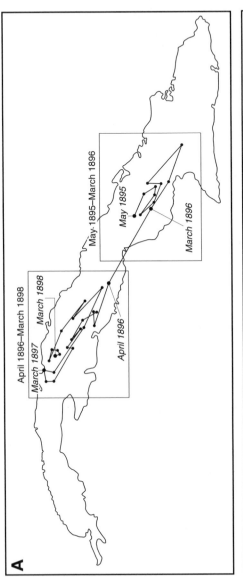

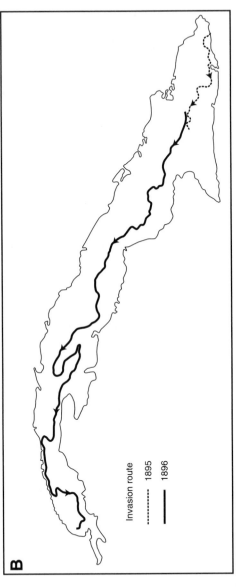

For the 38-month duration of the Cuban Insurrection prior to US military intervention in April 1898, the cause-specific death rate per 10,000 population for each of the seven cities was treated as a time series. As required for cross-correlation analysis, to ensure that the time series were stationary, all series were detrended by fitting linear regression models. Then any potential confounding effects of annual disease cycles driven by meteorological phenomena were eliminated by deseasonalizing the detrended series (Cliff and Haggett, 1988: 148–9). After detrending and deseasonalizing, the time series of death rates for each mortality category (all causes, infectious diseases, yellow fever, smallpox, and enteric fever) in each of the seven cities was systematically treated as the reference series in equation (6.A20) against which the remaining six series were compared by computing the CCF. This yielded 42 CCFs for analysis.

To examine whether the war-time associations differed from the associations that prevailed in peace, a parallel analysis was conducted on the time series of death rates per 10,000 population for the 61-month period (Jan. 1890–Jan. 1895) immediately prior to the onset of the insurrection.

CCF RESULTS, I: DEATHS FROM ALL CAUSES

For deaths from all causes, Figure 12.9 maps the principal results of the CCF analysis for the pre-war period (upper map) and the war period (lower map). The vectors link each city to those cities with which it shared the largest and second largest CCF values at lags $-6 \leq k \leq 6$. Reciprocal links mark in-phase ($k = 0$) associations, while out-of-phase associations ($k \neq 0$) are represented by unidirectional links. The values of the lag k (in months) are recorded on the vectors. Vector weights define the strength of the correlation, r_k, between the city pairs.

Table 12.2 lists the number of vectors which were statistically significant at the $p = 0.01$ level (two-tailed test) for sample sizes of 61 months (pre-war period) and 38 months (war period). Summary statistics for the set of vectors are also given in Table 12.2, including the median and average values of r_k (denoted $r_{k_{median}}$ and $\bar{r}_k$ respectively) and the average value of k (denoted $\bar{k}$), where k is the lag. Finally, to measure the association between a given series and all others, the maximum value of r_k between the reference series and each

---

Fig. 12.8. The spread of infectious diseases in the Cuban Insurrection

Notes: (A) Location of the geographical centre of mortality from infectious diseases. The location is based on the combined series of mortality from three infectious diseases (yellow fever, smallpox, and enteric fever) in seven Cuban cities. For each month of above-average mortality, May 1895–March 1898, the location of the centre is indicated by a circle. Vectors link the position of the mortality centre in successive months. (B) Invasion route followed by the Cuban *insurrectos* in the years 1895 and 1896.

Source: Smallman-Raynor and Cliff (1999, fig. 4, p. 343), with Fig. 12.8B originally redrawn from Thomas (1971: 318).

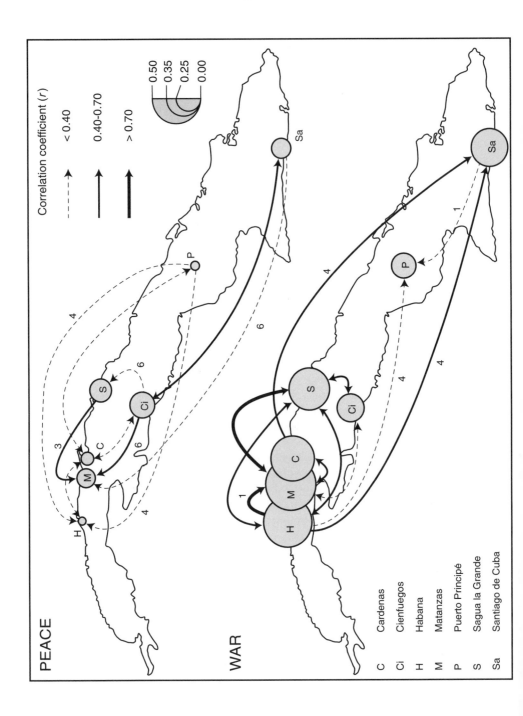

Table 12.2. Summary statistics of CCF analysis in Figs. 12.9 and 12.10

	Number of significant vectors[1]		$r_{k_{median}}$		$\bar{r}_k$		$\bar{k}$	
	1890–4	1895–8	1890–4	1895–8	1890–4	1895–8	1890–4	1895–8
All causes	4(40)	10(91)	0.31	0.59	0.34	0.59	2.07	0.93
Infectious diseases	5(56)	8(80)	0.36	0.41	0.44	0.45	3.21	3.64
Yellow fever	9(90)	8(89)	0.46	0.66	0.51	0.66	1.50	1.79
Smallpox	2(22)	7(100)	0.00	0.83	0.14	0.76	4.17	2.75
Enteric fever	4(57)	8(100)	0.36	0.56	0.35	0.57	3.08	2.75

Note: [1] Number of statistically significant vectors (as judged at the $p = 0.01$ level in a two–tailed test), expressed as a percentage proportion of all vectors, is shown in parentheses.
Source: Smallman-Raynor and Cliff (1999, table IV, p. 345).

of the comparison series was averaged across the six CCFs. For each reference series, the corresponding cities in Figure 12.9 are represented by a circle whose area is drawn proportional to this average maximum value of r_k; cities whose series are closely associated with all others appear as large circles, while cities which are weakly associated with all others appear as small circles.

Figure 12.9 and Table 12.2 reveal that the Cuban Insurrection was accompanied by a sharp rise in the association of the city mortality series. For the pre-war period, the upper map shows a weakly structured system with a preponderance of relatively low and statistically non-significant correlations ($r_{k_{median}} = 0.31$; $\bar{r}_k = 0.34$), out-of-phase ($k \neq 0$) associations, and a relatively long average lead/lag time ($\bar{k} = 2.07$). By contrast, the war period (lower map) is characterized by a strongly structured system with a preponderance of relatively high and statistically significant correlations ($r_{k_{median}} = 0.59$; $\bar{r}_k = 0.59$), in-phase ($k = 0$) associations, and a relatively low average lead/lag time ($\bar{k} = 0.93$).

Interpretation

One plausible interpretation of the changing association of the urban mortality series is that, during the pre-war period, the seven Cuban cities were only

◄────────────────────────────

Fig. 12.9. Spatial associations for mortality from all causes, Cuba, 1890–1898

Notes: The maps are based upon cross-correlations (CCFs) between the monthly series of mortality rates per 10,000 population in seven Cuban cities. Vectors link each city to those cities with which it shared the largest and second largest CCF values at lags $-6 \leq k \leq 6$. Reciprocal links mark in-phase ($k = 0$) associations, while out-of-phase associations ($k \neq 0$) are represented by (i) unidirectional links with (ii) the values of the lag k (in months) recorded on the vectors. Vector weights define the strength of the correlation, r_k, between the city pairs. On each map, cities are represented by a circle whose area is drawn proportional to the association of the corresponding mortality series with all others. (Upper map) Peacetime, January 1890–January 1895. (Lower map) Insurrection, February 1895–March 1898.
Source: Smallman-Raynor and Cliff (1999, fig. 5, p. 345).

weakly integrated in terms of the mechanisms that drove their mortality patterns. A principal effect of the war was to increase the epidemiological interdependence of the same cities, thereby creating a more highly integrated system of mortality. Such an effect is consistent with the high-level population mixing engendered by the Cuban Insurrection.

CCF RESULTS, II: INFECTIOUS DISEASES

Figure 12.10 repeats the analysis of Figure 12.9 for infectious diseases. Figure 12.10A maps the results for the combined series of mortality due to the three diseases in the pre-war period (upper map) and the war period (lower map), while the disaggregated results for each disease and time period are given in Figures 12.10B (yellow fever), 12.10C (smallpox), and 12.10D (enteric fever). Again, Table 12.2 gives the summary statistics (number of statistically significant correlations, $r_{k_{median}}$, $\bar{r}_k$, and $\bar{k}$) for each set of vectors.

The spatial associations illustrated in Figure 12.10 share a broad feature in common with the pattern for overall mortality in Figure 12.9. In each instance, there is a visual contrast between the (relatively) weakly structured systems of the pre-war period and the (relatively) strongly structured systems of the war period. The inter-period differences are confirmed in Table 12.2 by the systematic increase in the values of $r_{k_{median}}$ and $\bar{r}_k$ for all four mortality categories and the increase in the number of statistically significant correlations for three mortality categories (infectious diseases, smallpox, and enteric fever). However, increases are very modest in some instances and, together, Table 12.2 and Figure 12.10 identify important differences between the individual diseases. We consider each disease in turn.

1. *Yellow fever (Figure 12.10B)*. The preponderance of statistically significant correlations (Table 12.2) implies a relatively high degree of spatial association in both the pre-war and war periods. However, it is evident from Figure 12.10B that there was a fundamental switch from an island-wide system in the pre-war period to a system of intensive activity around a northwestern regional cell in the war period. For the constituent cities of this cell (Cardenas, Cienfuegos, Habana, Matanzas, and Sagua), the war was associated with a near-doubling of $\bar{r}_k$ (from 0.31 to 0.60) and a near-halving of $\bar{k}$ (2.00 to 1.10). These results are consistent with a simple model of spatial transmission

----

Fig. 12.10. Spatial associations for infectious diseases, Cuba, 1890–1898

Notes: The maps are based upon cross-correlations (CCFs) between the monthly series of mortality rates per 10,000 population in seven Cuban cities. (A) Combined series of mortality from three infectious diseases (yellow fever, smallpox, and enteric fever). (B) Yellow fever. (C) Smallpox. (D) Enteric fever. In each instance, the associations are mapped for the periods January 1890–January 1895 (upper map) and February 1895–March 1898 (lower map). See caption to Figure 12.9 for other mapping conventions.

Source: Smallman-Raynor and Cliff (1999, fig. 6, p. 346).

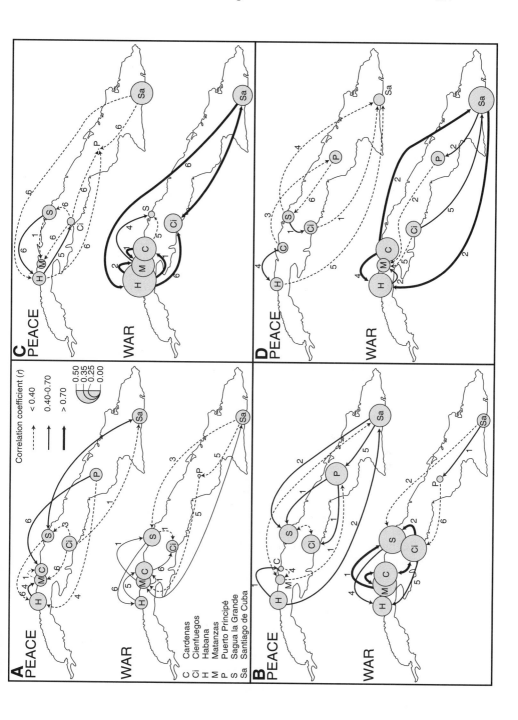

in which the war served to bolster the epidemiological integration of the cities of northwestern Cuba. The transmission of diseases between the cities accelerated (as judged by the reduction in the average lag, $\bar{k}$), and the geographically peripheral cities of central (Puerto Principé) and southeastern (Santiago) Cuba became epidemiologically decoupled from the main cell of disease activity.

2. *Smallpox (Figure 12.10C)*. The war dramatically increased the similarity in the mortality time series of the cities. In the pre-war period, Table 12.2 and Figure 12.10 show that spatial associations were essentially non-existent. Statistically significant correlations are few in number, the values of $r_{k_{median}}$ (= 0.00) and $\bar{r}_k$ (= 0.14) are correspondingly low, and the average lead/lag ($\bar{k}$ = 4.17) is long. In contrast, the war period was characterized by a highly structured and island-wide epidemiological system with many significant correlations, very high values of $r_{k_{median}}$ (= 0.83) and $\bar{r}_k$ (= 0.76), and a reduced average lead/lag time ($\bar{k}$ = 2.75). While the difference between war and peace may partly reflect the relative lack of smallpox activity in the years preceding the insurrection (see Fig. 12.7B), the results are again consistent with a simple model of spatial transmission in which the war was associated with marked epidemiological integration of the urban system, and accelerated disease transmission.

3. *Enteric fever (Figure 12.10D)*. Table 12.2 shows that the war period was associated with a doubling of the number of significant correlations, and a corresponding increase in the values of $r_{k_{median}}$ and $\bar{r}_k$. As for yellow fever and smallpox, these results are consistent with an increased epidemiological integration of the urban system in wartime. However, $\bar{k}$ displayed only a modest reduction between the two time periods. This implies that the war had little effect on the speed of the spatial transmission process.

12.3.4 Conclusion

To understand the epidemiological characteristics of late-nineteenth-century Habana, the USMHS Surgeon and Chief Quarantine Officer of Cuba, H. R. Carter, commented upon the need to isolate the 'normal course' of diseases in the years prior to 1895 from the 'abnormal' years that accompanied the insurrection (USMHS, 1900: 1840–54). Underpinning this need was a recognition that disease dynamics vary between war and peace. In the spirit of Chief Quarantine Officer Carter's advice, this section has examined the manner in which the spatial dynamics of three infectious diseases (yellow fever, smallpox, and enteric fever) altered as a consequence of the Cuban Insurrection. Four principal findings have emerged from our analysis. First, we have shown that the pre-war period was characterized by a settlement system that was only weakly integrated in terms of the causes of mortality. One principal effect of the insurrection was to increase the epidemiological interdependence of the

Table 12.3. Casualties in the British and Empire forces during the Malaya Campaign, 8 December 1941–15 February 1942

Contingent	Killed	Wounded	Missing & Prisoners	Total
British	307	96	37,894	38,297
Australian	516	1,364	1,919[1]	9,832[2]
Indian	340	807	62,591	63,738
Total	1,163	2,267	102,404	111,867[2]

Notes: [1] Missing only. [2] Balance includes 6,033 hospital admissions and deaths due to illnesses and accidents.
Source: Data from Crew (1957, tables 9–11, pp. 106–7).

settlements, creating a more highly integrated system of disease activity. This was caused by the increased population mixing engendered by the Cuban Insurrection. Secondly, the insurrection was associated with acceleration of the spatial processes of disease transmission. This is consistent with increased epidemiological integration and accords with the results of an earlier study of the spatial transmission of war epidemics (Smallman-Raynor and Cliff 1998*a*, 1998*b*). Thirdly, although the exact details vary by disease, both enhanced integration and increased velocity transcended the predisposition of the Spanish military to yellow fever and Cuban civilians to smallpox. It implies the operation of a common mechanism for both military and civil populations. Fourthly, the spatial course of epidemics in wartime was dictated by a shifting locus of hostilities, with the early involvement of the southeastern province of Oriente and a drift away from this initial focus as the insurrection progressed. In contrast, the pre-war period was characterized by a mortality centre that was rooted in the northwestern and central provinces of the country.

12.4 Asia: Prisoners of War, Forced Labour, and Disease in the Far East, 1942–1944

At 20.30 hours on Sunday 15 February 1942—with the Philippines, Hong Kong, and Malaya already in the hands of Japan—the British port of Singapore finally capitulated to the invading Japanese Army. The ten-week Malaya Campaign was over at a cost of some 112,000 casualties to the British and Empire forces (Table 12.3). For many tens of thousands of survivors of the Allied Malaya Command, an initial period of incarceration in Changi, Singapore Island, the principal prisoner of war (POW) camp in Japanese-held Southeast Asia, was followed from mid-1942 by employment as forced labour on the Burma–Thailand Railway. So began one of the most notorious and, in the collective conciousness of Allied POWs, enduring chapters in the

Asia–Pacific War.[9] In this section, we review patterns of disease among Allied POWs held captive in Changi camp (Sect. 12.4.1), before turning to the epidemiological experiences of one of the parties ('F' Force) dispatched from Changi to work on the line of the Burma–Thailand Railway (Sect. 12.4.2).

12.4.1 Changi Prisoner of War Camp, Singapore Island

The conditions that prevailed in Changi POW camp are reviewed by Havers (2000), while medical aspects of the incarceration are summarized by Crew (1957: 115–41). According to the latter source, deficiency diseases represented the gravest continuing threat to the health of the internees. The limited rations administered to the prisoners contributed to the steady malnutrition and, with a diet lacking in vitamin B complex, protein, and fat, beriberi and other deficiency diseases began to present as early as April 1942 (Crew, 1957: 137). Infectious diseases, too, spread widely in the camp. Among the British and Australian prisoners, a total of 55,445 hospital admissions were registered in the period February 1942–May 1944, of which dysentery and diarrhoea (19,935 admissions), malaria (6,950), and diphtheria (1,637) ranked among the leading illnesses. All told, there were 491 British and 138 Australian deaths in the POW hospital, with a further 58 among the Dutch prisoners (Crew, 1957: 134).

TIME SERIES OF INFECTIOUS DISEASES

The line traces in Figure 12.11 plot the monthly count of hospital admissions for the three leading infectious diseases (dysentery, diphtheria, and malaria) in selected contingents of the POW population in Changi camp, February 1942–May 1944.[10] Owing to the fragmentary nature of the available data, Figures 12.11A and 12.11B relate to dysentery and diphtheria in the combined population of British and Dutch POWs, while Figure 12.11C relates to malaria among British POWs alone. For reference, the bar charts on each graph plot the mean monthly strength of the entire POW population.

A striking feature of the bar charts in Figure 12.11 is the reduction in size of the POW population over the course of the observation period. In the early months of 1942, the average monthly strength of the camp was in excess of 50,000. Between May 1942 and May 1943, however, large numbers of prisoners were dispatched as working parties such that, by June 1943, the number of POWs in Changi had fallen to just 6,000. In December 1943 and January 1944, the remnants of these various parties began to return to Changi (Crew, 1957).

---

[9] The personal experiences of Allied POWs on the Burma–Thailand Railway have attracted a significant literature, of which Eric Lomax's *The Railway Man* (London: Vintage, 1996) is one recent contrbution.

[10] Data for the final month of the observation period in Fig. 12.11 (May 1944) includes information for the newly established POW hospital at Kranji.

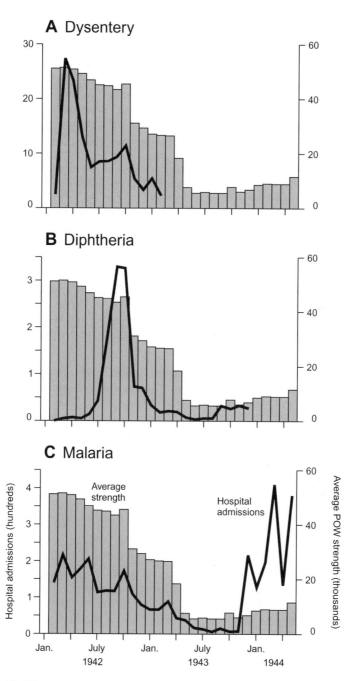

Fig. 12.11. Disease among Allied prisoners in Japanese prisoner of war camps, Singapore Island, February 1942–May 1944

Notes: Line traces plot the monthly count of hospital admissions as documented by Crew (1957) for Changi POW camp. (A) Dysentery in British and Dutch POWs. (B) Diphtheria in British and Dutch POWs. (C) Malaria in British POWs. For reference, the average monthly strength of POWs (all nationalities) is plotted on each graph as a bar chart. Note that data for the final month of the observation period (May 1944) includes internees in the POW hospital at Kranji.
Source: Data from Crew (1957, tables 13, 16, 17 and 18, pp. 133–6).

Dysentery (Figure 12.11A). Figure 12.11A shows that dysentery reached epidemic proportions in the months immediately following the establishment of Changi camp. At the height of the epidemic, in March and April 1942, over 5,000 British and Dutch POWs were admitted to hospital. Thereafter, the epidemic began to subside, but there was a secondary peak with the arrival of Dutch POWs from Java in October 1942. All told, a total of 195 dysentery deaths were recorded during the course of the epidemic (Crew, 1957: 134–5).

Diphtheria (Figure 12.11B). Diphtheria began to spread in the camp in June and July 1942, to reach epidemic proportions during August, September, and October. At the peak of the epidemic, the number of patients in the diphtheria block of the camp hospital stood at 846. By mid-January 1943, however, the number had slipped to 272 and, within a few months, the block was all but empty (Crew, 1957: 136).

Malaria (Figure 12.11C). As Figure 12.11C shows, malaria was common among POWs during 1942, but fell steadily with the falling strength of the prison population. From late 1943, however, a sudden and sustained upsurge coincided with the return of working parties from the various labour camps on the mainland (Crew, 1957: 134).

Other diseases. In addition to the diseases plotted in Figure 12.11, other infectious conditions also gained some prominence in the POW population. Sporadic cases of dengue were recorded shortly after the troops had congregated at Changi and, by May 1942, an epidemic (associated with 1,592 hospital cases) was in full force. Occasional deaths from pulmonary tuberculosis were also recorded in the camp hospital while, according to Crew (1957: 136), skin diseases were 'exceedingly prevalent' among the prisoners.

12.4.2 *'F' Force on the Burma–Thailand Railway*

Beginning in mid-1942, many thousands of Allied internees were transferred from Changi POW camp to work on the construction of the Burma–Thailand Railway. By the time the jungle railroad was finally completed, in mid-October 1943, a combination of brutality, exposure, malnutrition, and disease had claimed the lives of no less than 20 per cent of the 62,000 POWs employed on the line. According to the available records, mortality was especially high among the later working parties (including 'D' and 'F' Forces) which had been dispatched from Changi in March and April 1943 and whose period of employment coincided with the onset of the monsoon season (Kinvig, 2000). Here, we focus on the epidemiological experience of the ill-fated 'F' Force. Our examination draws on evidence originally included in *The History of 'F' Force*, a report prepared by the Commanding Officer and submitted to the War Department in February 1946 (Crew, 1957: 141–71).

Table 12.4. Record of mortality in 'F' Force dispatched from Changi prisoner of war camp, Singapore Island, to work on the construction of the Thailand–Burma Railway in 1943–1944

Nationality	Left Changi (Apr. 1943)	Died (Burma, Thailand, *en route* to Changi)	Escapees (fate unknown)	Missing	Unconfirmed death report	Alive (27 Apr. 1944)
Australian	3,662	1,058	0	0	0	2,604
British	3,336	2,029	5	1	1	1,300
Total	6,998	3,087	5	1	1	3,904

Source: Crew (1957, table 31, p. 164).

DISEASE AND MORTALITY IN 'F' FORCE

The tragedy of the 7,000-strong 'F' Force, consisting of approximately equal numbers of Australian and British POWs, is succinctly summarized by Crew (1957: 141):

In April 1943 . . . ['F' Force] was sent from Changi to Thailand. By the end of August 1943, 25 per cent. of the men were dead and 90 per cent. of the remainder were seriously ill. By December 1943, 40 per cent. of the whole force were dead. The survivors were returned to Changi. This move was completed in April 1944, by which time death had claimed 3,100, or 45 per cent. of the original 7,000.

Table 12.4 gives the bills of mortality for the Australian and British contingents of 'F' Force, while the map in Figure 12.12 shows the location of the construction camps in which the force was based in the period May–November 1943. The accompanying graphs plot, as line traces, the monthly death rate (per 1,000 survivors) from five leading causes of mortality in the force, May 1943–April 1944. Finally, the overall monthly mortality count (all causes) is plotted on each graph as a bar chart.

Cholera (Figure 12.12A). 'F' Force had scarcely reached Headquarters Camp (Shimo Nieke)—the culmination of a 300 km journey from the staging point at Bampong, Thailand, to their place of employment on the rail line—when Asiatic cholera appeared among the men.[11] The first case was diagnosed in the Australian contingent on 15 May 1943, with the disease spreading rapidly in the days and weeks that followed. The epidemic finally terminated in September, by which time almost 10 per cent. of 'F' Force had succumbed.

---

[11] Although instructions had been issued that all men of 'F' Force should be inoculated against cholera, only partial vaccination coverage was achieved prior to departure from Changi. See Crew (1957: 143).

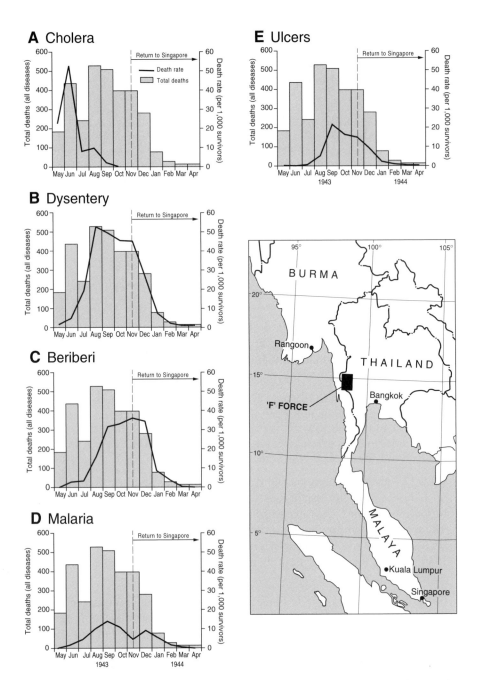

Fig. 12.12. Death rates from sample diseases in a party of Allied prisoners of war ('F' Force) engaged in the construction of the Burma–Thailand Railway, May 1943–April 1944

Notes: The monthly death rate (computed per 1,000 survivors at the beginning of the month) is plotted on each graph as a line trace. (A) Cholera. (B) Dysentery. (C) Beriberi. (D) Malaria. (E) Ulcers. Note that deaths attributed to multiple diseases have been included in more than one category in graphs A–E. For reference, the bar charts plot the total monthly count of deaths from all causes. The position of the main construction camps occupied by 'F' Force is indicated on the location map.

Source: Data from Crew (1957, table 32, p. 165).

Other diseases (Fig. 12.12B–E). Although the remaining graphs in Figure 12.12 display widely varying mortality rates, with dysentery (1,380 deaths)[12] and beriberi (864 deaths)[13] being implicated in the majority of deaths, all four curves share a common form: an extended period of relatively high mortality from August/September to November/December 1943. Only with the return to Singapore in late 1943 did mortality from the sample diseases begin to subside.

As judged by the disease histories of some other forces (including 'A' and 'D' Forces), the general epidemiological profile of 'F' Force was fairly typical of working parties in the vicinity of the Burma–Thailand border during 1943 (Crew, 1957: 168–71).

12.5 Europe: Civilian Epidemics and the World Wars

12.5.1 Tuberculosis as a War Pestilence

As we noted in Section 1.3.2, the early years of the twentieth century marked a watershed in the epidemiological history of war. Due partly to developments in the firepower of belligerent states and partly to improvements in military hygiene and disease control, the Russo-Japanese War (1904–5) and World War I signalled the start of an enduring temporal trend in which more soldiers died in battle than in military lazarets (Councell, 1941). At the same time, the great war pestilences which had racked the military and civil populations of earlier centuries—cholera, dysentery, plague, smallpox, typhoid, typhus, and yellow fever—were joined and, in some cases, supplanted by conditions such as cerebrospinal meningitis, respiratory tract infections, sexually transmitted infections, and tuberculosis as the most potent disease threats of war (see e.g. Lancaster, 1990: 314–40). Indeed, such were the developments that, in 1947, Marc Daniels could proclaim tuberculosis as 'the major health disaster of the Second World War' (Daniels, 1947: 201).

Against this background, the present subsection explores the impact of the world wars on tuberculosis activity in the civil population of Europe. Our consideration begins with a brief overview of the factors which may contribute to a wartime increase in tuberculosis. A geographical consideration of the epidemic ascendancy of tuberculosis in the European theatre is then followed by an examination of the spatial parameters that underpinned one prominent epidemiological feature of wartime Britain: the rise of pulmonary tuberculosis among young adult women in World War I.

---

[12] Including deaths for which the additional causes of beriberi (332), malaria (115), and ulcers (101) were also stated; see Crew (1957: 165).
[13] Including deaths for which the additional causes of dysentery (332), malaria (62), and ulcers (57) were also stated; see Crew (1957: 165).

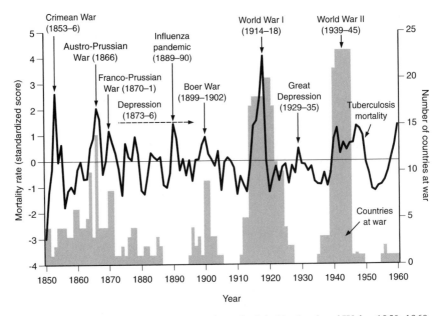

Fig. 12.13. Mortality from pulmonary tuberculosis in England and Wales, 1850–1960

Notes: The annual series of tuberculosis mortality, plotted as a line trace, has been detrended and is expressed in standard Normal score form. For reference, the number of European countries at war in each year is plotted as a bar chart.

Source: Smallman-Raynor and Cliff (2003, fig. 4.1, p. 74).

TUBERCULOSIS AND WAR

The signature of war can be deciphered in many past records of tuberculosis activity. By way of illustration, the line trace in Figure 12.13 is based on information included in the volumes of the Registrar-General's *Annual Report* and plots, in detrended form, the annual rate of mortality from pulmonary tuberculosis in England and Wales, 1850–1960. Wartime peaks in tuberculosis mortality reflect not only conflicts in which Great Britain held a military stake (Crimean War, South African War (Boer War), and the world wars), but also the overspill from continental European wars in which Britain maintained a non-belligerent status (Austro-Prussian War and Franco-Prussian War).[14]

---

[14] Although the years of the Austro-Prussian War (1866) and the Franco-Prussian War (1870–1) were accompanied by marked increases in mortality from pulmonary tuberculosis in England and Wales (Fig. 12.13), evidence for a direct epidemiological link with the conflicts is generally lacking. We note, however, that fugitives from the warring states played a role in the spread of other infectious diseases (most notably, smallpox in 1870–1) to, and within, England and Wales (see e.g. Rolleston, 1933). Under these circumstances, and by analogy with the international movements of tuberculous refugees in more recent conflicts, the mortality levels associated with the Austro-Prussian and Franco-Prussian Wars in Figure 12.13 may have been inflated—to a greater or lesser extent—by continental Europeans in search of refuge from the troubles.

TUBERCULOSIS AND THE WAR ENVIRONMENT

The aetiology, epidemiology, and clinical course of tuberculosis is outlined in Appendix 1A. Specific factors which may contribute to a wartime increase in tuberculosis activity, and which could account for past mortality fluctuations of the type shown in Figure 12.13 include a broad range of primary environmental influences on the transmission and host resistance to the tubercle bacillus (Johnston, 1993). The crowding of both military and civil populations provides conditions ripe for the aerosol transmission of the tubercle bacillus. Such crowding arises from the destruction of housing infrastructure, billeting, and close-quarter accommodation in military assembly and training camps, concentration and prison camps, refugee camps, hospitals, and air-raid shelters. Protein-calorie malnutrition, resulting from the disruption of agricultural production and the shredding of food supply lines, food rationing and distribution controls, is aetiologically linked to a reduction in human resistance to pre-existing or new tubercular infection. Additionally, as part of a general war effort, increased employment in munitions production and/or certain other 'dusty' industries may serve as a further stimulant to latent pulmonary infection. The physical exertion and mental stress that typically accompanies a war may also weaken resistance to infection, while the adverse consequences of disruption of tuberculosis control programmes, including the military requisition of dedicated hospital facilities and sanatoria, are illustrated by the experience of some European countries during World War I.[15]

WORLD CONFLICT AND TUBERCULOSIS: THE EUROPEAN THEATRE

The social, physical, and environmental conditions engendered by World War I (1914–18) and World War II (1939–45) had a severe, if geographically uneven, impact on tuberculosis activity in the European theatre of war (see e.g. Doull, 1945; Daniels, 1946, 1947; Long, 1948; Hoefnagels, 1950). By way of illustration, Figure 12.14 is based on information included in Alderson's (1981) *International Mortality Statistics* and plots the quinquennial series of mortality from all infectious diseases (Fig. 12.14A) and tuberculosis (Fig. 12.14B) in a 15-country sample of belligerent and non-belligerent European states, 1901–5 to 1961–5. The sample countries are categorized by belligerent status in Table 12.5.[16] For each category, the line traces in Figures 12.14A and B plot the corresponding mortality levels as an average standardized mortality ratio (SMR) over the constituent units.

---

[15] For overviews of the factors that may promote the occurrence of tuberculosis in wartime, with special reference to Europe during the world wars, see Leslie (1915–16), Heaf (1941–2), and Daniels (1947, 1949).

[16] The selection of European countries in Table 12.5 has been dictated by the availability of tuberculosis data. Unfortunately, information for several of the states most severely affected by World War I and/or World War II (including Germany, Poland, and Serbia) is either unavailable or too fragmentary to include in the present analysis.

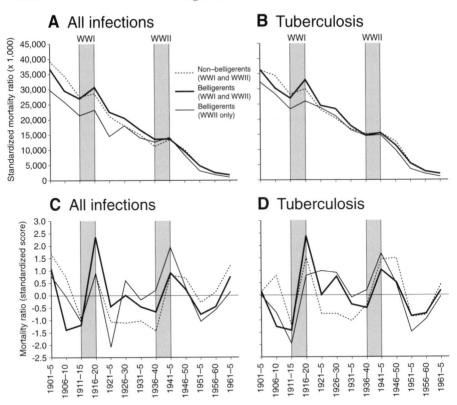

Fig. 12.14. Mortality from infectious diseases in Europe, 1901–1965

Notes: For sample European countries, grouped by belligerent status in World War I (1914–18) and World War II (1939–45), the upper graphs plot the average standardized mortality ratio (SMR, formed to a factor of 1,000) by quinquennial period, while the lower graphs plot the detrended series of SMRs (expressed in standard Normal score form). Graphs A and C, all infectious diseases. Graphs B and D, tuberculosis (all forms). Countries are categorized by belligerent status in Table 12.5.

Source: Smallman-Raynor and Cliff (2003, fig. 4.3, p. 83).

Figures 12.14A and B show that the wars produced temporary interruptions in a long-term downward trend in underlying mortality from infectious diseases. To examine the interruptions more closely, the series in Figures 12.14A and B are replotted in detrended form in Figures 12.14C (all infectious diseases) and D (tuberculosis). Formed in this manner, wartime mortality is manifested as major spikes of disease activity. Although the spikes are generally most pronounced for the belligerent states in a given war, it is also apparent that the epidemiological consequences of the conflicts spilled over to the non-belligerent states of Europe.

Table 12.5. Estimated impact of World War I and World War II on national-level records of tuberculosis mortality in sample European and non-European countries

Country	Percentage impact of war on recorded levels of tuberculosis mortality[1]			
	World War I		World War II	
	Increment	Decrement	Increment	Decrement
European countries				
Belligerents (WWI and WWII)				
Austria	**9.3**		No data	
Belgium	**7.9**		**21.7**	
Bulgaria		No data		−3.9
Czechoslovakia		No data	**0.7**	
France		No data	**22.0**	
Hungary		No data	**4.0**	
Italy	**10.3**		**16.6**	
United Kingdom				
England and Wales	**2.3**			−6.4
Scotland		−10.8		−0.4
Belligerents (WWII only)				
Denmark	**5.3**			−22.9
Finland[2]		No data	**11.3**	
Netherlands	**26.4**		**47.4**	
Non-belligerents (WWI and WWII)				
Eire		No data	**16.9**	
Spain	**7.4**		**1.3**	
Switzerland		−0.3		−6.1
Non-European countries				
Belligerents (WWI and WWII)				
Australia		−8.0		−6.3
Canada		−6.5		−7.4
USA		−4.7		−7.5

Notes: [1] Formed as a percentage estimate of the increment/decrement in tuberculosis mortality associated with World War I and World War II. [2] Not classified as an independent state in World War I.
Source: Smallman-Raynor and Cliff (2003, table 4.3, p. 85).

National Patterns

For each of the 15 European countries included in Figure 12.14, Table 12.5 gives a percentage estimate of the change in tuberculosis mortality associated with World War I and World War II.[17] Here, a relatively large and positive value indicates that the war period was associated with a proportionately large increment in tuberculosis mortality, while a relatively large and negative value

[17] The estimates have been formed by expressing the mortality rate for the war period as a percentage deviation from the average of the rates in the periods immediately preceding and following the war.

indicates a proportionately large decrement. For reference, parallel estimates are also given for three non-European members of the Allied forces (Australia, Canada, and the United States).

While Table 12.5 underscores the epidemiological impact of the wars in many European states, geographical variations are evident and reflect the relative severity of the wartime conditions (Heaf, 1941–2; Daniels, 1949). Among the belligerents of World War I the largest increments in tuberculosis mortality were recorded for the embattled states of Austria, Belgium, and Italy. Away from the scene of active hostilities, a more modest increment was recorded for England and Wales while, for Scotland, the long-term decline in tuberculosis mortality was largely unchecked by the war. Likewise, among the belligerents of World War II, stark increments in Italy and the occupied lands of northern Europe (Belgium, France, and the Netherlands) contrast with mortality decrements in such countries as Bulgaria, Denmark, and England and Wales. While the privations that contributed to these latter variations are outlined elsewhere (see e.g. Anonymous, 1944), three further features of Table 12.5 are also apparent:

(1) for many non-belligerent states, neutrality afforded little—if any— protection against the epidemiological consequences of the war. In this context, the experiences of Denmark, Spain, and the Netherlands in World War I and of Ireland in World War II are especially noteworthy;

(2) although comparative data are limited, evidence for countries such as Belgium, Italy, and the Netherlands suggests that the relative impact of war on tuberculosis activity was greater in World War II than World War I;

(3) away from the European theatre, the wars had but little effect on tuberculosis mortality in the belligerent states of Australia, Canada, and the United States.

CASE STUDY: ENGLAND AND WALES

While countries of continental Europe were to experience the worst excesses of the war-related increases in tuberculosis mortality (Table 12.5), the somewhat more modest but still marked experience of England and Wales is illustrated in Figure 12.15. Figure 12.15A relates to the period 1911–60 and plots, in both crude (broken line trace) and detrended (heavy line trace) form, the annual

→

Fig. 12.15. Annual series of tuberculosis mortality in England and Wales, 1911–1960

Notes: (A) Pulmonary tuberculosis. (B) Non-pulmonary tuberculosis. On each graph, the broken line trace plots the tuberculosis mortality rate (per 100,000 population), while the heavy line trace plots the detrended mortality rate (expressed as a standard score). The remaining graphs plot the detrended mortality rates for pulmonary and non-pulmonary tuberculosis for (C) males and (D) females.

Source: Smallman-Raynor and Cliff (2003, fig. 4.4, p. 86).

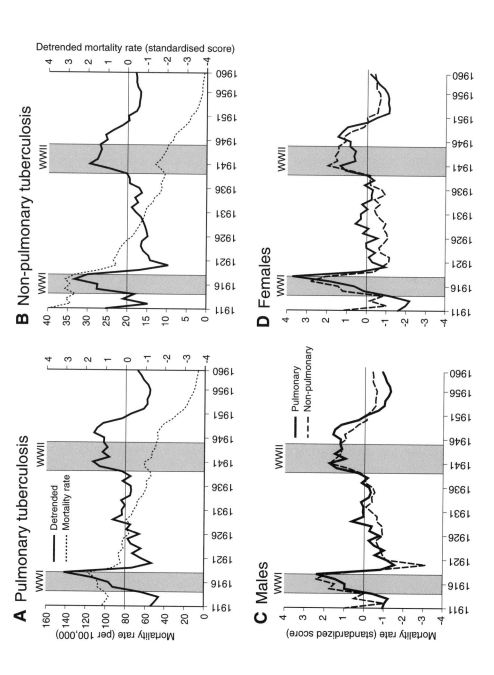

mortality rate per 100,000 for pulmonary tuberculosis. Figure 12.15B plots the equivalent information for non-pulmonary tuberculosis, while the remaining charts plot the detrended mortality rates for pulmonary and non-pulmonary tuberculosis in males (Fig. 12.15C) and females (Fig. 12.15D).

The detrended series in Figure 12.15 yield a common signal. Regardless of gender or disease site, World War I was accompanied by a steep rise in the mortality curve. This was followed by an abrupt fall at the end of the hostilities. Minor interruptions to the relative epidemiological calm of the inter-war years were then replaced, from the onset of World War II, by a second and more protracted recrudescence in tuberculosis mortality. High mortality levels continued into the post-war period, only beginning a decline in the late 1940s. The complex of factors which could account for the sustained post-war affects of World War II relative to World War I are uncertain but may relate in part to the adverse health consequences of the greater structural damage sustained in the second conflict (Daniels, 1947, 1949).

Tuberculosis Mortality in Females during World War I

One prominent epidemiological feature of tuberculosis in the civil population of wartime Britain was the disproportionate increase in active disease among young adult women in the early years of World War I. So, while the total number of tuberculosis-related deaths in England and Wales grew by about 7 per cent between 1914 and 1916, deaths among females aged 15 to 44 years grew by an average of about 12 per cent, with the largest increases in those aged 15 to 19 years (22%) and 20 to 24 years (14%) (Medical Research Council, 1942: 34). Spurred by speculation that the increases were attributable to working conditions associated with the wartime employment of females in munitions factories and other industries (see e.g. Registrar-General, 1918, p. lix), the results of a Medical Research Committee inquiry into the circumstances surrounding the mortality rise appeared in 1919 under the title *An Inquiry Into the Prevalence and Aetiology of Tuberculosis among Industrial Workers, with Special Reference to Female Munition Workers* (Medical Research Committee, 1919). While the report concluded that industrial employment had introduced a 'special factor' in the development of the disease (Medical Research Committee, 1919: 59), a geographical examination of the data collated by the authors of the *Inquiry* reveals that the wartime rise in tuberculosis mortality among young adult females was characterized by a distinctive spatial pattern.

Spatial patterns. To examine the pattern, Figure 12.16 is based on information included in the *Inquiry* and maps deaths from pulmonary tuberculosis in adult females (aged 15–45 years) for the year 1916. For the selected age–sex group and time period, each circle in Figure 12.16 represents one of the 106 county and metropolitan boroughs of England and Wales, with the area of each circle scaled to an index of proportionate mortality for pulmonary tuberculosis (formed as the ratio of deaths from pulmonary tuberculosis to deaths from all

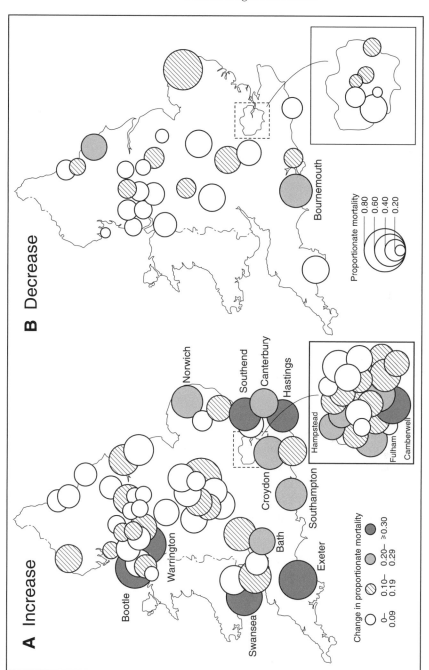

Fig. 12.16. World War I and pulmonary tuberculosis mortality in adult females (aged 15–45 years) in the county and metropolitan boroughs of England and Wales

Notes: Each borough is identified by a circle whose area is scaled to the proportionate mortality from pulmonary tuberculosis in 1916. Boroughs are distinguished according to the change in proportionate mortality between 1913 and 1916: (A) increase; (B) decrease. Circles are shaded according to the change (increment or decrement) in proportionate mortality.

Source: Smallman-Raynor and Cliff (2003, fig. 4.5, p. 88).

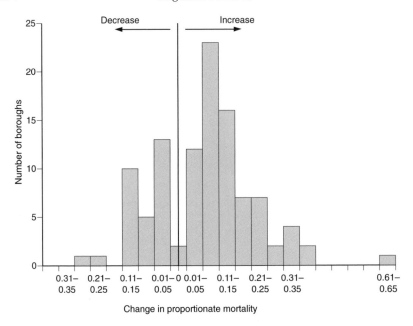

Fig. 12.17. Frequency distribution of the change in proportionate mortality from pulmonary tuberculosis in adult females (aged 15–45 years) in the county and metropolitan boroughs of England and Wales, 1913–1916

Source: Smallman-Raynor and Cliff (2003, fig. 4.6, p. 89).

other causes) in the corresponding boroughs.[18] Set against the pre-war base year of 1913, the maps identify boroughs which recorded an increase (map A) and a decrease (map B) in proportionate mortality in the period 1913–16. For a given borough, the change in proportionate mortality is indicated by the choropleth shading. Finally, Figure 12.17 plots the frequency distribution of boroughs by change in proportionate mortality, 1913–16.

While Figures 12.16 and 12.17 confirm the general tendency for a wartime increase in proportionate mortality, inspection of Figure 12.16A reveals a marked geographical pattern to the increase. In contrast to the boroughs of central and northern England, which are characterized by modest (0.10–0.19) or low (<0.10) increments to a relatively high background level of proportionate mortality, the largest increments (>0.20) are recorded in boroughs of southern England and Wales. With the notable exception of two northwestern towns (Warrington and Bootle), both adjacent to the port of Liverpool, the largest increments are identified in coastal/port towns, cities, and proximal settlements

---

[18] As noted by the authors of the *Inquiry*, the formation of proportionate mortalities (rather than mortality rates) overcomes the difficulties associated with wartime population movements and related uncertainties regarding the size of the female population in a given borough.

Table 12.6. World War I and proportionate mortality from respiratory tuberculosis, females (aged 15–45 years), in the industrial and non-industrial county and metropolitan boroughs of England and Wales

Time period	Average proportionate mortality from respiratory tuberculosis	
	Industrial boroughs	Non-industrial boroughs
Pre-war (1913)	0.40	0.39
War (1916)	0.47	0.47
Wartime change (1913–16)	0.07	0.08

of South Wales (Swansea), southern (Bath, Exeter, and Southampton), and southeastern (Brighton, Hastings, Canterbury, and Southend) England. In addition, large increments are also identified in some boroughs of East Anglia (Norwich) and metropolitan London.

Possible explanations. Although the authors of the *Inquiry* concluded that the wartime increase in tuberculosis mortality was linked to industrial employment (Medical Research Committee, 1919: 24), they emphasized that the association between the changes in proportionate mortality plotted in Figure 12.16 and the industrial status of the 106 boroughs was 'not very striking' (ibid. 15). The evidence presented in Table 12.6 concurs with their viewpoint. The table is based on the industrial/non-industrial categorization of boroughs adopted by the *Inquiry* and gives the average proportionate mortality for pulmonary tuberculosis in 1913 and 1916. For both categories of borough, the proportionate mortalities and their associated increases over the observation period are virtually identical.

While the results in Table 12.6 may reflect the need for a more detailed classification of industrial employment structure, we note that most of the boroughs identified as having recorded large increments in proportionate mortality—including Bath, Brighton, Canterbury, Exeter, Hastings, Southampton, and Southend, as well as the London boroughs of Camberwell and Hampstead—were classified by the *Inquiry* as non-industrial centres. Thus, subject to instabilities associated with small disease counts in the less populous centres, other factors may account for the distinctive spatial pattern in Figure 12.16. Although these factors could include mechanisms such as selective migration, it is noteworthy that the broad geographical pattern mapped in Figure 12.16A, with the larger relative increases in proportionate mortality centred on the southern half of the country, is analogous to the pattern exhibited by contemporary epidemics of other infectious diseases.

For example, cerebrospinal meningitis spread widely with the southerly flux of both military and civil populations in the early part of World War I (Reece, 1916). Further research is required to determine whether the same wartime population flux, centred on the settlements of southern England and Wales, contributed to the development of the tuberculosis pattern in Figure 12.16.

THE ENDURING ASSOCIATION OF TUBERCULOSIS AND WAR

Globally, no less than 350 wars, revolutions, and coups d'état have been staged in the half-century since World War II (Brogan, 1992; Arnold, 1995). Most of these clashes have centred on developing countries. Many have been of limited extent and severity, and a bloodless few had little or no discernible affect on the health of the countries involved. But many others shattered economies and infrastructure, as well as leaving thousands or millions of dead, homeless, or displaced people in their wake (Levy and Sidel, 1997). As far as the epidemiological evidence permits, such conflicts, like their pre-1945 counterparts, have typically been accompanied by a pronounced—sometimes dramatic and often protracted—increase in tubercular infection and disease (Bahr *et al.*, 1991; Rybka and Punga, 1996; Pavlović *et al.*, 1998).

As regards Europe, the international flight of refugees, asylum seekers, and other fugitives from modern conflicts has served to carry the tuberculosis problem beyond the borders of warring states, sometimes into territories where background levels of tuberculosis activity are relatively low (Black and Healing, 1993; Rieder *et al.*, 1994; Fengler, 1995). Thus, beginning with the Slovenian and Croatian Wars of Independence in the summer of 1991, almost a decade of fighting in the former Yugoslavia spawned the largest international movement of European refugees since World War II. In the years 1991–3 alone, an estimated 512,000 Bosnian and Croatian refugees entered the countries of Western Europe, with tuberculosis prominent among the anticipated health problems of these people (Black and Healing, 1993). Tuberculosis screening by the recipient countries has underscored such health concerns (Rieder *et al.*, 1994), with exceptionally high levels of tubercular disease among Bosnian medical evacuees assigned to the United Kingdom serving to illustrate the problem (Black and Healing, 1993).

In an optimistic conclusion to his review of the spread of tuberculosis in Europe during World War II, Marc Daniels argued that the means for the elimination of tuberculosis were already in place. 'Given a long enough respite from mutual massacre there is no reason why this disease . . . should not be almost eradicated before this century is out' (Daniels, 1949: 1140). Unfortunately, recent events have dashed such optimism and the epidemiological consequences of war, so far as tuberculosis is concerned, endure into a new century.

12.5.2   The Serbian Typhus Epidemic, 1914–1915

The great epidemics of typhus fever that spread in Eastern Europe during World War I (1914–18) and in its aftermath rank among the most severe outbreaks of the disease in modern times. With epidemic transmission fuelled by the continuous flux of soldiers, POWs, and refugees, and with railways serving as efficient conduits in the spatial propagation of the disease, typhus fever diffused widely in the region. In Congress Poland and Galicia, over 431,000 cases of typhus fever were recorded from 1916 to 1919 (Goodall, 1920) while, in revolutionary Russia, 5 million or more fell victim to the disease between 1917 and 1922 (Zinsser, 1935; Patterson, 1993c). Elsewhere, typhus fever struck Austria, Bosnia and Herzegovina, Hungary, Romania, and Serbia, along with the Baltic states of Estonia, Latvia, and Lithuania (Councell, 1941).

In this subsection, we examine one of the earliest and most severe of the typhus epidemics that spread as a consequence of World War I: the Serbian epidemic of 1914–15. The disease first appeared in Serbia during the latter months of 1914 and, in conjunction with a concurrent epidemic of louse-borne relapsing fever, is estimated to have resulted in some 120,000 military and civilian deaths. Our account of the Serbian typhus epidemic draws on epidemiological information gathered by William Hunter, Colonel-in-Charge of the British Military Sanitary Mission to Serbia in 1915, and published in the *Proceedings of the Royal Society of Medicine* in 1920 (Hunter, 1920). An overview of the nature of typhus fever, along with relapsing fever, is given in Appendix 1A.

ORIGIN AND GEOGRAPHICAL SPREAD

The origins of the Serbian typhus epidemic are reviewed by Strong *et al.* (1920: 18–20). In connection with the retreat of the Austro-Hungarian Army from northern Serbia in December 1914, cases of typhus and relapsing fever began to appear in the Serbian Army, their Austrian prisoners, and the local civil population. The initial focus of the outbreak was the town of Valyevo, situated near the Bosnian frontier (Fig. 12.18). When the Serbians had abandoned Valyevo in the face of the Austrian advance, the town—like the rest of Serbia—was apparently free from typhus fever. But, when the Serbian Army returned to Valyevo in the latter weeks of 1914, they found 3,000 Austrian sick and wounded, some of whom were suffering from typhus and relapsing fevers. After an initial period of concentration, the Austrian prisoners from Valyevo and elsewhere—approximately 40,000 in number—were redistributed across Serbia. Typhus and relapsing fevers followed the redistribution so that, by January 1915, the diseases had been seeded across the country (Strong *et al.*, 1920).

From these putative beginnings, Figure 12.19 is based on five-day counts of hospital patients and plots the number of recorded cases of typhus fever in 42

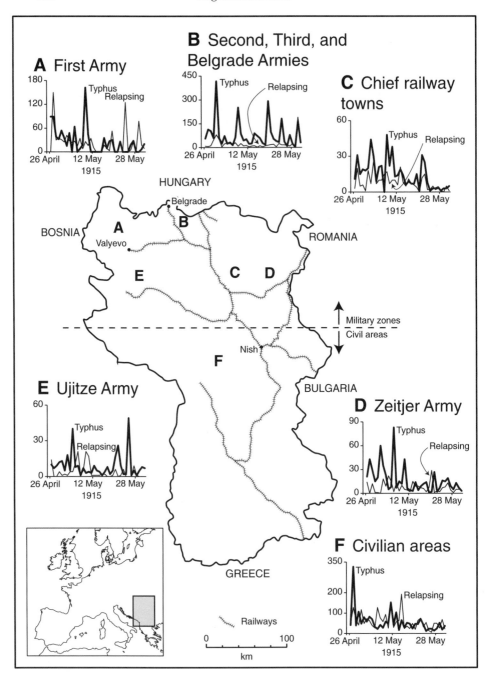

Fig. 12.18. Typhus and relapsing fever in the military and civilian areas of Serbia, 1915

Notes: Graphs plot the daily count of hospital admissions for typhus fever and relapsing fever in military (northern) zones and civilian (southern) areas of Serbia, 26 April to 31 May. For each graph, A–F, corresponding letter codes are used to identify locations on the accompanying map.
Source: Based on data in Hunter (1920, tables H and K, pp. 62–5).

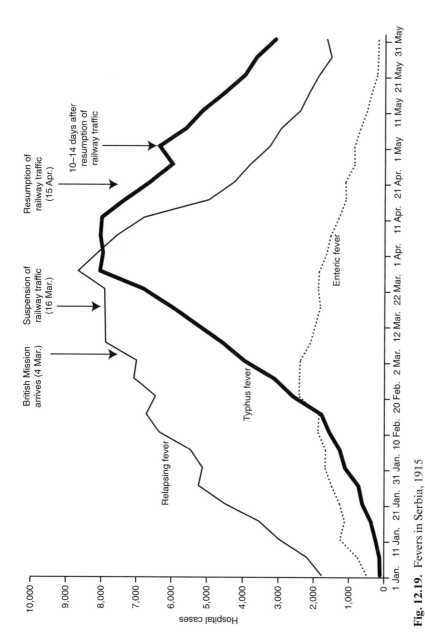

Fig. 12.19. Fevers in Serbia, 1915

Notes: Line traces plot the number of cases of typhus, relapsing, and enteric fever in hospital by five-day period, 1 January to 31 May.
Source: Based on data in Hunter (1920, table I, p. 58).

towns of Serbia, January–May 1915. The corresponding series for relapsing fever and enteric fever are also plotted while, for reference, principal events in the epidemic control of typhus are indicated. As the graph shows, typhus fever spread rapidly in February, reaching an extended peak in late March and early April. Thereafter, the epidemic began to recede, eventually terminating in June (Soubbotitch, 1918; Hunter, 1920).

Hospital Conditions: Eyewitness Testimony

Graphic accounts of the conditions that prevailed in Serbia at the height of the typhus epidemic are provided by members of the British Military Sanitary Mission which was dispatched to assist in the control of the outbreak in early March 1915. Writing of his arrival in Serbia on 4 March, Hunter (1920: 42–3) commented that:

I knew little then, that within a few days I was to be amidst conditions in which I was to see not 1,000 [typhus] cases in a year, but 1,000 cases in a day; to find a maximum not of 2,500 cases a year, but 4,000 cases in the hospitals at the same time, rapidly rising to over 8,000 in the course of the next three weeks, plus an unknown number among the civilian population of Serbia, probably three to four times as many, of whom there was no information.

New cases of typhus fever entered the hospitals at a rate of up to 1,000 to 1,500 a day, with the mortality rate reaching 40 per cent in March (Hunter, 1920). Conditions in the hospitals were appalling. On 7 March, for example, the 200-bed hospital at Nish (Fig. 12.18) had two doctors to treat some 700 fever patients:

Groups of thirty, forty, fifty and sixty cases of typhus, relapsing and typhoid patients all mixed together, lay in ill-ventilated rooms, close together on wooden boards, in some cases three or four in two or three beds, with one blanket covering the whole, many of them on the floor; and some of them under the beds and in the passages between the beds (ibid. 49).

There were no nurses in the hospital. Austrian prisoners acted as attendants, while arrangements for disinfection, washing, bathing, and the supply of clean linen and bedding were entirely lacking. Under such circumstances, the patients infected each other in hospital and, on their discharge, carried disease to the outside world (ibid.).

TYPHUS CONTROL: THE SUSPENSION OF RAILWAY TRAFFIC

To assist in the control of typhus and relapsing fevers, the British Military Sanitary Mission implemented a series of preventive strategies, of which disinfection and quarantine played a central role. Among the novel methods of cleansing and disinfection, Hunter (1920) lists the formation of the 'English sanitary disinfecting train', along with the construction and use of railway van disinfectors and douche baths (Pl. 12.2). Especially prominent among the

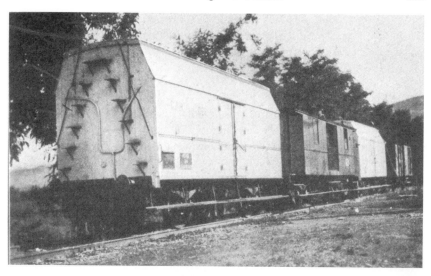

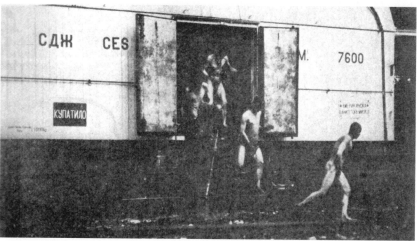

Pl. 12.2. Railway van steam bathing and disinfecting unit in Serbia, 1915
Source: Strong *et al.* (1920, pl. XII, fig. 1 and pl. XIII, fig. 1, between pp. 32–3).

control strategies, however, was the temporary suspension of passenger rail traffic, the cancellation of all military leave, and the construction of a quarantine and disinfecting station on the railway immediately behind the chief armies. In this manner, it was hoped to halt the transmission of disease between the northern (military) zones and the southern (civil) areas of the country; the division between the military zones and civil areas is indicated in Figure 12.18 by the broken horizontal line.

As Figure 12.19 shows, the month-long suspension of passenger rail traffic (16 Mar.–14 Apr.) produced a plateau and subsequent fall in the typhus curve, but with a discernible rise in disease activity some 10 to 14 days after travel resumed.

Resumption of Rail Traffic: Impact on Spatial Disease Transmission

For each of the six military (north) zones and civil (south) areas of Serbia, the graphs in Figure 12.18 plot the daily number of hospital admissions for typhus fever and relapsing fever in the period following the resumption of rail traffic, 26 April–31 May 1915. For each graph, A–F, corresponding letter codes are used to identify locations on the accompanying map.

Method: cross-correlation analysis. To examine the impact of the resumption of rail traffic on the spatial transmission of typhus fever in the set of six military zones and civil areas, cross-correlation functions (CCFs; see Sect. 6.7.3) were computed between each pair of daily series of typhus admissions in Figure 12.18. For the purposes of comparison, a parallel analysis was conducted for the daily series of admissions for relapsing fever.

Results. The principal results of the CCF analysis are mapped in Figure 12.20 for typhus fever (Fig. 12.20A) and relapsing fever (Fig. 12.20B). On each map, geographical units are indicated by a circle whose area is drawn proportional to the number of disease-specific (typhus fever and relapsing fever) hospital admissions during the observation period. Vectors link each unit to those units with which it shared the largest and second largest CCF values at daily lags $-12 \leq k \leq 12$. Reciprocal links mark in-phase ($k = 0$) associations, while out-of-phase associations ($k \neq 0$) are represented by unidirectional links with the values of k (in days) recorded on the vectors. Vector directions mark the implied direction of disease transmission, while vector weights define the strength of the correlation, r_k, between the units.

Figure 12.20 draws a sharp distinction between (i) the comparatively strongly structured system for typhus fever (Fig. 12.20A) characterized by a preponderance of relatively high correlations and (ii) the comparatively weakly structured system for relapsing fever (Fig. 12.20B) characterized by a preponderance of modest correlations. The maps imply that the resumption of rail

----

Fig. 12.20. Spatial associations for typhus and relapsing fever in Serbia, 1915

Notes: The maps are based upon cross-correlations (CCFs) between the daily series of hospital admissions for typhus fever (A) and relapsing fever (B) in six military and civilian areas of Serbia. The associations relate to the time interval after the resumption of railway traffic, 26 April to 31 May. On each map, geographical units are indicated by a circle whose area is drawn proportional to the total number of hospital admissions during the observation period. Vectors link each unit to those units with which it shared the largest and second largest CCF values at lags $-12 \leq k \leq 12$. Reciprocal links mark in-phase ($k = 0$) associations, while out-of-phase associations ($k \neq 0$) are represented by (i) unidirectional links with (ii) the values of k (in days) recorded on the vectors. Vector weights define the strength of the correlation, r_k, between the units.

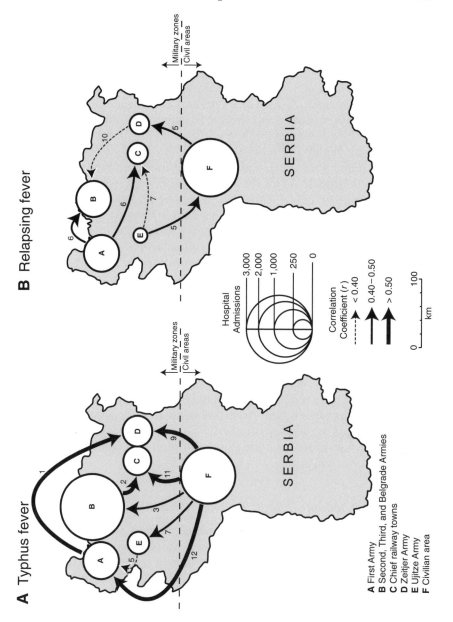

A Typhus fever

B Relapsing fever

SERBIA

Military zones
Civil areas

Hospital
Admissions
3,000
2,000
1,000
250
0

Correlation
Coefficient (*r*)
< 0.40
0.40–0.50
> 0.50

0   100
km

A First Army
B Second, Third, and Belgrade Armies
C Chief railway towns
D Zeitjer Army
E Ujitje Army
F Civilian area

traffic had a more marked impact upon the spatial transmission of typhus fever than it did upon relapsing fever.

Further features of Figure 12.20, relating to differences in the implied direction of disease transmission, are also evident:

(1) Typhus fever (Fig. 12.20A). The many bonds linking the civil area (F) to the military zones (A–E), with the military zones lagging the civil area by several days or more, imply that the resumption of rail traffic was associated with a dominant south → north (civil → military) flow of typhus infection. Within the subsystem of military zones, the bonds linking zones A and B to zones C and D are suggestive of a secondary (easterly) flux of the disease among the military zones;

(2) Relapsing fever (Fig. 12.20B). The several bonds linking the northwestern military zones (A and E) to other units in the system (military zones B and C and civil area F) imply that the resumption of rail traffic was associated with a general easterly and southerly spread of relapsing fever. The pattern is complex and some evidence for northerly transmission is provided by the link between civil area F and the northeastern military zone D.

Conclusions. In his consideration of the spread of typhus fever and relapsing fever in Serbia, Hunter (1920: 61) proposed that the resumption of passenger rail traffic had the effect of kindling two discrete transmission pathways, namely: (i) a southerly flux of typhus fever from the northern military zones; and (ii) a northerly flux of relapsing fever from the southern civil area. Instead, the results in Figure 12.20 suggest that Hunter's proposed transmission pathway (i) was in fact reversed—from civil to military zones rather than from military to civil. For pathway (ii), the CCF analysis suggests an important east–west corridor as well as north–south diffusion of typhus resulting from the resumption of rail traffic.

12.5.3 Pandemic Influenza in England and Wales, 1918–1919

Case studies of the Spanish influenza pandemic of 1918–19 have already been provided for US Army camps (Sect. 7.4.1) and the islands of the South Pacific (Sect. 11.3). In this subsection, our consideration of the pandemic turns to the spread of influenza within the civil settlement system of England and Wales (Johnson, 2001; Bowley, 2001). As the Local Government Board (1919: 4) note, influenza had first appeared in Britain in the early summer of 1918, amid growing apprehension over the possible importation of a host of infectious diseases—typhus fever, smallpox, dysentery, malaria, and trench fever— with soldiers, refugees, and others from war-torn Europe. In the event, major epidemics of the anticipated diseases never materialized. Influenza, on the other hand, spread widely in a civil population that had been subject to almost four years of wartime privations, strain, and, as part of the general war effort,

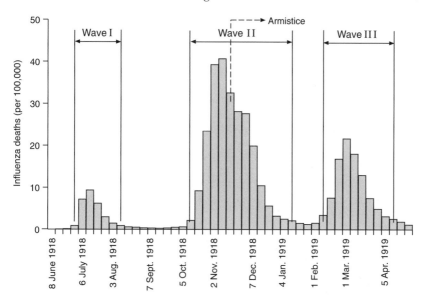

Fig. 12.21. Weekly influenza death rate (per 100,000 population), London and the county boroughs of England and Wales, June 1918–April 1919

Note: The time intervals associated with Waves I, II, and III of the epidemic are indicated.
Source: Smallman-Raynor *et al.* (2002, fig. 1, p. 457).

geographical upheaval to the most populous urban and industrial areas of the country. The spatial transmission of the epidemic, based on a study of the weekly count of reported influenza deaths in London and the 82 county boroughs of England and Wales (Local Government Board, 1919: 24–7), is examined by Smallman-Raynor *et al.* (2002) and we draw on their account here. Additional sources of information include Copeman (1920) and Parsons *et al.* (1922).

THE EPIDEMIC WAVES IN ENGLAND AND WALES

Figure 12.21 is taken from Smallman-Raynor *et al.* (2002) and plots the weekly influenza death rate per 100,000 population in London and the county boroughs of England and Wales, June 1918–April 1919. Consistent with the evidence for the global pandemic (Sect. 11.3.1), Figure 12.21 shows that the epidemic in England and Wales spread as three waves of infection. To define the duration of each wave, the aggregate weekly series of influenza mortality rates was first reworked as standard scores. Following Smallman-Raynor and Cliff (1998a), a sustained weekly score in excess of 0.5 standard deviations below the zero mean, with an additional calendar week at the beginning ('lead-in') and end ('tail-out') of each phase, was used to define the wave periods.

Table 12.7. Influenza in London and the county boroughs of England and Wales, June 1918–April 1919

Phase	Period			Reported deaths[2]	Peak week[1]
	Start[1]	End[1]	Duration (weeks)		
Epidemic	29 June 1918	12 Apr. 1919	42	64,759 (381.9)	9 Nov. 1918
Wave I	29 June 1918	10 Aug. 1918	7	4,894 (28.9)	13 July 1918
Wave II	12 Oct. 1918	11 Jan. 1919	14	41,857 (246.9)	9 Nov. 1918
Wave II	8 Feb. 1919	12 Apr. 1919	10	16,693 (98.4)	1 Mar. 1919

Notes: [1] Specified as the last day of the calendar week. [2] Reported deaths per 100,000 population are given in parentheses.
Source: Smallman-Raynor *et al.* (2002, table II, p. 457).

Specified in this manner, Table 12.7 gives the duration of each wave (designated as Waves I, II, and III), along with summary information on the number of reported deaths and the week of peak mortality. The wave intervals are marked on Figure 12.21.

Spread Patterns

The exact source of the 1918–19 influenza epidemic in the urban system of England and Wales is not known, although an introduction of the virus with military personnel on sick or home leave from the Western Front is generally suspected.[19] Sporadic outbreaks of the disease had occurred among British soldiers in France as early as April 1918, to be followed by a more general dissemination among the troops from the end of May (Macpherson *et al.*, 1922–3, i. 174–5). At about the same time, the Grand Fleet was assailed by influenza at its Scottish naval stations of Scapa and Rosyth while, by the start of June, the Scottish connection had been reinforced by outbreaks of an influenza-like disease in the civil population of Glasgow (Local Government Board, 1919: 7). As for England and Wales, the apparent epidemiological silence was broken when, on Saturday 22 June, *The Times* informed readers that a type of influenza 'similar to that reported in Spain' had appeared on the streets of Birmingham.[20] Certainly Birmingham was the first provincial city to display a sudden and sustained increase in recorded influenza mortality with accompanying deaths in nearby Coventry and Wolverhampton, Manchester, the port

[19] On the possibility that the causative agent (manifesting as 'purulent bronchitis') was present in both the civil and military populations of England and Wales long before the epidemic outbreak of June 1918, see Abrahams *et al.* (1917), Allen (1917), Ministry of Health (1920), Oxford *et al.* (1999), and Oxford (2000). See also Sect. 11.3.1.

[20] *The Times* (London) 1918: 22 June, p. 6.

cities of Liverpool, London, and Middlesborough and, soon thereafter, all urban centres of the country (Local Government Board, 1919: 7–32).[21]

Spatial patterns of wave progression. Against this background, the maps in Figure 12.22 chart the spread of Waves I (Fig. 12.22A), II (Fig. 12.22B), and III (Fig. 12.22C). Each of 83 geographical units (London and the 82 county boroughs) is represented in Figure 12.22 by a circle, with each circle shaded according to the week of the infection wave in which an influenza death was first registered. Geographical units in which influenza deaths were recorded in the week immediately preceding the onset of each wave (i.e. possible seed locations) have been shaded black.[22] As a backdrop to the point distributions, linear trend surfaces (Haggett *et al.*, 1977: 379–84), fitted for the average time to death in each wave,[23] show the main trends in wave progression. The implied direction of wave progression is indicated on each map by a vector.

A prominent feature of Figure 12.22 is the between-wave switch in the implied direction of epidemic progression, represented by a southward (Wave I) ⇒ northward (Wave II) ⇒ southward (Wave III) sequence of influenza transmission. We consider each wave in turn.

1. *Wave I (June–August 1918).* Consistent with contemporary reports,[24] the black circles in Figure 12.22A indicate that influenza was circulating and causing deaths in major ports and inland cities of northern England (Liverpool, Manchester, and Middlesbrough), the industrial West Midlands (Birmingham, Coventry, and Wolverhampton), and London at the onset of Wave I. From these putative index locations, the subsequent spread pattern was characterized by the rapid appearance of influenza deaths in the proximal county boroughs of central and northern England and Metropolitan London during weeks 1–2, and a relatively delayed appearance of influenza deaths in central-southern and south coastal settlements in subsequent weeks. Consistent with these broad timings, the surface in Figure 12.22A depicts a southerly drift of the infection wave.

2. *Wave II (October 1918–January 1919).* Although the black circles in Figure 12.22B confirm that influenza was present in urban centres across England and Wales at the onset of Wave II, the early involvement of southern localities (most notably, the seaports of Portsmouth and Cardiff) distinguishes this from the previous wave. This may be attributed to the early and heavy

---

[21] In summarizing the earliest evidence for the epidemic prevalence of Wave I, the Registrar-General (1920: 12) identified the Lancashire towns of Bacup and Rawtenstall to have been 'the first areas to have suffered a really serious mortality', although 'no definite evidence can be found . . . that this or any other locality can claim the doubtful distinction of being the first affected in the country'.

[22] Interpretation of the possible seed locations in Fig. 12.22 must proceed with caution. For Wave III, at least, the many black circles in Fig. 12.22C almost certainly reflect the geographically widespread nature of influenza mortality (albeit at a relatively low level) at the onset of the wave, rather than an apparently simultaneous and early introduction of a novel virus to these locations.

[23] *Average time to death* is calculated in the same manner as *average time to infection* (App. 6A.2), but with x_t in equation 6.A3 formed as the number of reported deaths (rather than cases) in time t.

[24] See e.g. *The Times* (London) 1918: 22 June, p. 6; 26 June, p. 7; 2 July, p. 3; 3 July, p. 3.

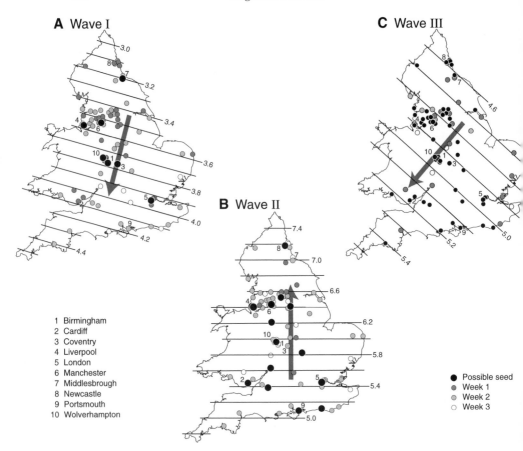

Fig. 12.22. The spread of influenza in London and the county boroughs of England and Wales, June 1918–April 1919

Notes: (A) Wave I, June–August 1918. (B) Wave II, October 1918–January 1919. (C) Wave III, February–April 1919. Geographical units are represented by circles, shaded according to the week of the corresponding wave in which the first influenza deaths were recorded; boroughs in which influenza deaths were recorded in the week immediately preceding the onset of a given wave are defined as seed locations. Linear trend surfaces for the expected time to death are plotted for each wave; numbers attached to the trend surfaces are in weeks.

Source: Smallman-Raynor *et al*. (2002, fig. 2, p. 459).

seeding of some south coastal settlements by naval personnel, among whom outbreaks of severe influenza had occurred at Portsmouth and elsewhere in August and September (Local Government Board, 1919: 8). However, Figure 12.22B also illustrates a relatively delayed appearance of influenza deaths in many localities of central and northern England. Linked to the early involvement of south coast settlements, this implies a northerly drift of the infection wave captured by the trend surface.

3. *Wave III (February–April 1919)*. While the many black circles in Figure 12.22C reflect the geographical ubiquity of influenza at the onset of Wave III, the surface suggests a dominant southward drift—albeit with a westward inflection—of the epidemic wave. Wave III marks a return to the broad spatial pattern of epidemic transmission identified in Figure 12.22A for Wave I.

Diffusion Processes

Using the method of autocorrelation on graphs (Sect. 6.4.2), Smallman-Raynor *et al.* (2002) demonstrate that the spread of Waves I to III was driven by a clearly defined process of spatial contagion. While the strength and timing of the process varied between the waves and was periodically bolstered by hierarchical components, the finding is consistent with the suggestion that epidemic transmission advanced so rapidly that purely hierarchical effects played but a minor role in the diffusion of the disease (Patterson and Pyle, 1991: 21).

LOCAL-AREA STUDIES: INFLUENZA IN CAMBRIDGE, 1918–1919

Among the several local-area studies to be included in the Ministry of Health's (1920) *Report on the Pandemic of Influenza*, Copeman's study of influenza in the borough of Cambridge is especially valuable because the data cover morbidity and mortality, as well as spanning the town, the colleges of the university, and the military contingent billeted in the town. As Copeman (1920: 388) commented:

The university population appeared to offer specially favourable material for such investigation [into the pandemic], owing to the fact that it consists in large measure of young adults on whom elsewhere the incidence of influenza had been specially marked during the past year. Moreover, in addition to the graduate and undergraduate population, there are, at present, 400 junior naval officers, exclusive of staff officers and batmen, who went into residence at Cambridge for a period of six months from January 31st, 1919, rooms being allocated to them in certain of the colleges, more particularly Trinity, Caius, King's, Magdalene, Pembroke, and Peterhouse . . . 40 military officers attending a course of instruction were also in residence in Sidney Sussex, while prior to the end of December, and for at least two years previously, there had also been at least 2,000 military cadets in residence, the length of stay of each individual cadet having been about 6 months.

To examine the spread of influenza in these various civil and military populations, Copeman drew not only on the local disease reports of physicians, but he also undertook a questionnaire survey of influenza activity in the colleges. All told, the survey yielded information on the influenza experience of 1,766 college members.

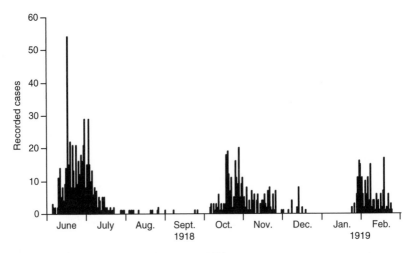

Fig. 12.23. Influenza in Cambridge, 1918–1919

Notes: Daily count of influenza cases treated at the First Eastern General Hospital, Cambridge, June 1918–February 1919. Cases are plotted according to the day of disease onset.
Source: Smallman-Raynor *et al.* (2002, fig. 4, p. 465), redrawn from Copeman (1920, charts I and II, facing p. 392).

Origin of the Epidemic in Cambridge

Figure 12.23 is based on the information collated by Copeman and plots the daily count of influenza cases reported by the First Eastern General Hospital in Cambridge, June 1918–March 1919. Comparison of this chart with Figure 12.21 shows that the 1,014 hospital cases recorded in Cambridge are distributed in the same three waves found nationally. As to the source of the disease, military personnel were the first to be affected. Influenza broke out among the military cadets at the beginning of June 1918, while the subsequent advent of the disease among the naval officers is summarized by Copeman (1920: 396):

it appears probable that the infection originated . . . with one of these officers who journeyed to Cambridge by himself, being apparently ill at the time. Although, like the cadets, distributed over the various colleges, the naval officers had ample opportunity of meeting one another, not only in their rooms but at lectures, with the result that an explosive outbreak of influenza occurred among them within a few days of their advent at the University, of so serious a character, that within about a week as many as 90 had been admitted to the First Eastern General Hospital . . . it may be noted that, at the same time, there were practically no cases of influenza among either the university or town population.

Copeman's conclusions included the following:

Wave severity. Mirroring the national picture, the second wave (Oct.–Nov. 1918) was the most severe as far as the borough was concerned. Among the colleges, there were 1,746 cases: 691 prior to 1918, 423 from July to September, 447 from October to December, and 185 from January to March 1918–19. Fatalities were low in the university population.

Age incidence. Incidence of the disease was mainly among young adults. Older persons largely escaped attack.

Quarantine. While the source of the infection was probably returning soldiers, influenza soon invaded the infant school populations in St Paul's, East Road and Sturton Street (Romsey and Sturton Towns in Fig. 12.24). On 22 October 1918, Copeman (1920: 440) noted,

it was decided to close the whole of the schools . . . in the borough, and at the same time steps were taken to have the Sunday schools closed also . . . A request made to managers of the cinemas and theatre to exclude children was immediately acquiesced in, and persons known to be arranging public meetings . . . were at once communicated with and the meetings abandoned for the time.

Closure of schools and abandonment of public meetings was historically a common quarantine device (see e.g. Cliff *et al.*, 1993: 416–17).

Diffusion Process

Figure 12.24 maps the diffusion process associated with the principal wave of the epidemic in Cambridge (Wave II). The vectors link the parishes of Cambridge on the basis of dates of the first report of influenza. New Town, adjacent to the railway station, was first affected. This is consistent with the believed source of the virus among naval cadets. From there, the infection spread anti-clockwise through the working-class areas of Cambridge in Sturton and Romsey Towns where railway and college staff lived, to arrive in the historic centre and the Cambridge colleges. From there, the disease spun out into another working-class area which housed college staff around the Newmarket Road. The centrifugal diffusion continued north and west into suburban Cambridge and finally swept anticlockwise out through Newnham, Cherry Hinton (including modern Trumpington), and Romsey, to finish finally in Old Chesterton. It is a classic contagious diffusion process based upon the intimate relationship between town and university. The overall attack rate was around 23 per cent.

Age of Attack

Figure 12.25 shows the age distribution of mortality rates usually found in a normal epidemic year (Fig. 12.25A), an influenza year (Fig. 12.25B), and a pandemic year associated with virus shift (Fig. 12.25C). In a normal year, mortality is concentrated among the young and the elderly and there is a deficit in the teens and early adult years. In years in which widespread influenza is found (Fig. 12.25B), the age distribution of mortality is the same as in a normal year but at a higher level. In pandemic years (Fig. 12.25C), teenagers and mature

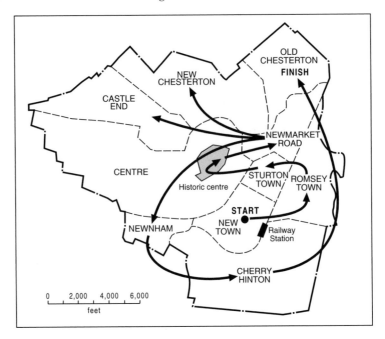

Fig. 12.24. Spread of Wave II of the 'Spanish' influenza epidemic in the Borough of Cambridge, 1918

Notes: Vectors trace the time-ordered sequence of first appearance of influenza (as judged by influenza deaths) in the districts of Cambridge, October–November 1918. According to Copeman (1920: 396), the first influenza death was recorded in New Town (marked 'start' on the map) on 1 October 1918, to be followed by Romsey Town (13 Oct.), Sturton Town (17 Oct.), Centre (18 Oct.), Newmarket Road (21 Oct.), Castle End, New Chesterton, and Newnham (all on 25 Oct.), Cherry Hinton (28 Oct.) and, finally, Old Chesterton (marked 'finish' on the map) on 17 November.
Source: Smallman-Raynor *et al.* (2002, fig. 5, p. 466), based on information in Copeman (1920: 396).

adults are heavily affected, with mortality rates among young adults equalling or exceeding those among the elderly. Figure 12.25D plots the age distribution of mortality in Cambridge. Consistent with the discussion in Section 11.3.3, the graph clearly shows the heavy mortality in young adults, and the continuing high rates in the mature years characteristic of pandemic years shown in Figure 12.25C.

Conclusion

Set within the national context, the local-level study of influenza in a single unit of the urban system (the Borough of Cambridge) provides detailed insights into the manner by which the disease entered and spread within the districts of

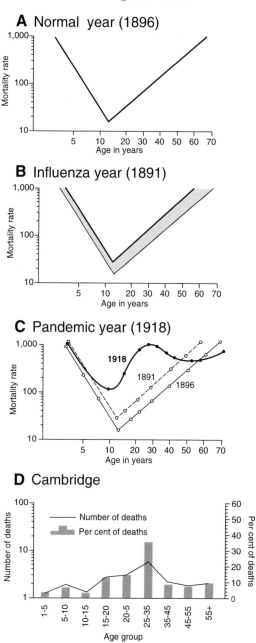

Fig. 12.25. Age distribution of mortality from influenza

Notes: Line traces plot the age distribution of mortality in a normal epidemic year (A), an influenza year (B), and a pandemic year associated with virus shift (C). (D) plots the distribution experienced in Cambridge during the 1918–19 pandemic.

Source: Smallman-Raynor *et al.* (2002, fig. 6, p. 467).

one provincial city. In particular, Cambridge serves to underscore the pivotal role of highly mobile military populations, both in the initial introduction of the influenza virus and in the localized 'supercharging' of disease transmission. Additionally, the Cambridge example highlights the special characteristics of pandemic influenza in terms of the ages of those attacked: high rates were experienced across the age spectrum, but especially in the 15 to 35 group, a feature also seen nationally and internationally (Langford, 2002).

SPANISH INFLUENZA AND ENCEPHALITIS LETHARGICA, 1918–1926

The global pandemic of encephalitis lethargica (von Economo's disease) that spread with, and in the aftermath of, the Spanish influenza pandemic of 1918–19 ranks as one of the more mysterious disease events of the early twentieth century (see Abrahamson, 1935; Ravenholt and Foege, 1982; and Ravenholt, 1993). While epidemics of encephalitic disease have historically occurred in conjunction with major waves of influenza activity, the 1918–26 pandemic of encephalitis lethargica was—like the influenza with which it appeared—characterized by an unusual virulence. The clinical course of the disease is reviewed by Ravenholt (1993) and reflected a diffuse involvement of the brain and the spinal cord. Disease onset was characterized by fever, with progressive lethargy, somnolence, and a range of other signs and symptoms including the disturbance of eye movements, headache, muscular weakness, delirium, and disablement. Lethargy varied in duration, from just a few days to weeks and months, terminating with death from comatose respiratory failure. The median interval from the onset of encephalitis to death was 14 days. The death rate associated with the acute stage of the disease was about 30 per cent, while a number of survivors developed parkinsonism in later years.

Although contemporary observers puzzled over the seemingly inconsistent temporal relationship between influenza and encephalitis lethargica (see e.g. Parsons *et al.*, 1922: 22–4), an aetiological link between the two diseases now seems evident (Ravenholt and Foege, 1982; Ravenholt 1993). Among the lines of evidence, Ravenholt and Foege (1982: 862) note that:

(i) both pandemics were globally distributed, were closely related in time, and only one aetiological agent (swine influenza virus) has yet been identified;

(ii) at all geographical scales, epidemics of influenzal pneumonia typically preceded epidemics of encephalitis lethargica;

(iii) during the early part of the encephalitis lethargica pandemic, many cases reported a previous episode of clinical influenza.

On the basis of available evidence, it appears that encephalitis lethargica was not transmissible from person to person (Ravenholt, 1993).

England and Wales

The first reports of encephalitis lethargica in England and Wales can be traced to London and Sheffield, where a previously unknown disease had appeared in March and early April 1918 (Harris, 1918; Hall, 1918). Prior to June 1918, the disease was spatially concentrated in the Eastern and Midlands counties. By the end of the year, the west of England had become involved. Describing the geographical spread of the disease at this time, Parsons *et al.* (1922: 12) observed:

Not by any steady advance in one direction . . . but in a seemingly haphazard way has encephalitis lethargica completed its invasion of this country, and the manner in which the disease here has skipped from place to place suggests in miniature some of its jumps from country to country which have been observed on the continent.

The temporal course of the epidemic in England and Wales is plotted on a monthly basis for the period January 1919–January 1922 in Figure 12.26B; for reference, charts 12.26A and 12.26C plot the monthly incidence of two other diseases with nervous system involvement, cerebrospinal meningitis and acute poliomyelitis. As Figure 12.26B shows, encephalitis lethargica occurred throughout the seasons but with a general tendency to peak in the late winter months (January and February) of the reporting years. Here, the upsurge in reported disease activity in the winter of 1920–1 is especially prominent. While this latter flare-up may be a reporting artefact associated with the anticipated publication of the Ministry of Health's *Memorandum on Encephalitis Lethargica*, a parallel increase in disease notifications was also observed for some other countries of Northern Europe (Parsons *et al.*, 1922; Ravenholt and Foege, 1982).

City Districts of Bristol

During the interval covered by Figure 12.26, encephalitis lethargica was primarily concentrated in the large cities and industrial centres of England and Wales. Of all the provincial cities, Bristol was distinguished in these years as having both the highest incidence and rate of disease activity. According to available records, the first case of encephalitis lethargica was identified in the city on 18 December 1918, with the disease appearing more generally in the early months of 1919 (Parsons *et al.*, 1922).

The local incidence of encephalitis lethargica (expressed as a rate per 10,000 population), January 1919–September 1921, is mapped for the city districts of Bristol in Figure 12.27. As the map shows, the most severely afflicted districts were located to the south of the River Avon: Knowle (5.0 per 10,000) and Bedminster (4.6 per 10,000). Generally lower rates were recorded to the north of the river, with the lowest rates (≤2.0 per 10,000) in Central Bristol and the western districts of Clifton and Westbury-on-Trym. The local geographical pattern of encephalitis lethargica in Bristol mirrored a more general, country-

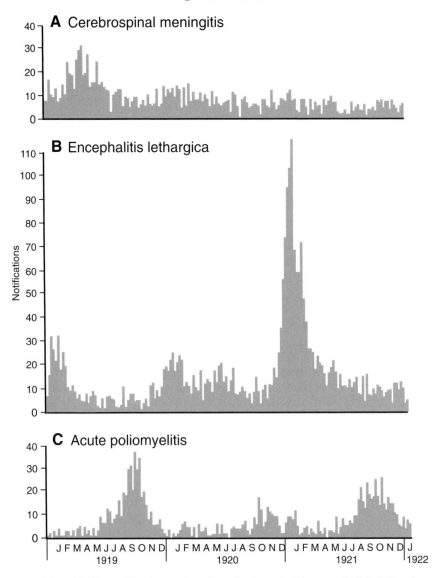

Fig. 12.26. Weekly notifications of cerebrospinal meningitis, encephalitis lethargica, and acute poliomyelitis in England and Wales, 1919–1921

Notes: Encephalitis lethargica was subject to notification in England and Wales as from 1 January 1919.

Source: Redrawn from Parsons *et al.* (1922, chart III, facing p. 26).

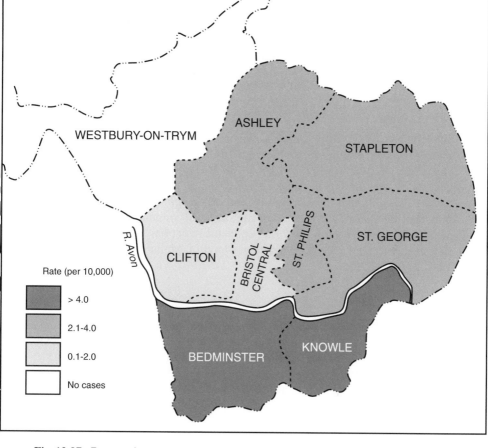

Fig. 12.27. Reported case rate (per 10,000 population) for encephalitis lethargica in the city districts of Bristol, UK, January 1919–September 1921

Source: Based on Parsons *et al.* (1922, facing p. 15).

wide, phenomenon: the tendency for the highest disease rates to occur in the most densely populated localities (Parsons *et al.*, 1922).

12.5.4 Service Personnel, Civilians, and Epidemic Poliomyelitis in Malta, 1942–1943

As Paul (1971: 346) notes, prior to the outbreak of World War II there was little intimation that poliomyelitis—a disease largely restricted to infants and children—was of military significance. Between 1920 and 1940, however, there had been a gradual and perceptible shift in the incidence of poliomyelitis among older age groups. The first indication of the military importance of the disease was the recovery, in 1941, of strains of poliovirus from the CNS tissue of fatal cases of an unidentified disease which had been attacking British soldiers in Egypt (Caughey and Porteous, 1946). Elsewhere, outbreaks of poliomyelitis were recorded among the British forces in India (McAlpine, 1945; Illingworth, 1945), while US forces in the Pacific experienced an explosive outbreak of the disease shortly after landing on the Philippine Islands in late 1944 (Sabin, 1960). The wider threat of military exposure to poliovirus, with the risk of onwards transmission to isolated civilian communities, was recognized by contemporary observers. In their examination of the military experience of poliomyelitis in Egypt, van Rooyan and Morgan (1943: 716) warned readers of the *Edinbugh Medical Journal* that there was 'always a chance that although the disease may not attain epidemic proportions under one set of living conditions, if it did reach a closed community (e.g. an isolated island), all factors favourable for an epidemic may arise'. Such was the situation in the beleaguered Mediterranean island of Malta during the winter of 1942–3 (Fig. 12.28).

THE MALTESE EPIDEMIC OF 1942–1943

Malta was no stranger to poliomyelitis. As Figure 12.29 shows, a steady trickle of paralytic cases had been reported each year from 1920. But the epidemic of 1942–3 overshadowed all previous experience of the disease on the island. During the course of the epidemic, almost 3 per cent of children aged 3 years or less were stricken by poliomyelitis (Seddon *et al.*, 1945), with further major outbreaks in the years that followed.

Origin and Spread of the Epidemic

Wyatt (1993) notes that some of the epidemics in Figure 12.29, such as those of 1945–6 and 1947–8, were caused by virulent strains of polioviruses imported from Egypt by Maltese natives. As regards the 1942–3 epidemic, some connection with the Allied relief of Malta and, in particular, the arrival of an overnight flight of about 250 RAF personnel in late 1942 is generally

——————————————————————————————▶

Fig. 12.28. Poliomyelitis in Malta and Gozo, November 1942–March 1943

Notes: Geographical distribution of a sample of 450 cases of paralytic poliomyelitis recorded among native civilians and British service personnel.
Source: Redrawn from Seddon *et al.* (1945, fig. 6, p. 13).

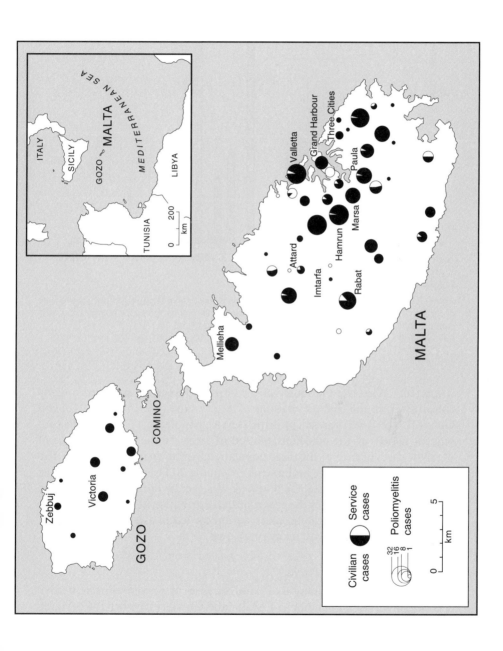

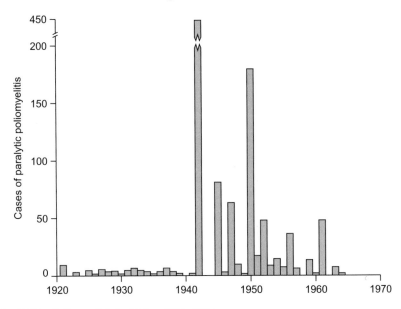

Fig. 12.29. Poliomyelitis in Malta, 1920–1964

Notes: Notified cases of paralytic poliomyelitis. Cases are counted from July of one year to June of the next to emphasize the epidemics. From the late 1950s, poliovirus vaccine was systematically administered leading to elimination of the disease from the island.
Source: Cliff *et al.* (2000, fig. 8.27, p. 425), originally from Wyatt (1993, fig. VIII.110.1, p. 943).

suspected.[25] Whatever the source of the virus, the epidemic appeared roughly concurrently in the civil populations of Malta (first case 15 Nov. 1942) and Gozo (21 Nov.) and the resident British service population (27 Nov.). The subsequent course of the epidemic, plotted in terms of the daily incidence of paralytic cases in each of the three populations, is shown in Figure 12.30. The epidemic reached its peak in the week beginning 20 December and, with the exception of sporadic cases, the outbreak was over by the following February (Seddon *et al.*, 1945). As for the geographical distribution of poliomyelitis, Figure 12.28 shows that paralytic cases were recorded in almost every town of Malta and Gozo, along with many rural areas.

Morbidity and Mortality Profiles

Table 12.8 gives the distribution of paralytic cases of poliomyelitis in the civil and British service populations of Malta and Gozo, November 1942–March

[25] A connection with Egypt, or North Africa and the Near East more generally, has not been established for the 1942–3 epidemic. It is noteworthy, however, that 106 cases of poliomyelitis were reported among British and Dominion service personnel in Egypt, Palestine, and Syria during 1941–2, with a highly virulent strain of poliovirus isolated from a fatal case in Egypt in May 1942; see Paul (1971: 349).

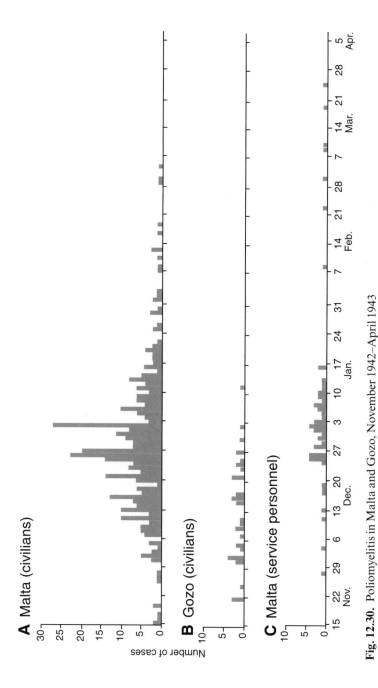

Fig. 12.30. Poliomyelitis in Malta and Gozo, November 1942–April 1943

Note: Notified cases of paralytic poliomyelitis are plotted by day of onset for the civil populations of Malta (A) and Gozo (B) and for British service personnel (C).

Source: Redrawn from Seddon *et al.* (1945, fig. 2, p. 5).

Table 12.8. Paralytic poliomyelitis in Malta and Gozo,
November 1942–March 1943

Population	Cases	Deaths
Civilians		
Malta	384	15[1]
Gozo	42	
British services		
Malta	57[2]	11
Total	483	26

Notes: [1] Poliomyelitis may have been a contributory factor in a further 11 fatalities. [2] Royal Navy, 2 cases; Army, 27 cases; Royal Air Force, 28 cases.
Source: Seddon *et al.* (1945, tables II and V, pp. 3, 8).

1943. As the table indicates, a total of 483 cases were reported during the epidemic, of which 426 were civilians and 57 were members of the British Army, Navy, and Air Force. While the majority of civilian cases occurred in children aged below 5 years, and the associated case-fatality rate was relatively low (3.5%), a case-fatality rate of 19.3 per cent was recorded for the (adult) service cases. As the *British Medical Journal* commented in later years,

The age distribution of the civilian and service cases suggests that the causal strain of virus must have differed only slightly from the usual endemic Maltese strain, for its successful attacks were confined to the more susceptible civilian age groups. On the other hand, the high incidence and severity of the disease in the service cases suggest that the strain differed greatly from that usually endemic in the British Isles. (Anonymous, 1945*b*: 774)

Although it is probable that British service personnel had immunity to strains of poliovirus that were prevalent in Britain, it would seem that such immunity afforded only limited protection against the virus encountered in Malta during the winter of 1942–3.

Environmental Factors Contributing to Spread

Further factors that may have contributed to the epidemic transmission of poliomyelitis in Malta in 1942–3 are reviewed by Seddon *et al.* (1945) and include a series of unusual environmental circumstances. At the time of the epidemic, the island had been subject to over two years of intense aerial bombardment by Italian and German forces, resulting in widespread destruction of housing and infrastructure. The sewer system was damaged, water provision was partially disrupted, and overcrowding in underground quarters was rife. A year-long blockade (Oct. 1941–Nov. 1942) served to intensify the problem of under-nutrition and malnutrition on the island while, from November 1942, raw sewage was used to manure food crops (Cassar, 1964: 558–68). Dysentery and typhoid fever began to spread widely in the latter half of 1942 and, although there is no evidence that food or water supplies were a source of poliovirus (Seddon *et al.*, 1945), it seems likely that insanitary living conditions contributed to the epidemic spread of poliomyelitis at this time.

CONCLUSIONS

In addition to the role of war as a factor in the generation of environmental conditions conducive to the spread of infectious diseases, the Maltese experience of poliomyelitis in World War II illustrates the intersection of several themes discussed in this and previous chapters: (i) the role of military personnel in the introduction of disease agents to civil populations (Sect. 8.3); (ii) the role of war in the emergence of apparently 'new' strains of disease agents for which military and/or civil populations have little, or no, acquired immunity (Ch. 9); (iii) the potentially explosive spread of war epidemics in island communities (Ch. 11); and (iv) differential patterns of disease susceptibility among soldiers and civilians in specific geographical locations (Sect. 12.3).

12.6 Conclusion to Part III

In Part III of this book, regional case studies have been used to illustrate a series of repeating themes in the geography of war and disease, 1850–1990. Drawing on a small sample of the several hundred documented wars, revolutions, and insurrections in the period, we have selected case studies—including, where possible, examples from both the nineteenth and twentieth centuries— which are both intrinsically interesting and which illustrate the core issues involved. Within these broad parameters, our choice of war has been conditioned by the richness of the disease records available for a dozen or so national and international conflicts (Table III.A). For many other conflicts, the disease records are too fragmentary to allow systematic analysis while, for yet others, relevant information is simply not available for examination.

An important feature of the 140-year time period under analysis was the decline in the relative importance of infectious diseases as a cause of morbidity and mortality in fighting forces (Ch. 4). The specific agents of many bacterial diseases and some viral diseases had been identified by the onset of World War II, while advances in vaccination, chemotherapy, and military hygiene contributed significantly to disease prevention, treatment, and control. However, as the case studies have shown, infectious diseases still had the potential to incapacitate large bodies of men when, as in the Korean and Vietnam Wars, front-line troops were deployed in unfamiliar epidemiological environments. As for civil populations, numerous examples—from the smallpox epidemic which accompanied the Franco-Prussian War in the late nineteenth century to the HIV/AIDS epidemic that spread in Uganda during the late twentieth century—underscore the enduring epidemiological threat of war to non-combatants.

Taken together, Parts II and III of this book have traced the historical association of war and disease from the days of ancient Greece and Rome to the brink of the present day. In the next and final chapter, we turn to the epidemiological consequences of wars and war-like events on the cusp of the new millennium.

Appendix 12A

Yellow Fever, Smallpox, and Enteric Fever in Cuba (Section 12.3)

This appendix places the general pattern of susceptibility to the three diseases examined in Section 12.3 (yellow fever, smallpox, and enteric fever) within the epidemiological context of late-nineteenth-century Cuba. An outline of the nature of each disease is provided in Appendix 1A.

Yellow Fever

Although the history of yellow fever in Cuba can be traced to the early seventeenth century (epidemic visitations were recorded in 1620, the 1640s, and the 1650s), evidence of the disease prior to the mid-eighteenth century is scant and the historical record points to the establishment of the island as an endemic focus in the years after 1761 (USMHS, 1896*b*: 387–9; Augustin, 1909). Certainly by the 1850s, yellow fever was a permanent resident of Habana City, with the disease prevailing on an annual basis in the port cities of Cardenas, Cienfuegos, Matanzas, Sagua la Grande, and Santiago de Cuba (USMHS, 1896*b*: 390–2; 1900: 1840–54). In these settlements, the occurrence of the disease was strongly seasonal. Transmission of the virus is dependent on warm and wet conditions conducive to the activity of the mosquito vector; disease occurrence in Cuban cities was usually greatest in June–December (the yellow fever season), with a marked low in January–May (USMHS, 1900: 1840–54; see Fig. 12.7A). In the acclimatized urban populations, yellow fever was typically a mild infection of childhood; a single exposure to the virus transferred lifelong immunity and epidemics were rare. Rather, severe epidemics awaited the wartime influx of large numbers of unacclimatized troops, and attendant civilians, from the Spanish mainland (USMHS, 1896*b*: 385–439; 1900: 1841–54).

Smallpox

In contrast to yellow fever, which was endemic to the island, nineteenth-century Cuba lacked the conditions necessary to maintain smallpox in endemic form. So, of the 13 smallpox epidemics to strike the island in that century, an external source of the virus is either known or strongly suspected. As a consequence, each epidemic was separated by an extended disease-free period, and this was accompanied by a systematic increase in the number of susceptibles. On each reintroduction to the island, smallpox virus spread rapidly through the civil population (Hopkins, 1983; Fenner *et al.*, 1988). In contrast, the bulk of Spanish soldiers in the insurrection of 1895–8 were vaccinated prior to, or soon after, their arrival on the island and the disease was of lesser significance in this population (USMHS, 1896*a*: 1061).

Enteric Fever

Given the insanitary conditions that prevailed in the larger settlements of late-nineteenth-century Cuba, coupled with the potentially long carrier state for typhoid fever (up to one in 20 untreated infectives will be permanent carriers of *Salmonella typhi*), it is not surprising that enteric fever was an endemic infection, at least in Habana City. Here, the disease displayed a weak seasonal pattern with a peak mortality in the summer months (see Fig. 12.7C). But, whereas prior exposure to yellow fever and small-pox viruses confers lifelong immunity on the victim, a prior bout of typhoid or para-typhoid fever offers only relative immunity that can be overcome by ingestion of a sufficiently large dose of bacilli. Under these circumstances, neither Cuban civilians nor Spanish soldiers could be considered immune to enteric fever.

PART IV

Prospects

13

War and Disease: Recent Trends and Future Threats

Yet the poor fellows think they are safe! They think that the war is over!
Only the dead have seen the end of war.

George Santayana, *Soliloquies in England*
(Soliloquy 25, 'Tipperary', 1924)[1]

---

[1] The line 'Only the dead have seen the end of war' was later used by General Douglas MacArthur at his Farewell Speech to the Corps of Cadets at West Point, 12 May 1962. MacArthur attributed the line to Plato.

13.1 Introduction

In the foregoing chapters, we have focused on the intersection of war and infectious disease over the 140-year period from 1850. We have examined long-term trends in disease activity in civil, military, and displaced populations (Chs. 3–5), outlined some of the analytical approaches used to describe the spread of war epidemics (Ch. 6), and we have explored in a regional context recurring themes at the interface of war and infectious disease (Chs. 7–12). In this concluding chapter, we examine the epidemiological consequences of wars and war-like events in the years since 1990. We begin in Section 13.2 by reviewing the empirical evidence for the spread of diseases in association with three recent conflicts: the Gulf War (1990–1); the Bosnian Civil War (1992–5); and Afghanistan and the 'War on Terrorism' (2001–). In Section 13.3, we examine the role of war both as an obstacle to disease eradication and to disease-control strategies while, in Section 13.4, we focus on biological weapons as one of the foremost threats to global security in the modern world. Finally, in Section 13.5, we isolate a series of further war-related issues (militarism; economic sanctions; international peacekeeping; disease re-emergence; and post-combat syndromes) that—given the balance of probabilities—are likely to be of continuing epidemiological significance in the current century.

13.2 Late-Twentieth and Early Twenty-First-Century Conflicts

As we enter a new millennium, there is an undercurrent of academic thought that nuclear weaponary and the end of the Cold War have rendered war obsolete; that war is, and will be, increasingly supplanted by economic competition between states and regions (see e.g. Black, 2000). Yet it is clear from Figure 13.1 that wars—of greater or lesser intensity—have continued to increase, rather than decrease, in number over the last few decades. This increase has remained largely focused in the less developed regions of the world (van der Wusten, 1985; Brogan, 1992; Arnold, 1995). By way of illustration, Figure 13.2 delimits the global pattern of conflict in the year 2000. As the map shows, levels of conflict intensity were highest in some of the poorest of the world's regions—in Sub-Saharan Africa, Central and South Asia (Murray *et al.*, 2002). In the words of John Keegan (1994: 14),

Have-nots against haves, haves against haves, haves against have-nots; that is war's history. Now our conscience is assailed by the pitiful and profitless phenomenon of war between have-nots and have-nots . . . Now war is exclusively an occupation for the poor alone. There are, commentators tell us, thirty wars in progress in the world. They are taking place—where? In the world's remote, resourceless, unproductive places: in Bosnia, the poorest part of Europe, in the Caucasus, the poorest part of the old

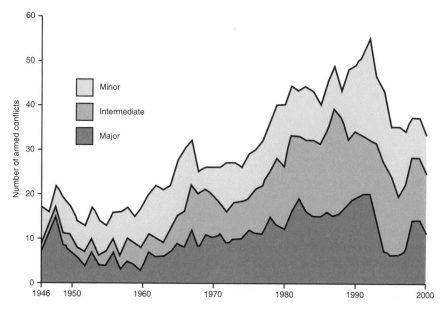

Fig. 13.1. Number of armed conflicts by year, 1946–2000

Notes: Line traces plot the annual number of conflicts by level of intensity. Minor conflicts, ≥25 deaths per year, but <1,000 accumulated deaths. Intermediate conflicts, ≥25 deaths per year and ≥1,000 accumulated deaths, but <1,000 deaths in a given year. Major conflicts, ≥1,000 deaths per year.

Source: Redrawn from Stewart (2002, fig. 1, p. 342), originally from Gleditsch *et al.* (2001, fig. 1, p. 8).

Soviet Union, in Cambodia, one of the poorest parts of Asia, in Angola, Mozambique, Somalia, Rwanda, some of the poorest parts of a continent by definition by poor. War, once a struggle over riches, or the proud vocation of peoples rich themselves, is now the calling of the wretched of the earth.

SOME RECENT TRENDS IN THE WAGING OF WAR

From the gamut of military, strategic, and other war-related developments of recent decades, van Creveld (1991) and UNHCR (2000) isolate three salient trends in modern conflicts: (i) the increasing involvement of non-state organizations; (ii) the increasing operation of 'low-intensity' conflicts; and (iii) the increasing involvement of civil populations. We briefly consider each trend in turn.

Non-state Organizations and Warfare

Over the last 50 years, there has been a growing tendency for the state to lose its monopoly over armed violence. Consistent with the patterns in Figure

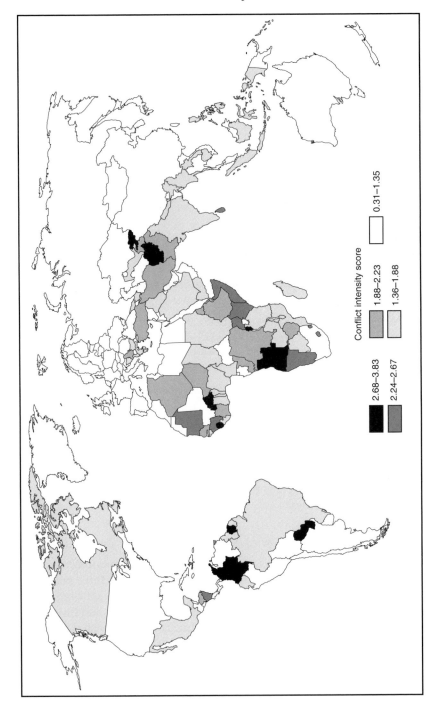

Fig. 13.2. Intensity of military conflict by country, 2000

Notes: Conflict intensity is measured according to the number of media reports of external and internal military conflict targeted at each country.

Source: Redrawn from Murray *et al.* (2002, fig. 2, p. 347).

1.3, the practice of wars conducted between states—interstate conflicts fought by regular armies—has been replaced by conflicts in which one or more of the combatants is a non-state organization. Guerrillas, terrorists, and rebels now rank among the principal combatants in many wars. Moreover, since the early 1990s and the decline of Superpower support for conflict in developing countries, sponsorship for wars has increasingly come from non-state organizations. As a consequence, ideologically based loyalities of minority groups, extremist factions, fundamentalist movements, and other non-state organizations are now viewed as an important motivating factor for war.

Low-Intensity Conflicts

The increasing involvement of non-state organizations has been associated with a rise in so-called 'low-intensity conflict' as a strategy of modern warfare. Low-intensity conflict emerged as an aspect of US military doctrine after the Vietnam War and can be defined as war at the 'grass-roots' level, involving not only military engagement but also political, economic, and psychological warfare (Garfield, 1989). Taking examples of wars from the 1980s, Garfield (1989) identifies three types of low-intensity conflict: (1) classic counter-insurgency, as practised in El Salvdaor; (2) active defence against potential insurgencies, as in Guatemala and Honduras; and (3) pro-insurgency, as conducted by proxy armies in Nicaragua, Angola, and Mozambique.

Civilians and Warfare

As low intensity conflicts have come to dominate the warscape, so the manner of fighting has changed. In particular, combatants have become increasingly intermingled with civilians. The combatants do not amount to armies as traditionally understood and the enemy is increasingly dispersed. Further, as demonstrated by the genocide in Rwanda (Central Africa) and Bosnia–Herzegovina (Europe) during the 1990s, civilians are viewed as legitimate targets in such wars. As a consequence, civilians have represented a rising proportion of war casualties so that, by the 1990s, they constituted an estimated 90 per cent of all war deaths (Table 1.10).

With these developments in mind, the following subsections examine the health impacts of selected wars and associated military operations in the late twentieth and early twenty-first centuries: the Gulf War, 1990–1 (Sect. 13.2.1); the Bosnian Civil War, 1992–5 (13.2.2); and Afganistan in the era of Operation Enduring Freedom, 2001–2 (13.2.3).

13.2.1 The Gulf War

On 2 August 1990, Iraqi forces overran the defences of neighbouring Kuwait. Four days later, on 6 August, United Nations (UN) Security Council Resolution 661 served to impose a worldwide embargo on trade with Iraq.

Thereafter, a six-month build-up of US, British, Canadian, and other coalition forces in the Persian Gulf region (Operation Desert Shield) was followed, from 17 January 1991, by a five-week aerial bombing campaign and subsequently a four-day ground assault on Iraq (Operation Desert Storm). With the Iraqi Republican Guard routed in the vicinity of Basra, Southern Iraq, on 27 February, and with the immediate collapse of all remaining Iraqi military opposition, a ceasefire in the Gulf War was agreed on 28 February (Kohn, 1999).

CIVIL POPULATION OF IRAQ

All told, the coalition forces dropped an estimated 80,000 tons of explosives on Iraq, resulting in the death of some 2,500 to 3,000 civilians. This death toll was, however, overshadowed by war and post-war mortality arising partly from the extensive destruction of life-sustaining civilian infrastructure (most especially, electricity-generating plants) and partly from economic and trade sanctions. Mass population displacement in the aftermath of the war, both in the north (Kurds) and south (Shiite muslims) of the country, further added to the plight of the civil population (Hoskins, 1997).

Morbidity and Mortality

Well over 100,000 Iraqi civilians are estimated to have died as a consequence of the health impacts of the war and associated sanctions in 1991. Epidemics of a range of infectious diseases including cholera, typhoid, hepatitis A, malaria, measles, and poliomyelitis contributed to the mortality. The situation was compounded by shortages of medicines and medical care. Many medical facilities were damaged or totally destroyed during the war, while economic sanctions were associated with shortages of all types of medicines and medical paraphernalia such as anaesthetics, vaccines, and surgical equipment (Hoskins, 1997).

Immunization services. Immunization services were suspended between January and March 1991. Refrigerated and frozen vaccines were ruined as a conssquence of electricity cuts, while the only syringe factory was destroyed during a coalition bombing raid. With immunization services unable to re-establish themselves until late 1991, vaccine-preventable diseases surged and, although subsequent immunization campaigns reduced the risk of major epidemics by the mid-1990s, implementation of the WHO Expanded Programme on Immunization (EPI) remained considerably weakened (Hoskins, 1997).

Undernutrition/malnutrition. Poor sanitation and contaminated water supplies promoted diarrhoea as a leading cause of death in children. Crowding and exposure also gave rise to a post-war upsurge in acute respiratory infections, with malnutrition and micronutrient deficiencies serving to complicate the clinical picture. By early 1991, supplies of essential foodstuffs such as wheat, rice, vegetable oil, and sugar had become scarce, resulting in an acute food deficit during the war and in its aftermath. In June 1991, for example, UNICEF reported a sharp rise in moderate and severe malnutrition among children aged under 5 years, with a corresponding increase in mortality from 43 per 1,000 (pre-war) to 129 per 1,000 (1991, post-war) (Ascherio *et al.*, 1992; Hoskins, 1997). Several years on, in 1996, the estimated mortality rate for children aged under 5 years still stood at 87 per 1,000 (Garfield and Leu, 2000).

COALITION FORCES: NON-BATTLE MORTALITY AMONG
US MILITARY PERSONNEL

Table 13.1 is taken from the study of Writer *et al.* (1996) and gives cause-specific counts of non-battle deaths among all US military personnel[2] deployed to the Persian Gulf during the preparatory (Operation Desert Shield) and combat (Operation Desert Storm) phases of the Gulf War, 1 August 1990–31 July 1991.[3] For reference, the table also gives the equivalent information for non-deployed US forces. When examined as a rate (expressed per 100,000 person-years), non-battle mortality for deployed forces (84.95 per 100,000) was moderately higher than for non-deployed forces (73.38 per 100,000), with the increment largely attributable to raised levels of unintentional injuries associated with aircraft, explosions, and other (non-specified) sources. For all other major categories of mortality in Table 13.1 (illness, self-inflicted, homicide, and unknown), death rates were lower in deployed than non-deployed forces.

When compared with the military campaigns described in the foregoing chapters of this book, a remarkable feature of Table 13.1 is the solitary confirmed death from infectious disease in the US Gulf forces—and this in over 0.26 million person-years of deployment. Such a statistic is testament to the advances in military medicine and hygiene over the past century.

ENVIRONMENTAL IMPACTS OF THE WAR

As described by Hoskins (1997), the environmental impacts of the Gulf War were wide-ranging. During the course of the war, some 4 million barrels of oil were spilt into the Persian Gulf, affecting not only wildlife and marine biology but, also, the production of potable water by coastal desalinization plants. Up to 500 oil fires were purposely ignited in Kuwait by departing Iraqi forces, resulting in the high-level release of sulphur dioxide, nitrogen oxide, and many other pollutants, including known carcinogens such as benzene, into the atmosphere. Coalition attacks on Iraqi chemical facilities and weapons stockpiles may have accounted for the wartime detection of chemical releases in the region, while coalition weapons were responsible for the scattering of some

[2] Including US Army, Air Force, Navy, and Marine Corps personnel.
[3] In addition to the 225 non-battle-related deaths recorded for US forces deployed to the Persian Gulf in Table 13.1, 147 US troops died as a direct result of trauma sustained during Operation Desert Storm (Writer *et al.*, 1996).

Table 13.1. Mortality from non-battle causes in US military personnel deployed to the Persian Gulf, and in non-deployed US forces, 1 August 1990–31 July 1991

	Deaths (rate per 100,000 person-years)		
	Deployed	Non-deployed	Total
All non-battle-related deaths	225 (84.95)	1,397 (73.38)	1,622 (74.79)
Unintentional injury	183 (69.09)	784 (41.18)	967 (44.59)
Motor vehicle	62 (23.41)	439 (23.06)	501 (23.10)
Motorcycle	0 (0.00)	65 (3.41)	65 (3.00)
Aircraft	47 (17.74)	104 (5.46)	151 (6.96)
Explosions	18 (6.80)	1 (0.05)	19 (0.88)
Other	56 (21.14)	175 (9.19)	231 (10.65)
Illness	30 (11.33)	264 (13.87)	294 (13.56)
Cardiovascular	2 (0.76)	69 (3.62)	71 (3.27)
Unexpected/undefined[1]	21 (7.93)	102 (5.36)	123 (5.67)
Cancer	0 (0.00)	28 (1.47)	28 (1.29)
Infectious disease	1 (0.38)	11 (0.58)	12 (0.55)
Other	6 (2.27)	54 (2.84)	60 (2.76)
Self-inflicted	10 (3.78)	206 (10.82)	216 (9.96)
Gunshot	10 (3.78)	120 (6.30)	130 (5.99)
Hanging/asphyxiation	0 (0.00)	54 (2.84)	54 (2.49)
Other	0 (0.00)	32 (1.68)	32 (1.48)
Homicide	1 (0.38)	102 (5.36)	103 (4.75)
Gunshot	1 (0.38)	67 (3.52)	68 (3.14)
Other	0 (0.00)	35 (1.84)	35 (1.61)
Unknown	1 (0.38)	41 (2.15)	42 (1.96)

Note: [1] Includes deaths for which there was no apparent preceding illness or injury and deaths attributed to cardiac or respiratory failure and other causes on casualty reports.
Source: Writer *et al.* (1996, table 1, p. 119).

40–300 tons of depleted uranium in Iraq and Kuwait. Unexploded ordnance remains a potential source of traumatic injury and death in the Gulf region.

13.2.2 Former Yugoslavia: Evidence from Bosnia–Herzegovina

On 25 June 1991, Croatia and Slovenia issued a joint declaration of independence from the Federal Republic of Yugoslavia. The ensuing wars of Croatian and Slovenian Independence, the Bosnian Civil War, and subsequently the Kosovo Uprisings, served to shatter state economies and infrastructure, leaving many tens of thousands dead, and generating the largest movement of European refugees since World War II. In this subsection, we examine the intersection of war and infectious disease in the former Yugoslavia, taking Bosnia–Herzegovina—the locus of Serb–Croat–Muslim hostilities in the Bosnian Civil War—as our geographical frame of reference. Figure 13.3 serves as a location map for the discussion.

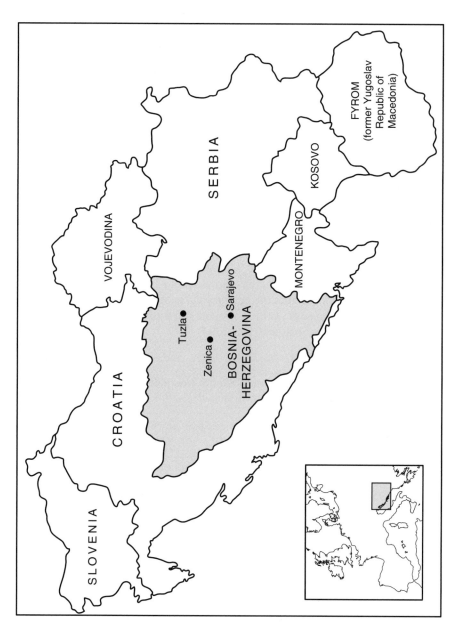

Fig. 13.3. Location map of the republics of the former Yugoslavia

EVIDENCE FROM BOSNIA–HERZEGOVINA

The Bosnian Civil War (1992–5) was the most brutal of the several conflicts to wrack Yugoslavia in the 1990s. Notorious for the genocide ('ethnic cleansing') and other violations of human rights that came to characterize the conflict, the hostilities left up to 250,000 dead, 2 million displaced, and several dozen (including the Bosnian Serb leader, Radovan Karadic) indicted by the UN as suspected war criminals. The physical damage inflicted by the war was estimated at US$20–40 billion. Many settlements were partially or completely destroyed while, some two years after the agreement of the Dayton peace accords (14 Dec. 1995), Bosnia–Herzegovina's GDP still remained at less than 50 per cent of its pre-war level (Alderslade *et al.*, 1996; Heritage, 2000).

Enteric Diseases

The early months of the Bosnian Civil War were associated with a marked increase in levels of enteric disease activity (Arnautovic *et al.*, 1994; Puvacic and Weinberg, 1994; Telalbasic *et al.*, 1994). By way of illustration, Table 13.2 gives the recorded incidence (per 100,000 population) of hepatitis A, diarrhoea, and dysentery in three locations of central Bosnia (Sarajevo City, Zenica City, and Tuzla Region) during sample months of the pre-war (1990–2) and war (1993) periods. As the table shows, explosive increases in enteric disease activity were recorded in the besieged cities of Sarajevo and Zenica in 1993, reflecting the collapse of sanitary systems and freshwater supplies during the bombardment of these places (CDC, 1993).

Table 13.2. Incidence rate of selected enteric diseases in sample locations of central Bosnia, 1990–1993

Location/time period	Disease incidence (per 100,000 population)		
	Hepatitis A	Diarrhoea	Dysentery
Sarajevo City			
1992 (Jan.–June)	0.9	13.2	0.3
1993 (Jan.–June)	5.1	94.9	4.0
Change	+560%	+719%	+1,250%
Zenica City			
1990–1 (May–July)	0.4	10.3	0.3
1993 (May–July)	4.6	83.9	4.4
Change	+1,210%	+815%	+1,692%
Tuzla Region			
1992	0.5	6.5	0.5
1993 (Jan.–June)	1.9	9.3	0.4
Change	+358%	+43%	−10%

Source: CDC (1993, table 1, p. 980).

Childhood Infections

The period covered by Table 13.2 was associated with a curtailment of routine immunization against such childhood infections as measles, mumps, rubella, and whooping cough. Between June 1991 and July 1993, for example, just 33 per cent of children aged 13 to 25 months were vaccinated against measles, compared with 90 to 95 per cent in 1990. Under such circumstances, the documented reduction in the wartime activity of measles and other vaccine-preventable diseases almost certainly reflects a breakdown of public health surveillance for these diseases (CDC, 1993; Puvacic and Weinberg, 1994).

Other Infectious Diseases: HFRS

Bosnia–Herzegovina and other Balkan states have been recognized as endemic foci of hantaviruses, the causative agents of haemorrhagic fever with renal syndrome (HFRS), since the 1950s (Trencséni and Keleti, 1971; Gligić *et al.*, 1989). Details of the nature of HFRS are given in Section 9.4.2 but, just prior to the unrest of the 1990s, significant outbreaks of the disease had been documented in Bosnia–Herzgovina in 1986 (Gligić *et al.*, 1989) and 1989 (Markotić *et al.*, 1994). By the mid-1990s, the environmental conditions engendered by the Bosnian Civil War were again favourable to the spread of HFRS.

The Tuzla outbreak. Hukic *et al.* (1996) note that, prior to the war, HFRS occurred in sporadic form in the vicinity of Tuzla (Fig. 13.3). Between 1995 and 1996, however, over 300 patients with HFRS were admitted to Tuzla hospital. With reference to Table 9.5, patients displayed evidence of infection with both Puumala- and Hantaan-like viruses, indicating that the Tuzla outbreak was associated with at least two serotypes of hantavirus. Factors which may have contributed to the spread of the disease in the region included an apparent increase in the abundance of small rodents which, in turn, was associated with the presence of military camps, inadequate waste disposal, and a general breakdown in hygiene and sanitary conditions. Additional factors, including the increased levels of human–rodent contact arising as a consequence of mass population displacement, may have further contributed to the spread of the disease (Hukic *et al.*, 1996).

HFRS in Sarajevo. Sporadic cases of HFRS were reported from Sarajevo during the siege of the city (Fig. 13.3). Clement *et al.* (1994), for example, document a case of the disease in a Canadian worker at the UN headquarters. Infection was probably acquired from rodents within the UN building. Later, in 1995–6, an HFRS-like disease began to appear in soldiers engaged in the de-blockade of the city. As in Tuzla, investigation of several dozen suspected patients at the city's war hospital revealed evidence of infection with both Puumala and Hantaan viruses (Beslagic *et al.*, 1996).

Conclusions

Notwithstanding the foregoing evidence, it is generally acknowledged that levels of infectious disease activity in Bosnia–Herzegovina were lower than those recorded during similar periods of war and civil unrest in developing countries (CDC, 1993; Alderslade *et al.*, 1996). Factors which may have contributed to the relative containment of infectious diseases in Bosnia–Herzegovina included: (i) residence of the majority of displaced persons in private houses rather than refugee camps; (ii) the continued function of some elements of local public health systems; (iii) the health-related efforts of UN agencies and non-governmental organizations (NGOs); (iv) high pre-war levels of immunization against vaccine-preventable diseases; and (v) the maintenance of a relatively high standard of hygiene by a well-educated and resourceful population (CDC, 1993).

13.2.3 Afghanistan, Operation Enduring Freedom, and the 'War on Terrorism'

On 7 October 2001—less than a month after the 11 September attacks on the World Trade Center and the Pentagon—US bombing missions in Afghanistan signalled the commencement of Operation Enduring Freedom. With the al-Qa'eda terrorist network and the supporting Taliban regime as the primary targets of attack, the initial air and sea campaign was accompanied by a build-up of US, British, and other Coalition troops in neighbouring Pakistan and Tajikistan. In late November, with the Taliban in retreat, with the Coalition-backed forces of the Northern Alliance in the ascendancy, and with provisional plans for a multi-ethnic power-sharing agreement in place, conventional ground troops began to move into southern Afghanistan.

CIVIL POPULATION

Operation Enduring Freedom is the most recent phase in an armed conflict that, after some 23 years, has left Afghanistan 'in the midst of an overwhelming humanitarian crisis' (Sharp *et al.*, 2002, p. S215). By 2002, sustained hostilities, politicial instability, and long-term socio-economic neglect, all compounded by severe drought, food shortages, and the human rights abuses of successive leaderships, had resulted in a set of health indicators that were among the poorest in the world. The average life expectancy was 46 years, the infant mortality rate (IMR) 165 per 1,000 live births, and the maternal mortality rate 1,700 per 10,000 live births. An estimated 5 million people—representing approximately 20 per cent of the Afghan population—were internally or internationally displaced, while virtually all health care was supplied by international relief agencies (Bhutta, 2002; Brundtland, 2002; Sharp *et al.*, 2002).

Health and Disease in the Winter of 2001–2

Although data are generally lacking, several infectious diseases were identified by the World Health Organization (WHO) as posing a special danger to the

Table 13.3. Endemic infectious diseases of military and non-military importance in Afghanistan and proximal states of central Asia

Military importance	Non-military importance
Anthrax	Diphtheria
Arboviral diseases	Echinococcal infections
Diarrhoeal diseases	Leprosy
Leishmaniasis	Measles
Leptospirosis	Poliomyelitis
Malaria	Tetanus
Rabies	
Respiratory diseases	
Rickettsial disease and	
relapsing fever	
Tuberculosis	
Typhoid fever	
Viral hepatitis	

Source: Based on information in Wallace *et al.* (2002).

civil population of Afghanistan in the winter of 2001–2: acute respiratory infections; diarrhoeal diseases; measles; and drug-resistant *Plasmodium falciparum* malaria. Risk factors for these diseases included: undernutrition and malnutrition; large-scale population migration; crowding in emergency relief camps; inadequate shelter and sanitation; low levels of immunization coverage for common childhood infections; and lack of access to health-care services. In addition to the significant, but seemingly less urgent, disease threats of cutaneous leishmaniasis and tuberculosis, the near-universal problems of war-related physical and psychological trauma further added to the plight of the Afghan people in the winter of 2001–2 (Sharp *et al.*, 2002).

COALITION FORCES

As Wallace *et al.* (2002, p. S172) note, past military deployments in Afghanistan have been associated with extraordinarily high levels of infectious disease activity. For example, during the Soviet military occupation of 1979–89, annual attack rates of infectious diseases exceeded 50 per cent, with viral hepatitis, typhoid fever, dysentery, and respiratory tract infections (RTIs) ranking as the most common ailments.[4] Additional diseases of potential significance to western military forces are listed in Table 13.3 and include leishmaniasis, malaria, and plague, among other conditions. At the time of writing,

---

[4] According to Sharp *et al.* (2002, p. S217), 415,932 Soviet personnel were admitted to hospital for 'serious illnesses', of which 115,308 were for infectious hepatitis and 31,080 for typhoid. The remainder included cases of plague, malaria, cholera, diphtheria, meningitis, dysentery, pneumonia, typhus, and paratyphus among other infectious conditions.

however, publicly documented instances of infectious diseases in the US-led Coalition forces had been largely restricted to outbreaks of gastrointestinal complaints.

Norwalk-Like Virus (NLV) Disease in British Troops

In mid-May 2002, 29 cases of an acute gastrointestinal illness, characterized by vomiting, diarrhoea, and fever, were identified among British military personnel at Bagram airfield. Most of the cases were attached to the 34 Field Hospital. The hospital was immediately closed to non-gastrointestinal patients and some 300 British troops were placed in quarantine. Medical repatriation of ten patients to England[5] resulted in secondary cases of the disease among attendant medical personnel on military flights (two cases) and close contacts of the patients (one case). Two unconfirmed cases of the disease were also recorded among personnel who had unloaded an aircraft used for repatriation. Subsequent studies revealed the causative agent of the disease to be Norwalk-like virus (NLV)—a commonly recognized cause of disability in recent military deployments.[6] Importation of the virus to Afghanistan by British military personnel is suspected (Ahmad, 2002; CDC, 2002).

13.3 War, Disease Eradication, and Control

13.3.1 Conflict and the Global Poliomyelitis Eradication Campaign

In Section 3.6.1 we noted how, in 1988, the Forty-First World Health Assembly committed WHO to the global eradication of poliomyelitis. Although tremendous strides towards the achievement of this goal were made during the 1990s (Fig. 3.19), wars in Central America, South Asia, and Sub-Saharan Africa have consistently posed one of the single greatest obstacles to the effective implementation of the eradication strategy (Fig. 13.4). In some countries, the war-related disruption of immunization services has triggered major outbreaks of poliomyelitis and other vaccine-preventable diseases. In the Russian Federation, for example, outbreaks of poliomyelitis in Chechnya during the mid-1990s were consequent upon three years of severe disruption to the health services. Likewise, in Iraq, an outbreak of poliomyelitis in 1999 was associated with continuing unrest in the north of the country. Other current or recent conflicts in Afghanistan, Angola, Democratic Republic of Congo, Liberia, Sierra Leone, Somalia, Sudan, and Tajikistan have also presented major obstacles to the eradication initiative, while refugee movements continue to result

---

[5] An additional case was flown to Germany.
[6] According to CDC (2002), for example, NLV was one of the most common causes of disability among coalition troops during the Gulf War; see McCarthy *et al.* (2000).

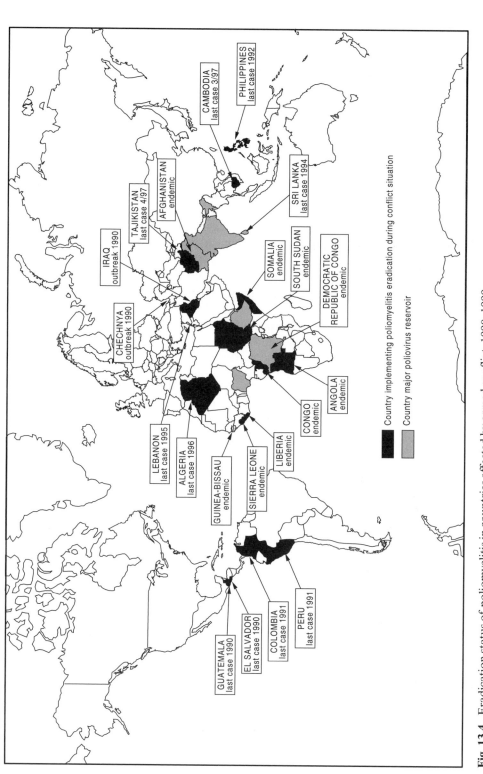

Fig. 13.4. Eradication status of poliomyelitis in countries affected by armed conflict, 1990–1999

Source: Redrawn from Tangermann *et al.* (2000, fig. 1, p. 331).

in the sub-optimal immunization coverage of susceptible populations (Bush, 2000; Tangermann *et al.*, 2000).

The south-central African state of Angola (Fig. 13.4) provides a dramatic example of the role of conflict as an obstacle to poliomyelitis eradication. In 1999—over a decade into the global eradication campaign—the Angolan capital province of Luanda hosted one of the largest epidemics of polio-myelitis ever recorded in Africa. Details of the origin and course of the epidemic are provided elsewhere (Valente *et al.*, 2000), but we note here that several factors related to the long-running Angolan Civil War (1975–) contributed to the explosive outbreak of poliomyelitis depicted in Figure 13.5:

(i) the sudden and unplanned influx of some 800,000 war-displaced people into Luanda in December 1998;

(ii) the origin of many of the war-displaced in parts of the country which, on account of hostilities, had not been reached by routine immuniza-tion or national immunization days (NIDs) and which had a corres-pondingly low vaccination coverage for poliomyelitis;

(iii) the settlement of many of the war-displaced in densely populated and insanitary municipalities of Luanda, thereby providing conditions suit-able for the spread of poliovirus.

In response to the outbreak, an emergency poliomyelitis vaccination cam-paign was implemented in Luanda on 17–18 April 1999. This resulted in the vaccination of 634,368 children. Emergency vaccination was also undertaken elsewhere in the country while, in the aftermath of the epidemic, national immunization days were held on 12–13 June, 17–18 July, and 21–2 August 1999. Geographical coverage of the latter, however, was again limited by hos-tilities. As Valente *et al.* (2000: 339) note, 'If continuous access in all districts for acute flaccid paralysis surveillance and supplemental immunizations cannot be assured, the current war in Angola may threaten global poliomyelitis eradication'.

13.3.2 Ceasefires, 'Periods of Tranquillity', and Disease Control

Ceasefires and 'periods of tranquillity' have occasionally been negotiated between hostile factions to allow the implementation of disease control and eradication initiatives in warring states. Indeed, such health-inspired breaks in fighting are increasingly being viewed not only as a means of permitting the delivery of disease intervention measures but also as an informal channel of communication and peace brokering (Bush, 2000). Examples of states in which ceasefires and periods of tranquillity have been negotiated for the purposes of

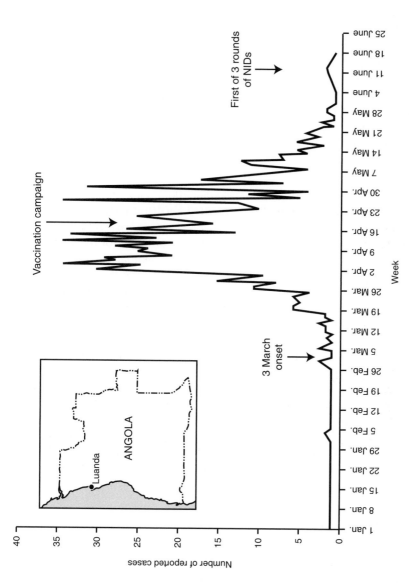

Fig. 13.5. Epidemic poliomyelitis in Luanda Province, Angola, January–June 1999

Notes: The graph plots the reported incidence of acute flaccid paralysis (AFP) by week of onset of paralysis. NIDs = National Immunization Days.

Source: Redrawn from Valente *et al.* (2000, fig. 2, p. 341).

the implementation of health initiatives include Afghanistan, Angola, El Salavdor, Lebanon, and Sudan (CDC, 1995; Tangermann *et al.*, 2000).

Sudan: The 'Guinea Worm Ceasefire'

On 27 March 1995, the Sudanese government announced a two-month cease-fire in the southern sector of the country, primarily to allow accelerated efforts in the eradication of dracunculiasis (Guinea worm), but also to promote the treatment of other diseases, to administer vaccines, and to distribute vitamin A. The so-called 'Guinea worm ceasefire' resulted in the visit of health teams to 2,028 villages, allowing improved monitoring of dracunculiasis, mass oral treatment of onchoceriasis, the intensification of efforts to eradicate poliomyelitis, and the delivery of vaccines for such WHO EPI target diseases as measles (CDC, 1995).

13.4 Biological Warfare and Bioterrorism

Biological weapons are generally regarded as representing one of the foremost threats to global security in the twenty-first century. Biological weapons are relatively inexpensive to produce and transport, and have the capacity for immense destruction over wide areas. In addition, the capability has been developed for pathogen delivery via a number of weapons systems including long-range missiles, dispersers on manned and drone aircraft, bombs and bomblets. Once the secret preserve of a handful of leading states, advanced bioweapons technology is increasingly finding its way to lesser state powers, non-state organizations, and others who have been attracted by the potential destructiveness of such weapons (Dando, 1994; Henderson, 2000). Recent events in Japan and the United States have served as a warning to the global community that, some day, the advanced technologies may well be exploited. 'The history of weapons development', Henderson (2000: 64) remarks, 'tells us that weapons that have been produced, for whatever reason, will eventually be used. One would hope that the history of biological weapons might be the exception to the rule, but it would be hazardous to believe that.'

13.4.1 Biological Weapons: Definitions and Disease Agents

The World Health Organization (1970: 12) defines biological weapons as 'those that depend for their effects on multiplication within the target organism, and are intended for use in war to cause disease or death in man, animals, or plants'. Although a large number of viruses, bacteria, rickettsiae, fungi, and protozoa have been posited as possible agents in biological weapons (Table 13.4), a series of factors (including cultivation and effective dispersal, transmission dynam-ics, environmental stability, infectious dose size, and availability of prophylac-

Table 13.4. Sample biological entities identified by the World Health Organization (WHO) for possible development in weapons

Disease (*disease agent*)[1]	Mortality
Bacteria	
Anthrax (*Bacillus anthracis*) [A22]	*c.*100% (inhalational)
Brucellosis (*Brucella spp.*) [A23]	<2%
Glanders (*Burkholderia mallei*) [A24.0]	*c.*95%
Tularaemia (*Franciscella tularensis*) [A21]	up to 5%
Cholera (*Vibrio cholerae*) [A00]	up to 80%
Plague (*Yersinia pestis*) [A20]	*c.*100% (pneumonic)
Fungi	
Coccidioidomycosis (*Coccidioides immitis*) [B38]	low
Rickettsiae	
Q fever (*Coxiella burnetii*) [A78]	low
Typhus fever (*Rickettsia prowazekii*) [A75]	up to 70%
Rocky Mountain spotted fever (*Rickettsia rickettsii*) [A77.0]	up to 80%
Viruses	
Chikungunya [A92.0]	very low
Crimean–Congo haemorrhagic fever [A98.0]	up to 50%
Dengue [A90/91]	very low (non-haemorrhagic cases)
Eastern equine encephalomyelitis [A83.2]	up to 80%
Influenza [J10, 11]	usually low
Japanese encephalitis [A83.0]	up to 50% (encephalitis cases)
Marburg virus disease [A98.4]	25%
Tick-borne encephalitis [A84.0]	up to 40%
Smallpox [B03]	up to 30%
Venezuelan equine encephalitis [A92.2]	low
Western equine encephalomyelitis [A83.1]	3–15%
Yellow fever [A95]	up to 40%

Note: [1] ICD-10 code for each disease given in square parentheses.
Source: Based on World Health Organization (1970) and Dando (1994, table 2.2, p. 31).

tic and therapeutic measures) suggests that relatively few agents have strategic potential. As far as present-day developments are concerned, comparative biological advantage—including ease of agent production, resistance to destruction, and the potential for aerosol dispersal—appears to favour the smallpox virus and the anthrax bacillus (*Bacillus anthracis*) over many other candidates (Henderson, 1999, 2000). As described in Appendix 1A, smallpox spreads naturally from person to person; routine vaccination ceased on the eradication of the disease in the late 1970s, with waning levels of global immunity in the ensuing years. Under such circumstances, smallpox bioweapons have the potential to spark pandemic transmission of the viral agent. Anthrax poses a rather different threat. If released as a fine-particle aerosol, the anthrax bacillus can

Table 13.5. Estimates of casualties resulting from a hypothetical biological attack with agents of selected diseases

Disease agent	Downwind reach (km)	Casualties[1]	
		Number of deaths	Number incapacitated
Rift Valley fever	1	400	35,000
Tick-borne encephalitis	1	9,500	35,000
Typhus	5	19,000	85,000
Brucellosis	10	500	125,000
Q fever	>20	150	125,000
Tularemia	>20	30,000	125,000
Anthrax[2]	>20	95,000	125,000

Notes: [1] Casualty estimates based on the release of 50 kg of agent by aircraft along a 2 km line, upwind of a population centre of 500,000. [2] Inhalational (pulmonary) anthrax.
Source: WHO estimates, reproduced from Christopher *et al.* (1997, table 2, p. 415).

spread on air currents for in excess of 50 miles, infecting humans and animals as it diffuses (Henderson, 2000).

CASUALTY SIMULATIONS

Table 13.5 gives WHO estimates of the likely number of casualties arising from a hypothetical biological attack with sample disease agents. Estimates are based on the release of 50 kg of each agent from an aircraft along a 2 km line, upwind of a population centre of 500,000. Although all the disease agents in Table 13.5 have the potential to incapacitate many tens of thousands of people, anthrax—in pulmonary or inhalational form—is distinguished by an exceptionally high mortality over an extended downwind reach.

13.4.2 Historical Dimensions of Biological Warfare

The history of biological warfare is reviewed by Christopher *et al.* (1997), Gould and Connell (1997), and Henderson (2000) among others. While the deliberate deployment of diseased cadavers, animal carcasses, and other infective materials as weapons of war can be traced to classical times, the strategic planning and scientific development of biological weapons—contingent on advances in microbiology—is a phenomenon of the last 100 years. During World War I, the Germans are alleged to have developed a biological warfare programme with the specific intent of contaminating Allied livestock and animal feed with the agents of anthrax and glanders. Notwithstanding efforts to control the use of biological weapons under the 1925 Geneva Protocol, the first viable programme of biological warfare emerged with the establishment of Japan's notorious germ warfare unit, Detachment 731, in the 1930s. By the end of World War II, Japanese forces are reputed to have deployed a range of biological entities (including the agents of plague, typhoid, cholera, and dysentery) in the war against China (Christopher *et al.*, 1997; Gould and Connell, 1997).

POST-WORLD WAR II DEVELOPMENTS

In the aftermath of World War II, a number of countries—including Belgium, Britain, Canada, the United States, and the Soviet Union—pursued offensive biological weapons programmes. Such were the developments that, by the late 1960s, the United States alone had stockpiled a large biological arsenal of lethal agents (including *B. anthracis* and botulinum toxin), incapacitating agents (including *Brucella suis* and Venezuelan equine encephalitis virus), and anti-crop agents (including rice blast and rye stem rust). Under the Nixon administration, however, the US programme was terminated in 1969–70, with the reputed destruction of the entire biological arsenal by February 1973 (Christopher *et al.*, 1997).

USSR: Sverdlovsk Anthrax Outbreak

While the 1972 Biological and Toxic Weapons Convention prohibited the possession, development, and stockpiling of pathogens or toxins in excess of the quantities required for 'peaceful purposes', several signatories to the Convention continued to participate in outlawed activities. For example, during the 1970s and 1980s, the former USSR is reputed to have solved many technical problems in bioweapons development including the production of antibiotic-resistant microbes, the preparation of microbes for aerosol dissemination, and pathogen delivery in missiles and warheads. The developments were not without incident. In April and May 1979, an anthrax outbreak occurred among people who lived and worked up to 4 km downwind of a military establishment in the Soviet city of Sverdlovsk; an outbreak was also recorded in livestock along an extended axis of the human epidemic zone for a distance of some 50 km (Meselson *et al.*, 1994) (Pl. 13.1). All told, inhalational anthrax was associated with 77 human cases and 66 deaths—the largest epidemic of inhalational anthrax ever documented. In 1992, after years of international dispute over the matter, President Yeltsin conceded that the epidemic was the result of an unintential release of anthrax spores from the Sverdlovsk biological facility (Christopher *et al.*, 1997; Gould and Connell, 1997).

Developments in the 1990s: Evidence from Iraq

Although a number of countries (including China, Cuba, India, Iran, Israel, Libya, North Korea, Russia, and Syria) are either known, or suspected, to have contributed to the international proliferation of biological weapons in the late

A

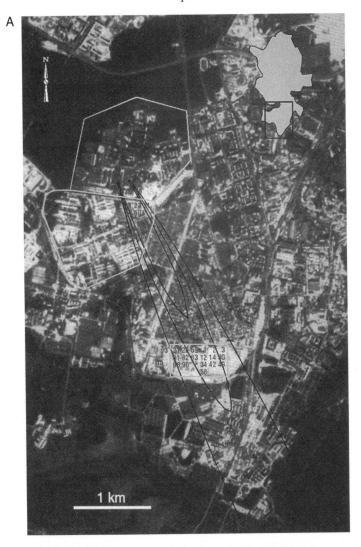

Pl. 13.1. Geographical spread of anthrax associated with the airborne escape of spores from the military microbiology facility at Sverdlovsk, former USSR, April–May 1979

Notes: Sverdlovsk is a city of about 1.2 million, situated 1,400 km to the east of Moscow. During April and May 1979, an outbreak of anthrax occurred among humans and livestock in a zone extending downwind from the city's military facility. All told, the outbreak among humans was associated with a documented 66 deaths from inhalational anthrax—the largest recorded epidemic in history. (A) Satellite photograph showing the probable location of patients at time of exposure to anthrax in early April 1979 (numbers), along with calculated contours of constant anthrax dosage (black lines). (B) Villages (letter coded) where livestock died of anthrax in April 1979, with calculated contours of constant anthrax dosage (black lines).

Source: Reprinted with permission from Meselson *et al.*, SCIENCE 266: 1202–8 (1994) (Figs. 2, 3).

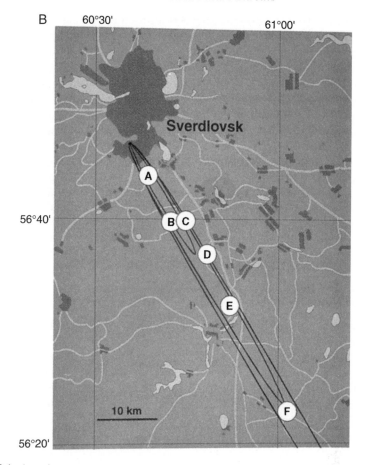

Pl. 13.1. (*cont.*)

twentieth century, the Iraqi programme has been subject to the closest scrutiny by the international community in recent years. In the aftermath of the Gulf War (Sect. 13.2.1), UN weapons inspectors in Iraq uncovered evidence of offensive biological programmes involving *B. anthracis*, rotavirus, and camel pox virus among other disease agents. Pathogen production and storage included 20,000 litres of botulinum toxin and 8,000 litres of anthrax spore suspension, with the capability for long-range delivery in the warheads of SCUD missiles (Gould and Connell, 1997; Henderson, 1999).

13.4.3 Bioterrorism in the United States

Recent years have been marked by an escalating concern over the threat of bioterrorism in the United States (Hughes, 1999; Tucker, 1999). Prior to the late 1990s, the FBI typically investigated a dozen cases each year involving the acquisition or use of biological, chemical, and nuclear materials. The number of investigations grew to 74 in 1997 and 181 in 1998. While some 80 per cent of the investigations were associated with hoaxes, a number were concerned with failed attacks. As regards the nature of the perpetrators, religious fundamentalism emerged as a motivating factor from the mid-1990s, while general civil populations and symbolic buildings and/or organizations were the most common (threatened or intended) targets of attack. As Tucker (1999: 503) warns:

the historical record suggests that future incidents of bioterrorism will probably involve hoaxes and relatively small-scale attacks, such as food contamination. Nevertheless, the diffusion of dual-based technologies relevant to the production of biological and toxin agents, and the potential availability of scientists and engineers formerly employed in sophisticated biological warfare programs such as those of the Soviet Union and South Africa, suggest that the technical barriers to mass-casualty terrorism are eroding.

BIOTERRORIST-RELATED ANTHRAX IN THE UNITED STATES, 2001

In the days and weeks that followed the atrocities of 11 September 2001, the civil population of the United States became the target for terrorist attacks with *B. anthracis*, the causative agent of anthrax. The nature of anthrax is outlined in Appendix 13A but, prior to 2001, the inhalational form of the disease in the United States had been entirely restricted to people with occupational exposure to anthrax spores. On 2 October 2001, however, the Florida Department of Health was notified of a possible case of inhalational anthrax in an office worker from Palm Beach County. The case history of the patient—a photographic editor with a Florida newspaper—revealed exposure to a suspicious (powder-containing) letter on 19 September; the patient succumbed on 5 October (Bush *et al.*, 2001). By 7 November, a further 21 cases of confirmed or suspected bioterrorist-related anthrax had been identified in the United States (CDC, 2001*c*). The distribution of cases by form of disease (cutaneous or inhalational anthrax), status of infection (confirmed or suspected), and geographical location (city or state) is given in Table 13.6; for reference, Figure 13.6 plots the cases by day of symptom onset.

As Figure 13.6 shows, the case distribution was characterized by two temporally discrete periods of activity: (i) late September/early October (nine cases) which, with the exception of two cases of inhalational anthrax in Florida, was centred on the northeastern states of New York and New Jersey; and (ii) mid-to-late October (13 cases), dominated by cases of inhalational anthrax in the District of Columbia and New Jersey. As regards exposure to *B. anthracis*, one or more cases in each of the four geographical clusters had direct or indirect contact with contaminated letters and/or postal facilities:

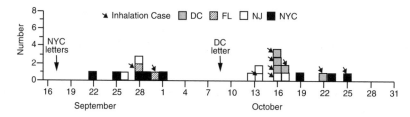

Fig. 13.6. Cases of bioterrorism-related anthrax by day of onset, United States, September–October 2001

Notes: Cases are geo-coded according to the place of work of patients. The postmarked dates of *B. anthracis*-contaminated letters sent to New York City and the District of Columbia are indicated for reference.
Source: Based on CDC (2001*b*, fig. 1, p. 941).

Table 13.6. Cases of bioterrorism-related anthrax in the United States (status: 7 November 2001)

	Florida	New York City	DC	New Jersey	Total
Inhalational					
Confirmed	2	1	5	2	10
Suspected	0	0	0	0	0
Cutaneous					
Confirmed	0	4	0	3	7
Suspected	0	3	0	2	5
Total	2	8	5	7	22

Source: CDC (2001*c*, table 1, p. 973).

(1) *Florida* (two cases). Both cases were employed at the same establishment and are believed to have been exposed to contaminated letters or packages in mid-September.

(2) *New York City* (eight cases). One of the earliest cases was a female who handled a letter postmarked 18 September and which was subsequently found to be contaminated with *B. anthracis* (CDC, 2001*b*).

(3) *New Jersey* (seven cases). Five of the cases worked at postal facilities through which contaminated mail bound for New York City and Washington, DC is either known or suspected to have passed (CDC, 2001*b*).

(4) *District of Columbia* (five cases). On 15 October, a staff member in the office of a US Senator was exposed to the contents of a letter contaminated with *B. anthracis*. Subsequent studies identified cases of

inhalational anthrax among workers at the Brentwood Mail Processing and Distribution Center and in the US State Department mail-sorting facility. Environmental sampling revealed the Brentwood postal facility to be widely contaminated with *B. anthracis* (CDC, 2001*a*, 2001*b*, 2001*f*).

The strain of *B. anthracis* used in the various attacks was subsequently identified as one commonly found in laboratories and, although processed for the purposes of aerosolization, the bacillus had not been engineered to enhance virulence.

International Assistance

Between 12 October and 13 November 2001, the US Centers for Disease Control and Prevention (CDC) received requests from 66 countries for advice, guidance, or assistance in the response to bioterrorism-related anthrax attacks. The majority of requests were from Central and South American countries. Although two overseas isolates were confirmed by CDC as *B. anthracis*, the origin of the infection was readily inferred: both isolates were recovered from the outer surfaces of diplomatic mail sent via the infected US State Department mail-sorting facility to the US Embassy in Peru (CDC, 2001*d*).

13.5 Further Issues

13.5.1 Militarism and Civil Health

In recent decades, 'militarism'—broadly defined as an 'aggressive tendency to prepare for war'[7] and encompassing the social, economic, and psychological dimensions of the acquisition, production, stockpiling, and use of arms—has had far-reaching implications for the health of civil populations (Levy and Sidel, 1997; Sidel, 2000). The impact has been particularly acute in developing countries where, since 1945, the vast majority of wars have been staged and where, according to available statistics, relative levels of arms expenditure have been disproportionately high (Levy and Sidel, 1997). Aside from the obvious effects of weapons usage on civil populations, Kiefer (1992) classifies the impact of militarism on the health profiles of developing countries under five broad headings: (i) diversion of resources; (ii) suppression of dissent; (iii) military classism; (iv) environmental damage; and (v) crime and terrorism. We consider headings (i) to (v) in turn.

   (i) *Diversion of resources.* Within a given country, there is an obvious trade-off between military and health expenditure and, by implication,

---

[7] The cited definition is one of three definitions of militarism offered by Kiefer (1992: 719), the others being 'the leadership of society by a military class' and 'the tendency to use military strategy in dealing with problems'.

the well-being of the people (Sidel, 1988). Indeed, the socio-economic effects of the diversion of finite resources to military concerns are well documented and include interruptions—of greater or lesser magnitude and duration—to national economic development, along with depriva-tion in such areas as nutrition, housing, education, and health service provision (Levy and Sidel, 1997). Woolhandler and Himmelstein (1985), for example, document a strong and positive association between one measure of socio-economic development (the infant mortality ratio, IMR) and levels of national military expenditure, with additional evidence that an increase in military expenditure presages a poor record of improvement in the IMR (see, however, Skrabanek, 1985).

(ii) *Suppression of dissent.* The control of scarce health resources is viewed as a core element of power in many militaristic states, with health-care personnel and facilities often perceived as legitimate targets for mili-tary operations. Kiefer (1992) suggests that the destruction of health resources provides one means of suppressing dissent and asserting political control over local populations.

(iii) *Military classism.* In some less developed countries, a military career is viewed as a means of upward social mobility, with the corruption and extortion of military elites serving to siphon off resources that would otherwise be made available to the civil population (Kiefer, 1992).

(iv) *Environmental damage.* Weapons testing, defoliation, bomb cratering, burning, oil spills, and fires, among other military impacts on the en-vironment, may serve to disrupt ecosystems, pollute water supplies, destroy crops, and force the abandonment of land. In turn, environ-mental changes may have a direct impact on infectious disease trans-mission (Levy *et al.*, 1997; Austin and Bruch, 2000).

(v) *Crime and terrorism.* Militarism is commonly associated with a black market in weapons which, in turn, is directly or indirectly linked to such crimes as drug running and banditry. Former soldiers, military desert-ers, and those with access to 'legal' military supplies may engage in the covert trade of weapons, representing a major source of arms for ter-rorist groups and other organizations worldwide (Kiefer, 1992).

FUTURE OUTLOOK

Despite official efforts to curb the international arms trade during the 1990s, Kiefer (1992: 723) argues that the economic and political developments of the late twentieth century will continue to fuel the militarization of developing countries:

First, the liberalization and the decentralization of the Soviet Union and former War-saw Pact countries . . . is likely to reduce the need for massive military expenditures in the industrial countries . . . this is leading arms manufacturers in those countries to look toward the Third World as a major market. Second . . . the growing dependence of the industrial economies on Third World labor, commodities, and markets creates an incentive for militarily advanced nations to establish hegemony, by arms transfers and/or war, in less developed nations.

The net effect will be the continued diversion of finite funds from such spheres as health to arms expediture.

13.5.2 Health Impacts of Economic Sanctions

In recent years, economic sanctions have increasingly been used as an adjunct, or alternative, to military intervention in states that are (or have been) in violation of international policies or laws (Levy and Sidel, 1997; Albright, 2000). Late-twentieth-century examples of UN and other internationally mandated sanctions include those directed against Haiti, Iraq, Rwanda, South Africa, and the states of the former Yugoslavia, while Cuba, Iran, Nicaragua, and Panama have been the subject of unilateral US sanctions. In some instances, the sanctions have been of limited scope and have had correspondingly little— if any—discernible impact on the domestic economies of the targeted countries. In other instances, such as Iraq in the 1990s (Sect. 13.2.1), however, comprehensive sanctions and embargoes have served to stymie economic activities, blocking access to foodstuffs, medicines, and medical products and resulting in an apparent deterioration in the health and well-being of the civil populations involved (Gibbons and Garfield, 1999; Morin and Miles, 2000). In the present section, we draw on evidence from the Caribbean island of Cuba to illustrate the health repercussions of economic sanctions and embargoes in the late twentieth century.

US SANCTIONS AND CUBA

The United States imposed a unilateral trade embargo on Cuba in 1961, shortly after the accession of Fidel Castro as communist leader of the island republic. Since that time, the US embargo against Cuba has become the longest-running trade embargo in modern history (Garfield and Santana, 1997). For many years, the sanctions had little impact on the economic fortunes of the island. Shored up by the Soviet Union and the other members of the COMECON/CMEA[8] trading association, the Cuban economy grew at a rate of about 2 to 4 per cent per annum in the 25 years to 1989. However, the dissolution of the Soviet bloc served to rupture Cuba's established patterns of international trade while, in 1992, more restrictive trade sanctions were imposed by the United States. These events were to have a deleterious effect on the economy of Cuba:

[8] Council for Mutual Economic Aid (COMECON)/Community for Mutual Economic Assistance (CMEA).

It was reported that in 1992 the loss of markets, credits, and favourable terms of trade through CMEA dropped the dollar value of this commerce by 93 per cent compared to 1988. The ability to import goods dropped to $2.2 billion in 1992, leaving Cuba with a 73 per cent decline in productive activity and a 45 per cent drop in GNP. (Garfield, in Levy and Sidel, 1997: 157)

Public Health Impacts

The economic decline was accompanied by a sharp reduction in the nutritional status of the population. The importation of foodstuffs fell by an estimated 50 per cent, while the calorific intake of adult Cuban males reduced from 3,100 (1989) to 1,863 (1994) as a daily average. Epidemics of vitamin B-related deficiency diseases began to appear while, as a general index of socio-economic dislocation, the early 1990s were associated with a perceptible increase in the proportion of low birthweight babies. Sanitary conditions began to decline and the provision of potable water became a more general problem for the authorities (Garfield and Santana, 1997; Barry, 2000).

Infectious diseases. Declining nutritional levels and deteriorating sanitary conditions were accompanied by an upsurge in infectious and parasitic diseases. So, for example, the reported rate of tuberculosis activity increased from 5.5 per 100,000 (1990) to 15.3 per 100,000 (1994), with the lack of medicines contributing to a sharp rise in deaths from tubercular diseases. As regards other infectious conditions, mortality from diarrhoeal diseases increased by 152 per cent between 1989 and 1993. Mortality from influenza and pneumonia increased by 77 per cent during the same interval. Although much of the initial increase in mortality was concentrated in older age groups (≥ 65 years), deteriorating health conditions and medical infrastructure began to affect other population groups by 1994. Nevertheless, for young children (<2 years), the health authorities succeeded in maintaining over 90 per cent immunization coverage for WHO EPI target diseases such as diphtheria, measles, and pertussis while, in 1993, Cuba was the first country to be certified free of wild poliovirus (Garfield and Santana, 1997; Barry, 2000).

Non-infectious conditions. Increases in mortality among those aged ≥ 65 years were identified for such non-infectious categories as suicide, unintentional injuries, asthma, and heart disease. In addition, essential medicines and medical products for the treatment and/or prevention of chronic diseases, including certain childhood cancers, were either restricted under the embargo, or proved inordinately expensive in their direct and shipping costs (Garfield and Santana, 1997; Barry, 2000).

Conclusions

In reviewing the health status of Cuba in the mid-1990s, Garfield and Santana (1997: 19) concluded that:

The medical system is still able to provide near universal coverage and to ensure the continuance of low mortality among those under 65 years of age even in the face of rising health threats. Yet despite the highly efficient use of health goods, these goods can no longer be stretched to meet the needs of the entire population. Preferential access to essential goods for women and children is exemplary but has resulted in the creation of new vulnerable groups among adult men and the elderly. By reducing access to medicines and medical supplies from other countries and preventing their purchase from US firms, the embargo contributes to this rise in morbidity and mortality.

Under the Trade Sanctions Reform and Export Enhancement Act of 2000, the US Congress passed legislation that eased restrictions on existing trade sanctions and which permitted the sale of certain medicines and foodstuffs to Cuba. The impact of this legislation on the health and well-being of the civil population of the island awaits examination.

13.5.3 UN Peacekeeping Forces

One major development in global military activity over the past half-century has been the international deployment of armed forces to oversee, to maintain, and increasingly to create the conditions of peace in ceasefires and armistices (Renner, 1997). Under the auspices of the UN Peacekeeping Operations, Seet and Burnham (2000) list no fewer than 49 peacekeeping missions in the 50 years to 1998. These missions are plotted, by year of operation, as the bar chart in Figure 13.7. In the period prior to 1990, the UN undertook only 18 different peacekeeping missions. But, with the end of the Cold War, the number of missions spiralled so that a total of 42 different missions in well over 30 countries of Africa, the Americas, Asia, Europe, and Oceania were operational at some stage during the 1990s.

MORTALITY TRENDS

As the line trace in Figure 13.7 shows, late-twentieth-century developments in peacekeeping duties were associated with a disturbing trend: an upsurge in the number of deaths among UN personnel. Indeed, as Seet and Burnham (2000) note, more peacekeepers died in the post-Cold War period (807 deaths) than in the preceding 40 years of peacekeeping missions (752 deaths). The majority of deaths recorded among the peacekeepers were attributable to unintentional violence (accidents, 41%) and hostile acts (36%). But 23 per cent of the deaths were classified in the category 'illness/other' (Seet and Burnham, 2000).

INFECTIOUS DISEASES

Table 13.7 lists the occurrence of infectious diseases and disease agents in sample UN and NATO peacekeeping operations, 1956–96. Among the more noteworthy events were outbreaks of hepatitis A among multinational forces in Gaza and the Lebanon in the 1950s to 1970s, cutaneous leishmanisasis among

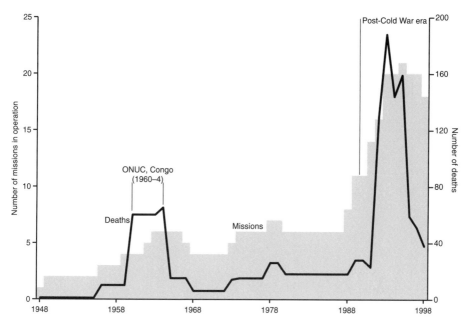

Fig. 13.7. United Nations peacekeeping missions, 1948–1998

Notes: The bar chart plots the number of peacekeeping missions in operation during a given year. The line trace plots the annual number of deaths in UN peacekeeping forces. Following Seet and Burnham (2000), the mortality count has been formed by assuming that deaths were equally distributed throughout the period of a given mission. For reference, the end of the Cold War has been set at 1990. The period associated with the United Nations Mission in Congo (ONUC), 1960–4, is indicated.

Source: Data from Seet and Burnham (2000, table 1, p. 600).

Fijian and other troops in Egypt during 1983–4, and dengue fever among US troops stationed in Somalia and Haiti in the early and mid-1990s. Although the outbreaks documented in Table 13.7 were generally small and deaths were few in number, Adams *et al.* (1997) note that the spread of such infectious diseases represents a potentially serious drain on peacekeeping personnel.

13.5.4 War-Associated Disease Emergence and Re-emergence: An Enduring Problem

As we observed in Chapter 9, wars have been associated with the emergence and re-emergence of infectious diseases throughout much of human history. And, as the recognized range of infectious disease agents has accelerated towards the twenty-first century, so wars have continued to play a leading role in the emergence complex (see e.g. Goma Epidemiology Group, 1995; Raoult *et al.*, 1998; Smith *et al.*, 1998). In the present section, we draw on the recent

Table 13.7. Some infectious diseases and disease agents documented in a sample of UN and NATO peacekeeping operations, 1950–2000

Year	Nationality of troops	Disease / infection	Cases	Reference
UN Expeditionary Force in Gaza 1956–62	Multinational	Hepatitis A	207	Hesla (1992)
UN Interim Force in Lebanon 1978	Multinational	Hepatitis A	83	Hesla (1992)
Multinational Force and Observers, Sinai Desert (Egypt) 1983–84	Fijian	Cutaneous leishmaniasis	63[1]	Norton *et al.* (1992); Fryauff *et al.* (1993)
UN Peacekeeping Force in Cyprus 1985	Swedish	Sandfly fever	8[2]	Eitrem *et al.* (1990)
UN Transition Assistance Group, Namibia 1989–90	Multinational	Respiratory tract infection	2,593[3]	Steffen *et al.* (1992)
UN Transition Authority Cambodia, Cambodia 1992–93	Multinational	HIV	7[4]	Soeprapto *et al.* (1995)
Operation Restore Hope, Somalia 1992–93	US	Dengue fever	14	Kanesa-thasan *et al.* (1994)
Operation Uphold Democracy, Haiti 1994 (19 Sept.–4 Nov.)	US	Dengue fever and other febrile diseases	106	CDC (1994*b*)
UN Mission in Haiti 1995	Bangladeshi	Hepatitis E[5]	4	Drabick *et al.* (1997)
Operation Resolute, Bosnia–Herzegovina 1995–96 (19 weeks) 1996	British British	Enteric disease Rubella	1,139[6] 4	Croft and Creamer (1997) Adams *et al.* (1997)

Notes: [1] Fifteen further cases were recorded among Australian/New Zealander (1), British (1), Colombian (6), Dutch (1), Italian (1), US (2), and Uruguayan (3) peacekeepers. [2] Results from prevalence study sample. [3] Study cohort. [4] Outpatient consultations, Apr. 1989–Mar. 1990. [5] Infection imported from Bangladesh to Haiti. [6] Data for entire 19-week period; an 'explosive' outbreak of gastrointestinal disease was recorded during week 2 of operations.

examples of visceral leishmaniasis (Sudan, Africa) and diphtheria (Tajikistan, Central Asia) to illustrate the enduring role of conflict as a facilitating factor in the process of disease emergence and re-emergence.

VISCERAL LEISHMANIASIS AND CIVIL WAR IN SOUTHERN SUDAN

Visceral leishmaniasis (kala-azar) is a zoonotic disease of tropical Africa and Asia caused by protozoa of the *Leishmania donovani* complex. The protozoa are transmitted from animals to man by species of sandfly (pre-dominantly *Phlebotomus*). In visceral leishmaniasis, unlike cutaneous and mucocutaneous forms of the disease, cells are infected beyond the subcutaneous and mucosal tissue. Symptoms include fever, diarrhoea, wasting, and enlargement of the abdomen, liver, and spleen. For untreated cases of the disease, two-year mortality rates of up to 95 per cent have been reported (Allison, 1993).

Emergence in Western Upper Nile, Southern Sudan

Prior to the mid-1980s, visceral leishmaniasis in the African state of Sudan appeared to be largely restricted to the eastern sector of the country, close to the border with Ethiopia (see Fig. 13.8A). Beginning in October 1988, however, medical teams in the Sudanese capital, Khartoum, began to notice an increase in the incidence of visceral leishmaniasis among war-displaced people originating from the purportedly disease-free southern province of western Upper Nile. Subsequent investigations in the province revealed an epidemic of devastating proportions. By the mid-1990s, an estimated 100,000 people—representing probably one-third of the resident population of western Upper Nile—had died of the disease (Seaman *et al.*, 1996). The source of the infection in the province is unknown, although Perea *et al.* (1991) have postulated importation with soldiers recruited and/or trained in the endemic east of Sudan. These soldiers were subsequently deployed as a consequence of the south's long-running civil war.

Diffusion patterns. Whatever the source of the epidemic in western Upper Nile, intra-provincial population movements in response to war and food shortages appear to have played an integral role in the local spread of the disease (Perea *et al.*, 1991; Seaman *et al.*, 1996). The diffusion pattern, based on the timing of intense disease activity in the various districts of the province, is plotted by the vectors in Figure 13.8B. As the map indicates, the epidemic first peaked in the southern sector of Jikany district in 1988–9, spreading onwards to western, northern, and southern districts in the years that followed.

Mortality rates. The proportional circles in Figure 13.8B plot the estimated population of sample districts at the time of appearance of visceral leishmaniasis. The shaded sectors provide percentage estimates of associated mortality in the years that followed. As the map shows, mortality from visceral

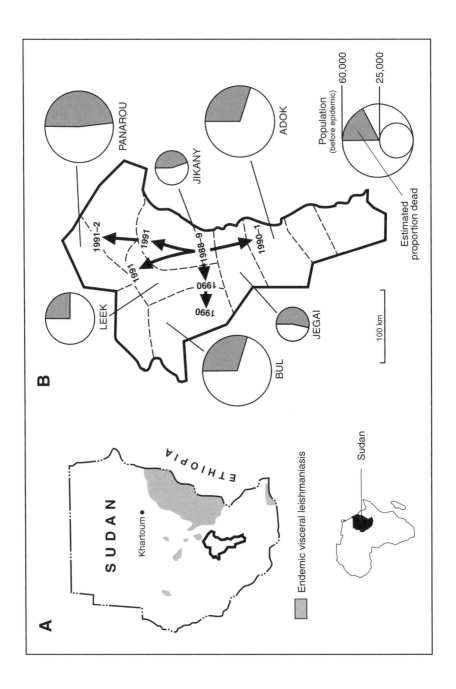

leishmaniasis is believed to have exceeded 25 per cent in all the sample districts, reaching highs of 48 per cent (Panarou) and 56 per cent (Jegai).

Outlook. A separate epidemic of visceral leishmaniasis was observed in the province of eastern Upper Nile in 1994. Hundreds are known to have died before the outbreak was identified. As Seaman *et al.* (1996: 871) note, the war-associated disruption of agriculture, relief, and disease-control programmes has ensured that the 'age-old cycle of war, famine and infectious disease is still part of the way of life among the threatened cultures of southern Sudan'. The epidemic has been a human tragedy of major proportions with conditions of war and famine continuing to favour the establishment of new endemic foci in the region.

DIPHTHERIA IN THE FORMER SOVIET UNION

Beginning in 1992–3, the Newly Independent States (NIS) of the former Soviet Union experienced the largest epidemic of diphtheria to strike the industrialized world for over 30 years (Vitek and Wharton, 1998). Between 1958 and the late 1970s, universal childhood immunization had reduced diph-theria activity in the Soviet Union to a level where national elimination was thought attainable. From 1977, however, diphtheria gradually began to re-emerge, spreading explosively after the collapse of the Soviet Union in 1991. Factors which may have contributed to the re-emergence and spread of the dis-ease in the 1990s are summarized in Table 13.8 and include such considerations as the flight of refugees from wars and civil unrest in Georgia and Tajikistan, the widespread breakdown of public health measures, and, in particular, reduced levels of immunization coverage (Vitek and Wharton, 1998; Dittmann *et al.*, 2000).

Civil War and Diphtheria in Tajikistan

Although all of the Newly Independent States were affected by the diphtheria epidemic, recorded levels of disease activity were highest in the state of

◄────────────────────────────────────

Fig. 13.8. Emergence of visceral leishmaniasis in western Upper Nile, southern Sudan, 1984–1994

Notes: (A) Areas of endemic visceral leishmaniasis in Sudan. The location of western Upper Nile, situated to the southwest of the main endemic area, is indicated by the heavy border. (B) Epidem-ic spread of visceral leishmaniasis in western Upper Nile during the 1980s and 1990s. Vectors trace the routes of disease diffusion while dates mark periods of intense disease activity in various areas of the province. Proportional circles provide estimates of district populations at the time of arrival of visceral leishmaniasis. Shaded sectors give the estimated percentage proportion of the popula-tion that subsequently died of the disease. The southernmost districts of the province were unaf-fected by the epidemic during the time interval under consideration.
Source: Based on information in Seaman *et al.* (1996, fig. 1, p. 863 and table 4, p. 870).

Table 13.8. Factors contributing to the re-emergence of diphtheria in the Newly Independent States (NIS) of the former Soviet Union, 1990–1996

1. Technology and industry
   Population of susceptible adults
2. Human demographics and behaviour
   Population resistance to vaccinating children
   Changes in childhood vaccination schedule
   High levels of militarization
   Decreased social controls, increased travel
3. Microbial adaptation and change
   Change in biotype or emergence of epidemic clones
4. Economic development and land use
   Highly crowded and intense urbanization, substandard housing
5. Breakdown of public health measures
   Decreased immunization in Central Asia and Caucasus
6. International travel and land use
   Repatriation of Russian population from republics
   Refugees from Tajikistan, refugees in Georgia

Source: Vitek and Wharton (1998, table 3, p. 548).

Tajikistan (Fig. 13.9) where, by the mid-1990s, several years of civil war had given rise to a dire socio-economic and humanitarian crisis (Keshavjee and Becerra, 2000). Immunization services were totally disrupted; vaccines, medicines, and equipment were in short supply, while many qualified medical personnel (including epidemiologists and infectious disease specialists) had abandoned the country's collapsing health-care system (Keshavjee and Becerra, 2000; Usmanov *et al.*, 2000).

Figure 13.9A maps the annual course of the diphtheria epidemic in the oblasts of Tajikistan, 1991–5. According to Usmanov *et al.* (2000), the disease was probably introduced from neighbouring Afghanistan in 1992–3. Thereafter, diphtheria spread across the whole of the country. At the peak of the epidemic, in 1994–5 (Fig. 13.9B), Tajikistan recorded a diphtheria rate of 105.8 per 100,000, to be compared to the rate of 50.2 per 100,000 for the second-ranked state (Russia) and the aggregate rate of 30.0 per 100,000 for the NIS (Vitek and Wharton, 1998). Only from October 1995, with the implementation of national immunization days for diphtheria, an intensive public information campaign, contact identification, immunization, and other remedial control

→

Fig. 13.9. Diphtheria in Tajikistan, 1991–1997

Notes: Maps (A) plot the annual diphtheria rate (per 100,000) by oblast, 1991–5. For reference, graph (B) traces the monthly count of reported diphtheria cases in Tajikistan, January 1993–August 1997.

Source: Redrawn from Usmanov *et al.* (2000, figs. 3 and 4, p. S89–90).

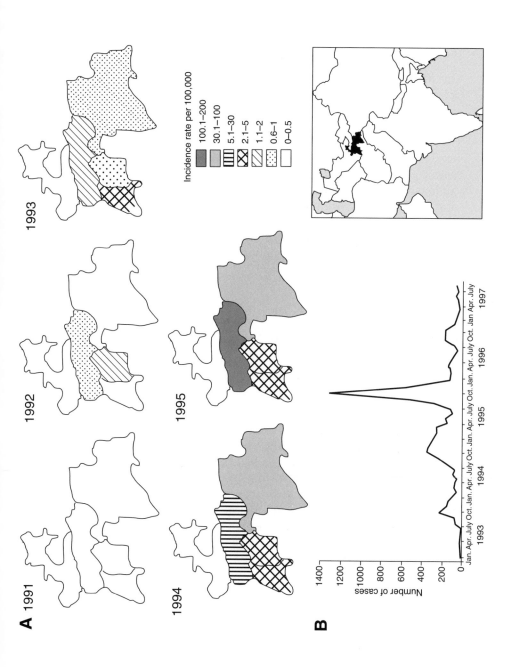

efforts, did the diphtheria epidemic in Tajikistan begin to wane (Usmanov *et al.*, 2000).

13.5.5 Post-combat Syndromes

One marked feature of many past wars has been the development among the veteran populations of debilitating syndromes characterized by a complex of signs and symptoms. In a review of these so-called *post-combat syndromes*, Hyams *et al.* (1996) have identified a series of examples—from the American Civil War (Da Costa syndrome) to the Gulf War (Gulf War syndrome)—that have variously manifested as fatigue or exhaustion, shortness of breath, headache, diarrhoea, dizziness, disturbed sleep, and forgetfulness (Table 13.9). Although not listed in Table 13.9, evidence is also accumulating of other, chronic fatigue-like, syndromes in veterans of such mid-nineteenth-century conflicts as the Crimean War and the Indian Mutiny (Jones and Wessely, 1999; Wessely *et al.*, 2001). Today, ill-defined maladies appear to be emerging among veterans of recent UN operations in Croatia, Cambodia, and Kosovo (Wessely *et al.*, 2001).

TYPES OF POST-COMBAT SYNDROME

In their historical examination of the medical records of British servicemen, Jones *et al.* (2002) used cluster analysis to identify similarities in the attributes of post-combat syndromes since the late nineteenth century. Three types of syndrome were identified, with each corresponding to a particular period of war history:

(1) A *debility syndrome*, without psychological or cognitive symptoms. This syndrome was primarily associated with conflicts of the nineteenth and early twentieth centuries (the Victorian campaigns, the South African War of 1899–1902, and World War I);

(2) A *somatic syndrome* focused on the heart. This syndrome was primarily associated with the early twentieth century (World War I), with additional evidence for the South African War and World War II;

(3) A *neuropsychiatric syndrome* with a range of somatic symptoms. This syndrome was primarily associated with conflicts of the mid- and late twentieth century, including World War II and the Gulf War.

The temporally shifting nature of post-combat syndromes, (1)→(2)→(3), appears to be related to developments in medical knowledge, the nature of warfare, and the cultural underpinnings of the era under consideration. As Jones *et al.* (2002: 323–4) conclude:

Post-combat syndromes have arisen from all major wars over the past century, and we can predict that they will continue to appear after future conflicts. What cannot be accurately forecast is their form, as they are moulded by the changing nature of health

Table 13.9. Symptoms commonly associated with war-related medical and psychological illnesses

Symptom	War and illness[1]					
	US Civil War Da Costa syndrome	World War I Effort syndrome	World War II Combat stress reaction	Vietnam War Agent Orange exposure	Vietnam and other wars Post-traumatic stress disorder (PTSD)	Gulf War Gulf War syndrome
Fatigue/exhaustion	+	+	+	+	+	+
Shortness of breath	+	+	+		+	+
Palpitations/tachycardia	+	+	+		+	
Precordial pain	+	+			+	
Headache	+	+	+	+	+	+
Muscle and joint pain				+	+	+
Diarrhoea	+		+	+	+	+
Excessive sweating	+	+	+	+		
Dizziness	+	+	+	+	+	
Fainting	+	+	+			
Disturbed sleep	+	+	+	+	+	+
Forgetfulness		+	+	+	+	+
Difficulty concentrating		+	+	+	+	+

Note: ¹ + indicates a commonly reported symptom.
Source: Hyams *et al.* (1996, table 1, p. 399).

fears and warfare . . . If each new post-combat syndrome is not interpreted as a unique or novel illness but as part of an understandable pattern of normal responses to the physical and psychological stress of war, then it may be managed in a more effective manner.

LATE-TWENTIETH-CENTURY CONFLICTS: GULF WAR SYNDROME

Shortly after the cessation of hostilities in the Gulf War (Sect. 13.2.1), veterans from the United States and subsequently Britain and Canada began to present with an unexplained set of illnesses which included fatigue, headache, diarrhoea, chest pain and shortness of breath, sleep disturbance, difficulty concentrating, and forgetfulness (Table 13.9). Gathered together under the rubric of 'Gulf War syndrome', more than 25,000 US, British, and Canadian veterans had developed the illnesses by the mid-1990s. At the same time, preliminary reports suggested the raised incidence of congenital defects among children born to Gulf War veterans (Hyams *et al.*, 1996; Wessely *et al.*, 2001).

POSSIBLE EXPLANATIONS

Although no new or unique syndrome has yet been formally identified among Gulf War veterans (Wessely *et al.*, 2001; Shapiro *et al.*, 2002), considerable speculation has surrounded possible factors, over and above the psychological dimensions of active combat, which may have adversely affected the symptomatic health of large numbers of servicemen. Particular attention has focused on the side-effects of measures undertaken to protect the combatants from the threat of chemical and biological warfare including multiple vaccinations against such biological agents as plague and anthrax (UK troops) and anthrax and botulism (US troops). Various other factors, including troop exposures to depleted uranium, organophosphate pesticides, nerve agents (sarin), and the toxins released by oil fires, have all been mooted in the aetiology of Gulf War-related illnesses (Wessely *et al.*, 2001). As Hoskins (1997: 276–7) notes, 'If Gulf War syndrome is the result of exposure to a toxic environmental contaminant, there may be, in the Gulf Region itself, many more thousands of civilian victims of this illness'.

13.6 Conclusion: The Future Disease Burden of Conflict

Since 1974, and despite many obstacles and setbacks, the World Health Organization's *Expanded Programme On Immunization* has been leading the world's peoples towards vastly reduced levels of incidence for many vaccine-preventable diseases (Keja and Henderson, 1984; Cutts *et al.*, 1991). In the early 1970s, fewer than 5 per cent of the world's children were vaccinated at all. By 1990, a tremendous public health effort had made it possible to reach almost 80 per cent of children born each year and to vaccinate them against six target diseases: diphtheria, tetanus, whooping cough (pertussis), poliomyelitis, tuberculosis, and measles. Vaccines which brought about the global eradication of smallpox in the late 1970s (Fenner *et al.*, 1988) have now controlled the transmission of poliomyelitis to the point that—hopefully—the disease may soon be eradicated. Other infectious diseases may follow in a more distant future.

But once war walks the stage, prospects for disease control, let alone eradication, become much bleaker. As we have shown in this book, past wars have fuelled catastrophic infections in both military and civil populations and, while the nature of warfare has changed, the link between war and disease remains as strong as ever. Although the huge loss of life from infections among soldiers has largely disappeared as a result of vaccination, the breakdown of hygiene, heath-care surveillance, and vaccination programmes during wars means that familiar infectious enemies rapidly re-establish themselves opportunistically in civil populations. Leading contenders are the various diarrhoeas, cholera, and dysentery among all age groups, old epidemic agents such as diphtheria and measles among children who escape routine vaccination, and sicknesses such as tuberculosis and the pneumonias among adults and the elderly. In addition, war remains an effective vehicle for spreading newly emerging infections such as HIV. To this glum tale, fresh threats posed by bioterrorism and post-combat syndromes must be added.

What does the future hold? Table 13.10 is based on the findings of the Global Burden of Disease Study (Murray and Lopez, 1996) and gives world regional estimates of the number of violent deaths due to war in 1990, along with baseline projections to the year 2020. Several features of the table are noteworthy:

(i) overall, 502,000 people are estimated to have died as a direct consequence of war in 1990, representing about 1 per cent of the 50.47 million deaths in that year;

(ii) geographically, the majority of war deaths in 1990 were concentrated in two world regions—Sub-Saharan Africa (268,000 deaths) and the states of the Middle Eastern Crescent (169,000 deaths);

(iii) by 2020, the annual burden of war mortality is projected to exceed 1 million, with Sub-Saharan Africa (630,000 deaths) and the Middle Eastern Crescent (336,000 deaths) remaining as the principal foci of war deaths;

(iv) the approximate doubling of war mortality between 1990 and 2020 is predicted to result in a modest rise in the ranking of war as a global cause of death, from rank 20 (1990) to rank 15 (2020) (see Fig. 13.10A).

However, estimates of the absolute number of deaths arising from war reveal little of the broader, non-fatal, disabling effects of armed conflict and in which disease plays a major role. So Table 13.10 also gives the estimated Disability-Adjusted Life Years (DALYs) for war in 1990 and 2020. Here, DALYs have

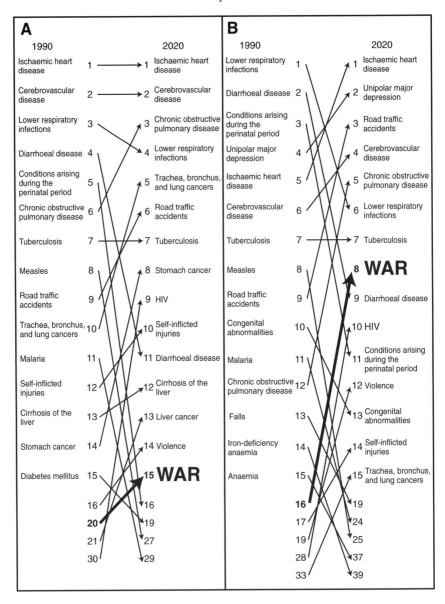

Fig. 13.10. Change in rank order of the 15 leading causes of disease and disability in the world, estimated for 1990 and 2020

Notes: (A) Rank order as defined by deaths. (B) Rank order as defined by Disability-Adjusted Life Years (DALYs). DALYs have been formed as the sum of (i) years of life lost due to premature mortality and (ii) years lived with disability. In all instances, the rank ordering of war is based on death and disability arising from the direct effects of conflict.

Source: Redrawn from Murray and Lopez (1996, figs. 7.9 and 7.12, pp. 361, 375).

Table 13.10. Estimated burden of conflict, 1990 and 2020

Region	Deaths (1,000s)		DALYs[1] (1,000s)	
	1990	2020[2]	1990	2020[2]
EME[3]	<1	<1	2	2
FSE[4]	29	29	1,149	1,123
Asia				
India	3	5	119	171
China	1	1	26	26
Other	15	21	593	789
Sub-Saharan Africa	268	630	10,698	25,192
Latin America and Caribbean	17	25	689	931
MEC[5]	169	336	6,744	13,080
Total	502	1,047	20,020	41,314

Notes: [1] Disability-Adjusted Life Years. [2] Baseline scenario. [3] Established Market Economies (Western Europe and North America). [4] Formerly Socialist Economies of Europe (Eastern Europe and Russia). [5] Middle Eastern Crescent (North Africa and Middle East).
Source: Data from Murray and Lopez (1996, tables 6a–h, 9a–h, 16a–h, 17a–h, pp. 433–64, 541–72, 760–91, 796–827).

been formed as the sum of (i) estimated years of life lost due to premature mortality resulting from war and (ii) estimated years of life lived with disability resulting from war. When viewed in this manner, the more general burden of war on human suffering becomes apparent. Within a global ranking of the direct causes of death and disability, Figure 13.10B sadly shows that war is projected to rise from rank 16 (20.02 million DALYs) to rank 8 (41.31 million DALYs) in the three decades to 2020. War-associated disease, like the poor, is likely always to be with us.

Appendix 13A

Anthrax (Section 13.4.3)

Anthrax is a disease principally of herbivorous mammals caused by the bacterium *Bacillus anthracis*. Humans generally acquire the infection through direct or indirect exposure to infected animals or animal products. Three human forms of anthrax are generally recognized: (i) *cutaneous anthrax*, acquired when the bacterium enters the skin through a cut or abrasion; (ii) *gastrointestinal tract anthrax*, acquired by the ingestion of contaminated food; and (iii) *inhalational anthrax*, acquired by the inhalation of airborne anthrax spores. All three human forms of anthrax are potentially lethal, although discussions of anthrax bioweapons have centred on the particular lethality of inhalational anthrax.

Inhalational Anthrax

A typical incubation period of one to six days gives way to a non-specific illness characterized by influenza-like symptoms. A brief remission is then followed by rapid deterioration with high fever, dyspnoea, cyanosis, and shock then follows. Haemorrhagic meningitis may be seen in up to 50 per cent of cases. Death is universal in all untreated cases and in approximately 95 per cent of cases for which treatment is started more than two days after symptom onset (Cieslak and Eitzen, 1999).

Vaccines and Therapies

Anthrax vaccines are available for both animals and humans. However, human vaccines are generally restricted to high-risk groups including the military and those at risk of occupational exposure. Antibiotic therapy is effective if delivered before or immediately after the onset of illness, while antibiotics can also be effective in the prophylactic treatment of those who are suspected of having been exposed to anthrax spores.

EPILOGUE

Pes is the chief of al the worldes welthe,
And to the heaven it ledeth ek the weie;
Pes is of soule and lif the mannes helthe,
Of pestilence and dothe the were aweie.

John Gower, *To Henry IV*

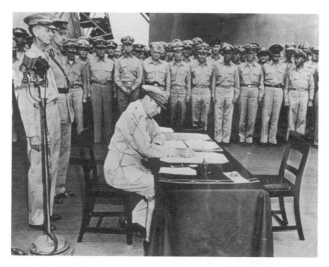

General Douglas MacArthur signing the Instrument of Surrender between the Allied Forces and Japan which concluded World War II, *USS Missouri*, 2 September 1945.

Source: Museum of World War II, Natick, Massachusetts.

REFERENCES

Numbers in square brackets after references indicate the sections in the text where the item is cited.

A

Aaby, P., Bukh, J., Lisse, I. M., and Smits, A. J. (1986). 'Severe measles in Sunderland, 1885: A European–African comparison of causes of severe infection'. *International Journal of Epidemiology*, 15: 101–7. [12.2.4]

Abrahams, A., Hallows, N. F., Eyre, J. W. H., and French, H. (1917). 'Purulent bronchitis: its influenzal and pneumococcal bacteriology'. *Lancet*, 1: 377–82. [12.5.3]

Abrahamson, I. (1935). *Lethargic Encephalitis*. New York. [12.5.3]

Adams, M. S., Croft, A. M., Winfield, D. A., and Richards, R. (1997). 'An outbreak of rubella in British troops in Bosnia'. *Epidemiology and Infection*, 118: 253–7. [13.5.3]

Adamson, B. (1980). 'Death from disease in Ancient Mesopotamia'. In: B. Alster (ed.), *Death in Mesopotamia: Papers Read at the XXVIᵉ Rencontre Assyriologique Internationale*. Copenhagen: Akademisk Forlag, 187. [2.2]

Ahmad, K. (2002). 'Norwalk-like virus attacks troops in Afghanistan'. *Lancet Infectious Diseases*, 2: 391. [13.2.3]

Ahuja, D. V., and Coons, S. A. (1968). 'Interactive graphics in data processing: geometry for construction and display'. *IBM System Journal*, 7: 188–205. [6.6.2, Appendix 6A.5]

AIDS Control Programme, Ugandan Ministry of Health (1990). 'Situational summary report on clinical AIDS in Uganda'. *AIDS Surveillance Report*, Fourth Quarter, 1–11. [10.4.2]

Albright, M. K. (2000). 'Economic sanctions and public health: a view from the Department of State'. *Annals of Internal Medicine*, 132: 155–7. [13.5.2]

Alderslade, R., Hess, G., and Larusdottir, J. (1996). 'Sustaining, protecting and promoting public health in Bosnia and Herzegovina'. *World Health Statistics Quarterly*, 49: 185–8. [13.2.2]

Alderson, M. (1981). *International Mortality Statistics*. London: Macmillan. [Appendix 1B, 3.1, 3.3, 3.3.2, 3.3.3, 3.4.4, 12.5.1]

Alexander, J. T. (1980). *Bubonic Plague in Early Modern Russia: Public Health and Urban Disaster*. Baltimore: The Johns Hopkins University Press. [1.1, 2.4.4]

Alger, R. A. (1901). *The Spanish-American War*. New York: Harper and Bros. [7.3.3]

Allen, R. W. (1917). 'Purulent bronchitis: its influenzal and pneumococcal bacteriology'. *Lancet*, 2: 509–10. [12.5.3]

Allison, M. J. (1993). 'Leishmaniasis'. In: Kiple (1993), 832–4. [13.5.4]

Allukian, M., and Atwood, L. (1997). 'Public health and the Vietnam War'. In: B. S. Levy and V. W. Sidel (eds.), *War and Public Health*. Oxford: Oxford University Press, 215–37. [1.4.3, 9.5]

Anderson, G. W. (1947). 'A German atlas of epidemic diseases'. *Geographical Review*, 37: 307–22. [6.1]

Anigstein, L., and Bader, M. N. (1943). 'Investigations on rickettsial diseases in Texas. Part 4. Experimental study of Bullis fever'. *Texas Reports on Biology and Medicine*, 1: 389–409. [7.4.2]

Ankrah, E. M. (1989). 'AIDS: methodological problems in studying its prevention and spread'. *Social Science and Medicine*, 29: 265–76. [10.4.2]

Anonymous (1854*a*). 'The war'. *Lancet*, 1: 301–2. [8.2.3]

——(1854*b*). 'Cholera in the Black Sea Fleet'. *Medical Times and Gazette*, 2: 350–1. [8.2.5]

——(1867). 'The climate of New Zealand'. *Lancet*, 2: 651. [11.2.2]

——(1939*a*). 'Epidemiological aspects of A.R. evacuation schemes'. *Medical Officer*, 61: 174. [5.5.1]

——(1939*b*). 'Town into country'. *Lancet*, 1: 605. [5.5.1, 5.5.4]

——(1939*c*). 'Measles: precautionary measures in reception areas'. *British Medical Journal*, 2: 934. [5.5.1]

——(1939*d*), 'Epidemiological notes: infectious diseases and evacuation'. *British Medical Journal*, 2: 792. [5.5.1, 5.5.3]

——(1939*e*). 'Evacuated children: small-pox and diphtheria prophylaxis'. *British Medical Journal*, 2: 934–5. [5.5.1]

——(1940). [Untitled]. *British Medical Journal*, 1: 660–1. [5.5.1]

——(1942*a*). 'Jaundice following yellow fever vaccination'. *Journal of the American Medical Association*, 119: 1110. [7.4.2]

——(1942*b*). 'The outbreak of jaundice in the army'. *Journal of the American Medical Association*, 120: 51–3. [7.4.2]

——(1943). [Untitled]. *Journal of the American Medical Association*, 123: 579. [7.4.2]

——(1944). 'Nutrition in enemy occupied Europe'. *Journal of the American Medical Association*, 124: 251. [12.5.1]

——(1945*a*). 'Atypical pneumonia. By the Commission on Acute Respiratory Diseases'. *American Journal of the Medical Sciences*, 209: 55–8. [Introduction to Part III, 7.4.2]

——(1945*b*). 'Poliomyelitis in Malta'. *British Medical Journal*, 1: 773–4. [12.5.4]

——(1953). 'Government services'. *Journal of the American Medical Association*, 152: 1448–50. [9.4]

Armenian, H. K. (1989). 'Perceptions from epidemiologic research in an endemic war'. *Social Science and Medicine*, 28: 643–7. [1.4.3, 5.6.3]

——Halabi, S. S., and Khlat, M. (1989). 'Epidemiology of primary health problems in Beirut'. *Journal of Epidemiology and Community Health*, 43: 315–18. [5.6.3]

Army Medical Department (1858). *The Medical and Surgical History of the British Army which Served in Turkey and the Crimea during the War against Russia in the Years 1854–55–56*, i and ii. London: Harrison and Sons. [1.4.1, 1.4.3, Appendix 1B, 8, 8.2.1, 8.2.2, 8.2.3, 8.2.4, 8.2.5, Appendix 8A]

Arnautovic, A., Celik, S., and Preljevic, S. B. (1994). 'Specifičnosti prevencije zaraznih bolesti u toku agresije na Republiku'. *Medicinski Arhiv*, 48: 73–6. [13.2.2]

Arnold, G. (1995). *Wars in the Third World since 1945* (2nd edn.). London: Cassell. [12.5.1, 13.2]

Arrizabalaga, J. (1993). 'Syphilis'. In: Kiple (1993), 1025–33. [2.3.3, Appendix 10A]

Ascherio, A., Chase, R., Coté, T., Dehaes, G., Hoskins, E., Laaouej, J., Passey, M., Qaderi, S., Shuqaidef, S., Smith, M. C., and Zaidi, S. (1992). 'Effect of the Gulf War on infant and child mortality in Iraq'. *New England Journal of Medicine*, 327: 931–6. [13.2.1]

Ashford, M.-W., and Huet-Vaughn, Y. (1997). 'The impact of war on women'. In: B. S. Levy and V. W. Sidel (eds.), *War and Public Health*. Oxford: Oxford University Press, 186–96. [10.1]

Augustin, G. (1909). *History of Yellow Fever*. New Orleans: Searcy and Pfaff. [Appendix 12A]

Austin, B. (1993). *1812: The March on Moscow*. London: Greenhill Books. [2.4.5]

Austin, J. E., and Bruch, C. E. (2000). *The Environmental Consequences of War: Legal, Economic and Scientific Pespectives*. Cambridge: Cambridge University Press. [13.5.1]

Ayers, G. (1971). *England's First State Hospitals and the Metropolitan Asylums Board, 1867–1930*. London: Wellcome Institute of the History of Medicine. [8.3.4]

B

Bahr, G., de L. Costello, A. M., Alahdab, Y., and Stanford, J. (1991). 'Epidemic tuberculosis in north Lebanon'. *Lancet*, 337: 983–4. [5.6.3, 12.5.1]

Bancroft, W. H., and Lemon, S. M. (1984). 'Hepatitis A from the military perspective'. In: R. J. Gerety (ed.), *Hepatitis A*. Orlando: Academic Press, 81–100. [7.4.2]

Bannister, B. A. (ed.) (1991). *Report of a Think Tank on the Potential Effects of Global Warming and Population Increase on the Epidemiology of Infectious Diseases*. Colindale: Public Health Laboratory Service. [3.5.3]

Barker, A. J. (1970). *The Vainglorious War, 1854–56*. London: Weidenfeld & Nicolson. [8.2.1]

Barrett, F. A. (2000). *Disease and Geography: The History of an Idea*. York: Canada, Geographical Monographs, York University, 23. [6.1]

Barrett, O., Skrzypek, G., Datel, D., and Goldstein, J. D. (1969). 'Malaria imported to the United States from Vietnam: chemoprophylaxis evaluated in returning soldiers'. *American Journal of Tropical Medicine and Hygiene*, 18: 495–9. [9.5.3]

Barry, M. (2000). 'Effect of the US embargo and economic decline on health in Cuba'. *Annals of Internal Medicine*, 132: 151–4. [13.5.2]

Bartlett, M. S. (1957). 'Measles periodicity and community size'. *Journal of the Royal Statistical Society A*, 120: 48–70. [6.7.1]

Barua, D., and Greenough, W. B. (eds.) (1992). *Cholera*. New York: Plenum Medical. [8.2.3]

Batchelor, C. A. (1995). 'Stateless persons: some gaps in international protection'. *International Journal of Refugee Law*, 7: 232–59. [5.2.2]

Baum, S. G. (2000). '*Mycoplasma pneumoniae* and atypical pneumonia'. In: Mandell *et al.* (2000), 2018–27. [7.4.2]

Bayne-Jones, S. (1968). *The Evolution of Preventive Medicine in the United States Army, 1607–1939*. Washington: US Government Printing Office. [2.6.2, 7.1, 7.3, 7.3.5, 7.4.1, 8.1]

Beadle, C., and Hoffman, S. L. (1993). 'History of malaria in the United States naval forces at war: World War I through the Vietnam conflict'. *Clinical Infectious Diseases*, 16: 320–9. [1.1, 2.2, 9.5.1, 11.4.2]

Bean, W. B. (1982). *Walter Reed: A Biography*. Charlottesville, Va.: University Press of Virginia. [7.3.2]

Benenson, A. S. (ed.) (1990). *Control of Communicable Diseases in Man* (5th edn.). Washington: American Public Health Association. [1.3.2, Appendix 1A, 3.5.2]

——(1997). 'Smallpox'. In: Evans and Kaslow (1997), 861–4. [Appendix 1A]

Benjamin, B. (1968). *Health and Vital Statistics*. London: Allen and Unwin. [3.3.1]

Bennett, J. V., Holmberg, S. D., Rogers, M. F., and Solomon, S. L. (1987). 'Infectious and parasitic diseases'. In: R. W. Amler and H. B. Dull (eds.), *Closing the Gap: The Burden of Unnecessary Diseases*. Oxford: Oxford University Press, 102–14. [3.5.1]

Bentley, N. (ed.) (1966). *Russell's Despatches from the Crimea, 1854–1856*. London: Deutsch. [8.2.1]

Berg, S. W. (1984). 'Sexually transmitted diseases in the military'. In: K. K. Holmes, A. Mardh, F. Sparling, and J. Wiesner (eds.), *Sexually Transmitted Diseases*. New York: McGraw-Hill Book Company, 90–9. [10.1, 10.3.1, 10.4.2]

Berkley, S., Okware, S., and Naamara, W. (1989). 'Surveillance for AIDS in Uganda'. *AIDS*, 3: 79–85. [10.4.2]

Beslagic, E., Cengic, D., Beslagic, R., and Hamzic, S. (1996). 'Seroloska potvrda epidemije hemoragicne groznice u toku deblokade Sarajeva'. *Medicinski Arhiv*, 50: 89–91. [13.2.2]

Bhutta, Z. A. (2002). 'Children of war: the real casualties of the Afghan conflict'. *British Medical Journal*, 324: 349–52. [3.2.3]

Bise, G., and Coninx, R. (1997). 'Epidemic typhus in a prison in Burundi'. *Transactions of the Royal Society of Tropical Medicine and Hygiene*, 91: 133–4. [5.7]

Black, F. L. (1984). 'Measles'. In: A. S. Evans (ed.), *Viral Infections of Humans: Epidemiology and Control* (2nd edn.). New York: Plenum, 397–418. [4.5.1]

——(1997). 'Measles'. In: Evans and Kaslow (1997), 507–29. [Appendix 1A]

Black, J. (2000). *War: Past, Present and Future*. Stroud: Sutton Publishing. [13.2]

Black, M. E., and Healing, T. D. (1993). 'Communicable diseases in former Yugoslavia and in refugees arriving in the United Kingdom'. *Communicable Disease Report. CDC Review*, 21: R87–90. [12.5.1]

Blewitt, B. (1951). ' "Q" fever: a new disease in armies'. *Journal of the Royal Army Medical Corps*, 97: 377–88. [8.4.1]

Bloomfield, A. L. (1958). *A Bibliography of Internal Medicine: Communicable Diseases*. Chicago: University of Chicago Press. [4.4.1]

Bodart, G. (1916). *Losses of Life in Modern Wars: Austria-Hungary; France*. Oxford: Clarendon Press. [1.2.5, 1.3.1, Appendix 1B, 2.4.5]

Boehnhardt, H. (1942). 'Eine eigentümliche Fiebererkrangkung in Bessarabien'. *Deutsche Militärarzt*, 7: 291–4. [8.4]

Bonham-Carter, V. (ed.) (1968). *Surgeon in the Crimea: The Experiences of George Lawson, Recorded in Letters to His Family, 1854–1855*. London: Constable. [8.2.1]

Bordley, J., and Harvey, A. (1976). *Two Centuries of American Medicine, 1776–1976*. Philadelphia: W. B. Saunders Co. [7.3.2]

Botas, J., Tavores, L., Carvalho, C., Feliciano, H., and Antunes, F. (1989). 'HIV-2 infection: Some clinical and epidemiological aspects in Portugal'. *Proceedings of the V International Conference on AIDS*, Montreal, 4–9 June, Abstract M.A.P.77. [10.4.2]

Bourdelais, P., and Raulot, J.-Y. (1978). 'La marche du choléra en France: 1832 et 1854'. *Annales Économies, Sociétés, Civilisations*, 33: 125–42. [8.2.3]

Bouvier, M., Pittet, D., Loutan, L., and Starobinski, M. (1990). 'Airport malarias: a mini-epidemic in Switzerland'. *Schweizerin Medizin Wochenschreiber*, 120: 1217–22. [3.5.3]

Bowley, H. (2001). 'The Geographical Aspects of the "Spanish" Influenza Pandemic in England and Wales, 1918–1919'. Unpublished BA dissertation, School of Geography, University of Nottingham. [12.5.3]

Box, G. E., Jenkins, G. M., and Reinsel, G. C. (1994). *Time Series Analysis: Forecasting and Control.* Englewood Cliffs, NJ: Prentice Hall. [5.5.3]

Bradley, D. J. (1988). 'The scope of travel medicine'. In: R. Steffen, H. O. Lobel, J. Haworth, and D. J. Bradley (eds.), *Travel Medicine: Proceedings of the First Conference on International Travel Medicine*, Zurich, Switzerland, Apr. 1988. Berlin: Springer Verlag, 1–9. [3.5.3]

Brecke, P. (1999). 'Simulation of the steps to war: classification of violent conflicts, a necessary prerequisite'. *Simulation*, 72: 52–8. [1.2.1, 1.2.2, 1.2.3]

Bridges, J. R. (1973). 'A study of malaria rates in the Que Son Mountains of Vietnam'. *Military Medicine*, 138: 413–17. [9.5.1]

Brock, T. D. (ed.) (1990). *Microorganisms: From Smallpox to Lyme Disease.* New York: Freeman. [2.3.3]

Brogan, P. (1992). *World Conflicts* (2nd edn.). London: Bloomsbury. [1.2.3, 11.1, 12.5.1, 13.2]

Brooks, S. (1966). *Civil War Medicine.* Springfield: Charles C. Thomas. [4.3.2, 7.2.3]

Brown, J. W., Hein, G. E., Ellman, P., and Joules, H. (1943). 'Discussion on atypical pneumonia'. *Proceedings of the Royal Society of Medicine, Section of Medicine*, 36: 385–90. [7.4.2]

Brown, V., Reilley, B., Ferrir, M.-C., Gabaldon, J., and Manoncourt, S. (1997). 'Cholera outbreak during massive influx of Rwandan returnees in November, 1996'. *Lancet*, 349: 212. [5.7]

Brundtland, G. H. (2002). 'Afghanistan: rebuilding a health system'. *Journal of the American Medical Association*, 287: 2354. [13.2.3]

Bryceson, A., Tomkins, A., Ridley, D., Warhurst, D., Goldstone, A., Bayliss, G., Toswill, J., and Parry, J. (1988). 'HIV-2-associated AIDS in the 1970s'. *Lancet*, 2: 22. [10.4.2]

Bulmer, E. (1945). 'B.L.A. medicine'. *British Medical Journal*, 2: 873–6. [8.4]

Bureau of Hygiene and Tropical Diseases (1989). 'Screening in Cuba'. *AIDS Newsletter*, 4: 6 (Item 304). [10.4.2]

——(1990). 'Zimbabwean military'. *AIDS Newsletter*, 5: 9 (Item 265). [10.4.2]

Burnet, F. M. (1979). 'Portraits of viruses: influenza virus A'. *Intervirology*, 11: 201–14. [11.3]

Bush, K. (2000). 'Polio, war and peace'. *Bulletin of the World Health Organization*, 78: 281–2. [13.3.1, 13.3.2]

Bush, L. M., Abrams, B. H., Beall, A., and Johnson, C. C. (2001). 'Index case of fatal inhalational anthrax due to bioterrorism in the United States'. *New England Journal of Medicine*, 345: 1607–10. [13.4.3]

Butler, A. G. (1938). *The Australian Army Medical Services in the War of 1914–18*, i (2nd edn.). Melbourne: Australian War Memorial. [4.4.1]

——(1940). *The Australian Army Medical Services in the War of 1914–18*, ii. Melbourne: Australian War Memorial. [4.4.1]

——(1943). *The Australian Army Medical Services in the War of 1914–1918*, iii. Melbourne: Australian War Memorial. [4.4.1, Introduction to Part III]

Butler, T. (2000). 'Yersinia species, including plague'. In: Mandell *et al.* (2000), 2406–14. [Appendix 1A]

C

Campbell, T. A., Strong, S., Grier, G. S., and Lutz, R. J. (1943). 'Primary atypical pneumonia: a report of 200 cases at Fort Eustis, Virginia'. *Journal of the American Medical Association*, 122, 723–9. [7.4.2]

Cantlie, N. (1974). *A History of the Army Medical Department* (2 vols.). Edinburgh and London: Churchill Livingstone. [2.4.4, 2.5.2, 2.6.2, 8.1, 8.2.1, 8.2.2]

Carlson, J. R., and Hammond, W. (1999). 'The English sweating sickness (1485–c.1551): a new perspective on disease etiology'. *Journal of the History of Medicine and Allied Sciences*, 54: 23–54. [2.3.3]

Carmichael, A. G. (1993*a*). 'Bubonic plague'. In: Kiple (1993), 628–31. [Appendix 1A, 2.3.1]

——(1993*b*). 'Plague of Athens'. In: Kiple (1993), 934–7. [2.2]

——(1993*c*). 'History of public health and sanitation in the West before 1700'. In: Kiple (1993), 192–200. [3.6]

Carr, W. (1991). *The Origins of the Wars of German Unification*. London: Longman. [8.3.1]

Carson, D. A. (1944). 'Observations on dengue'. *United States Naval Medical Bulletin*, 42: 1081–4. [11.4.2]

Carson, T. E., and Johnson, D. W. (1973). 'Venereal disease in the military, with special reference to incidence and management in Southeast Asia'. In: L. Nicholas (ed.), *Sexually Transmitted Diseases*. Springfield, Ill.: Charles C. Thomas, 105–39. [10.1, 10.3.1]

Carswell, J. W. (1987). 'HIV-infection in healthy persons in Uganda'. *AIDS*, 1: 223–7. [10.4.2]

——Lloyd, G., and Howells, J. (1989). 'Prevalence of HIV-1 infection in East African lorry drivers'. *AIDS*, 3: 759–61. [10.4.2]

——Sewankambo, N., Lloyd, G., and Downing, R. G. (1986). 'How long has the AIDS virus been in Uganda?' *Lancet*, 1: 1217. [10.4.2]

Caselli, G. (1991). 'Health transition and cause-specific mortality'. In: Schofield *et al.* (1991), 68–96. [3.4.1]

Cash, P. (1976). 'The Canadian military campaign of 1775–1776: medical problems and effects of disease'. *Journal of the American Medical Association*, 236: 52–6. [2.6.2]

Cassar, P. (1964). *Medical History of Malta*. London: Wellcome Institute for the History of Medicine. [12.5.4]

Castiglioni, A. (1947). *A History of Medicine* (2nd edn.). London: Routledge and Kegan Paul. [1.1, 2.2]

Cates, W. Jr. (1998). 'Syphilis'. In: Evans and Brachman (1998), 713–32. [Appendix 10A]

Caughey, J. E., and Porteous, W. M. (1946). 'An epidemic of poliomyelitis occurring among troops in the Middle East'. *Medical Journal of Australia*, 1: 5–10. [12.5.4]

Cavanaugh, D. C., Dangerfield, H. G., Hunter, D. H., Joy, R. J. T., Marshall, J. D., Quy, D. V., Vivona, F., and Winter, E. (1968). 'Some observations on the current plague outbreak in the Republic of Vietnam'. *American Journal of Public Health*, 58: 742–52. [9.5.2]

CDC (1990). *Prevalence of HIV-1 Antibody in Civilian Applicants for Military Service, October 1985–December 1989.* Selected tables prepared by the Division of HIV/AIDS. Atlanta: Centers for Disease Control and Prevention. [Appendix 1A, 4.6.2]

——(1993). 'Status of public health—Bosnia and Herzegovina, August–September 1993'. *Morbidity and Mortality Weekly Report*, 42: 973, 979–82. [13.2.2]

——(1994a). 'Health status of displaced persons following civil war—Burundi, December 1993–January 1994'. *Morbidity and Mortality Weekly Report*, 43: 701–3. [5.7]

——(1994b). 'Dengue fever among US military personnel—Haiti, September–November, 1994'. *Morbidity and Mortality Weekly Report*, 43: 845–8. [13.5.3]

——(1995). 'Implementation of health initiatives during a cease-fire—Sudan, 1995'. *Morbidity and Mortality Weekly Report*, 44: 433–6. [13.3.2]

——(1998). 'Cholera outbreak among Rwandan refugees—Democratic Republic of Congo, April 1997'. *Morbidity and Mortality Weekly Report*, 47: 389–91. [5.7]

——(2001a). 'Update: investigation of bioterrorism-related anthrax and interim guidelines for exposure management and antimicrobial therapy, October 2001'. *Morbidity and Mortality Weekly Report*, 50: 909–19. [13.4.3]

——(2001b). 'Update: investigation of bioterrorism-related anthrax and interim guidelines for clinical evaluation of persons with possible anthrax'. *Morbidity and Mortality Weekly Report*, 50: 941–8. [13.4.3]

——(2001c). 'Update: investigation of bioterrorism-related anthrax and adverse events from antimicrobial prophylaxis'. *Morbidity and Mortality Weekly Report*, 50: 973–6. [13.4.3]

——(2001d). 'Update: investigation of bioterrorism-related anthrax, 2001'. *Morbidity and Mortality Weekly Report*, 50: 1008–10. [13.4.3]

——(2001e). 'Surveillance of mortality during a refugee crisis—Guinea, January–May 2001'. *Morbidity and Mortality Weekly Report*, 50: 1029–32. [5.4.1]

——(2001f). 'Evaluation of *Bacillus anthracis* contamination inside the Brentwood Mail Processing and Distribution Center—District of Columbia, October 2001'. *Morbidity and Mortality Weekly Report*, 50: 1129–33. [13.4.3]

——(2002). 'Outbreak of acute gastroenteritis associated with Norwalk-like viruses among British military personnel—Afghanistan, May 2002'. *Morbidity and Mortality Weekly Report*, 51: 477–9. [13.2.3]

Census Office, Uganda. (1982). *Report of the 1980 Population Census: Volume 1. The Provisional Results by Administrative Areas.* Kampala: Ministry of Planning and Economic Development. [10.4.2]

Chadwick, F. E. (1911). *The Relations of the United States and Spain: The Spanish–American War.* New York: C. Scribner's Sons. [7.3.1]

Chalmers, A. K. (1930). *The Health of Glasgow 1818–1925: An Outline.* Glasgow: Glasgow Corporation. [12.2.4]

Chanteau, S., Ratsifasoamanana, L., Rasoamanana, B., Rahalison, L., Randriambelosoa, J., Roux, J., and Rabeson, D. (1998). 'Plague, a reemerging disease in Madagascar'. *Emerging Infectious Diseases*, 4: 101–4. [9.2.1]

Charlton, J., and Murphy, M. (eds.) (1997). *The Health of Adult Britain 1841–1994*, i. London: The Stationary Office. [3.2.2]

Chatfield, C. (1980). *The Analysis of Time Series: An Introduction* (2nd edn.). London: Chapman and Hall. [5.5.3]

Chelala, C. A. (1990). 'Central America: the cost of war'. *Lancet*, 335: 153–4. [10.4.2]

Chimni, B. S. (2000). *International Refugee Law: A Reader*. New Delhi: Sage. [5.2.2]

Chipman, N. P. (1911). *The Tragedy of Andersonville: Trial of Captain Henry Wirz, the Prison Keeper*. Sacramento: N. P. Chipman. [7.2.2]

Christie, A. B. (1987). *Infectious Diseases: Epidemiology and Clinical Practice*, i. New York: Churchill Livingstone. [4.4.1]

Christopher, G. W., Cieslak, T. J., Pavlin, J. A., and Eitzen, E. M. (1997). 'Biological warfare: a historical perspective'. *Journal of the American Medical Association*, 278: 412–17. [2.3.3, 2.6.2, 13.4.1, 13.4.2]

Cieslak, T. J., and Eitzen, E. M. (1999). 'Clinical and epidemiologic principles of anthrax'. *Emerging Infectious Diseases*, 5: 552–5. [Appendix 13A]

Cioffi-Revilla, C. (1996). 'Origins and evolution of war and politics'. *International Studies Quarterly*, 40: 1–22. [1.2.1]

Cirillo, V. J. (2000). 'Fever and reform: the typhoid epidemic in the Spanish–American War'. *Journal of the History of Medicine and Allied Sciences*, 55: 363–97. [7.3]

Clausewitz, K. von (1976). *On War*, ed. and trans. by M. Howard and P. Paret. Princeton: Princeton University Press. [1.2.1]

Clement, J., McKenna, P., Avsic-Zupanc, T., and Skinner, C. R. (1994). 'Rat-transmitted hantavirus disease in Sarajevo'. *Lancet*, 344: 131. [13.2.2]

Cliff, A. D., and Haggett, P. (1988). *Atlas of Disease Distributions: Analytic Approaches to Epidemiological Data*. Oxford: Blackwell Reference. [2.4.6, 4.6.1, 4.6.2, 5.3.1, 5.5.4, 6.6, 8.2.3, 10.4.1, 12.3.3]

——— (1989). 'Spatial aspects of epidemic control'. *Progress in Human Geography*, 13: 313–47. [4.4.1]

——— and Ord, J. K. (1986). *Spatial Aspects of Influenza Epidemics*. London: Pion. [1.3.2, 3.4.2]

——— ——— and Versey, G. R. (1981). *Spatial Diffusion: An Historical Geography of Epidemics in an Island Community*. Cambridge: Cambridge University Press. [1.3.2, 7.3.4, 8.3.3, 11.1, 11.5, 12.2.4]

——— and Smallman-Raynor, M. (1993). *Measles: An Historical Geography of a Major Human Viral Disease from Global Expansion to Local Retreat, 1840–1990*. Oxford: Blackwell. [2.6.1, 3.5.3, 4.3, 4.3.1, 4.3.2, 4.4.1, 4.5.1, 11.2, 12.2.4, 12.5.3]

——— ——— (1998). *Deciphering Global Epidemics: Analytical Approaches to the Disease Records of World Cities, 1888–1912*. Cambridge: Cambridge University Press. [1.3.2, 1.4.1, 1.4.2, 2.3.3, 3.2.2, 3.3.3, 3.4.1, 3.4.2, 3.4.3, 3.5, 3.5.1, 3.5.3, 3.6.1, 5.5.3]

——— ——— (2000). *Island Epidemics*. Oxford: Oxford University Press. [2.3.1, Introduction to Part III, Appendix 6A.2, 8.2.5, 10.5, 11.1, 11.2, 11.2.1, 11.3.2, 11.5, 12.5.4]

——— and Ord, J. K. (1981). *Spatial Processes: Models and Applications*. London: Pion. [Appendix 6A.1, 10.4.2]

Cole, R., and MacCallum, W. G. (1918). 'Pneumonia at a base hospital'. *Journal of the American Medical Association*, 70: 1146–56. [4.4.1]

Collins, S. D. (1930). 'The influenza epidemic of 1928–1929 with comparative data for 1918–1919'. *American Journal of Public Health*, 20: 119–29. [11.3]

Collis, W. R. F. (1945). 'Belsen camp: a preliminary report'. *British Medical Journal*, 1: 814–16. [8.4]

Comstock, G. W., and O'Brien, R. J. (1998). 'Tuberculosis'. In: Evans and Brachman (1998), 777–804. [Appendix 1A]

Conacher, J. B. (1987). *Britain and the Crimea, 1855–56: Problems of War and Peace.* London: Macmillan. [8.2.1]

Cook, G. C. (2001). 'Influence of diarrhoeal disease on military and naval campaigns'. *Journal of the Royal Society of Medicine*, 94: 95–7. [1.3.2]

Cook, N. D. (1981). *Demographic Collapse: Indian Peru, 1520–1620.* Cambridge: Cambridge University Press. [2.6.1]

——(1998). *Born to Die: Disease and New World Conquest, 1492–1650.* Cambridge: Cambridge University Press. [2.6.1]

Cooper, B. C., and Kiple, K. F. (1993). 'Yellow fever'. In: Kiple (1993), 1100–7. [Appendix 1A]

Cooter, R. (1993). 'War and modern medicine'. In: W. F. Bynum and R. Porter (eds.), *Companion Encyclopedia of the History of Medicine*, ii. London: Routledge. [1.3.1]

Copeman, S. M. (1920). 'Report on incidence of influenza in the University and Borough of Cambridge and in the Friends' School, Saffron Waldon'. In: Ministry of Health, *Report on the Pandemic of Influenza, 1918–19.* Reports on Public Health and Medical Subjects, No. 5. London: HMSO, appendix I, 388–444. [Appendix 1B, 12.5.3]

Corbett, P. E. (1962). 'Laws of war'. *Encyclopaedia Britannica*, xiii: 807–13. [1.2.4]

Cornish, W. R. (1871). 'The origin of the smallpox epidemic'. *Lancet*, 2490: 703. [8.3.1]

Costagliola, D., Laporte, A., Chevret, S., and Valleron, A. J. (1990). 'Incubation time for AIDS among homosexual men and pediatric cases'. *Proceedings of the VI International Conference on AIDS*, San Francisco, 20–4 June, Abstract Th.C.661. [10.4.2]

Councell, C. E. (1941). 'War and infectious disease'. *Public Health Reports*, 56: 548–73. [1.3.2, 5.5.1, 8.4, 12.5.1, 12.5.2]

Cowley, R. G. (1970). 'Implications of the Vietnam War for tuberculosis in the United States'. *Archives of Environmental Health*, 21: 479–80. [9.5, 9.5.3]

Crawfurd, R. (1914). *Plague and Pestilence in Literature and Art.* Oxford: Clarendon Press. [1.1, 2.2, 2.4.5]

Creighton, C. (1965). *A History of Epidemics in Britain* (2 vols.). London: Frank Cass and Co. Ltd. [1.1, 2, 2.3.1, 2.3.3, 2.4.3, 2.4.4, 2.4.5, 2.6.2]

Crew, F. A. E. (1956). *The Army Medical Services: Campaigns*, i. A. S. MacNalty (ed.), *History of the Second World War: United Kingdom Medical Series.* London: HMSO. [8.4]

——(1957). *The Army Medical Services: Campaigns*, ii. A. S. MacNalty (ed.), *History of the Second World War: United Kingdom Medical Series.* London: HMSO. [8.4, 12.4, 12.4.1, 12.4.2]

Croft, A. M. J., and Creamer, I. S. (1997). 'Health data from Operation Resolute (Bosnia). Part 1: primary care data'. *Journal of the Royal Army Medical Corps*, 143: 13–18. [13.5.3]

Crompton, D. W. T., and Savioli, L. (1993). 'Terrestrial parasitic infections and urbanization'. *Bulletin of the World Health Organization*, 71: 1–7. [3.5.3]

Crosby, A. W. (1967). 'Conquistador y pestilencia: the first New World pandemic and the fall of the great indian empires'. *Hispanic American Historical Review*, 47: 321–37. [2.6.1]

——(1986). *Ecological Imperialism: The Biological Expansion of Europe, 900–1900.* Cambridge: Cambridge University Press. [2.6.1]

——(1989). *America's Forgotten Pandemic: The Influenza of 1918.* Cambridge: Cambridge University Press. [7.4.1]

——(1993). 'Influenza'. In: Kiple (1993), 807–11. [11.3]

Crosby, T. L. (1986). *The Impact of Civilian Evacuation in the Second World War.* London: Croom Helm. [5.5.2]

Cumpston, J. H. L. (1919). *Influenza and Maritime Quarantine in Australia.* Sydney: Commonwealth of Australia, Quarantine Service Publication, No. 18. [4.4.1, 11.1, 11.3.2, 11.5]

——and Lewis, M. J. (1989). *Health and Disease in Australia: A History.* Canberra: Australian Government Publishing Service. [11.2.1, 11.3.2]

Cunningham, H. H. (1958). *Doctors in Gray: The Confederate Medical Service.* Baton Rouge, La.: Louisiana State University Press. [4.3.2]

Currey, R. N., and Gibson, R. V. (1946). *Poems from India by Members of the Forces.* London: Oxford University Press. [5]

Curtin, P. D. (1989) *Death by Migration: Europe's Encounter with the Tropics in the Nineteenth Century.* New York: Cambridge University Press. [Appendix 1B, 2.6.2, 4.1, 4.2, 4.2.1, 4.2.2, 10.2, 10.2.1, 10.2.2]

——(1998). *Disease and Empire: The Health of European Troops in the Conquest of Africa.* Cambridge: Cambridge University Press. [12.2, 12.2.2]

Curtiss, J. S. (1979). *Russia's Crimean War.* Durham, NC: Duke University Press. [8.2.1]

Cutts, F. T., and Smith, G. (1994). *Vaccination and World Health.* London: Wiley. [3.6.1]

——Henderson, R. H., Clements, C. J., Chen, R. T., and Patriarca, P. A. (1991). 'Principles of measles control'. *Bulletin of the World Health Organization,* 69: 1–7. [13.6]

D

Dando, M. (1994). *Biological Warfare in the 21st Century: Biotechnology and the Proliferation of Biological Weapons.* London: Brassey's. [13.4, 13.4.1]

Daniels, M. (1946). 'Tuberculosis in Poland'. *Lancet,* 2: 537–40. [12.5.1]

——(1947). 'Tuberculosis in post–war Europe: an international problem'. *Tubercle,* 28: 201–10, 222, 233–8. [1.4.3, 12.5.1]

——(1949). 'Tuberculosis in Europe during and after the Second World War'. *British Medical Journal,* 2: 1065–72, 1135–40. [12.5.1]

de Bevoise, K. (1995). *Agents of the Apocalypse: Epidemic Disease in the Colonial Philippines.* Princeton: Princeton University Press. [1.1]

de Lalla, F., Rizzardini, G., Rinaldi, E., Santoro, D., Zeli, L., and Verga, G. (1990). 'HIV, HBV, delta-agent and treponema pallidum infections in two rural African areas'. *Transactions of the Royal Society of Tropical Medicine and Hygiene,* 84: 144–7. [10.4.2]

——— Santoro, D., and Galli, M. (1988). 'Rapid spread of HIV infection in a rural district of Central Africa'. *AIDS,* 2: 317. [10.4, 10.4.2]

Dear, I. C. B., and Foot, M. R. D. (1995). *The Oxford Companion of the Second World War.* Oxford: Oxford University Press. [11.4]

Debré, R., and Joannon, P. (1926). *La Rougeole: Epidémiologie, Immunologie, Prophylaxie.* Paris: Masson et Cie. [4.4.1]

DeMaio, J., and Zenilman, J. (1998). 'Gonococcal infections'. In: Evans and Brachman (1998), 285–304. [Appendix 10A]

Derbes, V. J. (1966). 'De Mussis and the great plague of 1348: a forgotten episode of bacteriological warfare'. *Journal of the American Medical Association*, 196: 59–62. [1.1, 2.3.3]

Derrick, E. H. (1937). 'Q fever, a new fever entity: clinical features, diagnosis and laboratory investigation'. *Medical Journal of Australia*, 2: 281–99. [9.1]

Desenclos, J. D., Michel, D., Tholly, F., Magdi, I., Pecoul, B., and Desve, G. (1990). 'Mortality trends among refugees in Honduras, 1984–1987'. *International Journal of Epidemiology*, 19: 367–73. [1.1, 5.4.1]

Deuel, R. E., Bawell, M. B., Matsumoto, M., and Sabin, A. B. (1950). 'Status and significance of inapparent infection with virus of Japanese B encephalitis in Korea and Okinawa in 1946'. *American Journal of Hygiene*, 51: 13–20. [9.4.1]

Dewing, H. B. (1914). *Procopius: History of the Wars, Books I and II.* London: William Heinemann. [2.3.1]

Dietrich, S. (1942). 'Der sogeannte katarrhalische Ikterus und die Hepatitis epidemica'. *Deutsche Medizinische Wochenschrift*, 68: 5–10. [8.4]

Dingle, J. H., Abernethy, T. J., Badger, G. F., Buddingh, G. J., Feller, A. E., Langmuir, A. D., Ruegsegger, J. M., and Wood, W. B., Jr. (1943). 'Primary acute pneumonia, etiology unknown'. *War Medicine*, 3: 223–48. [7.4.2]

Dittmann, S., Wharton, M., Vitek, C., Ciotti, M., Galazka, A., Guichard, S., Hardy, I., Kartoglu, U., Koyama, S., Kreysler, J., Martin, B., Mercer, D., Rønne, T., Roure, C., Steinglass, R., Strebel, P., Sutter, R., and Trostle, M. (2000). 'Successful control of epidemic diphtheria in the states of the former Union of Soviet Socialist Republics: lessons learned'. *Journal of Infectious Diseases*, 181 (suppl. 1), S10–22. [13.5.4]

Dobyns, H. F. (1963). 'An outline of Andean epidemic history to 1720'. *Bulletin of the History of Medicine*, 37: 493–515. [2.6.1]

Dols, M. W. (1977). *The Black Death in the Middle East.* Princeton: Princeton University Press. [2.3.1]

Dorling, D. (1995). *A New Social Atlas of Britain.* Chichester: John Wiley. [6.6]

Doull, J. A. (1945). 'Tuberculosis mortality in England and certain other countries during the present war'. *The Medical Officer*, 74: 153–5. [12.5.1]

Drabick, J. J., Gambel, J. M., Gouvea, V. S., Caudill, J. D., Sun, W., Hoke, C. H., and Innis, B. L. (1997). 'A cluster of acute hepatitis E infection in United Nations Bangladeshi peacekeepers in Haiti'. *American Journal of Tropical Medicine and Hygiene*, 57: 449–54. [13.5.3]

Dumas, S., and Vedel-Petersen, K. O. (1923). *Losses of Life Caused by War.* Oxford: Clarendon Press. [1.3.2, 8.2, 8.3.1, 11.1, 11.3]

Duncan, L. C. (1918). 'An epidemic of measles and pneumonia in the 31st Division, Camp Wheeler, Ga.' *The Military Surgeon*, 41: 1–13. [4.4.1]

Dunn, F. L. (1993). 'Malaria'. In: Kiple (1993), 855–62. [Appendix 1A]

E

Earle, R. (1996). ' "A grave for Europeans"? Disease, death, and the Spanish–American Revolutions'. *War in History*, 3: 371–83. [2.6.2]

Eckert, E. A. (2000). 'The retreat of plague from central Europe, 1640–1720: a geomedical approach'. *Bulletin of the History of Medicine*, 74: 1–28. [2.4.4]

Edward, Earl of Derby (1865). *The Iliad of Homer, Rendered into English Blank Verse by Edward, Earl of Derby. In Two Volumes* (5th edn.). London: John Murray. [1.1]

Eitrem, R., Vene, S., and Niklasson, B. (1990). 'Incidence of sand fly fever among Swedish United Nations soldiers in Cyprus during 1985'. *American Journal of Tropical Medicine and Hygiene*, 43: 207–11. [13.5.3]

Elias, C. J., Alexander, B. H., and Sokly, T. (1990). 'Infectious disease control in a long-term refugee camp: the role of epidemiologic surveillance and investigation'. *American Journal of Public Health*, 80: 824–8. [5.4.1]

Ell, S. R. (1996). 'Pilgrims, crusades and plagues'. In: M. Waserman and S. S. Kottek, *Health and Disease in the Holy Land: Studies in the History and Sociology of Medicine from Ancient Times to the Present*. Lampeter: The Edwin Mellen Press, 173–87. [2.3.2]

Englehorn, T. D., and Wellman, W. E. (1945). 'Filariasis in soldiers on an island in the South Pacific'. *American Journal of the Medical Sciences*, 209: 141–52. [11.4.2]

Erhardt, C., and Berlin, J. (eds.) (1974). *Mortality and Morbidity in the United States*. Cambridge, Mass.: Harvard University Press. [3.3.4]

Evans, A. S. (1982). *Viral Infections of Humans*. New York: Plenum. [1.3.2]

——and Brachman, P. S. (eds.) (1998). *Bacterial Infections of Humans: Epidemiology and Control* (3rd edn.). New York: Plenum Medical. [Appendix 1A]

——and Kaslow, R. A. (eds.) (1997). *Viral Infections of Humans: Epidemiology and Control* (4th edn.). New York: Plenum Medical. [Appendix 1A]

Ewan, C., Bryant, E., and Calvert, D. (1990). *Health Implications of Long Term Climate Change*. Canberra, ACT: National Health and Medical Research Council of Australia. [3.5.3]

F

Fawcett Commission (Committee of Ladies) (1901). 'Report on the concentration camps in South Africa by the Committee of Ladies appointed by the Secretary of State for War containing reports on the camps in Natal, the Orange River Colony and the Transvaal (1902)'. *Parliamentary Papers*, CD 893. [12.2.1, 12.2.3]

Feibel, R. (1968). 'What happened at Walcheren: the primary medical sources'. *Bulletin of the History of Medicine*, 42: 62–72. [2.4.5]

Feinstein, M., Yesner, R., and Marks, J. L. (1946). 'Epidemics of "Q" fever in troops returning from Italy in the spring of 1945. I. Clinical aspects of the epidemic at Camp Patrick Henry, Virginia'. *American Journal of Hygiene*, 44: 72–81. [8.4.1]

Felsenfeld, O. (1971). *Borrelia: Strains, Vectors, Human and Animal Borreliosis*. St Louis: Warren H. Green. [Appendix 1A]

Fengler J. D. (1995). 'Tuberkulose—Wiederkehr einer vergessenen Infektionskrankheit?' *Zeitschrift für Arztliche Fortbildung und Qualitätssicherung*, 89: 223–7. [12.5.1]

Fenner, F. (1986). 'The eradication of infectious diseases'. *South African Medical Journal*, 66 (suppl.), 35–9. [3.6.1]

——Henderson, D. A., Arita, I., Jesek, Z., and Ladnyi, I. D. (1988). *Smallpox and its Eradication*. Geneva: World Health Organization. [Appendix 1A, 3.6.1, 8.3.1, 8.3.3, 8.3.4, Appendix 12A, 13.6]

Fetter, B., and Kessler, S. (1996). 'Scars from a childhood disease'. *Social Science History*, 20: 593–611. [12.2.1]

Fine, E. M. (1993). 'Herd immunity: history, theory, practice'. *Epidemiological Reviews*, 15: 265–302. [3.5.3]

Fleming, A. F. (1988). 'AIDS in Africa: an update'. *AIDS-Forschung*, 3: 116–34. [10.4.2]

Flinn, M. W. (1981). *The European Demographic System, 1500–1820.* Brighton: Harvester. [3.4.1]

Foner, P. S. (1972). *The Spanish–Cuban–American War and the Birth of American Imperialism* (2 vols.). New York: Monthly Review Press. [7.3.1]

Forrest, J. A. (1939). 'Epidemiological aspects of the A.R. evacuation schemes'. *Medical Officer*, 61: 201. [5.5.1]

Fox, W. F. (1889). *Regimental Losses in the American Civil War, 1861–1865: A Treatise on the Extent and Nature of the Mortuary Losses in the Union Regiments, with Full and Exhaustive Statistics Compiled from the Official Records on File in the State Military Bureaus and at Washington.* Albany, NY: Albany Publishing Company. [1.4.1]

Frohman, C. E. (1965). *Rebels on the Lake: The Piracy, the Conspiracy, Prison Life.* Columbus: Ohio Historical Society. [7.2.2]

Fryauff, D. J., Modi, G. B., Mansour, N. S., Kreutzer, R. D., Soliman, S., and Youssef, F. G. (1993). 'Epidemiology of cutaneous leishmaniasis at a focus monitored by the Multinational Force and Observers in the northeastern Sinai Desert of Egypt'. *American Journal of Tropical Medicine and Hygiene*, 49: 598–607. [13.5.3]

Fuenfer, M. M. (1991). 'The United States Army Special Forces—Walter Reed Army Institute of Research Field Epidemiological Survey Team (Airborne), 1965–1968'. *Military Medicine*, 156: 96–9. [9.6]

Fulton, J. F. (1953). 'Medicine, warfare, and history'. *Journal of the American Medical Association*, 153: 482–8. [1.3.1]

G

Gajdusek, D. C. (1956). 'Hemorrhagic fevers in Asia: a problem in medical ecology'. *Geographical Review*, 45: 20–42. [9.1, 9.2.1, 9.4.1, 9.4.2, 9.6]

Galloway, P. R. (1985). 'Annual variations in deaths by age, deaths by cause, prices, and weather in London, 1670–1830'. *Population Studies*, 39: 487–505. [3.4.1]

——(1986). 'Long-term fluctuations in climate and population in the preindustrial era'. *Population and Development Review*, 12: 1–24. [3.4.1]

Gantenberg, R. (1939). 'Ruhr aus dem Feldzug in Polen 1939'. *Deutsche Medizinische Wochenschrift*, 65: 1789–93, 1820–5. [8.4]

Garfield, R. M. (1989). 'War-related changes in health and health services in Nicaragua'. *Social Science and Medicine*, 28: 669–76. [13.2]

——and Leu, C.-S. (2000). 'A multivariate method for estimating mortality rates among children under 5 years from health and social indicators in Iraq'. *International Journal of Epidemiology*, 29: 510–15. [13.2.1]

——and Neugut, A. I. (1991). 'Epidemiologic analysis of warfare: a historical review'. *Journal of the American Medical Association*, 266: 688–92. [1.2.5, 1.3.1]

————(1997). 'The human consequences of war'. In: B. S. Levy and V. W. Sidel, *War and Public Health.* New York: Oxford University Press, 27–38. [1.2.5]

——and Santana, S. (1997). 'The impact of the economic crisis and the US embargo on health in Cuba'. *American Journal of Public Health*, 87: 15–20. [13.5.2]

Garrison, F. H. (1917). *An Introduction to the History of Medicine, with Medical Chronology, Suggestions for Study and Bibliographic Data*. Philadelphia: W. B. Saunders Co. [2.3.3]

Gernsheim, H., and Gernsheim, A. (1954). *Roger Fenton: Photographer of the Crimean War: His Photographs and his Letters from the Crimea*. London: Secker and Warburg. [8.2.5]

Gibbons, E., and Garfield, R. (1999). 'The impact of economic sanctions on health and human rights in Haiti, 1991–1994'. *American Journal of Public Health*, 89: 1499–504. [13.5.2]

Gibson, J. J., Brodsky, R. E., and Schultz, M. G. (1974). 'Changing patterns of malaria in the United States'. *Journal of Infectious Diseases*, 130: 553–5. [9.5.3]

Gilbert, D. N., Moore, W. L., Hedberg, C. L., and Sanford, J. (1968). 'Potential medical problems in personnel returning from Vietnam'. *Annals of Internal Medicine*, 68: 662–78. [9.5.3]

Girdwood, R. H. (1950). 'The Burma Campaigns—1942–1945: clinical aspects'. *Journal of the Royal Army Medical Corps*, 94: 1–20. [9.3]

Gleditsch, N. P., Wallensteen, P., Eriksson, M., Sollenberg, M., and Strand, H. (2001). 'Armed conflict 1946–2000: a new dataset'. *Euroconference: Identifying Wars: Systematic Conflict Research and its Utility in Conflict Resolution and Prevention*, Uppsala, 8–9 June 2001. (Available at: http://www.pcr.uu.se/workpapers.html. Last viewed 12 Feb. 2003.) [13.2]

Glezen, W. P., and Couch, R. B. (1997). 'Influenza viruses'. In: Evans and Kaslow (1997), 473–505. [Appendix 1A]

Gligić, A., Obradović, M., Stojanović, R., Vujošević, N., Ovćarić, A., Frušic, M., Gibbs, C. J. Jr., Calisher, C. H., and Gajdusek, D. C. (1989). 'Epidemic hemorrhagic fever with renal syndrome in Yugoslavia, 1986'. *American Journal of Tropical Medicine and Hygiene*, 41: 102–8. [13.2.2]

Global Programme for Vaccines and Immunization, World Health Organization (1995). *Immunization Policy*. Geneva: World Health Organization. [3.6.1]

Glover, J. A. (1939–40). 'Evacuation: some epidemiological observations on the first four months'. *Proceedings of the Royal Society of Medicine, Section of Epidemiology and State Medicine*, 33: 399–412. [5.5, 5.5.1]

——(1940). 'Epidemiological aspects of evacuation'. *British Medical Journal*, 1: 629–31. [5.5, 5.5.1, 5.5.3]

Goldfrank, D. M. (1994). *The Origins of the Crimean War*. London: Longman. [8.2.1]

Goma Epidemiology Group (1995). 'Public health impact of Rwandan refugee crisis: what happened in Goma, Zaire, in July, 1994?' *Lancet*, 345: 339–44. [5.7, 13.5.4]

Gooch, B. D. (1956). 'A century of historiography on the origins of the Crimean War'. *American Historical Review*, 60: 33–58. [8.2.1]

——(ed.) (1969). *The Origins of the Crimean War*. Lexington, Mass.: Heath. [8.2.1]

Goodall, C. R. (1991). 'Procrustes methods and the statistical analysis of shape (with discussion)'. *Journal of the Royal Statistical Society*, B53, 285–340. [6.6.2]

Goodall, E. W. (1920). 'Typhus fever in Poland, 1916 to 1919'. *Proceedings of the Royal Society of Medicine, Section of Epidemiology and State Medicine*, 13: 261–76. [12.5.2]

Goodman, A. A., Weinberger, E. M., Lippincott, S. W., Marble, A., and Wright, W. H. (1945). 'Studies of filariasis in soldiers evacuated from the South Pacific'. *Annals of Internal Medicine*, 23: 823–6. [11.4.2]

Gottlieb, M., Schroff, R., Schanker, H. M., Weissman, J. D., Fan, T., Wolf, R. A., and Saxon, A. S. (1981). '*Pneumocystis carinii* pneumonia and mucosal candidiasis in previously healthy homosexual men: evidence of a new acquired cellular immunodeficiency'. *New England Journal of Medicine*, 305: 1425–32. [10.4.1]

Gould, R., and Connell, N. D. (1997). 'The public health effects of biological weapons'. In: B. S. Levy and V. W. Sidel (eds.), *War and Public Health*. Oxford: Oxford University Press, 98–116. [13.4.2]

Gower, J. C. (1975). 'Generalised Procrustes analysis'. *Psychometrika*, 40: 33–50. [6.6.2]

——(1985). 'Measures of similarity, dissimilarity and distance'. In: Kotz and Johnson (1985), 397–405. [Appendix 6A.4]

Grahl-Madsen, A. (1966). *The Status of Refugees in International Law. Volume I: Refugee Character*. Leiden: A. W. Sithoff. [5.2.2]

——(1972). *The Status of Refugees in International Law. Volume II: Asylum, Entry and Sojourn*. Leiden: A. W. Sithoff. [5.2.2]

Gray, G. C., Callahan, J. D., Hawksworth, A. W., Fisher, C. A., and Gaydos, J. C. (1999). 'Respiratory diseases among U.S. military personnel: countering emerging threats'. *Emerging Infectious Diseases*, 5: 379–85. [Introduction to Part III]

Greenberg, J. H. (1969). 'Public health problems relating to the Vietnam returnee'. *Journal of the American Medical Association*, 207: 697–702. [9.5.3]

Greenwood, B., and De Cock, K. (eds.) (1998). *New and Resurgent Infections: Detection and Management of Tomorrow's Infections*. Chichester: Wiley. [9.2.1]

Griffiths, J. T. (1945). 'A scrub typhus (tsutsugamushi) outbreak in Dutch New Guinea'. *Journal of Parasitology*, 31: 341–50. [11.4.2]

Grubler, A., and Nakicenovic, N. (1991). *Evolution of Transport Systems*. Vienna: IIASA Laxenburg. [3.5.3]

Guerra, F. (1978). 'The dispute over syphilis: Europe versus America'. *Clio Medica*, 13: 39–61. [2.3.3]

Gutmann, M. (1977). 'Putting crises in perspective: the impact of war on civilian populations in the seventeenth century'. *Annales de Démographie Historique*, 1: 101–28. [2.4.4]

Guttman, L. (1968). 'A general non-metric technique for finding the smallest coordinate space for a configuration of points'. *Psychometrika*, 33: 469–506. [Appendix 6A.4]

Guttstadt, A. (1873). 'Die Pocken-Epidemie in Preussen, insbesondere in Berlin 1870/72, nebst Beiträgen zur Beurtheilung der Impffrage'. *Zeitschrift des königlich Preussischen Statistichen Bureaus,* 13: 116–58. [1.4.1, 8.1, 8.3, 8.3.1, 8.3.2, 8.3.3]

H

Haggett, P. (1991). 'Some components of global environmental change'. In: Bannister (1991), 5–14. [3.5.3]

——(1992). 'Sauer's "Origins and Dispersals": its implications for the geography of disease'. *Transactions of the Institute of British Geographers*, 17: 387–98. [3.5.3]

——(1994). 'Geographical aspects of the emergence of infectious diseases'. *Geografiska Annaler*, 76B: 91–104. [3.5.3]

——(1995). 'Some epidemiological implications of increased international travel'. In: Proceedings, *Review of International Response to Epidemics and Application of Inter-*

national Health Regulations. Geneva: World Health Organization, WHO Document EMC/IHR/GEN/95.5. [3.5.3]

——(2000). *Geographical Structure of Epidemics*. Oxford: Oxford University Press. [6.7.1, 6.7.2]

——Cliff, A. D., and Frey, A. (1977). *Locational Analysis in Human Geography*. London: Edward Arnold. [12.5.3]

Hall, A. J. (1918). 'Note on an epidemic of toxic ophtherlmoplegia associated with acute asthenia and other nervous manifestations'. *Lancet*, 1: 568–9. [12.5.3]

Hall, R. (1993). *'Notifiable diseases surveillance, 1917–1991'*. Computer spreadsheet, Canberra: Department of Health, Housing, Local Government and Community Services. [3.2.1]

Halperin, S. W. (1973). 'The origins of the Franco-Prussian War revisited: Bismarck and the Hohenzollern candidature for the Spanish throne'. *Journal of Modern History*, 45: 83–91. [8.3.1]

Hamley, E. B. (1891). *The War in the Crimea*. London: Seeley. [8.2.1]

Hand, W. L. (2000). *'Haemophilus* species (including chancroid)'. In: Mandell *et al.* (2000), 2378–83. [Appendix 10A]

Hankins, C. A., Friedman, S. R., Zafar, T., and Strathdee, S. A. (2002). 'Transmission and prevention of HIV and sexually transmitted infections in war settings: implications for current and future armed conflicts'. *AIDS*, 16: 2245–52. [10.4]

Harden, V. A. (1993). 'Typhus, epidemic'. In: Kiple (1993), 1080–4. [Appendix 1A]

Hardy, A. (1993). 'Relapsing fever'. In: Kiple (1993), 967–70. [Appendix 1A]

Harper, P. A., Downs, W. G., Oman, P. W., and Levine, N. D. (1963). 'New Hebrides, Solomon Islands, Saint Matthias Group, and Ryukyu Islands'. In: J. B. Coates (ed.), *Medical Department, United States Army. Preventive Medicine in World War II. Volume VI: Communicable Diseases. Malaria*. Washington: US Government Printing Office, 399–495. [11.4.1, 11.4.2]

Harris, W. (1918). 'Acute infective ophthalmoplegia or botulism'. *Lancet*, 1: 568. [12.5.3]

Hart, T. A., and Hardenbergh, W. H. (1963). 'The Southwest Pacific area'. In: J. B. Coates (ed.), *Medical Department, United States Army. Preventive Medicine in World War II. Volume VI: Communicable Diseases. Malaria*. Washington: US Government Printing Office, 513–80. [11.4.2]

Havers, R. (2000). 'The Changi POW camp and the Burma–Thailand railway'. In: P. Towle, M. Kosuge, and Y. Kibata (eds.), *Japanese Prisoners of War*. London: Hambledon and London, 17–36. [12.4.1]

Hazlett, D. R. (1970). 'Scrub typhus in Vietnam: experience at the 8th Field Hospital'. *Military Medicine*, 135: 31–4. [9.3]

Heaf, F. (1941–2). 'Prevention of tuberculosis in war-time'. *British Journal of Tuberculosis*, 35–6: 127–33. [12.5.1]

Health Organization, League of Nations (1931). *Health*. Geneva: Information Section, League of Nations. [1.4.2]

Health Section, League of Nations (1922). 'Introductory note'. *Epidemiological Intelligence: Eastern Europe in 1921*, E.I.1, 3. [1.4.2]

Heaton, L. D. (1963). *Internal Medicine in World War II, Volume II: Infectious Diseases*. Washington: Department of the Army. [4.4.1]

Hecker, J. F. C. (1859). *The Epidemics of the Middle Ages (Third Edition, Completed by the Author's Treatise on Child–Pilgrimages)*, trans. by B. G. Babington. London: Trübner & Co. [1.1, 2.3.3, 2.4.1]

Heer, F. (1998). *The Medieval World: Europe, 1100–1350*. London: Phoenix. [2.3.2]

Heiser, V. G. (1918). 'Barrack life and respiratory disease: some epidemiologic observations on the recent outbreak of influenza'. *Journal of the American Medical Association*, 71: 1909–11. [7.4.1]

Henderson, D. A. (1999). 'The looming threat of bioterrorism'. *Science*, 283: 1279–82. [13.4.1, 13.4.2]

——(2000). 'Weapons for the future'. *Lancet*, 354 (suppl. IV), 64. [13.4, 13.4.1, 13.4.2]

Henderson-Sellars, A., and Blong, R. J. (1989). *The Greenhouse Effect: Living in a Warmer Australia*. Kensington, Sydney: New South Wales University Press. [3.5.3]

Heng, M. B., and Key, P. J. (1995). 'Cambodian health in transition'. *British Medical Journal*, 311: 435–7. [1.4.3]

Hennock, P. (1998). 'Vaccination policy against smallpox, 1835–1914: a comparison of England with Prussia and Imperial Germany'. *Social History of Medicine*, 11: 49–71. [8.3.4]

Heritage, A. (ed.) (2000). *Dorling Kindersley World Desk Reference* (3rd edn.). London: Dorling Kindersley. [13.2.2]

Herrick, A. B., Crocker, S. B., Harrison, S. A., John, H. J., MacKnight, S. R., and Nyrop, R. F. (eds.) (1969). *Area Handbook for Uganda*. Washington: US Government Printing Office. [10.4.2]

Hesla, P. E. (1992). 'Hepatitis A in Norwegian troops'. *Vaccine*, 10 (suppl. 1), S80–1. [13.5.3]

Hilan, R. (1993). 'The effects on economic development in Syria of a just and long-lasting peace'. In: S. Fischer, D. Rodrik, and E. Tuma (eds.), *The Economics of Middle East Peace: Views From the Region*. Cambridge, Mass.: MIT Press, 55–79. [5.6.3]

Hinrichsen, J. (1944). 'Venereal disease in the major armies and navies of the world'. *American Journal of Syphilis, Gonorrhea, and Venereal Diseases*, 28: 736–72. [Introduction to Part III, 10, 10.1, 10.2, 10.2.1, 10.3.1]

——(1945a). 'Venereal disease in the major armies and navies of the world'. *American Journal of Syphilis, Gonorrhea, and Venereal Diseases*, 29: 80–124. [10.1, 10.2.1]

——(1945b). 'Venereal disease in the major armies and navies of the world'. *American Journal of Syphilis, Gonorrhea, and Venereal Diseases*, 29: 229–67. [10.1, 10.2.1, 10.2.2]

Hirsch, A. (1883). *Handbook of Geographical and Historical Pathology* (3 vols.). trans. from 2nd German edn. by C. Creighton. London: New Sydenham Society. [1.1, 1.3.2, 2.4.1, 2.4.2, 2.4.4, 2.4.5, 2.4.6, 8.2.3, 8.3.1, 11.2.2]

Hirst, F. L. (1953). *The Conquest of Plague*. Oxford: Clarendon Press. [2.2]

Hobhouse E. (1901). *Report of a Visit to the Camps of Women and Children in the Cape and Orange River Colonies*. London: Friars Printing Association Ltd. [12.2.1]

——(1902). *The Brunt of the War, and Where it Fell*. London: Methuen. [12.2.1]

Hoefnagels, L. H. A. (1950). 'Tuberculosis in Holland'. *Tubercle*, 31: 198–209. [12.5.1]

Hoehn, K. (ed.) (1937). *Ulmer Bilder-Chronik*, iv. Ulm: Verlag. [1.3.2]

Hoff, E. C. (ed.) (1955–69). *United States: Army Medical Service: Preventive Medicine in World War II*. Washington: US Army, Surgeon General's Office. [1.4.1]

——(ed.) (1958). United States. *Army Medical Service. Preventive Medicine in World War II: Volume IV. Communicable Diseases Transmitted Chiefly through Respiratory and Alimentary Tracts*. Washington: US Government Printing Office. [4.4.1, 4.5.1]

Holladay, A. J. (1986). 'The Thucydides syndrome: another view'. *New England Journal of Medicine*, 315: 1170–3. [2.2]

Hooper, E. (1990). *Slim: A Reporter's Own Story of AIDS in East Africa*. London: Bodley Head. [10.4.2]

Hopkins, D. R. (1983). *Princes and Peasants: Smallpox in History*. Chicago and London: University of Chicago Press. [1.1, 2.6.2, Appendix 12A]

Hoskins, E. (1997). 'Public health and the Persian Gulf War'. In: B. S. Levy and V. W. Sidel (eds.), *War and Public Health*. New York: Oxford University Press, 254–78. [13.2.1, 13.5.5]

Howard, M. (1961). *The Franco-Prussian War: The German Invasion of France, 1870–1871*. London: Methuen. [8.3.1]

Howard, M. R. (1991). 'Medical aspects of Sir John Moore's Corunna Campaign, 1808–1809'. *Journal of the Royal Society of Medicine*, 84: 299–302. [2.4.5]

——(1999). 'Walcheren 1809: a medical catastrophe'. *British Medical Journal*, 319: 1642–5. [2.4.5]

Huerkamp, C. (1985). 'The history of smallpox vaccination in Germany: a first step in the medicalization of the general public'. *Journal of Contemporary History*, 20: 617–35. [8.3.4]

Hughes, J. M. (1999). 'The emerging threat of bioterrorism'. *Emerging Infectious Diseases*, 5: 494–5. [13.4.3]

Hukic, M., Kurt, A., Torstensson, S., Lundkvist, Å., Wiger, D., and Niklasson, B. (1996). 'Haemorrhagic fever with renal syndrome in north-east Bosnia'. *Lancet*, 347: 56–7. [13.2.2]

Hulse, E. V. (1971). 'Joshua's curse and the abandonment of ancient Jericho: schistosomiasis as a possible medical explanation'. *Medical History*, 15: 376–86. [2.2]

Hunt, C. W. (1989). 'Migrant labour and sexually transmitted disease: AIDS in Africa'. *Journal of Health and Social Behaviour*, 30: 353–73. [10.4.2]

Hunter, G. W. (1953). 'Local health hazards among US Army troops returning from Korea'. *American Journal of Public Health and the Nation's Health*, 43: 1408–17. [9.4, 9.4.1]

Hunter, R. (1991) 'The English sweating sickness, with particular reference to the 1551 outbreak in Chester'. *Reviews of Infectious Diseases*, 13: 303–6. [1.1, 2.3.3]

Hunter, W. (1920). 'The Serbia epidemics of typhus and relapsing fever in 1915: the origin, course, and preventive measures employed for their arrest'. *Proceedings of the Royal Society of Medicine, Section of Epidemiology and State Medicine*, 13: 29–158. [12.5.2]

Hyams, K. C., Wignall, F. S., and Roswell, R. (1996). 'War syndromes and their evaluation: from the U.S. Civil War to the Persian Gulf War'. *Annals of Internal Medicine*, 125: 398–405. [13.5.5]

Hymes, K. B., Cheung, T., Greene, J. B., Prose, N. S., Marcus, A., Ballard, H., William, D. C., and Laubenstein, L. J. (1981). 'Kaposi's sarcoma in homosexual men—a report of eight cases'. *Lancet*, 2: 598–600. [10.4.1]

I

ICRC (1950). *Internal and Contagious Diseases in Prisoner of War and Civilian Internee Camps during the Second World War*. Geneva: Medical Division, International Committee of the Red Cross. [1.4.2, 10.3.2]

Illingworth, R. S. (1945). 'Poliomyelitis and meningismus: a hundred cases'. *Journal of the Royal Army Medical Corps*, 84: 210–17. [12.5.4]

Ingham, F. J. (1953). 'Discussion on military medical problems in Korea: army health problems'. *Proceedings of the Royal Society of Medicine, United Services Section*, 46: 1041–6. [9.4]

Intergovernmental Panel on Climatic Change (1990). *Scientific Assessment of Climate Change: Report Prepared for IPCC by Working Group 1*. Geneva: World Meteorological Organization. [3.5.3]

Irons, E. N., and Armstrong, H. E. (1947). 'Scrub typhus in Dutch New Guinea'. *Annals of Internal Medicine*, 26: 201–20. [11.4.2]

J

Jackson, T. (1999). *The Boer War*. London: Channel 4 Books, Macmillan Ltd. [12.2]

Jacobi, J., Kreyenberg, G., and Dörschel, W. (1943). 'Erfahrungen bei ueber 600 Kranken mit hepatitis epidemica'. *Deutsche Militärarzt*, 8: 479–86. [8.4]

James, L. (1981). *Crimea 1854–56: The War with Russia from Contemporary Photographs*. New York: Van Nostrand Reinhold. [8.2.5]

Johnson, N. P. A. S. (2001). 'Aspects of the Historical Geography of the 1918–19 Influenza Pandemic in Britain'. Unpublished Ph.D. thesis, Department of Geography, University of Cambridge. [12.5.3]

—— and Mueller, J. (2002). 'Updating the accounts: global mortality of the 1918–1920 "Spanish" influenza pandemic'. *Bulletin of the History of Medicine*, 76: 105–15. [11.3, 11.3.4]

Johnston, W. D. (1993). 'Tuberculosis'. In: Kiple (1993), 1059–68. [Appendix 1A, 12.5.1]

Jones, E., and Wessely, S. (1999). 'Chronic fatigue syndrome after the Crimean War and the Indian Mutiny'. *British Medical Journal*, 319: 1645–7. [13.5.5]

—— Hodgins-Vermaas, R., McCartney, H., Everitt, B., Beech, C., Poynter, D., Palmer, I., Hyams, K., and Wessely, S. (2002). 'Post-combat syndromes from the Boer war to the Gulf war: a cluster analysis of their nature and attribution'. *British Medical Journal*, 324: 321–4. [13.5.5]

Jones, W. S. (1969). 'Chinese liaison detail'. In: J. H. Stone (ed.), *Crisis Fleeting: Original Reports on Military Medicine in India and Burma in the Second World War*. Washington: US Government Printing Office, 69–134. [9.3.1]

Jordan, E. O. (1927). *Epidemic Influenza: A Survey*. Chicago: American Medical Association. [11.3]

Jowett, B. (1900). *Thucydides: Volume I: Essay on Inscriptions and Books 1–III* (2nd edn., rev.). Oxford: Clarendon Press. [2.2, 5.2]

Joy, R. J. T. (1999). 'Malaria in American troops in the South and Southwest Pacific in World War II'. *Medical History*, 43: 192–207. [11.4.2]

K

Kalipeni, E., and Oppong, J. (1998). 'The refugee crisis in Africa and implications for health and disease: a political ecology approach'. *Social Science and Medicine*, 46: 1637–53. [5.1, 5.2.3, 5.4]

Kanesa-thasan, N., Iacono-Connors, L., Magill, A., Smoak, B., Vaughn, D., Dubois, D., Burrous, J., and Hoke, C. (1994). 'Dengue serotypes 2 and 3 in US forces in Somalia'. *Lancet*, 343: 678. [13.5.3]

Kawamura, A., Tanaka, H., and Tamura, A. (eds.) (1995). *Tsutsugamushi Disease*. Tokyo: University of Tokyo Press. [9.3]

Keegan, J. (1989). *The Second World War*. London: Hutchinson. [10.3]

——(1994). *A Brief History of Warfare—Past, Present and Future*. The Sixth Wellington Lecture. Southampton: University of Southampton. [13.2]

Keja, J., and Henderson, R. (1984). 'The Expanded Programme on Immunization: global overview'. World Health Organization Second Conference on Immunization Policies, Karlovy Vary, 10–12 Dec. [13.6]

Kempthorne, G. A. (1930). 'The Egyptian Campaign of 1801'. *Journal of the Royal Army Medical Corps*, 55: 217–30. [2.4.5]

Keshavjee, S., and Becerra, M. C. (2000). 'Disintegrating health services and resurgent tuberculosis in post-Soviet Tajikistan: an example of structural violence'. *Journal of the American Medical Association*, 283: 1201. [9.1, 13.5.4]

Kessler S. (1999*a*). 'Brutal truth behind "sacred history"'. *Cape Argus Post (South Africa)*, 2 Feb.: 15. [12.2.2]

——(1999*b*). 'Graves hide suffering of blacks in Boer War'. *Daily Telegraph*, 22 Apr.: 23. [12.2.2]

Keusch, G. T., and Bennish, M. L. (1998). 'Shigellosis'. In: Evans and Brachman (1998), 631–56. [Appendix 1A]

Khlat, M., and Khoury, M. (1991). 'Inbreeding and diseases: demographic, genetic and inbreeding perspectives'. *Epidemiological Reviews*, 13: 28–41. [3.5.3]

Kiefer, C. W. (1992). 'Militarism and world health'. *Social Science and Medicine*, 34: 719–24. [13.5.1]

Kilbourne, E. D. (1987). *Influenza*. New York: Plenum. [Appendix 1A, 11.3]

Kim-Farley, R. J. (1993). 'Measles'. In: Kiple (1993), 871–5. [Appendix 1A]

Kinglake, A. W. (1863). *The Invasion of the Crimea: Its Origin, and an Account of its Progress down to the Death of Lord Raglan* (8 vols.). Edinburgh and London: W. Blackwood and Sons. [8.2.1]

Kinlen, L. J., and John, S. M. (1994). 'Wartime evacuation and mortality from childhood leukaemia in England and Wales in 1945–9'. *British Medical Journal*, 309: 1197–202. [5.5.5]

Kinvig, C. (2000). 'Allied POWs and the Burma–Thailand railway'. In: P. Towle, M. Kosuge, and Y. Kibata (eds.), *Japanese Prisoners of War*. London: Hambledon and London, 37–57. [12.4.2]

Kiple, K. F. (ed.) (1993). *The Cambridge World History of Human Disease*. Cambridge: Cambridge University Press. [Appendix 1A]

Kirby, P. R. (1965). *Sir Andrew Smith, M. D., K. C. B.: His Life, Letters and Works*. Cape Town: A. A. Balkema. [8.2.2]

Kohn, G. C. (1998). *Encyclopedia of Plague and Pestilence*. Ware, Herts.: Wordsworth. [1.1, 2.2, 2.3.1, 2.3.2, 2.3.3, 2.4.4, 2.4.5, 2.4.6, 2.5.1, 2.6.2, 9.5.2, 11.1]

——(1999). *Dictionary of Wars* (rev. edn.). New York: Checkmark. [1.2.3, 1.3.3, 2.1, 13.2.1]

Kohn, S., and Meyendorff, A. F. (1932). *The Cost of the War to Russia: The Vital Statistics of European Russia during the World War, 1914–1917*. Carnegie Endowment for International Peace. New Haven: Yale University Press. [4.4.1]

Kotz, S., and Johnson, N. L. (eds.) (1985). *Encyclopaedia of the Statistical Sciences*, v. New York: John Wiley and Sons, Inc. [Appendix 8B]

Krause, R. M. (ed.) (1998). *Emerging Infections: Biomedical Research Reports.* San Diego: Academic Press. [9.2.1]

Kreidberg, M. A., and Henry, M. G. (1975). *History of Military Mobilization in the United States Army, 1775–1945.* Westport, Conn.: Greenwood Press. [7.1, 7.2.2, 7.3.1, 7.3.3, 7.3.5, 7.4.1]

Krogstad, D. J. (2000). 'Plasmodium species (malaria)'. In: Mandell *et al.* (2000), 2817–31. [Appendix 1A]

Kruskal, J. B. (1964*a*). 'Multidimensional scaling by optimizing goodness of fit to a nonmetric hypothesis'. *Psychometrika*, 29: 1–27. [Appendix 6A.4]

——(1964*b*). 'Nonmetric multidimensional scaling: a numerical method'. *Psychometrika*, 29: 115–29. [Appendix 6A.4]

Kuhn, H. W., and Kuenne, R. E. (1962). 'An efficient algorithm for the numerical solution of the generalised Weber problem in spatial economics'. *Journal of Regional Science*, 4: 21–33. [Appendix 6A.3]

Kunitz, S. J. (1986). 'Mortality since Malthus'. In: D. Coleman and R. Schofield (eds.), *The State of Population Theory*. Oxford: Blackwell. [3.4.1]

——(1991). 'The personal physician and the decline of mortality'. In: Schofield *et al.* (1991), 248–62. [3.4.1]

Kunz, E. (1973). 'The refugee in flight: kinetic models and forms of displacement'. *International Migration Review*, 7: 125–46. [5.2.3]

——(1981). 'Exile and resettlement: refugee theory'. *International Migration Review*, 15: 42–51. [5.2.3]

L

Lambert, S. M. (1934). *The Depopulation of Pacific Races*. B.P.B.M. Special Publication 23, Honolulu. [11.3.4]

Lancaster, H. O. (1990). *Expectations of Life: A Study in the Demography, Statistics, and History of World Mortality.* New York: Springer-Verlag. [1.2.4, 1.2.5, 1.3.2, 1.4.1, 2.4.2, 3.4.2, 3.4.3, 4.1, 4.3.1, 4.4.1, 8.4, 12.5.1]

Landers, J. (1993). *Death and the Metropolis: Studies in the Demographic History of London 1670–1830.* Cambridge: Cambridge University Press. [3.4.1]

Langford, C. (2002). 'The age pattern of mortality in the 1918–19 influenza pandemic: an attempted explanation based on data for England and Wales'. *Medical History*, 46: 1–20. [11.3, 12.5.3]

Larson, A. (1990). 'The social epidemiology of Africa's AIDS epidemic'. *African Affairs*, 89: 5–25. [10.4.2]

LeBaron, C. W., and Taylor, D. W. (1993). 'Typhoid Fever'. In: Kiple (1993), 1071–7. [Appendix 1A]

Lederberg, J. (1998). 'Emerging infections: an evolutionary perspective'. *Emerging Infectious Diseases*, 4: 366–71. [9.2.1]

——Shope, R. E., and Oaks, S. C. (eds.) (1992). *Emerging Infections: Microbial Threats to Health in the United States.* Washington: National Academy Press. [3.5.2, 9.2.1, 9.5, 9.5.3]

Lee, H. W. (1989). 'Hemorrhagic fever with renal syndrome in Korea'. *Reviews of Infectious Diseases*, 11 (suppl. 4), S864–76. [9.4.2]

——and Dalrymple, J. M. (1989). *Manual of Hemorrhagic Fever with Renal Syndrome*. Seoul: WHO Collaborating Centre for Virus Reference and Research (Haemorrhagic Fever with Renal Syndrome), Institute for Viral Diseases, Korea University. [9.4.2]

Leishman, A. W. D. (1944). 'An outbreak of smallpox in British troops with a note on the use of sulphathiazole in treatment'. *Journal of the Royal Army Medical Corps*, 82: 58–62. [9.3]

——and Kelsall, A. R. (1944). 'A year of military medicine in India'. *Lancet*, 2: 231–5. [9.3]

Le Goff, J. (1988). *Medieval Civilization, 400–1500*. Oxford: Basil Blackwell. [2.3.2]

Leslie, R. M. (1915–16). 'Tuberculosis and the war'. *British Journal of Tuberculosis*, 9–10: 71–7. [12.5.1]

Levie, H. S. (1986). *The Code of International Armed Conflict*, i. London: Oceana Publications. [1.2.4]

Levine, M. M. (1998). 'Typhoid fever'. In: Evans and Brachman (1998), 839–58. [Appendix 1A]

Levy, B. S., and Sidel, V. W. (1997). 'The impact of military activities on civilian populations'. In: B. S. Levy and V. W. Sidel, *War and Public Health*. New York: Oxford University Press, 149–67. [12.5.1, 13.5.1, 13.5.2]

——Shahi, G. S., and Lee, C. (1997). 'The environmental consequences of war'. In: B. S. Levy and V. W. Sidel (eds.), *War and Public Health*. Oxford: Oxford University Press, 51–62. [13.5.1]

Lilienfield, L. S., Rose, J. C., and Corn, M. (1986). 'UNRWA and the health of Palestinian refugees'. *New England Journal of Medicine*, 315: 595–600. [5.6.1, 5.6.2, 5.6.4]

Lincoln, A. F., and Sivertson, S. E. (1952). 'Acute phase of Japanese B encephalitis: two hundred and one cases in American soldiers, Korea, 1950'. *Journal of the American Medical Association*, 150: 268–73. [9.2.2, 9.4, 9.4.1]

Lingoes, J. C., and Roskam, E. E. (1973). 'A mathematical and empirical analysis of two multidimensional scaling algorithms'. *Psychometrika*, 38, monograph supplt. [Appendix 6A.4]

Local Government Board (1919). *Forty-Eighth Annual Report of the Local Government Board, 1918–1919: Supplement Containing the Report of the Medical Department for 1918–19*. London: HMSO. [Appendix 1B, 12.5.3]

Lodge, H. C. (1899). *The War with Spain*. New York: Harper and Brothers. [7.3.1]

Logan, W. P. D. (1950). 'Mortality in England and Wales from 1848–1947'. *Population Studies*, 4: 132–78. [3.2.2]

Long, E. R. (1948). 'Tuberculosis in Germany'. *Proceedings of the National Academy of Sciences, USA*, 34: 271–7. [12.5.1]

Lovell, W. G. (1992). 'Disease and depopulation in early colonial Guatemala'. In: N. D. Cook and W. G. Lovell (eds.), *'Secret Judgements of God': Old World Disease in Colonial Spanish America*. Norman, Okla.: University of Oklahoma Press, 49–83. [2.6.1]

Low, N., Davy Smith, G., Gorter, A., and Arauz, R. (1990). 'AIDS and migrant populations in Nicaragua'. *Lancet*, 336: 1593–4. [10.4.2]

Low-Beer, D., Smallman-Raynor, M., and Cliff, A. D. (forthcoming). 'Mortality during the South African War: the crossing of military and refugee disease histories'. *Social History of Medicine*. [12.2, 12.2.1, 12.2.2, 12.2.3]

Luby, J., Schultz, M. G., Nowosiwsky, T., and Kaiser, R. L. (1967). 'Introduced malaria at Fort Benning, Georgia, 1964–1965'. *American Journal of Tropical Medicine and Hygiene*, 16: 146–53. [9.5.3]

Lynch, C., Weed, F. W., and McAfee, L. (eds.) (1923–9). *The Official History Series for World War I: The Medical Department of the United States Army in the World War.* Washington: US Army, Surgeon General's Office. [1.4.1]

Lysons, D. (1895). *The Crimean War from First to Last.* London: J. Murray. [8.2.1]

M

McAlpine, D. (1945). 'Epidemiology of acute poliomyelitis in India command'. *Lancet*, 2: 130. [12.5.4]

McArthur, N. (1968). *Island Populations of the Pacific.* Canberra: Australian National University Press. [11.1, 11.2, 11.2.1, 11.2.2, 11.3.4, 11.5]

McCarthy, M., Estes, M. K., and Hyams, K. C. (2000). 'Norwalk-like virus infection in military forces: epidemic potential, sporadic disease, and the future direction of prevention and control efforts'. *Journal of Infectious Diseases*, 181: 387–91. [13.2.3]

——Hyams, K. C., El-Tigani El-Hag, A., El-Dabi, M. A., El-Sadig El-Tayeb, M., Khalid, I. O., George, J. F., Constantine, N. T., and Woody, J. N. (1989). 'HIV-1 and hepatitis B transmission in Sudan'. *AIDS*, 3: 725–9. [10.4, 10.4.2]

McCoy, O. R., and Sabin, A. B. (1964). 'Dengue'. In: J. B. Coates (ed.), *Medical Department, United States Army: Preventive Medicine in World War II: Volume VII: Communicable Diseases: Anthropodborne Diseases other than Malaria.* Washington: US Government Printing Office, 29–62. [11.4.2]

McElroy, J. (1879). *Andersonville: A Story of Rebel Military Prisons. Fifteen Months a Guest of the So-called Southern Confederacy, A Private Soldier's Experience in Richmond, Andersonville, Savannah, Millen, Blackshear and Florence.* Toledo: D. R. Locke. [7.2.2]

McEvedy, C. (1988). 'The bubonic plague'. *Scientific American*, 254: 3–12. [2.3.3]

McGrew, R. E. (1965). *Russia and the Cholera, 1823–1832.* Madison: University of Wisconsin Press. [1.1, 2.4.6]

McGuffie, T. H. (1947). 'The Walcheren Expedition and the Walcheren fever'. *English Historical Review*, 62: 191–202. [1.1, 2.4.5]

McKeown, T. (1976). *The Modern Rise of Population.* London: Edward Arnold. [3.4.1, 3.4.2]

Mackie, T. T. (1946). 'Observations on tsutsugamushi disease (scrub typhus) in Assam and Burma: preliminary report'. *Transactions of the Royal Society of Tropical Medicine and Hygiene*, 40: 15–56. [9.3.1, 9.6]

MacNalty, A. (1940). 'The public health in wartime'. *British Medical Journal*, 1: 333–6. [5.5.1]

——(ed.-in-chief) (1952–72). *History of the Second World War: United Kingdom Medical Series.* London: HMSO. [1.4.1]

McNeill, W. H. (1976). *Plagues and Peoples.* Oxford: Basil Blackwell. [2.2, 2.6.1]

McNinch, J. H. (1953). 'Far East Command Conference on Epidemic Hemorrhagic Fever: introduction'. *Annals of Internal Medicine*, 38: 53–60. [9.4, 9.4.2]

Macpherson, W. G., Herringham, W. P., Elliott, T. R., and Balfour, A. (eds.) (1922–3). *History of the Great War Based on Official Documents: Medical Services, Diseases of the War* (2 vols.). London: HMSO. [1.4.1, 4.4.1, 8.4, 9.1, 11.3.1, 12.5.3]

McQueen, H. (1975). ' "Spanish flu" 1919: political, medical and social aspects'. *Medical Journal of Australia*, 1: 565–70. [11.3.2]

McSherry, J. (1993). 'Dengue'. In: Kiple (1993), 660–4. [11.4.2]

Magee, J. C. (1941). 'Establishment of a board for the investigation of influenza and other epidemic diseases in the army'. *Journal of the American Medical Association*, 116: 512. [7.4.2]

Major, R. (1940). *War and Disease*. London: Hutchinson. [1.1, 1.3.1, 1.3.2, 2.2, 2.3.2, 2.4.5, 8.1, 8.4, 10.1]

Mandell, G. L., Bennett, J. E., and Dolin, R. (eds.) (2000). *Principles and Practice of Infectious Diseases*: ii. New York: Churchill Livingstone. [Appendix 1A]

Mann, J. M., Chin, J., Piot, P., and Quinn, T. C. (1988). 'The international epidemiology of AIDS'. *Scientific American*, 259: 60–9. [10.4.1]

Markotić, A., Sarcevic, A., and Hlaca, D. (1994). 'Znacaj brze dijagnostike hemoragicne groznice sa bubreznim sindromom (HFRS) u ratu'. *Medicinski Arhiv*, 48: 109–11. [13.2.2]

Marks, G., and Beatty, W. K. (1976). *Epidemics*. New York: Charles Scribner's Sons. [2.6.1]

Marriott, H. L. (1945). 'Medical problems of South-East Asia Command'. *Lancet*, 1: 679–84. [9.3]

—— Hill, I. G. W., Hawksley, J. C., and Bomford, R. R. (1946). 'Medical experiences of the war in the South-East Asia Command'. *Transactions of the Royal Society of Tropical Medicine and Hygiene*, 39: 461–84. [9.3]

Marrus, M. R. (1985). *The Unwanted: European Refugees in the Twentieth Century*. Oxford: Oxford University Press. [5.1, 5.2]

Marshall, I. H. (1954). 'Hemorrhagic fever. I. Epidemiology'. *American Journal of Tropical Medicine and Hygiene*, 3: 587–600. [9.4.2]

Marshall, J. D., Joy, R. J. T., Ai, N. V., Quy, D. V., Stockard, J. L., and Gibson, F. L. (1967). 'Plague in Vietnam 1965–66'. *American Journal of Epidemiology*, 86: 603–16. [9.2.2, 9.5.2]

Massey, D. (1999). 'Space–time, "science" and the relationship between physical geography and human geography'. *Transactions of the Institute of British Geographers, New Series*, 24: 261–76. [6.6]

Masur, H., Michelis, M. A., Greene, J. B., Onorato, I., Van de Stouwe, R. A., Holzman, R. S., Wormser, G., Brettman, L., Lange, M., Murray, H. W., and Cunningham-Rundles, S. (1981). 'An outbreak of community-acquired *Pneumocystis carinii* pneumonia: initial manifestations of cellular immune dysfunction'. *New England Journal of Medicine*, 305: 1431–8. [10.4.1]

Maxcy, K. F. (1973). 'Epidemiology'. *Encyclopaedia Britannica*, viii: 640–3. [1.3.2]

Mayda, J. (1962). 'Geneva Conventions'. *Encyclopaedia Britannica*, x: 114. [1.2.4]

Medical Department, United States Army (1960). *Preventive Medicine in World War II. Volume V: Communicable Diseases Transmitted through Contact or by Unknown Means*. Washington: US Government Printing Office. [10.3.1]

Medical Research Committee (1919). *An Inquiry into the Prevalence and Aetiology of Tuberculosis among Industrial Workers, with Special Reference to Female Munition Workers*. London: HMSO. [12.5.1]

—— (1942). *Report of the Committee on Tuberculosis in War-Time*. London: HMSO. [12.5.1]

Megaw, J. W. D. (1944). [Untitled]. *Bulletin of War Medicine*, 4: 734–5. [7.4.2]

—— (1945). 'Scrub typhus as a war disease'. *British Medical Journal*, 2: 109–12. [9.3.1]

Mellor, W. F. (ed.) (1972). *Casualties and Medical Statistics*: *History of the Second World War*: *United Kingdom Medical Series*. London: HMSO. [1.4.3, 4.5.1]

Meselson, M., Guillemin, J., Hugh-Jones, M., Langmuir, A., Popova, I., Shelokov, A., and Yampolskaya, O. (1994). 'The Sverdlovsk anthrax outbreak of 1979'. *Science*, 266: 1202–8. [13.4.2]

Millis, W. (1931). *The Martial Spirit*: *A Study of Our War with Spain*. Cambridge, Mass.: The Riverside Press. [7.3.1]

Ministère de la Guerre (1922). *Pandémie de Grippe du 1er Mai 1918 au 30 Avril 1919*. Paris: Imprimerie Nationale. [1.4.1]

——(1932). *Aperçu Statistique sur l'Évolution de la Morbidité et de la Mortalité Générales dans l'Armée et sur l'Évolution de la Morbidité et de la Mortalité Particulières à Certaines Maladies Contagieuses de 1862 Jusqu'à nos Jours*. Paris: Imprimerie Nationale. [10.2, 10.2.1]

Ministry of Health (1920). *Report on the Pandemic of Influenza, 1918–19*. Reports on Public Health and Medical Subjects, No. 4. London: HMSO. [7.4.1, 11.3, 11.3.1, 12.5.3]

——(1946). *On the State of the Public Health during Six Years of War*: *Twenty-First Report of the Chief Medical Officer*. London: HMSO. [5.5.1, 5.5.5]

Mitchell, B. R. (1998). *International Historical Statistics*: *Europe, 1750–1993* (4th edn.). Basingstoke: Macmillan. [8.3.1]

Mohammed Ali, O., Bwayo, J. J., Mutere, A. N., Jaoko, W., Plummer, F. A., and Kreiss, J. K. (1990). 'Sexual behaviour of long-distance truck drivers and their contribution to the spread of sexually transmitted diseases and HIV infection in East Africa'. *Proceedings of the VI International Conference on AIDS*, San Francisco, 20–4 June, Abstract F.C.729. [10.4.2]

Mollison, D. (1977). 'Spatial contact models for ecological and epidemic spread'. *Journal of the Royal Statistical Society B*, 39: 283–326. [Appendix 6A.2]

——(1991). 'Dependence of epidemic and population velocities on basic parameters'. *Mathematical Biosciences*, 107: 255–87. [Appendix 6A.2]

Morens, D. M., and Littman, R. J. (1992). 'Epidemiology of the Plague of Athens'. *Transactions of the American Philological Association*, 122: 271–304. [2.2]

Morin, K., and Miles, S. (2000). 'The health effects of economic sanctions and embargoes: the role of health professionals'. *Annals of Internal Medicine*, 132: 158–61. [13.5.2]

Morris, B. (1987). *The Birth of the Palestinian Refugee Problem, 1947–1949*. Cambridge: Cambridge University Press. [5.6]

Morse, S. S. (1995). 'Factors in the emergence of infectious diseases'. *Emerging Infectious Diseases*, 1: 7–15. [9.2.1]

Munro-Faure, A. D., Andrew, R., Missen, G. A. K., and Mackay-Dick, J. (1951). 'Scrub typhus in Korea'. *Journal of the Royal Army Medical Corps*, 97: 227–9. [9.3]

Munson, E. L. (1917). 'An epidemiological study of an outbreak of measles, Camp Wilson, Tex.'. *The Military Surgeon*, 11: 6–12. [4.4.1]

Murray, C. J. L., King, G., Lopez, A. D., Tomijima, N., and Krug, E. G. (2002). 'Armed conflict as a public health problem'. *British Medical Journal*, 324: 346–9. [1.3.1, 13.2]

——and Lopez, A. D. (1996). *Global Burden of Disease and Injury Series, Volume I*: *The Global Burden of Disease*: *A Comprehensive Assessment of Mortality and Disability from Diseases, Injuries, and Risk Factors in 1990 and Projected to 2020*. Harvard, Mass.: Harvard School of Public Health. [13.6]

N

Nathanson, N., and Nichol, S. (1998). 'Korean hemorrhagic fever and Hantavirus pulmonary syndrome: two examples of emerging hantaviral diseases'. In: Krause (1998), 365–74. [9.4.2]

Neel, S. (1973). *Vietnam Studies: Medical Support of the U.S. Army in Vietnam, 1965–1970*. Washington: US Government Printing Office. [9.2.1, 9.2.2, 9.5, 9.5.1, 9.5.2, 9.5.3]

Newman, L. M., Miguel, F., Jemusse, B. B., Macome, A. C., and Newman, R. D. (2001). 'HIV seroprevalence among military blood donors in Manica Province, Mozambique'. *International Journal of STD and AIDS*, 12: 225–8. [10.4.2]

N'Galy, B., and Ryder, R. W. (1988). 'Epidemiology of HIV infection in Africa'. *Journal of Acquired Immune Deficiency Syndromes*, 1: 551–8. [10.4.2]

Nickerson, H., and Wright, Q. (1962). 'War'. *Encyclopaedia Britannica*, 23: 321–36. [1.2, 1.2.2, 1.2.3]

Norton, S. A., Frankenburg, S., and Klau, S. N. (1992). 'Cutaneous leishmaniasis acquired during military service in the Middle East'. *Archives of Dermatology*, 128: 83–7. [13.5.3]

Nowosiwsky, T. (1967). 'The epidemic curve of *Plasmodium falciparum* malaria in a nonimmune population: American troops in Vietnam, 1965 and 1966'. *American Journal of Epidemiology*, 86: 461–7. [9.5.1]

O

O'Higgins, P., and Jones, N. (1999). *Morphologika: Tools for Shape Analysis*. University College London (Available at: http://evolution.anat.ucl.ac.uk/morph/helphtmls/morph.html. Last viewed 12 Feb. 2003.) [6.6.2]

Oficino del Censo de los Estados Unidos (1908). *Censo de la República de Cuba Bajo la Administración Provisional de los Estados Unidos*. Washington: US Government Printing Office. [12.3]

Offner, J. (1992). *An Unwanted War: The Diplomacy of the United States and Spain over Cuba, 1895–1898*. London: University of North Carolina Press. [7.3.1]

Ogden, P. E. (1984). *Migration and Geographical Change*. Cambridge: Cambridge University Press. [3.4.4]

Ollivier, E. (1913). *The Franco-Prussian War and its Hidden Causes*. London: Sir Isaac Pitman and Sons. [8.3.1]

Olson, E., Hames, C. S., Benenson, A. S., and Genovese, E. N. (1996). 'The Thucydides Syndrome: Ebola déjà vu? (or Ebola reemergent?)'. *Emerging Infectious Diseases*, 2: 155–6. [2.2]

Omara-Otunnu, A. (1987). *Politics and the Military in Uganda*. London: Macmillan Press. [10.4.2]

Ongom, V. L. (1970). 'Prevelance and incidence of venereal diseases in military communities in Uganda'. *East African Medical Journal*, 47: 479–83. [10.4.2]

Openshaw, S. (1984). *The Modifiable Areal Unit Problem Concepts and Techniques in Modern Geography*. Norwich: Geo Books. [6.6.2]

Oxford, J. S. (2000). 'Influenza A pandemics of the 20th century with special reference to 1918: virology, pathology and epidemiology'. *Reviews in Medical Virology*, 10: 119–33. [1.1, 9.2.1, 11.3, 11.3.1, 12.5.3]

Oxford, J. S., Sefton, A., Jackson, R., Johnson, N. P. A. S., and Daniels, R. S. (1999). 'Who's that lady'. *Nature Medicine*, 5: 1351–2. [11.3, 11.3.1, 12.5.3]

P

Padley, R., and Cole, M. (eds.) (1940). *Evacuation Survey: A Report to the Fabian Society*. London: Routledge. [5.5.1]

Pagès, G. (1970). *The Thirty Years War, 1618–1648*, trans. D. Maland and J. Hooper from the French, *La Guerre de Trente Ans*, Paris: Payot. Edinburgh: R. & R. Clark. [2.4.2]

Pakenham, T. (1979). *The Boer War*. London: George Weidenfeld & Nicolson Ltd. [12.2, 12.2.1, 12.2.2, 12.2.3, 12.2.4, 12.2.5]

Palha de Sousa, C., Barreto, J., de la Cruz, J., Barquet, L., Bomba, A., Chomera, L., Costa, P., Faustino, H., and Mondlane, C. (1989). 'The influence of war on HIV epidemic in Mozambique'. *Proceedings of V International Conference on AIDS*, Montreal, 4–9 June, Abstract Th.G.23. [1.1, 10.4, 10.4.2]

Palmer, A. (1987). *The Banner of Battle: The Story of the Crimean War*. London: Weidenfeld and Nicolson Ltd. [8.2.1]

Palmer, S. R. (1993). 'Q fever'. In: Kiple (1993), 957–61. [8.4, 8.4.1]

Pappas, J. (1943). 'The venereal disease problem, United States Army'. *Military Surgeon*, 93: 172–83. [10.1, 10.3.1]

Parish, H. J. (1968). *Victory with Vaccine: The Story of Immunization*. Edinburgh: E. & S. Livingstone. [4.7]

Parker, G. (1984). *The Thirty Years' War*. London: Routledge and Kegan Paul. [2.4.2]

Parsons, A. C., MacNalty, A. S., and Perdrau, J. R. (1922). *Report on Encephalitis Lethargica*. Reports on Public Health and Medical Subjects, No. 11. London: HMSO. [12.5.3]

Patterson, K. D. (1993a). 'Bacillary dysentery'. In: Kiple (1993), 604–6. [1.3.2, Appendix 1A]

——(1993b). 'Amebic dysentery'. In: Kiple (1993), 568–71. [1.3.2, Appendix 1A]

——(1993c). 'Typhus and its control in Russia, 1870–1940'. *Medical History*, 37: 361–81. [12.5.2]

——(1994). 'Cholera diffusion in Russia, 1823–1923'. *Social Science and Medicine*, 38: 1171–91. [2.4.6]

——and Pyle, G. F. (1991). 'The geography and mortality of the 1918 influenza pandemic'. *Bulletin of the History of Medicine*, 65: 4–21. [11.3, 11.3.1, 12.5.3]

Paul, J. R. (1971). *A History of Poliomyelitis*. New Haven: Yale University Press. [9.2.1, 12.5.4]

——and McClure, W. W. (1958). 'Epidemic hemorrhagic fever attack rates among United Nations troops during the Korean War'. *American Journal of Hygiene*, 68: 126–39. [9.2.2, 9.4.2]

Pavlović, M., Šimić, D., Krstić-Burić, M., Čorović, N., Živković, Ð., Rožman, A., and Peroš-Golubičić, T. (1998). 'Wartime migration and the incidence of tuberculosis in the Zagreb region, Croatia'. *The European Respiratory Journal*, 12: 1380–3. [12.5.1]

Pennington, D. H. (1989). *Europe in the Seventeenth Century* (2nd edn.). London: Longman. [2.4.2]

Perea, W. A., Ancelle, T., Moren, A., Nagelkerke, M., and Sondorp, E. (1991). 'Visceral leishmaniasis in southern Sudan'. *Transactions of the Royal Society of Tropical Medicine and Hygiene*, 85: 48–53. [13.5.4]

Peterson, W. (1975). *Population*. New York: Macmillan. [5.2.3]

Philip, C. B. (1948). 'Tsutsugamushi disease (scrub typhus) in World War II'. *Journal of Parasitology*, 34: 169–91. [1.1, 9.1, 9.2.1, 9.2.2, 9.3, 9.3.1, 9.6, 11.4.2]

——(1964). 'Scrub typhus and scrub itch'. In: Medical Department, United States Army, *Preventive Medicine in World War II. Volume VII: Communicable Diseases. Anthropodborne Diseases other than Malaria*. Washington: US Government Printing Office, 275–347. [9.3, 9.3.1, 11.4.2]

Piot, P., Plummer, F. A., Mhalu, F. S., Lamboray, J. L., Chin, J., and Mann, J. M. (1988). 'AIDS: an international perspective'. *Science*, 239: 573–9. [10.4.1]

——Taelman, H., Minlangu, K. B., Mbendi, N., Ndangi, K., Kalambayi, K., Bridts, C., Quinn, T. C., Feinsod, F. M., Wobin, O., Mazebo, P., Stevens, W., Mitchell, S., and McCormick, J. B. (1984). 'Acquired immunodeficiency syndrome in a heterosexual population in Zaire'. *Lancet*, 2: 65–9. [10.4.1]

Polišenský, J. V. (1971). *The Thirty Years War*. London: B. T. Batsford. [2.4.2]

Pollitzer, R. (1959). *Cholera*. Geneva: World Health Organization. [8.2.3]

Pon, E., McKee, K. T., Diniega, B. M., Merrell, B., Corwin, A., and Ksiazek, T. G. (1990). 'Outbreak of hemorrhagic fever with renal syndrome among U.S. marines in Korea'. *American Journal of Tropical Medicine and Hygiene*, 42: 612–19. [9.4.2]

Pool, D. I. (1973). 'The effects of the 1918 pandemic of influenza on the Maori population of New Zealand'. *Bulletin of the History of Medicine*, 47: 273–81. [11.3.3, 11.5]

——(1977). *The Maori Population of New Zealand, 1769–1971*. Auckland: Auckland University Press. [11.2.1, 11.2.2]

Porter, J. D. H., Gastellu-Etchegorry, M., Navarre, I., Lung, G., and Moren, A. (1990). 'Measles outbreaks in the Mozambican refugee camps in Malawi: the continued need for an effective vaccine'. *International Journal of Epidemiology*, 19: 1072–7. [5.4.1]

Poser, C. M. (1994). 'The dissemination of multiple sclerosis: a Viking saga? A historical essay'. *Annals of Neurology*, 36 (suppl.), S231–43. [2.3.1]

——(1995). 'Viking voyages: the origin of multiple sclerosis? An essay in medical history'. *Acta Neurologica Scandinavica*, 161 (suppl.), 11–22. [2.3.1]

Preston, S. H. (1976). *Mortality Patterns in National Populations with Special Reference to Recorded Causes of Death*. New York: Academic Press. [3.3.4, 3.4.1]

Price-Smith, A. T. (2002). *The Health of Nations: Infectious Disease, Environmental Change, and their Effects on National Security and Development*. Cambridge, Mass.: Massachusetts Institute of Technology. [9.2.1]

Prinzing, F. (1916). *Epidemics Resulting from Wars*. Oxford: Clarendon Press. [1.1, 1.3.2, 2.2, 2.3.2, 2.3.3, 2.4.1, 2.4.2, 2.4.4, 2.4.5, 2.4.6, 8.1, 8.2, 8.2.1, 8.2.3, 8.3.1, 8.3.2, 8.3.3, 8.3.4, 10.1]

Prothero, R. M. (1994). 'Forced movements of population and health hazards in tropical Africa'. *International Journal of Epidemiology*, 23: 657–64. [5.1, 5.4]

Pruitt, F. W., and Cleve, E. A. (1953). 'Epidemic hemorrhagic fever'. *American Journal of Medical Sciences*, 225: 660–8. [9.4.2]

Puryear, V. (1931). 'New light on the origins of the Crimean War'. *Journal of Modern History*, 3: 218–34. [8.2.1]

Puvacic, Z., and Weinberg, J. (1994). 'Impact of war on infectious disease in Bosnia-Hercegovina'. *British Medical Journal*, 309: 1207–8. [13.2.2]

Q

Quinn, T. C., Mann, J. M., Curran, J. W., and Piot, P. (1986). 'AIDS in Africa: an epidemiologic paradigm'. *Science*, 234: 955–63. [10.4.2]

R

Ramenofsky, A. R. (1987). *Vectors of Death: The Archaeology of European Contact*. Albuquerque: University of New Mexico Press. [2.6.1]

Raoult, D., Ndihokubwayo, J. B., Tissot-Dupont, H., Roux, V., Faugere, B., Abegbinni, R., and Birtles, R. J. (1998). 'Outbreak of epidemic typhus associated with trench fever in Burundi'. *Lancet*, 352: 353–8. [1.1, 5.4.1, 5.7, Introduction to Part III, 13.5.4]

Ravenholt, R. T. (1993). 'Encephalitis lethargica'. In: Kiple (1993), 708–12. [12.5.3]

——and Foege, W. H. (1982). '1918 influenza, encephalitis lethargica, parkinsonism'. *Lancet*, 2: 860–4. [12.5.3]

Reece, R. J. (1916). 'Report on cerebro-spinal fever and its epidemic prevalence among the civil population in England and Wales, with special reference to outbreaks in certain districts during the first six months of the year 1915'. In: Reports to the Local Government Board on Public Health and Medical Subjects (New Series, No. 110), *Reports on Cerebro-Spinal Fever*. London: HMSO, 73–114. [Part III (introduction), 12.5.1]

Reed, W., Vaughan, V. C., and Shakespeare, E. O. (1900). *Abstract of Report on the Origin and Spread of Typhoid Fever in US Military Camps during the Spanish War of 1898*. Washington: Government Printing Office. [7.3.2]

————(1904). *Report on the Origin and Spread of Typhoid Fever in US Military Camps during the Spanish War of 1898*, i and ii. Washington: Government Printing Office. [1.1, 1.4.1, 1.4.3, Appendix 1B, 7.1, 7.3, 7.3.1, 7.3.2, 7.3.3, 7.3.4]

Rees, J. (1854). 'Report on the recent outbreak of cholera in H. M. S. Britannia'. *Medical Times and Gazette*, 2: 609–10. [8.2.5]

Registrar-General (1918). *Seventy-Ninth Annual Report of the Registrar-General of Births, Deaths, and Marriages in England and Wales*. London: HMSO. [12.5.1]

——(1920). *Report on the Mortality from Influenza in England and Wales during the Epidemic of 1918–19: Supplement to the Eighty-First Annual Report of the Registrar-General of Births, Deaths, and Marriages in England and Wales*. London: HMSO. [12.5.3]

Reid, A. H., Fanning, T. G., Hultin, J. V., and Taubenberger, J. K. (1999). 'Origin and evolution of the 1918 "Spanish" influenza hemagluttinin gene'. *Proceedings of the National Academy of Sciences USA*, 96: 1651–5. [11.3.1]

Reid, D. D., Adelstein, A. M., and Logan, W. D. (1975). 'Percy Stocks: an appreciation'. *British Journal of Preventive and Social Medicine*, 29: 65–72. [5.5.1]

Reiley, C. G., and Russell, K. (1969). 'Observations on fevers of unknown origin in the Republic of Vietnam'. *Military Medicine*, 134: 36–42. [9.5.1]

Reister, F. A. (ed.) (1976). *Medical Statistics in World War II*. Washington: US Government Printing Office. [1.4.1, Appendix 1B, Part III (introduction), 7.4.2, 10.3.1, 11.4.1, 11.4.2]

Rendle Short, A. (1955). *The Bible and Modern Medicine: A Survey of Health and Healing in the Old and New Testaments*. London: Paternoster. [2.2]

Renner, M. (1997). 'Keeping peace and preventing war: the role of the United Nations'. In: B. S. Levy and V. W. Sidel (eds.), *War and Public Health*. New York: Oxford University Press, 360–74. [13.5.3]

Richardson, L. F. (1944). 'The distribution of wars in time'. *Journal of the Royal Statistical Society*, 107: 242–50. [1.2.1]

—— (1960). *Statistics of Deadly Quarrels*. Pittsburgh: Boxwood. [1.2.2, 1.3.3, 11.1]

Rieder, H. L., Zellweger, J.-P., Raviglione, M. C., Keizer, S. T., and Migliori, G. B. (1994). 'Tuberculosis control in Europe and international migration'. *The European Respiratory Journal*, 7: 1545–53. [12.5.1]

Risse, G. B. (1993). 'History of Western medicine from Hippocrates to germ theory'. In: Kiple (1993), 11–19. [1.3.2]

Robbins, F. C., Gauld, R. L., and Warner, F. B. (1946a). ' "Q" fever in the Mediterranean area: report of its occurrence in Allied troops. II. Epidemiology'. *American Journal of Hygiene*, 44: 23–50. [8.4.1]

—— and Ragan, C. A. (1946). ' "Q" fever in the Mediterranean area: report of its occurrence in Allied troops. I. Clinical features of the disease'. *American Journal of Hygiene*, 44: 6–22. [8.4.1]

—— and Rustigian, R. (1946). ' "Q" fever in the Mediterranean area: report of its occurrence in Allied troops. IV. A laboratory outbreak'. *American Journal of Hygiene*, 44: 64–71. [8.4.1]

—————— Snyder, M. J., and Smadel, J. E. (1946b). ' "Q" fever in the Mediterranean area: report of its occurrence in Allied troops. III. The aetiological agent'. *American Journal of Hygiene*, 44: 51–63. [8.4.1]

Roberts, A., and Guelff, R. (2000). *Documents on the Laws of War*. Oxford: Oxford University Press. [1.2.4]

Robinson, A. H. (1982). *Early Thematic Mapping in the History of Cartography*. Chicago: University of Chicago Press. [6.1]

Roemer, M. I. (1993). 'Internationalism in medicine and public health'. In: W. F. Bynum and R. Porter (eds.), *Encyclopaedia of the History of Medicine*, ii. London: Routledge, 1417–35. [3.6]

Rohlf, F., and Slice, D. E. (1990). 'Extensions of the Procrustes method for the optimal superimposition of landmarks'. *Systematic Zoology*, 39: 40–59. [6.6.2]

Rolleston, J. D. (1933). 'The smallpox pandemic of 1870–1874'. *Proceedings of the Royal Society of Medicine, Section of Epidemiology and State Medicine*, 27 (Part I), 177–92. [8.3.1, 12.5.1]

Rothenberg, R. B. (1993). 'Gonorrhea'. In: Kiple (1993), 756–63. [Part III (introduction)]

Royal Commission (1858). *Report of the Commissioners Appointed to Inquire into the Regulations Affecting the Sanitary Condition of the Army, The Organization of the Military Hospitals, and the Treatment of the Sick and Wounded, with Evidence and Appendix*. London: HMSO. [8.2.1]

Runciman, S. (1951–5). *A History of the Crusades*, i–iii. Cambridge: Cambridge University Press. [2.3.2]

Russell, J. C. (1972). 'Population in Europe 500–1500'. In: C. M. Cipolla (ed.), *The Fontana Economic History of Europe: The Middle Ages*. London: Fontana, 25–70. [2.3.1]

Russell, W. H. (1877). *The British Expedition to the Crimea* (new and rev. edn.). London: G. Routledge. [8.2.1]

Rybka, L. N., and Punga, V. V. (1996). 'Tuberkulez u bezhentsev iz dal'nego zarubezh'ia'. *Problemy Tuberkuleza*, 3: 12–14. [12.5.1]

S

Saah, A. J. (2000*a*). '*Rickettsia prowazekii* (epidemic or louse–borne typhus)'. In: Mandell *et al.* (2000), 2050–3. [Appendix 1A]

——(2000*b*). '*Orientia tsutsugamushi* (scrub typhus)'. In: Mandell *et al.* (2000), 2056–7. [9.3]

Sabin, A. B. (1960). 'Poliomyelitis'. In: Medical Department, United States Army (1960), 367–400. [12.5.4]

——Schlesinger, R. W., Ginder, W. R., and Matsumoto, M. (1947). 'Japanese B encephalitis in an American soldier in Korea'. *American Journal of Hygiene*, 46: 356–75. [9.4.1]

Sadik, T. (1991). *The State of World Population 1991*. New York: United Nations Population Fund. [3.5.3]

Saimot, A. G., Couland, J. P., Mechali, D. X., Matherson, S., Dazza, M. C., Rey, M. A., Brun-Vézinet, F., and Leibowitch, J. (1987). 'HIV-2/LAV-2 in Portuguese man with AIDS (Paris 1978)'. *Lancet*, 1: 688. [10.4.2]

Santos-Ferreira, M. O., Cohen, T., Lourenço, M. H., Alemida, M. J., Chamaret, S., and Montagnier, L. (1990). 'A study of seroprevalence of HIV-1 and HIV-2 in six provinces of People's Republic of Angola: clues to the spread of HIV infection'. *Journal of Acquired Immunodeficiency Syndromes*, 3: 780–6. [10.4, 10.4.2]

Sapero, J. J., and Butler, F. A. (1945). 'Highlights on epidemic diseases occurring in military forces in the early phases of the war in the South Pacific'. *Journal of the American Medical Association*, 127: 502–6. [11.4.2, 11.5]

Sartwell, E., and Smith, W. M. (1944). 'Epidemiological notes on meningococcal meningitis in the army'. *American Journal of Public Health*, 34: 40–9. [7.4.2]

Savitt, T. L. (1993). 'Filariasis'. In: Kiple (1993), 724–30. [11.4.2]

Schmaljohn, C., and Hjelle, B. (1997). 'Hantaviruses: a global disease problem'. *Emerging Infectious Diseases*, 3: 95–104. [9.4.2]

Schmid, G. (1985). 'The global distribution of Lyme disease'. *Reviews of Infectious Diseases*, 7: 41–50. [3.5.3]

Schmid, G. P. (1998). 'Chancroid'. In: Evans and Brachman (1998), 191–6. [Appendix 10A]

Schofield, R., and Reher, D. (1991). 'The decline of mortality in Europe'. In: Schofield *et al.* (1991), 1–17. [3.4.1, 3.4.2]

Schofield, R., Reher, D., and Bideau, A. (eds.) (1991). *The Decline of Mortality in Europe*. Oxford: Clarendon Press. [3.4.1]

Schulten, H., and Broglie (n/i) (1943). 'Ueber das Russische Kopfschmerzfieber. Eine neuartige Infektionskrankheit mit meningealen Reizerscheinungen'. *Münchener Medizinische Wochenschrift*, 90: 24–5. [8.4]

Seaman, J., Mercer, A. J., and Sondorp, E. (1996). 'The epidemic of visceral leishmaniasis in Western Upper Nile, Southern Sudan: course and impact from 1984 to 1994'.

International Journal of Epidemiology, 25: 862–71. [1.1, Part III (introduction), 9.1, 13.5.4]

Seas, C., and Gotuzzo, E. (2000). '*Vibrio cholerae*'. In: Mandell *et al.* (2000), 2266–72. [Appendix 1A]

Seddon, H. J., Agius, T., Bernstein, H. G. G., and Tunbridge, R. E. (1945). 'The poliomyelitis epidemic in Malta 1942–3'. *Quarterly Journal of Medicine, New Series*, 14: 1–26. [1.1, 12.5.4]

Seet, B., and Burnham, G. M. (2000). 'Fatality trends in United Nations peacekeeping operations, 1948–1998'. *Journal of the American Medical Association*, 284: 598–603. [13.5.3]

Sellars, A. W., and Sturm, E. (1919). 'The occurrence of the Pfeiffer bacillus in measles'. *Bulletin of the Johns Hopkins Hospital*, 30: 331–7. [4.4.1]

Serwadda, D., Mugerwa, R. D., Sewankambo, N. K., Lwegaba, A. L., Carswell, J. W., Kirya, G. D., Bayley, A. C., Downing, R. G., Tedder, R. S., Clayden, S. A., Weiss, R. A., and Dalgleish, A. G. (1985). 'Slim disease: a new disease in Uganda and its association with HTLV-III infection'. *Lancet*, 2: 849–52. [10.4.2]

Shafritz, J. M., Shafritz, T. J. A., and Robertson, D. B. (1989). *Dictionary of Military Science*. New York: Facts on File. [1.2.1]

Shapiro, S. E., Lasarev, M. R., and McCauley, L. (2002). 'Factor analysis of Gulf War illness: what does it add to our understanding of possible health effects of deployment?' *American Journal of Epidemiology*, 156: 578–85. [13.5.5]

Sharp, T. W., Burkle, F. M., Jr., Vaughn, A. F., Chotani, R., and Brennan, J. J. (2002). 'Challenges and opportunities for humanitarian relief in Afghanistan'. *Clinical Infectious Diseases*, 34 (suppl. 5), S215–28. [13.2.3]

Shears, P., Berry, A. M., Murphy, R., and Nabil, M. A. (1987). 'Epidemiologic assessment of the health and nutrition of Ethiopian refugees in emergency camps in Sudan'. *British Medical Journal*, 295: 314–18. [5.4.1, 5.4.2, 5.8]

Shepherd, J. (1991). *The Crimean Doctors: A History of the British Medical Services in the Crimean War* (2 vols.). Liverpool: Liverpool University Press. [8.1, 8.2, 8.2.1, 8.2.2]

Shope, R. E., and Meegan, J. M. (1997). 'Arboviruses'. In: Evans and Kaslow (1997), 151–83. [Appendix 1A]

Shortridge, K. F. (1999). 'The 1918 "Spanish" flu: pearls from swine?' *Nature Medicine*, 5: 384–5. [11.3.1]

Shrewsbury, J. F. D. (1950). 'The Plague of Athens'. *Bulletin of the History of Medicine*, 24: 1–25. [1.1, 2.2]

——(1964). *The Plague of the Philistines and other Medical-Historical Essays*. London: Victor Gollancz. [1.1, 1.3.2, 2.2]

Sidel, V. W. (1988). 'The arms race as a threat to health'. *Lancet*, 2: 442–4. [13.5.1]

——(2000). 'The impact of military preparedness and militarism on health and the environment'. In: J. E. Austin and C. E. Bruch, *The Environmental Consequences of War: Legal, Economic and Scientific Pespectives*. Cambridge: Cambridge University Press, 426–43. [13.5.1]

Siegal, F., Lopez, C., Hammer, G. S., Brown, A. E., Kornfield, S. J., Gold, J., Hassett, J., Hirschmann, Z., Cunningham-Rundles, C., Adelsberg, B. R., Purham, D. M., Siegal, M., Cunningham-Rundles, S., and Armstrong, D. (1981). 'Severe acquired immunodeficiency in male homosexuals manifested by chronic perianal ulcerative herpes simplex lesions'. *New England Journal of Medicine*, 305: 1439–44. [10.4.1]

Siegel, D., Baron, R., and Epstein, P. (1985). 'The epidemiology of aggression: health consequences of war in Nicaragua'. *Lancet*, 1: 1492–3. [1.4.3]

Simmons, J. S. (1943). 'The present state of the Army's health'. *Journal of the American Medical Association*, 122: 916–23. [7.4.2]

Simpson, R. J. S. (1911). *The Medical History of the War in South Africa: An Epidemiological Essay*. London: HMSO. [12.2, 12.2.1, 12.2.2]

Simpson, W. J. A. (1905). *A Treatise on Plague*. Cambridge: Cambridge University Press. [2.2]

Singer, J. D., and Small, M. (1972). *The Wages of War, 1816–1965: A Statistical Handbook*. New York: John Wiley & Sons. [1.2.2, 1.2.5, 11.1]

Skrabanek, P. (1985). 'Militarism and mortality'. *Lancet*, 2: 46. [13.5.1]

Smallman-Raynor, M., and Cliff, A. D. (1991). 'Civil war and the spread of AIDS in Central Africa'. *Epidemiology and Infection*, 107: 69–80. [10.4, 10.4.2]

————(1998*a*). 'The Philippines insurrection and the 1902–4 cholera epidemic: part I—epidemiological diffusion processes in war'. *Journal of Historical Geography*, 24: 69–89. [6.1, 6.2.1, 6.4.2, 11.5, 12.3.4, 12.5.3]

————(1998*b*). 'The Philippines insurrection and the 1902–4 cholera epidemic: part II—diffusion patterns in war and peace'. *Journal of Historical Geography*, 24: 188–210. [6.1, 6.2.2, 6.3.1, 6.4.2, 6.5.1, 6.7.2, 6.7.3, 12.3.4]

————(1999). 'The spatial dynamics of epidemics in war and peace: Cuba and the insurrection against Spain, 1895–98'. *Transactions of the Institute of British Geographers, New Series*, 24: 331–52. [11.5, 12.3, 12.3.1, 12.3.2, 12.3.3]

————(2000). 'The epidemiological legacy of war: the Philippine–American War and the diffusion of cholera in Batangas and La Laguna, southwest Luzón, 1902–4'. *War in History*, 7: 29–64. [6.1, 6.3.1, 6.5.2]

————(2001*a*). 'Epidemiological spaces: the use of multidimensional scaling to identify cholera diffusion processes in wake of the Philippines insurrection, 1899–1902'. *Transactions of the Institute of British Geographers, New Series*, 26: 288–305. [6.1, 6.2.1, 6.6.2]

————(2001*b*). 'Epidemic diffusion processes in a system of U.S. military camps: transfer diffusion and the spread of typhoid fever in the Spanish–American War, 1898'. *Annals of the Association of American Geographers*, 91: 71–91. [7.3, 7.3.1, 7.3.2, 7.3.3, 7.3.4]

————(2002). 'The geographical transmission of smallpox in the Franco-Prussian War: prisoner of war (POW) camps and their impact upon epidemic diffusion processes in the civil settlement system of Prussia, 1870–71'. *Medical History*, 46: 241–64. [8.3, 8.3.1, 8.3.3]

————(2003). 'War and disease: some perspectives on the spatial and temporal occurrence of tuberculosis in wartime'. In: M. Gandy and A. Zumla (eds.), *The Return of the White Plague: Global Poverty and the New Tuberculosis*. London: Verso, 70–92. [1.3.2, 12.5.1]

————(forthcoming). 'The geographical spread of cholera in the Crimean War: epidemic transmission in the camp systems of the British Army of the East, 1854–55'. *Journal of Historical Geography*. [8.2, 8.2.1, 8.2.2, 8.2.3, 8.2.4, 8.2.5, Appendix 8A]

————and Haggett, P. (1992). *London International Atlas of AIDS*. Oxford: Blackwell Reference. [4.6, 4.6.1, 10.1, 10.4, 10.4.1, 10.4.2]

——Johnson, N., and Cliff, A. D. (2002). 'The spatial anatomy of an epidemic: influenza in London and the county boroughs of England and Wales, 1918–19'. *Transactions of the Institute of British Geographers, New Series*, 27: 452–70. [12.5.3]

——Nettleton, C., and Cliff, A. D. (2003). 'Wartime evacuation and the spread of infectious diseases: epidemiological consequences of the dispersal of children from London during World War II'. *Journal of Historical Geography*, 29: 396–421. [5.5, 5.5.1, 5.5.2, 5.5.3, 5.5.4]

Smith, D. H., Pepin, J., and Stich, A. H. R. (1998). 'Human African trypanosomiasis: an emerging public health crisis'. *British Medical Bulletin*, 54: 341–55. [13.5.4]

Smith, G. L., Irving, W. L., McCauley, J. W., and Rowlands, D. J. (eds.) (2001). *New Challenges to Health: The Threat of Virus Infections*. Cambridge: Cambridge University Press. [9.2.1]

Smith, H. B., and Tirpak, D. (eds.) (1989). *Potential Effects of Global Climatic Change on the United States: Volume G. Health*. Washington: US Government Printing Office (Environmental Protection Agency, EPA 230-05-89-057). [3.5.3]

Smith, I. R. (1996). *The Origins of the South African War*. Harlow, Essex: Longman. [12.2, 12.2.5]

Smith, J. (1994). *The Spanish–American War: Conflict in the Caribbean and the Pacific 1895–1902*. Longman: London. [7.3.1]

Snow, J. (1855a). *On the Mode of Communication of Cholera* (2nd edn.). London: J. Churchill. [6.1, 8.2.1]

——(1855b). 'On the chief cause of the recent sickness and morbidity in the Crimea'. *Medical Times and Gazette*, 1: 457–8. [8.2.1, 8.2.5]

Soeprapto, W., Ertono, S., Hudoyo, H., Mascola, J., Porter, K., Gunawan, S., and Corwin, A. L. (1995). 'HIV and peacekeeping operations in Cambodia'. *Lancet*, 346: 1304–5. [13.5.3]

Sohn, Y. M. (2000). 'Japanese encephalitis immunization in South Korea: past, present and future'. *Emerging Infectious Diseases*, 6: 17–24. [9.4.1]

Soper, G. A. (1918). 'The pandemic in the army camps'. *Journal of the American Medical Association*, 71: 1899–909. [7.4.1, 11.3.1]

Sörensen, J. (1932). *The Saga of Fridtjof Nansen*. London: George Allen and Unwin. [5.2.1]

Sorokin, P. A. (1937). *Social and Cultural Dynamics*, iii: *Fluctuation of Social Relationships, War and Revolution*. New York: American Book Company. [1.2.5, 2.2]

Soubbotitch, V. (1918). 'A pandemic of typhus in Serbia in 1914 and 1915'. *Proceedings of the Royal Society of Medicine, Section of Epidemiology and State Medicine*, 11: 31–9. [1.1, 12.5.2]

Sparling, P. F., and Handsfield, H. H. (2000). '*Neisseria gonorrhoeae*'. In: Mandell *et al.* (2000), 2242–58. [Appendix 10A]

Spate, O. H. K. (1979, 1983, 1989). *The Pacific since Magellan. Volume I: The Spanish Lake. Volume II: Monopolists and Freebooters. Volume III: Paradise Found and Lost.* Canberra: Australian National University Press. [11.2.1]

Speck, R. S. (1993). 'Cholera'. In: Kiple (1993), 642–9. [Appendix 1A]

Spicer, A. J. (1978). 'Military significance of Q fever: a review'. *Journal of the Royal Society of Medicine*, 71: 762–7. [8.4.1]

Spies, S. B. (1977). *Methods of Barbarism? Robert and Kitchener and Civilians in the Boer Republics, January 1900–May 1902.* Cape Town, South Africa: Human and Rousseau. [12.2, 12.2.2, 12.2.3]

Stannard, D. E. (1992). *American Holocaust: Columbus and the Conquest of the New World.* Oxford: Oxford University Press. [2.6.1]

Steefel, L. (1962). *Bismark, the Hohenzollern Candidacy, and the Origins of the Franco-German War.* Cambridge, Mass.: Harvard University Press. [8.3.1]

Steffen, R., Desaules, M., Nagel, J., Vuillet, F., Schubarth, P., Jeanmaire, C.-H., and Huber, A. (1992). 'Epidemiological experience in the mission of the United Nations Transition Assistance Group (UNTAG) in Namibia'. *Bulletin of the World Health Organization,* 70: 129–33. [13.5.3]

Stein, M. L. (1999). *Interpolation of Spatial Data: Some Theory for Kriging.* New York: Springer. [Appendix 6A.3]

Steinberg, S. H. (1966). *The 'Thirty Years War' and the Conflict for European Hegemony.* London: Edward Arnold. [2.4.2]

Steiner, E. (1968). *Disease in the Civil War: Natural Biological Warfare in 1861–1865.* Springfield, Ill.: Charles C. Thomas. [7.2, 7.2.2]

——(1977). *Medical History of a Civil War Regiment: Disease in the Sixty-Fifth United States Colored Infantry.* Clayton, Miss.: Institute of Civil War Studies. [4.3.1, 4.3.2, 7.2.2]

Sternberg, T. H., Howard, E. B., Dewey, L. A., and Padget, P. (1960). 'Venereal diseases'. In: Medical Department, United States Army (1960), 139–331. [10.1, 10.3.1]

Stewart, F. (2002). 'Root causes of violent conflict in developing countries'. *British Medical Journal,* 324: 342–5. [13.2]

Stocks, P. (1940). 'The first seven months: a study of war-time mortality in London'. *Lancet,* 1: 725–9. [5.5.1, 5.5.3]

——(1941). 'Diphtheria and scarlet fever incidence during the dispersal of 1939–40'. *Journal of the Royal Statistical Society,* 104: 311–45. [5.5, 5.5.1, 5.5.4, 5.5.5]

——(1942). 'Measles and whooping-cough incidence before and during the dispersal of 1939–41'. *Journal of the Royal Statistical Society,* 105: 259–91. [5.5, 5.5.1]

Stokes, J. (1958). 'Measles'. In: Hoff (1958), 129–34. [4.5.1]

Stokes, J. F., and Miller, A. A. (1947). 'An outbreak of severe infective hepatitis in Burma'. *Quarterly Journal of Medicine, New Series,* 16: 211–36. [9.3]

Strong, R. P., Shattuck, G. C., Sellards, A. W., Zinsser, H., and Hopkins, J. G. (1920). *Typhus Fever with Particular Reference to the Serbian Epidemic.* Cambridge, Mass.: American Red Cross at the Harvard University Press. [12.5.2]

Stuart-Harris, C. H., Schild, G. C., and Oxford, J. S. (1985). *Influenza: The Viruses and the Disease* (2nd edn.). Baltimore: Edward Arnold. [11.3, 11.3.1]

Stuhlfauth, K. (1941). 'Die epidemische Gelbsucht. Gehäuftes Auftreten unter Soldaten und der Zivilbevölkering in Norwegen'. *Deutsche Militärarzt,* 6: 591–602. [8.4]

Surgeon-General's Office (1870–88). *The Medical and Surgical History of the War of the Rebellion (1861–65).* Washington: Government Printing Office. [1.4.1, Appendix 1B, 4.3.1, 7.2.1, 7.2.2, 7.2.3, 7.2.4, 7.2.5]

Swartzwelder, J. C. (1964). 'Filariasis bancrofti'. In: Medical Department, United States Army, *Preventive Medicine in World War II. Volume VII: Communicable Diseases. Anthropodborne Diseases Other than Malaria.* Washington: US Government Printing Office, 63–71. [11.4.2]

Szreter, S. (1988). 'The importance of social intervention in Britain's mortality decline, *c.*1850–1914: a reinterpretation of the role of public health'. *Social History of Medicine*, 1: 1–38. [3.4.1]

T

Tangermann, R. H., Hull, H. F., Jafari, H., Nkowane, B., Everts, H., and Aylward, R. B. (2000). 'Eradication of poliomyelitis in countries affected by conflict'. *Bulletin of the World Health Organization*, 78: 330–8. [1.1, 13.3.1, 13.3.2]

Tarlé, E. (1942). *Napoleon's Invasion of Russia, 1812.* London: Allen and Unwin. [2.4.5]

Taviner, M., Thwaites, G., and Gant, V. (1998). 'The English sweating sickness, 1485–1551: a viral pulmonary syndrome'. *Medical History*, 42: 96–9. [2.3.3]

Telalbasic, S., Cardaklija, Z., and Pinjo, F. (1994). 'Dijarealna oboljenja u hospital-iziranih pacijenata u toku prve godine rata'. *Medicinski Arhiv*, 48: 77–8. [13.2.2]

Terrell, J. (1986). *Prehistory in the Pacific Islands: A Study of Variation in Language, Customs and Human Biology.* Cambridge: Cambridge University Press. [11.2.1]

Thomas, H. (1971). *Cuba, or the Pursuit of Freedom.* London: Eyre and Spottiswoode. [12.3.2]

Thomas, H. M., Jr. (1943). 'Meningococcic meningitis and septicemia: report of an outbreak in Fourth Service Command during winter and spring of 1942–1943'. *Journal of the American Medical Association*, 123: 264–72. [7.4.2]

Thompson, A. G. G. (1939). 'Epidemiological aspects of the A.R. evacuation schemes'. *Medical Officer*, 61: 192. [5.5.1]

Thompson, A. W. S. (1946). 'Malaria control in mobile warfare: Italian Campaign 1943–1946'. *Journal of the Royal Army Medical Corps*, 86: 109–26. [8.4]

Thompson, H. (ed.) (1911). *The Photographic History of the Civil War. Volume Seven: Prisons and Hospitals.* New York: The Review of Reviews Co. [4.3.2, 7.2.2]

Thongcharoen, P. (1989). *Japanese Encephalitis Virus Encephalitis: An Overview.* Bangkok: Faculty of Tropical Medicine, Mahidol University. [9.4.1]

Thwaites, G., Taviner, M., and Gant, V. (1997). 'The English sweating sickness, 1485–1551'. *New England Journal of Medicine*, 336: 580–2. [2.3.3]

Titmuss, R. M. (1950). *Problems of Social Policy: History of the Second World War, United Kingdom Civil Series.* London: HMSO. [5.5, 5.5.1, 5.5.2]

Tobler, W. (1965). 'Computation of the correspondence of geographical patterns'. *Papers: Regional Science Association*, 15: 131–42. [6.6.2, Appendix 6A.5]

——(1976). 'Spatial interaction patterns'. *Journal of Environmental Systems*, 6: 271–301. [6.6.2]

Tomkins, S. M. (1992). 'The influenza epidemic of 1918–19 in Western Samoa'. *Journal of Pacific History*, 27: 181–97. [11.3.4]

Toole, M. J. (1997). 'Displaced persons and war'. In: B. S. Levy and V. W. Sidel (eds.), *War and Public Health.* New York: Oxford University Press, 197–212. [5.3.1, 5.4.1, 5.4.2, 5.8]

——Galson, S., and Brady, W. (1993). 'Are war and public health compatible?' *Lancet*, 342: 1193–6. [1.4.3]

——and Waldman, R. J. (1990). 'Prevention of excess mortality in refugee and displaced populations in developing countries'. *Journal of the American Medical Association*, 263: 3296–302. [5.3.1, 5.4.1, 5.8]

Trask, D. F. (1981). *The War with Spain in 1898*. New York: Macmillan. [7.3.1, 7.3.3]

Traub, R., and Wisseman, C. L. (1968). 'Ecological considerations in scrub typhus'. *Bulletin of the World Health Organization*, 39: 209–18. [9.3]

Trencséni, T., and Keleti, B. (1971). *Clinical Aspects and Epidemiology of Haemorrhagic Fever with Renal Syndrome: Analysis of Clinical and Epidemiological Experiences in Hungary*. Budapest: Akadémiai Kiadó. [9.4.2, 13.2.2]

Tsai, T. F. (2000). 'Flaviviruses (yellow fever, dengue, denge hemorrhagic fever, Japanese encephalitis, St Louis encephalitis, tick-borne encephalitis)'. In: Mandell *et al.* (2000), 1714–36. [9.4.1, 11.4.2]

Tucker, J. B. (1999). 'Historical trends related to bioterrorism: an empirical analysis'. *Emerging Infectious Diseases*, 5: 498–504. [13.4.3]

Tufte, E. R. (1983). *The Visual Display of Quantitative Information*. Cheshire, Conn.: Graphics Press. [2.4.5]

Tukey, J. W. (1962). 'The future of data analysis'. *Annals of Mathematical Statistics*, 33: 1–67. [10.4.2]

——(1977). *Exploratory Data Analysis*. Reading, Mass.: Addison-Wesley. [10.3.1]

U

UNAIDS (2002). *Report on the Global HIV/AIDS Epidemic 2002*. Geneva: UNAIDS [10.4.1]

UNHCR (2000). *The State of the World's Refugees 2000: Fifty Years of Humanitarian Action*. Oxford: Oxford University Press. [5.1, 5.2.1, 5.2.2, 5.3, 5.3.1, 5.3.2, 5.4, 5.6.1, 5.7, 13.2]

United States Army (1928). *The Medical Department of the United States Army in the World War: Volume ix: Communicable and Other Diseases*. Washington: Government Printing Office. [4.4.1, 7.3.5, 7.4.1]

UNRWA (2001*a*). *UNRWA Statistical Profile: General*. Vienna: UNRWA. (Available at: http://www.un.org/unrwa/pr/pdf/figures.pdf. Last viewed 17 Dec. 2001.) [5.6.1]

——(2001*b*). *Map of UNRWA's Area of Operations 2000*. Vienna: UNRWA. (Available at: http://www.un.org/unrwa/refugees/images/map.jpg. Last viewed 17 Dec. 2001.) [5.6]

——(2002). *UNRWA*. (Available at: http://www.un.org/unrwa. Last viewed 21 June 2002.) [5.6.1, 5.6.2, 5.6.4]

Urlanis, B. T. (1971). *Wars and Population*. Moscow: Progress. [1.2.2, 1.3.1, 1.3.2, 1.3.3, 1.4.1, 1.4.3]

US Army (1856). *Statistical Report on the Sickness and Mortality in the Army of the United States, Compiled from the Records of the Surgeon General's Office; Embracing a Period of Sixteen Years, from January, 1839, to January, 1855*. Washington: A. O. P. Nicholson. [1.4.1, Appendix 1B]

Usmanov, I., Favorov, M. O., and Chorba, T. L. (2000). 'Universal immunization: the diphtheria control strategy of choice in the Republic of Tajikistan, 1993–1997'. *Journal of Infectious Diseases*, 181 (suppl. 1): S86–93. [5.4.1, Part III (introduction), 13.5.4]

USMHS (1896*a*). *Public Health Reports.* Washington: Government Printing Office. [Appendix 12A]

——(1896*b*). *Annual Report of the Supervising Surgeon-General of the Marine Hospital Service for the Fiscal Year 1895.* Washington: Government Printing Office. [Appendix 12A]

——(1900). *Public Health Reports.* Washington: Government Printing Office. [12.3.4, Appendix 12A]

US War Department (1900). *Census of Cuba Taken under the Direction of the War Department, USA Bulletin No 1: Total Population by Provinces, Municipal Districts, Cities, and Wards.* Washington: Government Printing Office. [12.3]

——(1920). *Annual Reports 1919. Volume I. In Four Parts. Part II: Report of the Surgeon-General.* Washington: Government Printing Office. [7.4.1]

V

Valente, F., Otten, M., Balbina, F., Van de Weerdt, R., Chezzi, C., Eriki, P., Van-Dúnnen, J., and Okwo Bele, J.-M. (2000). 'Massive outbreak of poliomyelitis caused by type-3 wild poliovirus in Angola in 1999'. *Bulletin of the World Health Organization*, 78: 339–46. [13.3.1]

Vallin, J., and Meslé, F. (1988). *Les Causes de Décès en France de 1925 à 1978.* Paris: Colin. [3.4.2]

van Creveld, M. (1991). *On Future War.* London: Brassey's. [13.2]

Van Damme, W. (1995). 'Do refugees belong in camps? Experiences from Goma and Guinea'. *Lancet*, 346: 360–2. [5.4, 5.7]

Van de Perre, P., Rouvroy, D., Lepage, P., Bongaarts, J., Kestelyn, P., Kayihigi, J., Hekker, A. C., Butzlier, J. P., and Clumeck, N. (1984). 'Acquired immunodeficiency syndrome in Rwanda'. *Lancet*, 2: 62–5. [10.4.1]

van den Bosch, F., Metz, J. A. J., and Diekmann, O. (1990). 'The velocity of spatial population expansion'. *Journal of Mathematical Biology*, 28: 529–65. [Appendix 6A.2]

van der Wusten, H. (1985). 'The geography of conflict since 1945'. In: D. Pepper and A. Jenkins (eds.), *The Geography of Peace and War.* Oxford: Basil Blackwell, 13–28. [13.2]

van Ravenswaay, A. C., Erickson, G. C., Reh, E., Siekierski, J. M., Pottash, R. R., and Gumbiner, B. (1944). 'Clinical aspects of primary atypical pneumonia: a study based on 1,862 cases seen at the Station Hospital, Jefferson Barracks, Missouri, from June 1, 1942, to Aug. 10, 1943'. *Journal of the American Medical Association*, 124: 1–6. [7.4.2]

van Rooyen, C. E., and Morgan, A. D. (1943). 'Poliomyelitis: experimental work in Egypt'. *Edinburgh Medical Journal*, 50: 705–20. [12.5.4]

Vaughan, V. C. (1926). *A Doctor's Memories.* Indianapolis: The Bobbs-Merrill Co. [7.3.2]

Velimirovic, B. (1972). 'Plague in South-East Asia: a brief historical summary and present geographical distribution'. *Transactions of the Royal Society of Tropical Medicine and Hygiene*, 66: 479–504. [1.1, 9.1, 9.2.1, 9.2.2, 9.5.2]

Vella, E. E. (1984). 'Belsen: medical aspects of a World War II concentration camp'. *Journal of the Royal Army Medical Corps*, 130: 34–59. [8.4]

Vitek, C. R., and Wharton, M. (1998). 'Diphtheria in the former Soviet Union: reemergence of a pandemic disease'. *Emerging Infectious Diseases*, 4: 539–50. [13.5.4]

W

Walker, A. S. (1957). 'The island campaigns'. In: A. S. Walker (ed.), *Australia in the War of 1939–1945, Series 5 (Medical)*. Canberra: Australian War Memorial, 9 and 279. [4.5.2]
——(1961). 'Medical services of the R.A.N., and R.A.A.F.'. In: A. S. Walker (ed.), *Australia in the War of 1939–1945, Series 5 (Medical)*. Canberra: Australian War Memorial, 133. [4.5.2]
Wallace, M. R., Hale, B. R., Utz, G. C., Olson, P. E., Earhart, K. C., Thornton, S. A., and Hyams, K. C. (2002). 'Endemic infectious diseases of Afghanistan'. *Clinical Infectious Diseases*, 34 (suppl. 5): S171–207. [13.2.3]
Warwick, P. (1983). *Black People and the South African War 1899–1902*. Cambridge: Cambridge University Press. [12.2.1, 12.2.2]
Watts, S. (1997). *Epidemics and History: Disease, Power and Imperialism*. New Haven: Yale University Press. [2.3.2]
Wawer, M. J., Serwadda, D., Musgrave, S. D., Konde-Lule, J. K., Musagara, M., and Sewankambo, N. K. (1991). 'Dynamics of spread of HIV-1 infection in a rural district of Uganda'. *British Medical Journal*, 303: 1303–6. [10.4.2]
Webster, R. G. (1999). '1918 Spanish influenza: the secrets remain elusive'. *Proceedings of the National Academy of Sciences USA*, 96: 1164–6. [11.3.1]
Wedgwood, C. V. (1938). *The Thirty Years War*. London: Jonathan Cape. [2.4.2]
Welshman, J. (1999). 'Evacuation, hygiene and social policy: the Our Towns report of 1943'. *The Historical Journal*, 42: 781–807. [5.5]
Wessely, S., and the King's College Gulf War Research Unit (2001). 'Ten years on: what do we know about Gulf War syndrome?' *Clinical Medicine*, 1: 28–37. [13.5.5]
Willcox, P. H. A. (1948). 'Mite typhus fever in Assam and Burma, 1944–1946'. *Transactions of the Royal Society of Tropical Medicine and Hygiene*, 42: 171–89. [9.3.1]
Willcox, R. R. (1946). 'Venereal disease in British West Africa'. *British Journal of Venereal Disease*, 22: 63–75. [10.4.2]
Willemin, G., and Heacock, R. (1984). *International Organization and the Evolution of World Society, Volume 2: The International Committee of the Red Cross*. Boston: Martinus Nijhoff. [1.4.2]
Williams, B. (1989). 'Assessing the health impact of urbanization'. *World Health Statistics Quarterly*, 43: 145–52. [3.5.3]
Wilson, G. S., and Miles, A. A. (1946). *Topley and Wilson's Principles of Bacteriology and Immunity* (3rd edn.). London: Edward Arnold and Co. [2.2]
Wilson, H. W. (1900). *The Downfall of Spain: Naval History of the Spanish-American War*. Boston: Little, Brown and Co. [7.3.1]
Wiltse, C. M. (1965). *United States Army in World War I. The Technical Services. The Medical Department: Medical Service in the Mediterranean and Minor Theaters*. Washington: US Government Printing Office. [10.3.1]

Wiseman, D. J. (1986). 'Medicine in the Old Testament World'. In: B. Palmer (ed.), *Medicine and the Bible*. Exeter: The Paternoster Press, 13–42. [2.2]

Wood, A. H. (1938). *History and Geography of Tonga*. Auckland: Wilson and Horton, Ltd. [11.3.4]

Wood, C. S. (1978). 'Syphilis in anthropological perspective'. *Social Science and Medicine*, 12: 47–55. [2.3.3]

Wood, W. B. (1988). 'AIDS north and south: diffusion patterns of a global epidemic and a research agenda for geographers'. *Professional Geographer*, 40: 266–79. [10.4.2]

——(1994). 'Forced migration: local conflicts and international dilemmas'. *Annals of the Association of American Geographers*, 84: 607–34. [5.2.3]

Woodland, J. C., McDowell, M. M., and Richards, J. T. (1943). 'Bullis fever (Lone Star Fever—Tick Fever): An endemic disease observed at Brooke General Hospital, Fort Sam Houston, Texas'. *Journal of the American Medical Association*, 122: 1156–60. [7.4.2]

Woods, R., and Shelton, N. (1997). *An Atlas of Victorian Mortality*. Liverpool: Liverpool University Press. [3.4.1]

——and Woodward. J. (1984). 'Mortality, poverty and the environment'. In: R. Woods and J. Woodward (eds.), *Urban Disease and Mortality in Nineteenth Century England*. London: Batsford Academic, 19–36. [3.41]

Woodward, J. J. (1863). *Outlines of the Chief Camp Diseases of the United States Armies as Observed during the Present War*. Philadelphia: J. B. Lippincott & Co. [1.4.3, Part III (introduction)]

——(1964). *Outlines of the Chief Camp Diseases of the United States Armies, with an Introduction by Saul Jarcho*. New York: Hafner. [4.3.1, 4.3.2]

Woolhandler, S., and Himmelstein, D. U. (1985). 'Militarism and mortality: an international analysis of arms spending and infant death rates'. *Lancet*, 1: 1375–8. [13.5.1]

World Health Organization (1970). *Health Aspects of Chemical and Biological Weapons*. Geneva: WHO. [13.4.1]

——(1976). *World Health Statistics Annual, 1973–1976*. Geneva: World Health Organization. [1.4.2]

——(1984). 'Communicable disease surveillance: surveillance and monitoring project—Lebanon'. *Weekly Epidemiological Record*, 59: 120–2. [5.6.3]

——(1995*a*). *World Health Report 1995: Bridging the Gaps*. Geneva: World Health Organization. [3.5.1]

——(1995*b*). *International Travel and Health: Vaccination Requirements and Health Advice*. Geneva: World Health Organization. [3.5.3]

——(1997). 'A large outbreak of epidemic louse-borne typhus in Burundi'. *Weekly Epidemiological Record*, 72: 152–3. [5.7]

——(2001). *Global Polio Eradication: Progress 2000*. WHO/Polio/01.03. Geneva: WHO. [3.6.1]

Wright, Q. (1924). 'Changes in the conception of war'. *American Journal of International Law*, 18: 755–67. [1.2.1]

——(1965). *A Study of War* (2nd edn.). Chicago: University of Chicago Press. [1.2.1, 1.2.2, 1.2.3, 1.2.4, 2.1, 2.4.5]

Wrigley, E. A. (1969). *Population and History*. London: Weidenfeld and Nicolson. [3.3.4]

——and Schofield, R. S. (1989). *The Population History of England 1541–1871: A Reconstruction* (2nd edn.). London: Edward Arnold. [3.4.1]

Writer, J. V., DeFraites, F. R., and Brundage, J. F. (1996). 'Comparative mortality among US military personnel in the Persian Gulf region and worldwide during Operations Desert Shield and Desert Storm'. *Journal of the American Medical Association*, 275: 118–21. [13.2.1]

Wurm, K. (1940). 'Die Ruhr im polnischen Feldzug unter Berücksichtigung persönlicher Erfahrungen'. *Medizinische Klinik*, 36: 1183–5, 1209–11. [8.4]

Wyatt, H. V. (1993). 'Poliomyelitis'. In: Kiple (1993), 942–50. [12.5.4]

Wylie, J. A. H., and Collier, L. H. (1981). 'The English sweating sickness (Sudor Anglicus): a reappraisal'. *Journal of the History of Medicine and Allied Sciences*, 36: 425–45. [2.3.3]

Z

Zeiss, H. (ed.) (1942–5). *Seuchen Atlas.* Hrgs. im Auftrag des Chefs des Wehrmachtsanitätswesens. Gotha: Perthes. [6.1]

Zeligs, M. A., Legant, O., and Webster, E. H. (1944). 'Epidemic dengue: its abortion in a combat area'. *United States Naval Medical Bulletin*, 42: 856–60. [11.4.2]

Zijlstra, E. E., Siddig Ali, M., El-Hassan, A. M., El-Toum, I. A., Satti, M., Ghalib, H. W., Sondorp, E., and Winkler, A. (1991). 'Kala-azar in displaced people from southern Sudan: epidemiological, clinical and therapeutic findings'. *Transactions of the Royal Society of Tropical Medicine and Hygiene*, 85: 365–9. [5.4.1]

Zinsser, H. (1935). *Rats, Lice and History.* London: Routledge. [1.1, 1.3.2, 2.2, 2.3.2, 2.4.1, 2.4.2, 9.2.1, 12.5.2]

Zolberg, A., Suhrke, A., and Aguayo, S. (1989). *Escape from Violence: Conflict and the Refugee Crisis in the Developing World.* Oxford: Oxford University Press. [5.1, 5.2, 5.2.3]

INDEX